BIOLOGICAL BASIS OF SUBSTANCE ABUSE

BIOLOGICAL BASIS OF SUBSTANCE ABUSE

Edited by

Stanley G. Korenman

Jack D. Barchas

New York   Oxford
OXFORD UNIVERSITY PRESS
1993

Oxford University Press

Oxford   New York   Toronto
Delhi   Bombay   Calcutta   Madras   Karachi
Kuala Lumpur   Singapore   Hong Kong   Tokyo
Nairobi   Dar es Salaam   Cape Town
Melbourne   Auckland   Madrid

and associated companies in
Berlin   Ibadan

Library of Congress Cataloging-in-Publication Data
Biological basis of substance abuse /
edited by Stanley G. Korenman, Jack D. Barchas.
p.   cm.   Includes bibliographical references and index.
ISBN 0-19-507154-9
1. Drug abuse—Physiological aspects—congresses.
I. Korenman, Stanley G., 1933–
II. Barchas, Jack D., 1935–
[DNLM: 1. Brain—drug effects—congresses. 2. Receptors, Drug—
metabolism—congresses. 3. Substance Abuse—congresses.
WL 300 B6145] RM316.B56 1993 615'.78—dc20
DNLM/DLC   for Library of Congress   92-49780

9 8 7 6 5 4 3 2 1

Printed in the United States of America
on acid-free paper

Preface

The public recognizes substance abuse as one of the most severe problems affecting not only the health of individuals and families but also the well-being of society. Few issues cross so many disciplines. Substance abuse has its origins in both psychosocial and biological factors. Integration of findings from both spheres of research will be necessary to achieve a full understanding of its many ramifications and the ability to develop effective preventive and treatment programs.

Recent studies of the actions of drugs of abuse have led to the recognition that their biological effects have many elements in common, suggesting that studies of one may shed light on actions of the others. This volume surveys key aspects of current knowledge about the biological components of substance use and abuse, focusing on their effects on the brain. It provides examples of studies of different classes of drugs at different levels of integration.

Expanding knowledge about the actions of drugs of abuse has important ramifications for the neural and behavioral sciences. For example, knowledge of the agonists for the THC receptors and the consequences of their activation should improve our understanding of cognition; elucidation of reinforcement, a form of memory, will strengthen our understanding of the learning process; dissection of the stimuli leading to activation of the reward center in the nucleus accumbens and characterization of its efferent pathways will be instrumental in tying neural functions to behavior. Such findings could shed light not only on normal behavior but also on the biological basis of mental illness.

New therapeutic initiatives may follow improved understanding of drug action. For example, a number of agents that reverse the acute effects of opiates, alcohol and stimulants are in clinical use. More important is the need to develop treatments for the compulsive use of drugs. Such therapies may be derived from biological or psychological approaches or, as has become increasingly true of mental illness, a combination of both. For many elements of addiction, a biological solution may be required. The very existence of addiction to cocaine, heroin, nicotine, alcohol and other addicting drugs implies that the reward and reinforcement centers of the brain can be activated by chemicals with highly selective effects and suggests that other agents can be identified or synthesized to reverse aspects of this process. Pharmacological research has already yielded a broad range of agonists, antagonists, and modulators of some drugs of abuse. Substantial advances have been made in understanding the molecular sites of drug action, localizing drug effects in the brain and relating the molecular and cellular changes to addictive behavior. And progress is being made toward developing more effective therapies.

The editors of this volume focused on relationships among substances of abuse in signalling mechanisms, localization of receptors and processes by which they give pleasure and by which they institute reinforcement. These events were analyzed at multiple levels of integration, from molecules to whole organisms, utilizing a wide variety of investigative techniques. This approach succeeded in generating important unifying themes and avenues for further study. Therefore, we continued the same organizational theme in this volume, whose five sections represent levels of complexity in the study of drug abuse rather than drug types. We hope that the reader will benefit by these thematic juxtapositions.

Los Angeles, California   S.G.K.
March 1993   J.D.B.

Acknowledgments

The editors acknowledge financial support from the National Institute on Drug Abuse and the UCLA Program in Psychoneuroimmunology for support of the conference that was the progenitor of this volume. We would particularly like to thank Robert Schuster, then director of NIDA, and Carmen Clemente of the UCLA Brain Research Institute for their encouragement and suggestions. We also thank Jean Abbot from UCLA-Extension, Barbara Winfield-Smith, Marylee Wirganowicz, Anita Davis and Sharon Viosca for their administrative and editorial assistance, and Jeff Bonforte for his assistance in preparing the index.

Contents

Contributors

Mary E. Abood
Department of Pharmacology and
  Toxicology
Medical College of Virginia
Richmond, Virginia

Thomas G. Aigner
Biological Psychiatry Branch
Laboratory of Neuropsychology
National Institute of Mental Health
Bethesda, Maryland

Huda Akil
Mental Health Research Institute
University of Michigan
Ann Arbor, Michigan

Arthur Alterman
VA Addiction Research Center
University of Pennsylvania
Philadelphia, Pennsylvania

Jack D. Barchas
Dean of Neuroscience
UCLA School of Medicine
Los Angeles, California

Henri Begleiter
Neurodynamics of Laboratory
SUNY Health Science Center at
  Brooklyn
Brooklyn, New York

Dana Beitner-Johnson
Laboratory of Molecular Physiology
Departments of Psychiatry and
  Pharmacology
Yale University School of Medicine
Connecticut Mental Health Center
New Haven, Connecticut

Barbara Bennett
Department of Physiology and
  Pharmacology
Bowman-Gray School of Medicine
Winston-Salem, North Carolina

Magali Bertolucci
Department of Psychiatry and
  Biobehavioral Sciences
Neuropsychiatric Institute and UCLA
  School of Medicine
Los Angeles, California

Floyd E. Bloom
Department of Neuropharmacology
  Research Institute
Scripps Clinic
La Jolla, California

John Boja
Neuroscience Branch
N.I.D.A. Addiction Research Center
Baltimore, Maryland

Tom I. Bonner
Laboratory of Cell Biology
National Institute of Mental Health
Bethesda, Maryland

Mark S. Brodie
Department of Physiology and
  Biophysics
University of Illinois
College of Medicine
Chicago, Illinois

Michael J. Brownstein
Laboratory of Cell Biology
National Institute of Mental Health
Bethesda, Maryland

Benjamin S. Bunney
Departments of Psychology and
Pharmacology
Yale University School of Medicine
New Haven, Connecticut

F. Ivy Carroll
Research Triangle Institute
Research Triangle Park, North Carolina

Arthur K. Cho
Department of Pharmacology
UCLA School of Medicine
Los Angeles, California

C. Robert Cloninger
Department of Psychiatry
Washington University
St. Louis, Missouri

Sam A. Deadwyler
Department of Physiology and
Pharmacology
Bowman-Gray School of Medicine
Winston-Salem, North Carolina

Stephen H. Dinwiddie
Department of Psychiatry
Washington University
St. Louis, Missouri

Thomas V. Dunwiddie
Department of Pharmacology
University of Colorado Health Sciences
Center
VA Medical Research Services
Denver, Colorado

Steven I. Dworkin
Department of Physiology and
Pharmacology
Bowman-Gray School of Medicine
Winston-Salem, North Carolina

James H. Eberwine
Department of Pharmacology
University of Pennsylvania
School of Medicine
Philadelphia, Pennsylvania

Gaylord D. Ellison
Department of Psychology
UCLA
Los Angeles, California

Christopher J. Evans
Department of Psychiatry and
Biobehavioral Sciences
Neuropsychiatric Institute and UCLA
School of Medicine
Los Angeles, California

Kym F. Faull
Department of Psychiatry and
Biobehavioral Sciences
Neuropsychiatric Institute and UCLA
School of Medicine
Los Angeles, California

Frank H. Gawin
Department of Psychiatry
Stimulant Abuse Treatment and
Research
UCLA
Los Angeles, California

Xavier Guitart
Laboratory of Molecular Psychiatry
Departments of Psychiatry and
Pharmacology
Yale University School of Medicine
Connecticut Mental Health Center
New Haven, Connecticut

Robert Hampson
Department of Physiology and
Pharmacology
Bowman-Gray School of Medicine
Winston-Salem, North Carolina

Steven J. Henriksen
Department of Neuropharmacology
Scripps Clinic
La Jolla, California

Miles A. Herkenham
Section on Functional Neuroanatomy
National Institute of Mental Health
Bethesda, Maryland

James P. Herman
Mental Health Research Institute
University of Michigan
Ann Arbor, Michigan

Charles Heyser
Department of Physiology and
* Pharmacology*
Bowman-Gray School of Medicine
Winston-Salem, North Carolina

George F. Koob
Department of Neuropharmacology
Scripps Clinic
La Jolla, California

Stanley G. Korenman
Dean of Ethics
UCLA School of Medicine
Los Angeles, California

Michael J. Kuhar
Neuroscience Branch
N.I.D.A. Addiction Research Center
Baltimore, Maryland

Robert Lew
Neuroscience Branch
N.I.D.A. Addiction Research Center
Baltimore, Maryland

Stephen J. Lolait
Laboratory of Cell Biology
National Institute of Mental Health
Bethesda, Maryland

Charles W. Luetje
Division of Neuroscience
Baylor College of Medicine
Houston, Texas

A. Thomas McLellan
VA Addiction Research Center
University of Pennsylvania
Philadelphia, Pennsylvania

Nigel T. Maidment
Department of Psychiatry and
* Biobehavioral Sciences*
Neuropsychiatric Institute and UCLA
* School of Medicine*
Los Angeles, California

Robert C. Malenka
Departments of Psychiatry and
* Physiology*
University of California, San Francisco
San Francisco, California

Alfred Mansour
Mental Health Research Institute
University of Michigan
Ann Arbor, Michigan

Lisa A. Matsuda
Laboratory of Cell Biology
National Institute of Mental Health
Bethesda, Maryland

James H. Meador-Woodruff
Mental Health Research Institute
University of Michigan
Ann Arbor, Michigan

Nancy K. Mello
Alcohol and Drug Abuse Research
* Center*
Harvard Medical School—McLean
* Hospital*
Belmont, Massachusetts

Jack H. Mendelson
Alcohol and Drug Abuse Research
* Center*
Harvard Medical School—McLean
* Hospital*
Belmont, Massachusetts

Jian Mu
Department of Physiology and
* Pharmacology*
Bowman-Gray School of Medicine
Winston-Salem, North Carolina

Eric J. Nestler
Laboratory of Molecular Psychiatry
Departments of Psychiatry and
* Pharmacology*
Yale University School of Medicine
Connecticut Mental Health Center
New Haven, Connecticut

R.A. North
Vollum Institute
Oregon Health Sciences University
Portland, Oregon

Charles P. O'Brien
Philadelphia VA Medical Center
University of Pennsylvania
Philadelphia, Pennsylvania

Bert W. O'Malley
Department of Cell Biology
Baylor College of Medicine
Houston, Texas

James W. Patrick
Division of Neuroscience
Baylor College of Medicine
Houston, Texas

Robert N. Pechnick
Department of Pharmacology
The Brain Research Institute
UCLA School of Medicine
Los Angeles, California

Sakire Pöğün
Department of Physiology
Ege University School of Medicine
Bornova, Turkey

Bernice Porjesz
Neurodynamics Laboratory
SUNY Health Science Center at
Brooklyn
Brooklyn, New York

Robert M. Post
Biological Psychiatry Branch
Laboratory of Neuropsychology
National Institute of Mental Health
Bethesda, Maryland

Terry E. Robinson
Department of Psychology and
Neuroscience Program
University of Michigan
Ann Arbor, Michigan

Martin K.-H. Schäfer
Mental Health Research Institute
University of Michigan
Ann Arbor, Michigan

Ursula Scheffel
Division of Nuclear Medicine
Department of Radiology
The Johns Hopkins Medical Institutions
Baltimore, Maryland

Rabi Simantov
Neuroscience Branch
N.I.D.A. Addiction Research Center
Baltimore, Maryland

James E. Smith
Department of Physiology and
Pharmacology
Bowman-Gray School of Medicine
Winston-Salem, North Carolina

Keith A. Trujillo
Mental Health Research Institute
University of Michigan
Ann Arbor, Michigan

Roxanne Vaughan
Neuroscience Branch
N.I.D.A. Addiction Research Center
Baltimore, Maryland

Mark von Zastrow
Department of Psychiatry
Department of Molecular and Cellular
Physiology
Stanford University Medical Center
Stanford, California

Shao Wang
Department of Physiology and
Pharmacology
Bowman-Gray School of Medicine
Winston-Salem, North Carolina

Stanley J. Watson
Mental Health Research Institute
University of Michigan
Ann Arbor, Michigan

Susan R.B. Weiss
Laboratory of Neuropsychology
National Institute of Mental Health
Bethesda, Maryland

Francis J. White
Department of Psychiatry
Wayne State University
School of Medicine
Detroit, Michigan

BIOLOGICAL BASIS OF SUBSTANCE ABUSE

The Neurobiology of Addiction: An Integrative View

FLOYD E. BLOOM

INTEGRATIVE THINKING IN THE ANALYSIS OF ADDICTIVE DISEASES

Medical researchers are accustomed to the vertical reasoning approach to disease mechanisms (Blois, 1988). In that approach, physician-diagnosed signs and patient-perceived symptoms are explained in terms of the underlying pathophysiological processes within cells and their biochemical or molecular causes. This mode of reasoning can also be usefully applied to the addictions. The patient's or experimental subject's manifestations are primarily described in terms of drug-seeking behaviors, and the integrative tactic is to define the cellular manifestations of the drug-dependent and drug-craving state and the biochemical, molecular, and ultimately atomic means by which this state is produced.

This chapter examines not only the means by which use of drugs of abuse can result in the drug-dependent state (for references, see Koob & Bloom, 1988) but also two additional temporal phases critical to the problems of drug-addicted subjects: (1) the changes that occur with multiple drug exposures over prolonged periods, which produce the states of altered drug sensitivity termed tolerance and sensitization and (2) the residual long-term changes that persist despite prolonged periods of drug abstinence and that contribute to the phenomenon of drug craving.

HIERARCHICAL LEVELS OF RESEARCH IN THE NEUROSCIENCES

The strategies used to analyze addictive drugs in the CNS may be molecular, cellular, or behavioral (Bloom, 1988). The traditional focus for characterizing drugs that alter behavior has been the intensively exploited molecular level.

This work was supported by Alcohol Research Center Grant AA 06420. This chapter is RISC NP # 6796.

Molecular discoveries provide biochemical probes for identifying the appropriate neuronal sites and mechanisms, of drug action, as well as pharmacological tools to verify them.

Research at the cellular level determines which specific neurons and which of their most proximate synaptic connections underlie the effects of a given drug. The cellular level of addictive drug analysis exploits both molecular and behavioral leads to determine the most likely brain sites at which drug-induced behavioral changes can be analyzed and provides the initial clues to the nature of drug-neuron interactions in terms of interneuronal communication, i.e., excitation, inhibition, or more complex forms of synaptic interaction, (for references, see Koob & Bloom, 1988). The locus of the cells or cell systems central to a drug action has also been inferred from experimental lesions or stimulations of specific brain sites.

Research at the behavioral level centers on the integrative phenomena that link populations of neurons into extended specialized circuits, ensembles, or more pervasively distributed "systems" that accomplish tasks, such as sensing, moving, or "reinforcing." Such tasks include the complex but still poorly understood mechanisms of learning, reward, and reinforcement. This three-part strategical hierarchy's main deficiency is the degree to which it blurs the currently most obscure element; namely, the means by which events on the behavioral level can be linked to discrete cells and circuits, and vice versa.

Koob and I (1988) analyzed the literature to determine whether the molecular, cellular, and behavioral data on the acute and chronic effects of addictive drugs form an internally consistent sequential pattern in which molecular events generate cellular effects that in turn are linked to behavioral phenomena to explain the common features of drug dependence. Our focus was on both the acute initial effects of abused drugs on specific neurons and the change in these effects with continued drug exposure. From that analysis, we proposed a potential role for a specific limbic-extrapyramidal system that has been implicated in both the reinforcement and adaptive responses to all three drug classes.

Substantial progress has been made in analyzing the molecular and cellular actions of three major types of abused drugs: opiates, such as heroin and morphine; psychostimulants, such as cocaine and amphetamines, and alcoholic beverages (ethanol). Research has pinpointed likely neurotransmitter systems (and their circuits) that are involved in opiate and psychostimulant addictions and has emphasized the relative importance of several possible transmitters underlying the more complex actions of ethanol, the least potent of these three drug types but probably the most widely abused. Although those three types of drugs remain the centerpiece of drug abuse research at the experimental level, substantial inroads have been made in studying phencyclidine, nicotine, benzodiazepines, and tetrahydrocannabinoids as well (see Chapters 13, 14, 18, and 21).

EFFECTS ON DRUG-NAIVE BRAIN

Most of the data on the effects of drugs of abuse in experimental animals pertains to the acute effects of these drugs on drug-naive subjects. Such studies have tried to determine what effects are produced by these drugs when given either by systemic administration in doses that are meaningful in terms of self-administration routines or by local micromethods into brain regions in which the reinforcing actions are thought to take place. The relative success of these approaches for opiates and psychostimulants can be attributed to earlier work that established the structural substrate of endogenous neurotransmission sites on which these drugs manifest their responses. Similarly, the nature of the acute cellular effects of ethanol may still be unknown because of its multiple potential reinforcing and intoxicating effects (see Bloom, 1987).

The Acute Actions of Opioids are Mediated by Endogenous Opioid Peptide Receptors in the Nucleus Accumbens

Three separate lines of work were initiated after the discovery of the endogenous opioid peptides (Civelli et al., 1983; Comb et al., 1983a & b; Douglass et al., 1982; Suda et al., 1982) and provide the cornerstone of opiate neuropharmacology. The first two lines clarified the separate genetic origins of the opioid peptides and produced detailed maps of neuronal pathways containing one or another of the three opioid peptide genes (Akil et al., 1984; Bloom, 1983). The third line established the basic effects of opiates and opioid peptides on neurons throughout the CNS.

The mu class of opiate receptor subtype is considered to be the major class underlying opiate self-administration (Chavkin & Goldstein, 1986; Goldstein & Kalant, 1990; Wala et al., 1990). With few exceptions, studies of central neurons agree that mu receptors suppress spontaneous discharge with little or no effect on membrane polarization and result in reduced responsivity to amino acid excitation, which is accompanied by diminution of afferent synaptic potentials, both excitatory and inhibitory (Moore et al., 1988; Siggins & Zieglgänsberger, 1981; Siggins et al., 1982). In most cases, this set of effects result in reduced firing of mu-responsive neurons. However, in some cases, notably the hippocampal pyramidal neurons and those in other locales that are essential links in the addiction circuitry, the responsive units are inhibitory interneurons. As a result of their opiate-induced inhibition, the adjacent pyramidal cells (and other immediate target neurons under their tonic inhibitory control) are disinhibited (Siggins et al., 1988; Zieglgänsberger et al., 1979). When the disinhibited neurons discharge at high rates, important functional sequelae, such as electrographic seizures in the hippocampal formation, emerge (Henriksen et al., 1979).

An important exception to this general effect is the response of noradrenergic neurons of the nucleus locus ceruleus. North and Aghajanian and their colleagues (see Chapters 4 and 10 and Aghajanian, 1978; Andrade et al., 1983; Freedman & Aghajanian, 1985; Rasmussen & Aghajanian, 1989; Rasmussen et al., 1990) have shown that in the locus ceruleus, mu receptors activate a potassium channel, producing hyperpolarization; the mu-receptor-mediated signal transduction involves the direct regulation of the channel protein by a guanosine triphosphate (G-protein) mechanism (Aghajanian & Wang, 1986, 1987; Christie et al., 1987; North & Williams, 1983; Wang & Aghajanian, 1987; Williams & North, 1984, 1988). These two basic response site characteristics— a hyperpolarizing potassium channel regulated by a G-protein-coupled receptor—are also attributes shared by the responsive elements for cocaine (see Chapter 10).

Within these mapped opioid peptide-containing neuronal circuits, major attention has been focused on the nucleus accumbens (nACC), in which micro-injections of a nondiffusible analog of naloxone will effectively quench opiate self-administration in rats (see Chapter 22; Ettenberg et al., 1984). In confirmation of the generally depressant effects of mu-receptor-responsive neurons, Hakan and Henriksen (1989) recently reported two routes of mu-receptor-mediated suppression of activity on neurons of the nACC: a direct activation of the dopamine projection from the ventral tegmental area, (VTA) potentially mediated by a disinhibitory mechanism as described above (see Chapter 4), and a direct opioid-mediated inhibition of spontaneous activity even after the dopamine projection has been pharmacologically antagonized.

The Acute Reinforcing Actions of Cocaine are Mediated by the Dopaminergic Projection to Nucleus Accumbens

The neurobiological mediator of cocaine, as well as of amphetamine psycho-stimulants, seems to be the neurotransmitter dopamine (DA). According to the currently favored molecular view, it is the ability of cocaine to inhibit dopamine reuptake that produces the drug's effect(Ritz et al., 1987, 1988, 1990; also see Chapter 5). These data support the conclusion that cocaine augments do-paminergic neuron activity by prolonging the effects of neuronally released dopamine via blockade of the reuptake process that normally terminates local dopamine postsynaptic actions. Dopamine-containing neurons of the ventral tegmentum and their tracts, which innervate limbic and frontal cortex, are required for the acute reinforcing actions of cocaine and d-amphetamine (Koob & Bloom, 1988; Koob et al., 1984; Roberts et al., 1990; Strecker et al., 1982).

Recent studies have begun to define the cellular basis for cocaine actions within the dopamine system of neurons. White and colleagues (Einhorn et al., 1988; Henry et al., 1989; White & Wang, 1984a & b) showed that dopamine normally depresses the spontaneous activity of neurons of the nACC, which are innervated by dopaminergic neurons of the ventral tegmental area (VTA). Importantly, dopamine also inhibits the firing of VTA dopamine neurons at three- to tenfold greater potency than in the nucleus accumbens. Intravenous administration of cocaine produces potent inhibition of VTA cell firing, whereas local iontophoresis of cocaine directly into VTA had only modest direct effects (Einhorn et al., 1988). Significantly, localized cocaine administration increased and prolonged the inhibitory effects of iontophoretically applied DA (Einhorn et al., 1988; Lacey et al., 1990b; Uchimura & North, 1990; also see Chapter 10). This relationship of potency suggests that when dopamine neurons are active, the dopamine they release in the presence of cocaine will have greater effects on reducing dopamine cell firing than on dopamine released into the terminal fields within the nACC. This result is complicated, however, by the GABA-mediated reciprocal circuit from the nACC to the VTA (White & Wang, 1984a and b). When dopamine is released into the nACC, the normally active tonic GABA inhibition of VTA dopamine neurons is reduced, thereby releasing DA neurons to fire. In the presence of cocaine, this released DA remains extracellularly in a position to occupy DA receptors and to further depress GABA (and other) cell firing. Drugs affecting neuronal uptake of the other major brain monoamines, norepinephrine (NE) or serotonin (5-HT), did not potentiate DA effects. However, North and colleagues (see Lacey et al., 1990a) have recently shown that low doses of cocaine potentiate the depolarizing effects of 5-HT on nACC neurons, as well as the hyperpolarizing effects of dopamine on these cells. The dopamine effects here and on the dopamine neurons themselves are interpreted as activating on outward potassium current (Lacey et al., 1990b and c). Although it remains to be determined whether cocaine acts only on DA neurons in the VTA or on other DA sources as well, Koob and colleagues (see Koob & Bloom, 1988 for references) have demonstrated that chemical destruction of the dopaminergic terminals within the nACC is sufficient to quell cocaine self-administration in rats and that this treatment does not disrupt heroin self-administration (Koob et al., 1984; et al., 1982).

The Acute Actions of Ethanol are Mediated through Multiple Transmitter Systems and Multiple Mechanisms of Action

The two previous examples indicate the importance of a neuronal template in defining the basis for the molecular and cellular reinforcement actions of cocaine or opiate addiction in meaningful brain locations. No comparable template has yet been formulated for the actions of ethanol. The reinforcing properties of ethanol have been related to its ability to produce mild euphoria and to reduce perceived anxiety (see Koob & Bloom, 1988 for references). Historically, investigators studying the actions of alcohol on the brain interpreted their data as if alcohol were a lipid solvent that alters the general functions of neuronal membranes by altering the lipids (Goldstein, 1987). However, such an interpretation is difficult to reconcile with the relatively well-defined neuropsychopharmacological profile of ethanol, which, in addition to its potentially reinforcing euphoric and anxiolytic effects, also includes changes in motor coordination, arousal, and cognition. Furthermore, highly selective cellular effects of ethanol have recently been reported (see Koob & Bloom, 1988 for review; also Rabin et al., 1987; Shefner, 1990; Siggins et al., 1987a & b).

For example, locus ceruleus neurons (Aston et al., 1982) exhibit pronounced dose-dependent depression of responsiveness to sensory stimuli at ethanol doses lower than those required for depressing mean spontaneous discharge rates. More pertinent to ethanol's reinforcement actions, dopaminergic neurons of the VTA and substantia nigra are also activated in response to relatively low doses of systemic ethanol administration (Gessa et al., Mereu & Gessa, 1985; Mereu et al., 1984). The activation of the dopaminergic neurons by ethanol may also result from a disinhibitory mechanism, since neurons in the adjacent substantia nigra pars reticulata are depressed by systemic ethanol in what may be a GABA-based effect.

Henriksen (see Chapter 20) has examined in detail the apparent inconsistency between the biochemical and behavioral pharmacological observations favoring an action of ethanol that enhances GABA-mediated effects, and the electrophysiologic observations that have consistently failed to show such effects of ethanol on either exogenously administered GABA or GABA agonists (Mancillas et al., 1986; Siggins et al., 1987b) or on pathways considered to be GABA mediated (Siggins et al., 1987). His recent data with Stephenson (personal communication; also see Chapter 10) suggest that, in the presence of low intoxicating doses of ethanol, the excitability of these GABA-interneurons—at least in the hippocampal CA3 fields—is increased, thereby enhancing their inhibition of their target cells. This interpretation helps reconcile the cellular electrophysiology and behavioral pharmacology of the ethanol-GABA interaction. However, it does not explain the in vitro biochemical result of apparent enhancement of GABA-mediated chloride fluxes in subcellular fractions of brain homogenates enriched in "neurosynaptosomes" (Suzdak, et al., 1986, 1988). Those fractions are especialy problematic since most identified GABA terminals are located on neuronal perikarya, not on dendrites (Freund et al., 1983, 1989; Somogyi & Hodgson, 1985; Somogyi et al., 1984, 1985). Most recently, Lin et al. (1991) have raised the possibility that noradrenergic receptors must be occupied, at least within the cerebellum, for GABA responses to be enhanced, creating yet an additional mechanism of ethanol action ready for replication testing.

ADAPTIVE RESPONSES WITH CHRONIC DRUG EXPOSURE

An important aspect of the addictive state is the development of tolerance to the drug being abused. Animal studies have been especially useful in dissecting out the alternative explanations and sites at which tolerance may arise and in suggesting which sites and actions may merit further analysis. Traditional pharmacological explanations have focused on changes in the metabolism of the primary neurotransmitters or in alterations of their receptor mechanisms. Only a few such changes have been reported. Akil and colleagues (Bronstein et al., 1990) have recently reported that animals dependent on morphine show accumulation of a novel form of beta-endorphin that is shortened at its C-terminus; such peptides have previously been suggested to possess opioid antagonist actions (Suh et al., 1988; Tseng & Li, 1986). In addition, minor changes in dopamine receptor sensitivity (Einhorn et al., 1988; Henry et al., 1989) and in intracellular proteins that may be phosphorylated as a result of dopamine receptor activation (see Chapter 4) have also been reported within the dopamine neurons and their targets after chronic cocaine exposure.

Koob and I (1988) have taken an operational approach to the phenomenon of tolerance, which we have cast as an attempt by the body to return to homeostasis equivalent to the drug-free condition. Much evidence suggests that physical dependence and tolerance generally develop and decay with a similar time course, leading to the concept that, as the drug-taker reacts to the effects of the drug, adaptive "processes" are initiated to counter those effects, and they persist after the drug has been cleared from the brain, thereby leaving the opposing processes unopposed. Such notions of undefined opposing or adaptive "processes" have been previously proposed at all levels of drug abuse research (see Koob & Bloom, 1988, 1989 for references).

The undefined "opposing" process may not operate *within* the system manifesting the initial effects of the drug, but rather may be manifest *between* regulatory systems to restore a homeostasis akin to the drug-free situation (Fig. 1-1). The changes noted above for some opiate- and dopamine-related changes would fall within our definition of *within*-system adaptations.

Withdrawal Reveals the Adaptive Process in Operation Unopposed by Concurrent Drug Action

In this regard, it is of interest to consider the adaptive response of cerebellar Purkinje neurons to several days of continuous ethanol exposure (Rogers et al., 1980; Siggins, et al., 1987a & b). After 10 to 14 days of ethanol intoxication, cerebellar Purkinje cells show complete tolerance in that previously disrupted patterns of cell firing are now completely normal, despite continued intoxicating blood levels of alcohol. However, within 90 minutes of withdrawal from ethanol, Purkinje cell firing is significantly disrupted, and, the specific disruption can be reversed by re-establishing an intoxicating blood concentration of ethanol. The changed pattern of firing of Purkinje cells during withdrawal resembles their response to NE iontophoresis or locus ceruleus (LC) stimulation (Hoffer et al., 1971a & b; Siggins et al., 1971a & b). This finding suggests that LC hyperactivity may accompany ethanol withdrawal, as it does opiate tolerance and withdrawal (see Chapter 4). These data are starting points from which to document the adaptive molecular mechanisms that accompany continued exposure to the drug. Another possible example of between-systems adaptive mechanisms are the recent findings (Trujillo & Akil, 1991) that antagonism of the N-methyl-D-aspartate (glutamate) receptor by systemic administration of low doses of MK-801 for 3 days attenuates the concurrent development of morphine tolerance and dependence.

Sensitization: A Special Adaptive Process with Psychostimulant Drug Usage

Under certain circumstances, repeated exposures to amphetamine can result in progressive enhancement of the behavioral locomotion response, an adaptive sequence termed "sensitization" (see Chapter 24). The basis for this inconsistently found long-term effect has recently been examined by Le Moal and colleagues (Deminiere et al., 1989; Piazza et al., 1989, 1990; Rivet et al., 1989) as a consequence of individual subject stress-related reactivity. In their view, the sensitization response requires significant release of endogenous corticosteroids; these steroids then act on central dopaminergic neurons or receptive cells to enhance the effects of the stimulant drug. Similar phenomena have also been reported for human stimulant abusers (see Chapter 28). In the nucleus accumbens, neurons have been found to be significantly more responsive to dopamine after chronic exposure to cocaine (Henry et al., 1989), providing perhaps one basis for the sensitization response.

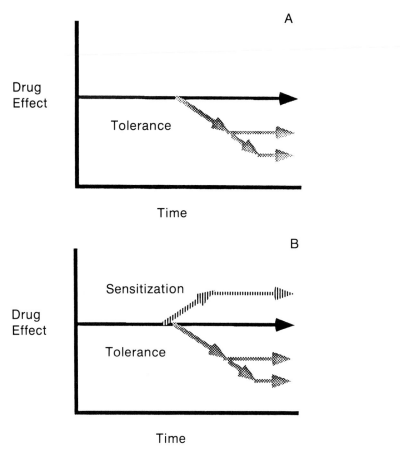

Figure 1-1. Composite schematic diagram of the loss of drug potency with continued exposure **(A)**, the appearance of the special sensitization response that occurs in some cases with psychostimulants **(B)**, and the operational "explanation" of tolerance by the emergence of unspecified adaptive or opposing mechanisms **(C)**.

THE NEUROSCIENCE OF DRUG CRAVING

Perhaps the least understood behavioral phenomenon of the pharmacology of addictive drugs is the molecular and cellular basis for the long-term craving that remains once there has been apparent functional recovery from the acute effects of withdrawal. During that recovery period, one could infer that addictive drug could have added negative reinforcing value simply by diminishing the adverse consequences of the withdrawal restabilization. Early experimental analysis of this effect has implicated the nucleus accumbens as a likely neural substrate for the disruptive aversive stimulus properties of opiate withdrawal (Koob et al., 1989). From the standpoint of efforts to define long-term "therapies" for addiction, understanding the basis for this residual craving must be an important objective.

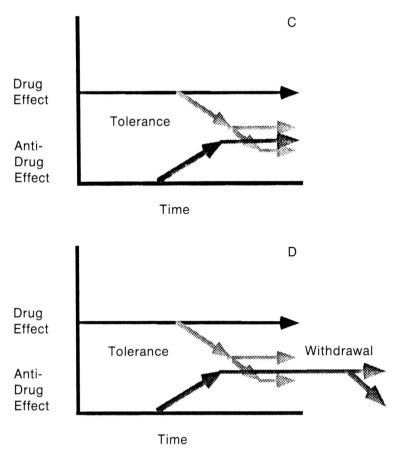

Figure 1-1 (*continued*)   (**D**), Residual opposing mechanisms persisting after the circulating drug levels decline to produce withdrawal; potentially some of these adaptive changes could persist still longer to account for the craving process.

CONCLUSIONS AND PERSPECTIVES

Based on the work of Wise (1988), the starting concept of drug craving may be seen as the drug-seeking motivation derived from the memory of past positive drug reinforcement. A critical body of knowledge related to this remembered reinforcement remains to be gathered, and at this stage major questions remain. What is the nature of drug discrimination mechanisms by which animals can identify stimulants and sedatives? Which neuronal systems that react to these drugs are responsible for self-administered drug reinforcements, and which initiate the adaptive or learned tolerance to these drugs (MacRae et al., 1987; Siegel, 1982; Siegel & Sado, 1986; Wenger et al., 1981). How do conditional environmental stimuli, associated with drug exposures, result in apparent adaptive tolerance under environmentally specific conditions? How do those conditional effects provide long-term associations by which drug reinforcements can be recalled to initiate craving?

As with every other heuristic body of knowledge within medical biology, so too the advent of rigorous approaches to the behavioral phenomena of addiction generates many more questions than answers. Nevertheless, such approaches are necessary to provide implementable answers to what makes some people more susceptible to addictive drug experimentation and what keeps them addicted against their volition.

REFERENCES

Aghajanian, G.K. (1978). Tolerance of locus coeruleus neurones to morphine and suppression of withdrawal response by clonidine. *Nature, 276*(5684), 186-188.

Aghajanian, G.K., & Y.Y. Wang (1986). Pertussis toxin blocks the outward currents evoked by opiate and alpha 2-agonists in locus coeruleus neurons. *Brain Res., 371*(2), 390-394.

Aghajanian, G.K., & Y.Y. Wang (1987). Common alpha 2- and opiate effector mechanisms in the locus coeruleus: Intracellular studies in brain slices." *Neuropharmacology, 26*(7B), 793-799.

Akil, H., Watson, S.J., et al. (1984). Endogenous opioids: Biology and function. *Annu. Rev. Neurosci., 7,* 223-255.

Andrade, R., Vandermaelen, C.P., et al. (1983). Morphine tolerance and dependence in the locus coeruleus: Single cell studies in brain slices. *Eur. J. Pharmacol., 91*(2-3), 161-169.

Aston, J.G., Foote, S.L., et al. (1982). Low doses of ethanol disrupt sensory responses of brain noradrenergic neurones. *Nature, 296*(5860), 857-860.

Blois, M.S. (1988). Medicine and the nature of vertical reasoning. N. Engl. J. Med., *318*(13), 847-851.

Bloom, F.E. (1983). The endorphins: A growing family of pharmacologically pertinent peptides. *Annu. Rev. Pharmacol. Toxicol., 23,* 151-170.

Bloom, F.E. (1987). The emerging pharmacology of ethanol. *J. Psychopharmacol. 1*(4), 227-236.

Bloom, F.E. (1988). Neurotransmitters: Past, present, and future directions. *Faseb. J., 2*(1), 32-41.

Bronstein, D.M., Przewlocki, R., et al. (1990). Effects of morphine treatment on proopiomelanocortin systems in rat brain. *Brain Res., 519*(1-2), 102-111.

Chavkin, C., & Goldstein, A. (1986). Brain chemistry and the addictions. *J. Subst. Abuse Treat., 3*(3), 157-61.

Christie, M.J., Williams, J.T., et al. (1987). Mechanisms of tolerance to opiates in locus coeruleus neurons. *Nida. Res. Monogr., 78,* 158-168.

Civelli, O., Birnberg, N., et al. (1983). Generation of diversity and evolution of opioid peptides. *Cold Spring Harb. Symp. Quant. Biol., 1,* 375-384.

Comb, M., Rosen, H., et al. (1983a). Regulation of opioid gene expression. *Peptides, 4*(5), 651-656.

Comb, M., Seeburg, P.H., et al. (1983b). Primary structure of the human proenkephalin gene. *DNA, 2*(3), 213-229.

Deminiere, J.M., Piazza, P.V., et al. (1989). Experimental approach to individual vulnerability to psychostimulant addiction. *Neurosci. Biobehav. Rev., 13*(2-3), 141-147.

Douglass, J., Cox, B., et al. (1982). Cloning and sequence analysis of cDNA for bovine adrenal preproenkephalin. *Nature, 295*(5846), 202-206.

Einhorn, L.C., Johansen, P.A., et al. (1988). Cocaine and central monoamingergic neurotransmission: A review of electrophysiological studies and comparison to amphetamine and antidepressants. *Life Sci., 42*(9), 949-968.

Ettenberg, A., Pettit, H.O., et al. (1984). Effects of opiate antagonists and their quaternary derivatives on heroin self-administration in the rat. *J. Pharmacol. Exp. Ther., 229*(2): 481-486.

Freedman, J.E., & Aghajanian, G.K. (1985). Opiate and alpha 2-adrenoceptor responses of rat and amygdaloid neurons: Co-localization and interactions during withdrawal." *J. Neurosci., 5*(11), 3016-3024.

Freund, T.F., Martin, K.A., et al. (1983). Glutamate decarboxylase-immunoreactive terminals of Golgi-impregnated axoaxonic cells and of presumed basket cells in synaptic contact with pyramidal neurons of the cat's visual cortex. *J. Comp. Neurol., 221*(3), 263-278.

Freund, T.F., Martin, K.A., et al. (1989). Arborisation pattern and postsynaptic targets of physiologically identified thalamocortical afferents in striate cortex of the macaque monkey. *J. Comp. Neurol., 289*(2), 315-336.

Gessa, G.L., Muntoni, F., et al. (1985). Low doses of ethanol inhibit the firing of neurons in the substantia, nigra, pars reticulata: A GABAergic effect? *Brain Res., 360*(1-2), 325-330.

Goldstein, A., & Kalant, H. (1990). Articles: Drug policy: Striking the right balance. *Science, 249*(4976), 1513-1521.

Goldstein, D.B. (1987). Ethanol-induced adaptation in biological membranes. *Ann. NY. Acad. Sci., 492*, 103-115.

Hakan, R.L., & Henriksen, S.J. (1989). Opiate influences on nucleus accumbens electrophysiology: Dopamine and non-dopamine mechanisms. *J. Neurosci., 9*(10): 3538-3546.

Henriksen, S.J., Bloom, F.E., et al. (1979). beta-Endorphin induces nonconvulsive limbic seizures. *Proc. Natl. Acad. Sci. USA., 76*(4), 2077-2080.

Henry, D.J., Greene, M.A., et al. (1989). Electrophysiological effects of cocaine in the mesoaccumbens dopamine system: Repeated administration. *J. Pharmacol. Exp. Ther., 251*(3), 833-839.

Hoffer, B.J., Siggins, G.R., et al. (1971a). Activation of a central noradrenergic projection to cerebellum. *Nature, 233*(5320), 481-483.

Hoffer, B.J., Siggins, G.R., et al. (1971b). Cyclic adenosine monophosphate and norepinephrine: Effect on Purkinje cells in rat cerebellar cortex. *Science, 174*(15), 1257-1259.

Koob, G.F., & Bloom, F.E. (1988). Cellular and molecular mechanisms of drug dependence. *Science, 242*(4879), 715-723.

Koob, G.F., & Bloom, F.E. (1989). Opponent process theory of motivation: Neurobiological evidence from studies of opiate dependence. *Neurosci. Biobehav. Rev., 13*(2-3): 135-140.

Koob, G.F., Pettit, H.O., et al. (1984). Destruction of dopamine in the nucleus accumbens selectively attenuates cocaine but not heroin self-administration in rats. *Psychopharmacology (Berlin), 84*(2), 167-173.

Koob, G.F., Wall, T.L., et al. (1989). Nucleus accumbens as a substrate for the aversive stimulus effects of opiate withdrawal. *Psychopharmacology (Berlin), 98*(4), 530-534.

Lacey, M.G., Mercuri, N.B., et al. (1990a). Actions of cocaine on rat dopaminergic neurones in vitro. *Br. J. Pharmacol., 99*(4), 731-735.

Lacey, M.G., P. Calabresi, et al. (1990b). Muscarine reduces inwardly rectifying potassium conductance in rat nucleus accumbens neurones. *J. Physiol., (London), 422*, 369-380.

Lacey, M.G., Calabresi, P., et al. (1990c). Potassium conductance increased by noradrenaline, opioids, somatostatin, and G-proteins: Whole-cell recording from guinea pig submucous neurons. *J. Neurosci., 10*(5), 1675-1682.

Lin, A.M.-Y., Freund, R.K., et al. (1991). Ethanol potentiation of GABA-induced electrophysiological responses in cerebellum: Requirement for catecholamine modulation. *Neurosci. Lett., 122*(1), 154-158.

MacRae, J.R., Scoles, M.T., et al. (1987). The contribution of Pavlovian conditioning to drug tolerance and dependence. *Br. J. Addict., 82*(4), 371-380.

Mancillas, J., Siggins, G.R., et al. (1986). Systemic ethanol: Selective enhancement of responses to acetylcholine and somatostatin in hippocampus. *Science, 231*(4734), 161-163.

Mereu, G., & Gessa, G.L. (1985). Low doses of ethanol activate dopaminergic neurons in the ventral tegmental area. *Brain Res., 348*(1), 201-203.

Mereu, G., Fadda, F., et al. (1984). Ethanol stimulates the firing rate of nigral dopaminergic neurons in unanesthetized rats. *Brain Res., 292*(1), 63-69.

Moore, S.D., Madamba, S.G., et al. (1988). Enkephalin analogues depress synaptic potentials in rat dentate granule cells recorded intracellularly in vitro. *Neurosci. Lett., 91*(1), 71-76.

North, R.A., and Williams, J.T. (1983). Opiate activation of potassium conductance inhibits calcium action potentials in rat locus coeruleus neurones. *Br. J. Pharmacol., 80*(2), 225-228.

Piazza, P.V., Deminiere, J.M., et al. (1989). Factors that predict individual vulnerability to amphetamine self-administration. *Science, 245*(4925), 1511-1513.

Piazza, P.V., Deminiere, J.M., et al. (1990). Stress- and pharmacologically-induced behavioral sensitization increases vulnerability to acquisition of amphetamine self-administration. *Brain Res., 514*(1), 22-26.

Rabin, R.A., Baker, R.C., & Dietrich, R.A. (1987). Specificity of the action of ethanol in the central nervous system: Behavioral effects. *Alcohol. Alcohol, 1*, 133-138.

Rasmussen, K., & Aghajanian, G.K. (1989). Withdrawal-induced activation of locus coeruleus neurons in opiate-dependent rats: Attenuation by lesions of the nucleus paragigantocellularis. *Brain Res., 505*(2), 346-350.

Rasmussen, K., Beitner, J.D.B., et al. (1990). Opiate withdrawal and the rat locus coeruleus: Behavioral, electrophysiological, and biochemical correlates. *J. Neurosci., 10*(7), 2308-2317.

Ritz, M.C., Lamb, R.J., et al. (1987). Cocaine receptors on dopamine transporters are related to self-administration of cocaine. *Science, 237*(4819), 1219-1223.

Ritz, M.C., Lamb, R.J., et al. (1988). Cocaine self-administration appears to be mediated by dopamine uptake inhibition. *Prog. Neuropsychopharmacol. Biol. Psychiatry, 12*(2-3), 233-239.

Ritz, M.C., Cone, E.J., et al. (1990). Cocaine inhibition of ligand binding at dopamine, norepinephrine and serotonin transporters: A structure-activity study. *Life Sci., 46*(9), 635-645.

Rivet, J.M., Stinus, L., et al. (1989). Behavioral sensitization to amphetamine is dependent on corticosteroid receptor activation. *Brain Res., 498*(1), 149-153.

Roberts, D.C., Koob, G.F., et al. (1980). Extinction and recovery of cocaine self-administration following 6-hydroxydopamine lesions of the nucleus accumbens. *Pharmacol. Biochem. Behav., 12*(5), 781-787.

Rogers, J., Siggins, G.R., et al. (1980). Physiological correlates of ethanol intoxication tolerance, and dependence in rat cerebellar Purkinje cells. *Brain Res., 196*(1), 183-198.

Shefner, S.A. (1990). Electrophysiological effects of ethanol on brain membranes. In *biochemistry and physiology of substance abuse* (pp. 25-53). Boca Raton, FL: CRC Press.

Siegel, S. (1982). Opioid expectation modifies opioid effects. *Fed. Proc., 41*(7), 2339-2343.

Siegel, S., & Sado, J.K. (1986). Attenuation of ethanol tolerance by a novel stimulus. *Psychopharmacology (Berlin), 88*(2), 258-261.

Siggins, G.R., & Zieglgänsberger, W. (1981). Morphine and opioid peptides reduce inhibitory synaptic potentials in hippocampal pyramidal cells in vitro without alteration of membrane potential. *Proc. Natl. Acad. Sci. USA., 78*(8), 5235-5239.

Siggins, G.R., Oliver, A.P., et al. (1971a). Studies on norepinephrine-containing afferents to Purkinje cells of art cerebellum. I. Localization of the fibers and their synapses. *Brain Res., 25*(3), 501-521.

Siggins, G.R., Hoffer, B.J., et al. (1971b). Activation of a central noradrenergic projection to cerebellum. *Nature, 233*(5320), 481-483.

Siggins, G.R., Bloom, F.E., et al. (1987a). Electrophysiological action of ethanol at the cellular level. *Alcohol, 4*(4), 331-337.

Siggins, G.R., Bloom, F.E., French, E.D., Madamba, S.G., Mancillas, J., Pittman, Q.J., & Rogers, J. (1987b). Electrophysiology of ethanol on central neurons. *Ann. NY. Acad. Sci., 492,* 350-366.

Siggins, G.R., McGinty, J.F., Chavkin, C., & Henriksen, S.J. (1982). The role of neuropeptides in the hippocampal formation. *Adv. Biochem. Psychopharmal., 33,* 413-422.

Somogyi, P., & Hodgson, A.J. (1985). Antisera to gamma-aminobutyric acid. III. Demonstration of GABA in Golgi-impregnated neurons and in conventional electron microscopic sections of cat striate cortex. *J. Histochem. Cytochem., 33*(3), 249-257.

Somogyi, P., Freund, T.F., & Kisvardy, Z.F. (1984). Different types of 3H-GABA accumulating neurons in the visual cortex of the rat. Characterization by combined autoradiography and Golgi impregnation. *Exp. Brain. Res., 54*(1), 45-56.

Somogyi, P., Hodgson, A.J., Chubb, I.W., Penke, B., & Erdei, A. (1985). Antisera to gamma-aminobutyric acid. II. Immunocytochemical application to the central nervous system. *J. Histochem. Cytochem., 33*(3), 240-248.

Strecker, R.E., Roberts, D.C., & Koob, G.F. (1982). Disruption of cocaine self-administration following 6-hydroxydopamine lesions of the ventral tegmental area in rats. *Pharmacol. Biochem. Behav., 17*(5), 901-904.

Suda, M., Nakao, K., Sakamoto, M., Yoshimasa, T., Morii, N., Yanaihara, N., Numa, S., & Imura, H.I. (1982). Cloning and sequence analysis of cDNA for bovine adrenal preproenkephalin. *Nature, 295*(5846), 202-206.

Suh, H.H., Tseng, L.F., & Li, C.H. (1988). Beta-endorphin-(1-27) antagonizes beta-endorphin- but not morphine-, D-Pen2-D-Pen5-enkephalin- and U50, 488H-induced analgesia in mice. *Neuropharmacology, 27*(9), 957-963.

Suzdak, P.D., Glowa, J.R., Crowley, J.N., Schwartz, R.D., Skolnick, P., & Paul, S.M. (1986). A selective imidazobenzodiazepine antagonist of ethanol in the rat. *Science, 234*(4781), 1243-1247.

Suzdak, P.D., Schwartz, R.D., et al. (1988). Alcohols stimulate gamma-aminobutyric acid receptor-mediated chloride uptake in brain vesicles: Correlation with intoxication potency. *Brain Res., 444*(2), 340-345.

Trujillo, K.A., & Akil, H. (1991). Inhibition of morphine tolerance and dependence by the NMDA antagonists MK801. *Science, 251*(1), 85-87.

Tseng, L.F., & Li, C.H. (1986). beta-Endorphin-(1-27) inhibits the spinal beta-endorphin-induced release of Met-enkephalin. *Int. J. Pept. Protein Res., 27*(4), 394-397.

Uchimura, N., & North, R.A. (1990). Actions of cocaine on rat dopaminergic neurones in vitro. *Br. J. Pharmacol., 99*(4), 731-735.

Wala, E.P., Sloan, J.W., & Martin, W.R. (1990). Drug abuse strategies. *Drug Alcohol Depend., 25*(2), 115-119.

Wang, Y.Y., & Aghajanian, G.K. (1987). Intracellular GTP gamma S restores the ability of morphine to hyperpolarize rat locus coeruleus neurons after blockade by pertussis toxin. *Brain Res., 436*(2), 396-401.

Wenger, J.R., Berlin, V., & Woods, S.C. (1981). Ethanol tolerance in the rat is learned. *Science, 213*(4507), 575-577.

White, F.J., & Wang, R.Y. (1984a). Electrophysiological evidence for A10 dopamine autoreceptor sensitivity following chronic d-amphetamine treatment. *Brain Res., 309,* 283-292.

White, F.J., & Wang, R.Y. (1984b). Interaction of cholecystokinin octapeptide and dopamine on nucleus accumbens neurons. *Brain Res., 300,* 161-166.

Williams, J.T., & North, R.A. (1984). Opiate-receptor interactions on single locus coeruleus neurones. *Mol. Pharmacol., 26*(3), 489-497.

Williams, J.T., North, R.A., et al. (1988). Inward rectification of resting and opiate-activated potassium currents in rat locus coeruleus neurons. *J. Neurosci., 8*(11), 4299-4306.

Wise, R.A. (1988). The neurobiology of craving: Implications for the understanding and treatment of addiction. *J. Abnorm. Psychol., 97*(2), 118-132.

Zieglgänsberger, W., French, E.D., & Siggins, G.R. (1979). Opioid peptides may excite hippocampal pyramidal neurons by inhibiting adjacent inhibitory interneurons. *Science, 205*(4404), 415-417.

I

CELL BIOLOGY

The importance of the familiar lock-and-key model of neuroregulators (ligands) and their receptors as a biological principle that facilitates understanding of basic processes is highlighted by the study of drugs of abuse. Processes that were completely without known mechanisms have been clarified with the discovery of the relevant receptor. Indeed, the search for receptors related to drugs of abuse has become important in revealing fundamental neurobiological processes. As the relevant receptors are cloned and their biology clarified, it is clear that we will learn much about tolerance, withdrawal and addiction.

Even before the discovery of endogenous opiates, the search for receptors for opiate drugs had begun to produce exciting results. Earlier pharmacological investigations involving neither protein chemistry nor molecular biology but careful classification of biological changes produced by drugs, led to a classification scheme that remains largely intact some decades later. The current status of the opiate systems is described by von Zastrow et al. Evans describes some of the implications of the current efforts to purify and study the molecular biology of the opiate receptors while Nestler and his colleagues demonstrate the importance of second messenger and phosphorylation mechanisms in the actions of opiates and cocaine.

In several systems, studies of receptors are still at an early stage. This applies to the cocaine receptor, for instance, which is discussed by Kuhar and colleagues. In another case, a whole receptor group was discovered without any knowledge of an endogenous ligand at the time of the discovery, as demonstrated by Matsuda et al. in the chapter on the THC receptor. While nicotine receptors have been well defined, their importance in the brain and their diversity are only now being clarified, as pointed out by Patrick and Luetje. This section closes with the powerful example of the steroid receptor superfamily, which is likely to serve as a model for other superfamilies relevant to drugs of abuse by O'Malley.

2

Molecular Mechanisms in Opiate Addiction: A Model for the Study of Substance Abuse

MARK von ZASTROW, MARY E. ABOOD,
JAMES H. EBERWINE, AND JACK D. BARCHAS

During the past two decades, since the discovery of the endogenous brain opioid systems, it has become possible to examine the biological mechanisms underlying opiate abuse and addiction. Consequently, clinical phenomena associated with abuse and addiction, which were refractory to biological understanding just two decades ago, are now becoming accessible to exploration at the cellular and molecular levels.

In this chapter we briefly outline some of these important advances in opioid biology. In doing so we have limited our scope to areas that, in our opinion, illustrate most clearly the emerging relationships between clinical phenomena and biological mechanisms in opiate addiction. For a thorough discussion of related aspects in this large field, the reader is referred to other chapters in this book and to additional review articles as cited in the text.

CLINICAL CHARACTERISTICS AND ETIOLOGY OF OPIATE ADDICTION

Opiate abuse and addiction have a complex and variable clinical presentation. Clinicians differ on a strict definition of the terms "abuse" and "addiction." In fact, opiate addiction is not recognized as a distinct clinical diagnosis in DSM-III-R (1987), the standard classification of mental disorders. Nevertheless, opiate addiction is a generally recognized clinical entity, and it is possible to identify three general phenomena that are typical of the opiate-addicted state. First, addicts exhibit *tolerance* to opiate drugs, such that they require increased opiate doses to achieve the same effect, as assessed by both subjective and objective criteria, than do opiate-naive subjects (Way et al., 1969). Second, opiate addicts exhibit drug *dependence;* that is, they crave continued administration of opiates and develop unpleasant physiological and psychological withdrawal symptoms if opiates are discontinued. Some consider opiate dependence as the sine qua non of opiate addiction; however, dependence develops in normal subjects after prolonged exposure to opiate drugs, and there is evidence that different brain circuitry is involved in producing dependence and reinforcement of repeated opiate ingestion (Bozarth & Wise, 1984). Third, opiate addicts exhibit some type of *cognitive and behavioral dysfunction* related to obtaining and ingesting opiate drugs. These cognitive and behavioral features have a heterogeneous presentation and include various "drug-seeking" behaviors (e.g., lying, stealing to support one's habit) and the apparent inability of the addict to recognize the negative consequences of drug use (so-called addict's denial). Cognitive and behavioral dysfunction is highly characteristic of opiate addiction, and it is so pervasive and robust that it may seem to be part of the addict's basic personality. Indeed, the extent to which this dysfunction results from pre-existing personality traits or from drug-induced dysfunction is open to debate (Miller, 1990). Addicts may manifest cognitive and behavioral dysfunction long after they have ceased the ingestion of opiate drugs; recognition of this dysfunction is a mainstay of modern relapse prevention efforts.

Attempts to understand the etiology of opiate addiction have traditionally invoked the influences of independent biological, psychological, and environmental factors. Such formulations emphasize the complexity of opiate addiction and are useful descriptively, but they do not account accurately for the consistent observation that apparently diverse etiologic factors are highly interrelated. For example, opiate tolerance is strongly determined by physiological mechanisms (biological influence), but it is also clear that psychological and environmental variables, such as the expectation and setting of drug ingestion, can affect a subject's level of drug tolerance. Opiate dependence as well seems to be strongly determined by physiological mechanisms, but withdrawal symptoms are influenced by psychological variables and can be precipitated by environmental cues (reviewed in Powell et al., 1990). Cognitive and behavioral features of opiate addiction, interpreted traditionally in psychological terms, can be understood on the basis of neurophysiological processes, including associative learning and the operation of brain reward circuitry (Koob & Bloom, 1988; Koob et al., 1989; Schaefer, 1988; see Chapter 1).

The remarkable interrelationship among these apparently diverse etiologic influences implies that opiate addiction can be understood most comprehensively by a neurobiological model. The complexity of opiate addiction results from the operation and perturbation of a limited number of biological mechanisms that fundamentally affect the function of the central nervous system (CNS). The CNS is the principal site at which diverse etiologic influences are integrated and intricate cognitive and behavioral patterns are generated. Although some phenomena observed in addiction, such as the gastrointestinal responses to opiate withdrawal (Chahl & Thornton, 1987), can be explained primarily by opiate effects on peripheral cells, addiction research has focused on the CNS as the principal site involved in the complex integration and processing underlying the clinical phenomena of opiate addiction. Understanding these fundamental biological mechanisms and the ways in which they affect neural processing is an important goal of modern addiction research.

OVERVIEW OF THE BIOLOGICAL SUBSTRATE OF OPIATE ADDICTION

The diversity of clinical presentation and etiologic influences involved in opiate addiction presages the complexity of the underlying neurobiology. Fully elucidating these biological mechanisms is an ambitious goal requiring a great deal more study; however, important inroads have been made that allow a glimpse at these mechanisms and suggest plausible hypotheses for directing further investigation. Seminal developments, which began approximately two decades ago and have formed the basis for essentially all current research into the biology of opiate addiction, were the discovery of the endogenous opioid peptides and receptors.

Opiate drugs were known, used, and abused for many centuries before it was recognized that these drugs interact with cellular receptors for endogenous opioid peptides. It is now appreciated that neurons present in the CNS use these endogenous opioid peptides as neurotransmitters and neuromodulators (reviewed in Kosterlitz et al., 1989). The diversity of endogenous opioid peptides and receptors found in the CNS is impressive (see Chapter 3). A large number of opioid peptides are produced by specific proteolytic cleavages and chemical modifications of three distinct polypeptide precursors (each encoded by a separate structural gene), and opioid-producing neurons are classified according to which precursor polypeptide they express (reviewed in Olson et al., 1990). The diversity of the opioid systems is also manifest at the level of opioid receptors. At least four subtypes of opioid receptor are expressed in the CNS and are distinguished according to how tightly they bind different opioid peptides. It is not yet known whether these receptor subtypes are encoded by separate structural genes or whether they differ by some type of chemical modification. The anatomical distribution of opioid neurons is highly organized, reflecting the organization of these neurons into distinct functional systems (reviewed in Mansour et al., 1988).

It was proposed two decades ago that opiate drugs exert their effects by interacting with endogenous opioid receptors. This hypothesis has been confirmed, and it is now generally believed that opioid receptors are the sole sites at which opiate drugs interact with the CNS (Kosterlitz et al., 1989). Therefore, a major focus in addiction research has been on the cellular effects mediated by the binding of opiate drugs to endogenous opioid receptors. Opioid receptors, like many other hormone and neurotransmitter receptors, are membrane proteins that transduce information across the plasma membrane by interacting with intracellular GTP-binding proteins (see Chapter 3, for an excellent discussion of the pertinent experimental evidence). GTP-binding proteins serve as intermediaries between receptors and intracellular signal transduction components. Binding of opioid peptide or opiate drug to opioid receptors modulates GTP-binding proteins (so-called G-proteins) that are coupled to these receptors, and these G-proteins subsequently modulate intracellular enzymes or ion channels. The result of this cascade is the conversion of extracellular information (receptor-ligand binding on the cell surface) to intracellular information (G-protein-mediated modulation of intracellular enzymes or membrane-bound ion channels). The molecular mechanisms underlying G-protein-coupled signal transduction are currently under intensive investigation (Ross, 1989).

Further appreciation of the complexity of opioid function in the CNS comes from the finding that opioid neurons communicate with nonopioid neurons. Opiate drugs, in addition to their direct effects on opioid receptor-bearing target cells, influence other neural systems by virtue of these interactions. For example, opiate drugs modulate catecholamine-producing neurons in the locus ceruleus (Rasmussen et al., 1990). Conversely, catecholamine-mediated signal transduction influences opioid peptide expression and release in the rat striatum (Abood et al., 1990; Llores-Cortes et al., 1990).

Clinical phenomena characteristic of opiate addiction do not occur acutely upon exposure of a subject to opiate drugs. Instead, addiction develops over an extended time period of prolonged or repeated drug administration. Therefore, addiction research has focused on examining the cellular effects of prolonged drug exposure.

Opiate drugs, like the endogenous opioid peptides, acutely affect receptor-mediated signal transduction events. Morphine, for example, stimulates mu and delta subtype opioid receptors, resulting in acute responses in signal transduction of receptor-bearing target cells that are similar to the response produced by endogenous opioid peptides. These acute responses include inhibition of adenylate cyclase (Sharma et al., 1977) and regulation of calcium channels (Hescheler et al., 1987) and potassium channels (Miyake et al., 1989). Prolonged exposure to opiate drugs results in a number of biochemical changes in target cells, which we refer to as *cellular adaptations* to distinguish them from acute effects on receptor-mediated signal transduction.

CELLULAR ADAPTATIONS TO OPIATE DRUGS

An impressive number of cellular adaptations to opiate drugs have been identified. As elaborated in the following discussion, these adaptations involve the regulation of a wide variety of subcellular components. In many cases the physiological roles of these adaptations are not clear. However, some cellular adaptations act to desensitize target cells to the continued presence of opiate drugs, suggesting a cellular basis for opiate tolerance observed clinically and in animal studies. Other cellular adaptations may predispose target cells to a transient period of hypersensitivity upon abrupt removal of opiate drug, suggesting a cellular correlate of opiate withdrawal.

Modulation of Opioid Receptors

Regulation of opioid receptors by prolonged exposure to opiate drugs has been observed in brain (Tao et al., 1987) and in transformed cells, and studies of transformed cell lines have provided rather detailed information about these regulatory phenomena. Transformed cells are derivatives of normal cell types, such as neuroblasts or glial cells, that have been transformed by tumor viruses or have been cultured from neoplastic tissue. Transformed cells can be grown indefinitely in culture, allowing the study of a large, uniform population of cells.

A number of investigators have focused on NG108-15 cells, a hybrid cell line produced by the fusion of transformed neuroblast cells with transformed glial cells (Hamprecht, 1977). These cells can be grown in culture and express delta opioid receptors that are coupled via inhibitory GTP-binding proteins to the regulation of adenylate cyclase and calcium channels (Hescheler et al., 1987; Sharma et al., 1977). Morphine, like enkephalin, binds opioid receptors in NG108 cells, thereby decreasing adenylate cyclase activity. Prolonged exposure of NG108 cells to opioid peptide or opiate agonist drugs results in desensitization of this response, so that the cells become less sensitive to the inhibitory effects of opiates and adenylate cyclase activity returns to baseline levels (Sharma et al., 1977).

Several receptor-based processes seem to contribute to this desensitization by altering receptor function and amount in target cells. One process is the functional uncoupling of opioid receptors from other signal transduction components, resulting in the impaired ability of receptors to modulate adenylate cyclase (Law et al., 1982). The molecular basis of this uncoupling is not known, although receptor phosphorylation has been suggested (Louie et al., 1988; Sibley et al., 1989).

Another receptor-based alteration involves the loss of receptor sites from target cells—the so-called downregulation of receptors. Cellular pathways and molecular mechanisms involved in downregulation of these receptors are not known, but internalization of receptors and transport to lysosomes are thought to occur (Law et al., 1984). Opioid peptides and certain opiate drugs induce receptor downregulation (Law et al., 1982). Other opiate drugs, such as levorphanol, do not induce downregulation. The ability of morphine to induce receptor downregulation in NG108 cells is less clear. In our hands, morphine induces some downregulation, but appears to have less efficacy than enkephalin (von Zastrow & Evans, 1990).

A third type of receptor-based regulation described quite recently involves a large and selective decrease in the affinity of opioid receptors for opioid peptides without a change in the binding of opiate alkaloid drugs. This finding is very interesting because it suggests that opiate drugs may not simply mimic endogenous opioid peptides, but may evade certain aspects of normal physiological regulation (see Chapter 3; Evans & von Zastrow, 1990).

Regulation of Production of Endogenous Opioid Peptides

Opioid peptides are produced via post-translational proteolysis and chemical modification of larger precursors (Olson et al., 1990). Consequently, there are numerous potential points at which biosynthesis could be regulated. Recent studies have identified dopaminergic regulation of opioid precursor mRNA levels (Abood et al., 1990) and opiate regulation of preproenkephalin expression in rat brain (Mocchetti et al., 1985; Tempel et al., 1990). These findings suggest that regulation of opioid peptide precursor gene expression, processing, and secretion may be important to opiate addiction. Further studies are needed to determine the importance of this type of regulation in the intact CNS.

Regulation of Other Components Involved in Signal Transduction

GTP-binding regulatory proteins (G-proteins) form a crucial link between receptor binding and intracellular signal transduction. Currently, this group of proteins is viewed as a system of components that integrate cellular signals received via a number of receptor systems (Ross, 1989). These proteins consist of three subunits (alpha, beta, and gamma) that, together with receptors, associate and dissociate conditionally in the signal transduction cycle. The beta and gamma subunits may be interchangeable among different G-proteins; alpha subunits are functionally distinct and have different binding specificities for receptors and second-messenger system proteins. There are at least five types of G-protein that differ in function and possess structurally distinct alpha subunits.

Within the field of opiate addiction research, three types of G-protein—G_s, G_i, and G_o—have been examined. Opioid receptors seem to interact with G_i and G_o, but no interaction with G_s has been demonstrated. Regulation of G-protein abundance could, because of their pivotal role as signal integrators, have a great impact on signal transduction in target cells. Recently, evidence that opiate drugs regulate G-proteins has been advanced. In rat locus ceruleus, morphine appears to regulate levels of G_i and G_o, as measured by pertussis toxin-catalyzed ribosylation. Toxin-catalyzed ribosylation is an indirect method for measuring levels of G-protein alpha subunits, as the alpha subunits of G_i and G_o are substrates for ADP-ribosylation catalyzed by pertussis toxin (Nestler et al., 1989). In NG108-15 cells, etorphine selectively increases G_s alpha subunit mRNA and protein levels, as measured by RNA blot hybridization and Western blotting using specific antisera (von Zastrow et al., 1991). It is curious that the G-protein type regulated in NG108 cells does not interact directly with opioid receptor. However, because G_s is expressed in limited amounts relative to other G-proteins present in cells, regulation of G_s expression could be a key control point for the modulation of cellular signal transduction (Gilman, 1987). It has been proposed that the opiate-induced increase in G_s may underlie the sensitization of adenylate cyclase that is observed upon removal of opiate agonist from NG108 cells and may be a cellular analog of opiate withdrawal observed clinically (Sharma et al., 1977; von Zastrow et al., 1991).

Tyrosine hydroxylase also appears to be regulated in cells by opiate drugs. Tyrosine hydroxylase is a phosphoprotein that functions as a key enzyme in the biosynthesis of catecholamines. In rat locus ceruleus, the major noradrenergic nucleus in brain, increased levels of tyrosine hydroxylase mRNA, antigen, phosphoprotein, and enzyme activity levels occur after chronic administration of morphine (see Chapter 4; Guitart et al., 1990). The regulation of tyrosine hydroxylase, like that of G_s, suggests potential ways in which functional modulation of nonopioid systems may be affected by opiate drugs.

Expression of the c-fos proto-oncogene also seems to be regulated as part of the cellular adaptation to opiates. The c-fos gene encodes a nuclear phosphoprotein (called Fos) that modulates expression of a variety of genes by binding to specific sites within the regulatory regions of these genes. It has been proposed that the fos protein thereby acts as a nuclear "third messenger" molecule that couples signal transduction events to the regulation of gene expression (Curran & Morgan, 1985). Expression of the c-fos gene can be induced by intracellular calcium and by cyclic AMP (Morgan & Curran, 1986). In the locus ceruleus and in other brain regions, morphine withdrawal is associated with increased expression of the c-fos gene (Hayward et al., 1990).

Regulation of Other Cellular Components

Other cellular components seem to be regulated in response to prolonged opiate exposure. In most cases, these components have not been characterized, and their physiological importance is unclear.

Many phosphoproteins can be detected in locus ceruleus preparations via biosynthetic labeling and two-dimensional gel electrophoresis. Prolonged morphine exposure seems to modulate levels of a number of these phosphoproteins, both in vivo and in tissue explants. Two of these proteins have been identified—one is tyrosine hydroxylase, and another may be a myelin basic protein (see Chapter 4).

A number of cDNA clones can be identified from an NG108-15 cell library, the abundance of which are regulated in response to prolonged treatment with opiate agonist. A similar screening approach suggests the existence of regulated transcripts in the brains of rats subjected to chronic morphine treatment (von Zastrow et al., 1991). The regulated genes have not yet been identified or characterized, so further study is necessary to evaluate the role that such regulation may play in opiate addiction.

CONCLUSION

The discovery of the endogenous opioid peptides and their receptors has opened the door to rapid advances in the biology of opiate addiction. A great deal has been learned about the cellular and molecular mechanisms underlying opiate action, and recent research has identified a variety of cellular adaptations that occur after prolonged exposure of target cells to opiate drug. These recent discoveries provide glimpses at mechanisms that may underlie the complex clinical phenomena of opiate addiction. With some trepidation, we suggest more specific roles that some of these cellular adaptations may play in opiate addiction:

> *Opiate tolerance:* Several cellular adaptations that involve opioid receptor-bearing cells directly may contribute to opiate tolerance. These adaptations include modulation of (1) receptor function, such as functional uncoupling of receptor from G-proteins, and of (2) the number of receptors expressed in target cells, such as by receptor downregulation, both of which could result in a diminished physiological response of cells to the continued administration of opiate drugs. Another adaptation that could

affect receptor-bearing cells directly is the regulation of the expression of signal-transducing G-proteins. Decreased expression of G_i or G_o could normalize the level of inhibitory signal transduction mediated by the G-protein system, whose inhibitory branch is hyperactive due to prolonged or repeated administration of opiate drugs. Alternatively, increased expression of G_s could compensate for this elevated inhibitory influence by increasing the tone of stimulatory signal transduction in cells. Other adaptations, such as regulation of tyrosine hydroxylase or opiate-regulated expression of various cellular genes, could also contribute to opiate tolerance, either by affecting the function of opioid receptor-bearing target cells directly or by affecting the function of other cells that interact with opioid systems in the CNS.

Opiate dependence: Many of the same mechanisms proposed to contribute to opiate tolerance could also function in producing opiate dependence, because regulation processes that compensate for the inhibitory influence of prolonged exposure of the CNS to opiate drugs could predispose the system to decompensation if opiate drugs are withdrawn. In this regard, the regulation of G_s by opiates is particularly interesting. Increased expression of stimulatory G-proteins by prolonged opiate administration could help the CNS achieve a stable equilibrium state, but this adaptation could result in hypersensitivity of the system upon opiate withdrawal. Such hypersensitivity has been observed in studies of transformed cells and may represent a cellular analog of opiate withdrawal observed clinically (Sharma et al., 1977).

Cognitive and behavioral dysfunction: It is more difficult, at present, to understand biological mechanisms underlying the cognitive and behavioral dysfunction observed in opiate addiction. One intriguing possibility is that cellular adaptations could modulate reward pathways in the CNS. As noted above and in Chapter 1, these pathways have been proposed to be important for behavioral reinforcement in addiction. Because catecholamines seem to be key neurotransmitters in brain reward circuitry, one might speculate that control of catecholamine biosynthesis, such as by regulation of tyrosine hydroxylase, could be involved. In addition to reward pathways, it is possible that opiate-induced cellular adaptations affect basic mechanisms in learning and memory. The strong cognitive and behavioral component of addiction observed clinically provides compelling impetus for investigation of this possibility. Trujillo and Akil (1991) have recently reported a very exciting finding that may be relevant to this idea. These investigators found that MK-801, an antagonist of NMDA receptors thought to be involved in learning and memory, inhibits the development of morphine tolerance and withdrawal phenomena in rats (Trujillo & Akil, 1991).

In summary, the past two decades have been a period of unprecedented discovery in opioid biology and mechanisms of addiction. Future investigations of cellular adaptations hold great promise for better understanding the biological mechanisms underlying opiate addiction. Elucidation of the molecular mechanisms controlling receptor number and function will provide additional insight and may identify target molecules for therapeutic intervention in the prevention of opiate tolerance. Further exploration of the role of G-protein regulation in opiate addiction may lead to exciting breakthroughs in understanding tolerance and dependence. Continued investigation of the effect of opiate drugs on cellular gene expression may provide greater insight into addiction phenomena by identifying heretofore unknown control points in cellular adaptation. Finally, correlating cellular mechanisms to clinical phenomena will be enormously important in determining the physiological and clinical importance of various cellular adaptations. Studies of opioid release and opiate effects in the intact CNS of experimental animals (Maidment et al., 1990) will be essential to the examination of cellular adaptations in the context of whole-animal physiology. Ultimately, correlations of cellular adaptations with in vivo function may be possible by noninvasive imaging techniques applied to human subjects.

REFERENCES

Abood, M.E., Eberwine, J.H., Erdelyi, E., & Evans, C.J. (1990). Regulation of both preproenkephalin mRNA and its derived opioids by haloperidol: A method for measurement of peptides and mRNA in the same tissue extract. *Brain Res. Mol. Brain Res., 8,* 243-248.

Bozarth, M.A., & Wise, R.A. (1984). Anatomically distinct opiate receptor fields mediate reward and physiological dependence. *Science, 224,* 516-520.

Chahl, L.A., & Thornton, C.A. (1987). Locomotor activity and contracture of isolated ileum precipitated by naloxone following treatment of guinea pigs with a single dose of morphine. *J. Pharmacy Pharmacol., 39,* 52-54.

Curran, T., & Morgan, J.I. (1985). Superinduction of c-fos by nerve growth factor in the presence of peripherally active benzodiazepines. *Science, 229,* 1265-1268.

Diagnostic and statistical manual of mental disorders (3rd ed. rev.). (1987). Washington DC: American Psychiatric Association.

Evans, C.J., & von Zastrow, M. (1990). A state of the delta opioid receptor that is blind to opioid peptides but retains high affinity for opiate alkaloids. In J.M. van Ree, A.H. Mulder, V.M. Wiegant, & T.B. van Wimersma Greidanus (Eds.), *New leads in opioid research* (pp. 159-161). Amsterdam: Excerpta Medica.

Gilman, A.G. (1987). G-proteins: Transducers of receptor-generated signals. *Annu. Rev. Biochem., 56,* 615-649.

Guitart, X., Hayward, M., Nisenbaum, L.K., Beitner-Johnson, D.B., Haycock, J.W., & Nestler, E.J. (1990). Identification of MARPP-58, a morphine- and cyclic AMP-regulated phosphoprotein of 58 kilodaltons, as tyrosine hydroxylase: Evidence for regulation of its expression by chronic morphine in rat locus ceruleus. *J. Neurosci., 10,* 2308-2317.

Hamprecht, B. (1977). Structural, electrophysiological, biochemical, and pharmacological properties of neuroblastoma-glioma cell hybrids in cell culture. *Int. Rev. Cytol.,* 99-165.

Hayward, M.D., Duman, R.S., & Nestler, E.J. (1990). Induction of the c-fos proto-oncogene during opiate withdrawal in the locus ceruleus and other regions of the rat brain. *Brain Res., 525,* 256-266.

Hescheler, J., Kameyama, M., Trautwein, W., & Schultz, G. (1987). The GTP-binding protein, N_o, regulates neuronal calcium channels. *Nature (London), 325,* 445-447.

Koob, G.F., & Bloom, F.E. (1988). Cellular and molecular mechanisms of drug dependence. *Science, 242,* 715-723.

Koob, G.F., Stinus, L., Le Moal, M., & Bloom, F.E. (1989). Opponent process theory of motivation: Neurobiologic evidence from studies of opiate dependence. *Neurosci. Biobehav. Rev., 13,* 135-140.

Kosterlitz, H.W., Corbett, A.D., & Patterson, S.J. (1989). Opioid receptors and ligands. *NIDA Res. Monogr., 95,* 159-166.

Law, P.-Y., Hom, D.S., & Loh, H.H. (1982). Loss of opiate receptor activity in neuroblastoma x glioma NG108-15 cells after chronic etorphine treatment: A multiple step process. *Mol. Pharmacol., 72,* 1-4.

Law, P.-Y., Hom, D.S., & Loh, H.H. (1984). Down-regulation of opiate receptor in neuroblastoma x glioma NG108-15 hybrid cells: Chloroquine promotes accumulation of tritiated enkephalin in the lysosomes. *J. Biol. Chem., 259,* 4096-4104.

Llorens-Cortes, C., Zini, S., Garbarg, M., & Schwartz, J.C. (1990). Changes in striatal enkephalin release following stimulation of dopaminergic or histaminergic receptors. In J.M. van Ree, A.H. Mulder, V.M. Wiegant, & T.B. van Wimersma Greidanus (Eds.), New leads in opioid research (pp. 234-236). Amsterdam: Excerpta Medica.

Louie, A.K., Zhan, J.N., Law, P.-Y., & Loh, H.H. (1988). Modification of opioid receptor activity by acid phosphatase in neuroblastoma x glioma NG108-15 hybrid cells. *Biochem. Biophys. Res. Comm., 152,* 1369-1375.

Maidment, N.T., Siddall, B.J., Rudolph, V.D., Erdelyi, E., & Evans, C.J. (1990). Microdialysis as a tool for studying the regulation of opioid peptide release in the rat basal ganglia in vivo. In J.M. van Ree, A.H. Mulder, V.M. Wiegant, & T.B. van Wimersma Greidanus (Eds.), *New leads in opioid research* (pp. 233-234). Amsterdam: Excerpta Medica.

Mansour, A., Khachaturian, H., Lewis, M.E., Akil, H., & Watson, S.J. (1988). Anatomy of CNS opioid receptors. *Trends Neurosci., 11,* 308-314.

Miller, L. (1990). Neuropsychodynamics of alcohol and addiction: Personality, psychopathology, and cognitive style. *J. Subst. Abuse Treat., 7,* 31-49.

Miyake, M., Christie, M.J., & North, R.A. (1989). Single potassium channels opened by opioids in rat locus ceruleus neurons. *Proc. Natl. Acad. Sci. USA., 86,* 3419-3422.

Mocchetti, I., Schwartz, J.P., & Costa, E. (1985). Use of mRNA hybridization and radioimmunoassay to study mechanisms of drug-induced accumulation of enkephalins in rat brain structures. *Mol. Pharmacol., 28,* 86-91.

Morgan, J.I., & Curran, T. (1986). Role of ion flux in the control of c-fos expression. *Nature, 322,* 552-555.

Nestler, E.J., Erods, J.J., Terwilliger, R., Duman, R.S., & Tallman, J.F. (1989). Regulation of G proteins by chronic morphine in the rat locus ceruleus. *Brain Res., 476,* 230-239.

Olson, G.A., Olson, R.D., & Kostin, A.J. (1990). Endogenous opiates: 1989. *Peptides, 11,* 1277-1304.

Powell, J., Gray, J.A., Bradley, B.P., Kasvikis, Y., Strang, J., Barrat, L., & Marks, I. (1990). The effects of exposure to drug-related cues in detoxified opiate addicts: A theoretical review and some new data. *Addictive Behav., 15,* 339-354.

Rasmussen, K., Beitner-Johnson, D.B., Krystal, J.H., Aghajanian, G.K., & Nestler,

E.J. (1990). Opiate withdrawal and the locus ceruleus: Behavioral, electrophysiologic, and biochemical correlates. *J. Neurosci., 10*, 2308-2317.

Ross, E.M. (1989). Signal sorting and amplification through G protein-coupled receptors. *Neuron, 3*, 141-152.

Schaefer, G.J. (1988). Opiate antagonists and rewarding brain stimulation. *Neurosci. Biobehav. Rev., 12*, 1-17.

Sharma, S.K., Klee, W.A., & Nirenberg, M. (1977). Opiate-dependent modulation of adenylate cyclase. *Proc. Natl. Acad. Sci. USA., 74*, 3365-3369.

Sibley, D.R., Benovic, J.L., Caron, M.G., & Lefkowitz, R.J. (1989). Regulation of transmembrane signalling by receptor phosphorylation. *Cell, 48*, 913-922.

Tao, P.L., Law, P.-Y., & Loh, H.H. (1987). Decrease in delta and mu opioid receptor binding capacity in rat brain after chronic etorphine treatment. *J. Pharmacol. Exp. Ther., 240*, 809-816.

Tempel, A., Kessler, J.A., & Zukin, R.S. (1990). Chronic naltrexone treatment increases expression of preproenkephalin and preprotachykinin mRNA in discrete brain regions. *J. Neurosci., 10*, 741-747.

Trujillo, K.A., & Akil, H. (1991). Inhibition of morphine tolerance and dependence by the NMDA receptor antagonist MK-801. *Science, 251*, 85-87.

von Zastrow, M., & Evans, C.J. (1990). Morphine blocks the peptide-selective binding change without blocking receptor downregulation. In J.M. van Ree, A.H. Mulder, V.M. Wiegant, & T.B. van Wimersma Greidanus (Eds.), *New leads in opioid research* (pp. 101-103). Amsterdam: Excerpta Medica.

von Zastrow, M., Barchas, J.D., & Eberwine, J.E. (1991). An approach to the molecular biology of opiate addiction: Identification of opiate-regulated transcripts. *NIDA Res. Symp.* (in press).

Way, E.L., Loh, H., & Shen, F.-H. (1969). Simultaneous quantitative assessment of morphine tolerance and physical dependence. *J. Pharmacol. Exp. Ther., 167*, 1-8.

3

Diversity Among the Opioid Receptors

CHRISTOPHER J. EVANS

In describing our current knowledge of opioid receptors and their role in the endogenous opioid system, I will take a somewhat different tack. In addition to categorizing the opioid system, as has been done in recent review articles, such as by Wollemann (1990), I would like to revel in its complexity, framing this perspective on opioid receptors with the question: Why might the evolutionary process have created such diversity within the vertebrate opioid system? We tend to categorize all opiates as pain killers or drugs that induce severe changes in psychological and physiological status that presumably trigger the potential for abuse. These perceptions are based on gross behavioral endpoints seen after the administration of alkaloid opiate drugs, such as morphine or heroin. However, opiates (the alkaloid ligands) and opioids (the peptide ligands) exhibit a broad and often conflicting spectrum of effects. For example, not all the endogenous opioid peptides induce simple analgesia. BAM18, a product of proenkephalin found in high concentrations in brain tissue (Evans et al., 1988), can actually block morphine analgesia and at low doses can result in hyperalgesia (Stevens et al., 1988). In this chapter I hope to highlight the potential of the endogenous opioid system as a diverse interneuronal communication system and to explain the numerous apparent contradictions in opiate and opioid pharmacology.

The first clue to the immense complexity and intricacy of the vertebrate endogenous opioid system emerged from opiate alkaloid structure/activity studies during the 1960s and 1970s. These studies synthesized libraries of analogs based on known opiate structures that were subsequently tested in bioassays. The data indicated that opiate effects could be divided into discrete subsets (Gilbert & Martin, 1976), a finding that led to the idea of multiple opiate receptors. During the 1970s and 1980s numerous receptors that interact with both opioid peptides and opiate alkaloids were described. As yet we do not have the structural data to identify the molecular basis of all the different receptors—the appropriate clones are eagerly awaited by the field. I initially attributed the claims of multiple opioid receptors not to differences in primary structure but to the cellular environment of the receptor and the second-messenger system to which it was coupled. This view may still have some merit.

However, in the case of many G-linked receptors—the class to which opiate receptors are considered to belong—diversity is generated by the expression of different genes that encode receptor proteins of different primary structure. Receptors binding serotonin, acetylcholine, and dopamine are examples of multiple G-protein-coupled receptors that are considered to bind single ligands (at last count 12 serotonin receptors had been cloned). With the refinement of binding assays and the tools of molecular biology it has become apparent that multiple receptors for bioactive molecules are the rule in mammalian CNS and not the exception.

What we know of the family of opioid receptors is gathered from ligand binding (generally performed on membrane fractions or tissue slices), electrophysiological studies, and bioassays. There are considerable limitations in the interpretation of results obtained using these techniques. For example, binding sites can be mimicked by enzymes, radioreceptor assays are often performed under nonphysiological conditions, and bioassays are often problematic due to ligand penetration or degradation. However, there is a general consensus based on results obtained by these methodologies that opioid receptors are heterogeneous. Inspired by the discovery of the enkephalins and extending the previous receptor designation by Gilbert and Martin (1976), Lord et al. (1977) described three major opioid receptor types: the mu, delta, kappa. The receptor groups were based upon the rank order of potency of different opioid peptides and opiate alkaloids in various binding and bioassays. As always, the story has become just a little more complex with the discovery of ligands with increased selectivity and more discriminating assays. In the last decade and a half, each of the major receptor groups has been subdivided, and a few extra types have been added to the literature. However, there is some controversy over a number of these receptors. Consequently, it is worthwhile to summarize briefly the binding proteins and receptors that have been characterized thus far.

DELTA OPIOID RECEPTOR(S)

Delta receptors are often considered tailored for met- and leu-enkephalin, and certainly of all the vertebrate endogenous opioids the enkephalins seem to possess the highest affinity for this receptor type. Deltorphans, a family of opioid peptides containing d-amino acids, that were recently isolated from frog skin (Erspamer et al. 1989) also have high affinity and selectivity for ∂ receptors. The receptors, according to bioassays and radioreceptor binding assays, dislikes C-terminal extensions present on many endogenous opioid peptides, especially those similar to dynorphin and BAM (Hurlbut et al., 1987). The selective ligands for delta receptors are the synthetic peptides (D-Pen^2, D-Pen^5) enkephalin and DTLET (Bochet et al., 1988; Knapp et al., 1989). The pentapeptide DADLE is often considered to be selective and does show high affinity for delta receptors, but it also binds well to mu receptors. Very recently a number of other selective delta ligands have been synthesized, and their bioactivities and binding results are suggestive of more than one delta receptor. With regard to second-messenger systems activated by delta agonists, electrophysiological studies have demonstrated coupling to both potassium and calcium channels (Gross et al., 1990; North et al., 1987), and the receptor has also been shown to couple to adenylate cyclase (Sharma et al., 1977).

Many studies of the delta opioid receptor have been performed on the neuroblastoma/glioma cell line NG108-15. The advantage of this cell line is that it is a homogeneous population of cells that contain only delta opioid receptors. However, the cell line is a cancer hybrid and may not be completely representative of the delta receptor in endogenous neurons with regard to G-protein coupling, lipid environment, post-translational processing, etc. Using a photoaffinity label based on DADLE, we have been able to selectively label a protein in membrane preparations of NG108-15 cells (Fig. 3-1). Our estimation of the molecular weight of the labeled protein is larger than that found using different delta affinity ligands (Bochet et al., 1988) and corresponds to a diffuse band running slightly below 60 Kd. The band is displaced by DADLE with an IC_{50} of about 2nM, and the labeling is blocked by alkaloid ligands, such as diprenorphine. If run on two-dimensional gels, there are at least three distinct bands (data not shown), the relative intensity of which can be altered by treatment with agonists. At present it is unclear whether the labeled material is indeed the receptor and, if it is, whether the multiply labeled bands are due to different phosphorylation states, products of differential post-translational processes, or subsets of delta receptors, due to different genes or splice products from the same gene.

There is evidence that delta opioid receptors in the NG108-15 cells interact with G_i2 (McKenzie & Milligan, 1990); specific antibodies to G_i2 interfere with the opioid-induced inhibition of adenylate cyclase in these cells, whereas antisera to G_i3 and G_o, the other major inhibitory G-proteins found in the NG108-15 cells, have no effect. The observation is indicative, but does not ensure that G_i2 will be the delta receptor transducer for cyclase inhibition in brain nor the only transducer in the NG108-15 cells. (Receptor/effector coupling is notoriously promiscuous, and the balance of second-messenger systems is delicate and interdependent.) A particularly elegant study (Taussig et al., 1992) demonstrated that transfection of a G_{oA} mutant rendered insensitive to pertussis toxin can rescue the function of opioid receptor signaling to potassium and calcium channels in the presence of toxin. Taken together, these data would suggest that delta receptors couple to channels via G_{oA} and to adenylate cyclase via G_i2.

Evans et al., 1992 and Kieffer et al. (1992) have isolated a cDNA clone that confers delta selective binding and functional coupling to adenylate cyclase in a fibroblast cell line (COS). The predicted protein sequence has homology with other G-protein coupled receptors, in particular the receptors binding somatostatin, angiotensin and interleukin-8. The cDNA clone recognizes a series of transcripts by Northern blot analysis which appear to derive from a single gene. However, it is at present unclear whether any of these transcripts encode distinct protein sequences and thus provide a molecular basis for pharmacological heterogeneity. This clone should provide the probes to study the regulation of delta receptors at the molecular level and lead to the identification of the other receptor subtypes.

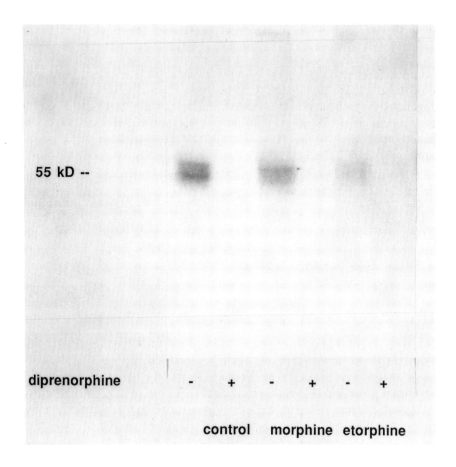

55 kD --

diprenorphine   -   +   -   +   -   +

control   morphine etorphine

Figure 3-1.   Confluent NG108-15 cells were either untreated (control) or treated for 18 hours with 100 μM morphine or 25 nM etorphine at 37°C in culture media. After the treatments the cells were harvested and a P_2membrane fraction prepared. Membranes (75 μg protein) were incubated in 50 mM HEPES/10 mM magnesium chloride at room temperature with [125]I Tyr.dAla.Gly AzidoPhe.dLeu (prepared in collaboration with Dr. Jacques Maddaluno) with or without 2 μM diphrenorphine. After washing at 4°C and photolysis to accomplish cross-linking, the samples were run on a SDS polyacrylamide reducing gel and then subjected to autoradiography. This study was done in collaboration with Dr. Mark von Zastrow.

MU OPIOID RECEPTOR(S)

The mu receptors are generally perceived as those favored by morphine. There has been a search for an "endogenous ligand" for these receptors since none of the naturally occurring opioid peptides is considered sufficiently "mu-selective." However, the enkephalins, beta-endorphin, metorphamide, and other proenkephalin products have a high affinity for these receptors. As discussed earlier, it is now well established that neurotransmitters can interact with different receptors. The conviction that there must be "selective" ligands for each of the receptors has diverted energy from understanding the interaction of patterns of endogenous ligands with opioid receptors. The finding of endogenous morphine, codeine, and other opiate alkaloids in mammals has implicated these alkaloids as potential endogenous mu ligands. However, at present the role of these alkaloid opiates in the vertebrate CNS is unclear, e.g., are they endogenously synthesized, are they stored in vesicles and under controlled release mechanisms? (see Chapter 17 for a discussion of issues related to endogenous morphinans). Interestingly, mu receptors are coupled to the same second-messenger systems as delta receptors, although each receptor may be coupled to different G-proteins—perhaps G_i2 for delta receptors and G_i1 for mu receptors (Harada et al., 1990). Recent evidence demonstrates that mu receptors can be coupled to adenylate cyclase in cell lines (Yu et al., 1990), and several earlier electrophysiological studies suggested coupling to both calcium and potassium channels (Gross et al., 1990; North et al., 1987). There has been considerable debate on subtypes of mu receptors (Paul et al., 1989), an issue that is hard to resolve without the structural data.

KAPPA OPIOID RECEPTOR(S)

The kappa receptors were originally defined by Gilbert and Martin (1976) as linked to physiological changes in which ketocyclazocine and related alkaloids were most active. However, with the discovery of the dynorphins, which have a high affinity for kappa receptors, a functional linkage of prodynorphin with kappa receptors has emerged. This linkage is supported, at least in the guinea pig hippocampus, by a study of Wagner et al. (1991). In a hippocampal slice preparation, antibodies to opioids derived from prodynorphin but not proenkephalin blocked the electrically induced displacement of $^3HU69,593$, a K_1 selective radioligand. However, the exclusive association of kappa receptors with prodynorphin may be misleading on two counts: (a) the localization of kappa receptors does not always reflect the localization of dynorphins (Herkenham, 1987) and (b) fragments of proenkephalin, such as BAM18 and metorphamide, have high affinity for kappa receptors and mimic many of the biological effects of dynorphins (Stevens et al., 1988; Weber et al., 1983). The discordance between kappa opioid receptor distribution and prodynorphin would perhaps be irrelevant if the dynorphins were stable to brain extracellular proteases; however, this is not the case, and dynorphin is degraded rapidly in the extracellular space (Young et al., 1987). There is evidence that the kappa receptors (like mu and delta receptors) can couple to both calcium channels and adenylate cyclase and the pharmacological evidence is accumulating for the anticipated multiplicity of kappa receptors (see Konkoy & Childers, 1991; Leslie, 1987; and Traynor, 1989 for reviews). Recently employing a strategy involving expression cloning and panning using a dynorphin analogue, a cDNA clone possessing distinct features of the G-protein receptor family was isolated and characterized (Xie et al., 1992). Cells transfected with the clone showed both opioid and opiate binding although the binding was low affinity and showed no selectivity for kappa ligands. The clone proved to be highly homologous with the neurokinin B (neuromedin K) receptor yet does not bind neurokinin B. At present it is unclear whether this is an opioid receptor—there remain some technical possibilities which could explain the low affinities, e.g., this cDNA clone may represent a truncated sequence or the recipient cells employed for expressing the clone may lack appropriate G-proteins or membrane components. Alternatively, the receptor may have a non-opioid endogenous ligand; possible candidates are one of the numerous peptides constituting the tachykinin family other than neurokinin B or mammalian FMRFamide analogues reported to be opioid antagonists (Yang & Majane, 1989).

EPSILON RECEPTOR

The high in vivo analgesic potency and the sensitivity of beta-endorphin in the rat vas deferens bioassay led to a search for a selective high-affinity binding site for this endogenous opioid peptide. Evidence has accumulated for such a site, which has been named the epsilon receptor. The epsilon receptor has had a somewhat controversial existence, undoubtedly because of the difficulties of working with beta-endorphin. One problem with the analysis of beta-endorphin binding is that the peptide is extremely sticky and requires special precautions to avoid nonspecific interactions. A recent binding study suggests that one of the kappa receptor subtypes corresponds to the epsilon receptor (Nock et al., 1990). This finding brings up the issue of receptor classification, a problem that even cloning may not solve.

OPIATE-BINDING PROTEINS

One strategy employed to isolate opiate receptors was chromatography, whereby opiate alkaloids were bound to solid supports and proteins from solubilized brain tissue isolated as a result of binding to the column. Using a morphine affinity column, this approach identified an opiate-binding protein from brain tissue. The protein was purified to homogeneity, and partial protein sequencing was employed to generate DNA probes to isolate a cDNA clone encoding the entire protein (Schofield et al., 1989). The predicted protein structure of this clone shows homology with the immunoglobulin superfamily, a group of proteins defined by distinct cysteine domains. The immunoglobulin superfamily includes many critical cell surface recognition molecules, such as immunoglobulins, the T-cell receptor, the major histocompatibility antigens, and neuronal associated proteins, e.g., NCAM. The morphine-binding protein has been named OBCAM, reflecting the homology within this family of proteins and the fact that it was purified based on opiate binding. Of some concern is the finding that the primary structure of OBCAM has no obvious membrane-spanning domains and no homology with the G-protein-coupled receptor family. However, membrane-binding domains may be present on alternative splice products, such as are found in immunoglobulin during B-cell maturation. This protein has been essentially overlooked as an opiate receptor candidate because of the structural constraints common to the G-protein receptor family. However, it is conceivable that the receptor is a complex of proteins, and OBCAM comprises a binding domain that is linked via a second protein to the G-protein. It remains to be seen how this protein will fit into the opiate receptor story.

SIGMA RECEPTORS

A number of synthetic opiate ligands are reported to interact with the sigma receptor. Two major sites are commonly quoted, the phencyclidine (PCP) and haloperidol-sensitive sites (for review, see Zukin & Zukin, 1988 and Chapter 18 this volume). Neither of these sites binds any of the endogenous opioid peptides, and an endogenous ligand has not thus far been characterized. The sigma receptor is not considered a classical opiate receptor because of the original definition of naloxone reversibility (Vaupel, 1983). This receptor awaits an endogenous ligand for a fuller understanding of its role in the CNS. A recent report suggests that the sigma receptor may be cytochrome oxidase P450 (Ross, 1990). This study is controversial and certainly questions the mechanism by which sigma receptor ligands could regulate phosphoinositol turnover (Brog & Beinfeld, 1990).

OPIOID RECEPTOR DISTRIBUTION

Receptor autoradiography utilizing radiolabeled opioid and opiate ligands is a useful method for the study of receptor anatomy, but several issues should be considered before interpreting the autoradiographic studies relating to the opioid system.

Autoradiography does not generally distinguish between internal and external receptors.

The slices for autoradiography are performed on euthanized tissue. Since euthanasia induces massive depolarization by Na/K pump immobilization and subsequent opioid peptide dumping (Maidment et al., 1991), it is conceivable that some receptors may be occupied with ligand and the receptor adaptation mechanisms for such an onslaught of agonist may result in impaired receptor binding in areas high in opioid peptide content.

In many studies the affinity of the binding sites is not addressed rigorously, and the pharmacology does not allow sufficient characterization of the binding sites.

The sensitivity of receptor autoradiography is dependent on the ligand characteristics; thus receptors may in fact be present in areas that appear to contain no positive signal. (We do not know how many receptors per cell are needed to induce "a significant biological response.")

Nonetheless, autoradiography is a very powerful technique for the analysis of receptors, and although the interpretation of results can sometimes be tricky, the technique promises much more information than "grind and bind" assays. Mansour et al. (1988) and Kuhar (1985) provide two thorough reviews of autoradiographic studies of opioid and opiate receptors. These articles address species variability and the problems of receptor autoradiography raised above. The conclusions from the studies are summarized as follows.

There seems to be considerable disparity between ligand and receptor distributions. The opioid system has never been characterized as either a neurotransmitter or neuromodulator system. The disparity between distributions would indicate that ligands have to travel to find their targets, which would favour the neuromodulator role (Herkenham, 1987). However, many of the opioid active processing products are extremely sensitive to extracellular proteolysis, suggesting they would have difficulty traveling. It would seem reasonable that the opioid system can act in either mode, depending on the stability of the processing products and the anatomy of the receptors and proteases. This aspect of the system is difficult to assess with biologically meaningful experiments.

Although there is a differential distribution in the relative densities of the major opioid receptor subtypes, there is sizeable overlap. It seems likely that many of the neurons can express more than one opiate receptor type. Indeed, in primary cultures of spinal cord, individual cells are found to express all combinations of mu, delta, and kappa receptors (Gross et al., 1990; Werz & Macdonald, 1982).

There is also considerable difference among species in the distribution of these receptors. This species variability in the endogenous opioid system is not restricted to the CNS and can also be observed in ligands present in the pituitary/adrenal axis (Evans et al., 1985). This lack of interspecies conservation in opioid system components is intriguing when considering the functional evolution of the endogenous opioid system.

EVIDENCE THAT OPIOID RECEPTORS ARE LINKED TO G-PROTEINS

It is important to review the data demonstrating that opioid receptors are coupled to their effector systems via G-proteins. Experiments in the early 1970s were unknowingly implying that opioid receptors couple to G-proteins although this receptor family was completely uncharacterized at this time. Collier and Roy in 1973 showed that opiates could inhibit prostaglandin E_1 or E_2 stimulation of adenylate cyclase. More recently, inhibition of adenylate cyclase by delta opiate receptors in the NG108-15 cell line and by mu receptors in SH-SY5Y cells was demonstrated (Yu et al., 1990). Binding assays also provided evidence of G-protein-coupled opiate receptors, and several groups demonstrated the sensitivity of opiate agonist binding to GTP and GTP analogs. An important experiment showed the dependence of GTP and sodium for the opiate-induced inhibition of cyclase in NG108-15 cells (Blume et al., 1979).

The role of GTP hydrolysis in the transmission process is intrinsic to the coupling of receptors to effector systems via G-proteins. Opiate inhibition of cyclase was demonstrated to involve the hydrolysis of GTP by Koski and Klee (1981). Perhaps the most powerful evidence comes from pertussis toxin, which ADP-ribosylates and inactivates the alpha subunits of inhibitory G-proteins. This potent bacterial toxin has proven to be an extremely useful diagnostic tool in opioid receptor pharmacology (e.g., Werling et al., 1989a). Pertussis toxin can abolish opioid actions, including those regulating adenylate cyclase and calcium and potassium channels. The evidence is thus heavily stacked in favor of the opioid receptors being members of, or associated with members of, the G-linked family of receptors.

FAMILY OF G-LINKED RECEPTORS

There are a number of excellent reviews of the structural characteristics of the G-protein-coupled receptor family (see O'Dowd et al., 1989). The members of the G_i, G_o, G_s, and transducin coupled receptors all have similar overall structural homology, including seven "apparent" membrane-spanning regions with considerable sequence interhomology. N-linked glycosylation consensus sequences are generally present on the N-terminal extracellular domain (this is not true of all receptors, e.g., the alpha$_{2B}$ adrenoreceptor). For the most part, the proteins appear to be in the molecular weight range of 40-60 Kd. It will be interesting to determine the necessary structural features for interaction with ligands and the conversion of the energy of agonist binding via conformational changes to activate the G-protein complex. These issues are currently being addressed for the cloned G-protein-coupled receptors using point mutation strategies and chimeric receptors.

Interestingly, the opiates are not the only substances of abuse that utilize receptor systems intimately involved with G-proteins. The major actions of cocaine are thought to be inhibition of uptake of dopamine and serotonin, transmitters that have receptors linked via G-proteins to intracellular second-messenger systems. The recently cloned THC receptor is linked to adenylate cyclase via pertussis-inactivated G-proteins. The possibility that there is a commonality in intracellular mechanisms concerning drug addiction is the subject of other chapters in this volume (see Chapter 4).

REGULATION OF OPIOID RECEPTORS

Studies attempting to detect changes in opioid receptors after exposure to opiate agonists and antagonists have employed whole-animal models, cell lines, particularly the NG108-15 line, and, to a more limited degree, electrophysiological and bioassays. Whole-animal studies are complicated by the multiplicity of receptors, ligand accessibility, and the interaction of nonopioid neuronal networks. However, these models are the most relevant to understanding drug-induced changes in abusers and patients on chronic opiate treatments. It is difficult to imagine that opiate tolerance and addiction processes are limited to effects on elements of the endogenous opioid system and do not perturb or are not perturbed by interfacing neuronal and co-localized neuronal systems.

A wealth of studies—many apparently contradictory—have examined receptor binding after chronic opiate agonist and antagonist treatment. From receptor autoradiographic analysis, it seems that chronic treatment with the opiate antagonist naltrexone can up regulate mu receptors in adult rats (Morris & Herz, 1989; Tempel et al., 1985). Interestingly, morphine treatment of adult rats also up regualtes mu receptors (Brady et al., 1989), a result that on the surface seems counterintuitive. One plausible explanation for this phenomenon is that after chronic morphine the receptors are uncoupled from their effector systems and the upregulation prepares the system for the subsequent neuronal shock of withdrawal. This explanation is consistent with the binding characteristics of brain membranes from chronically morphine-treated guinea pigs (Werling, et al. 1989b). With regard to delta receptors, etorphine and DADLE treatment of rats has been shown to decrease receptor numbers (Tao et al., 1987, 1988).

During development, mu receptors also seem to be sensitive to opiate ligands, but contrary to the adaptations observed in adults, morphine administration to pups is reported to downregulate striatal mu receptors (Tempel et al., 1988). A consistent theme in these regulation experiments is unclear and presumably reflects the fact that regulation of opioid systems may occur at multiple levels, i.e., translational/transcriptional level, post-translational modification level, second-messenger coupling, and compartmentalization.

Studies in the cell line NG108-15 have provided some interesting findings about the molecular adaptive mechanisms involved in acute and chronic opiate treatment. Whether these findings are entirely relevant to the in vivo situation is questionable, but the model does not have merit for dissecting possible molecular mechanisms for subsequent in vivo testing. Early studies (Sharma et al., 1975) demonstrated homeostatic mechanisms in the adenylate cyclase system induced by chronic treatment with morphine, a low-affinity agonist at the delta opioid receptors present on NG108-15 cells. The results are interesting in that acute morphine inhibits both basal and PGE-stimulated cyclase in both control and chronic morphine-treated cells. However, the inhibition of cAMP production is counteracted in the chronic morphine-treated cells by a compensatory increase in basal adenylate cyclase activity. In a separate set of experiments the PGE-stimulated adenylate cyclase activity was severely impaired by chronic pretreatment with etorphine—a high-affinity delta agonist—although, like the morphine tolerance, an upregulation of basal cyclase activity was observed (Griffin et al., 1985).

Two major opiate agonist-induced regulatory processes have been described in NG108-15 cells; namely, downregulation, in this instance defined as the loss of receptors from the cell surface, and desensitization, the loss of second-messenger responsiveness (Law et al., 1983). These two processes require different concentrations of agonist (a tenfold higher concentration is required for desensitization than downregulation), show different time courses (downregulation occurs much more slowly than desensitization), and can be differentiated on the basis of temperature (downregulation occurs at lower temperatures than desensitization).

Our group has recently reported a dramatic agonist-induced change in opioid peptide binding to delta opioid receptors in intact NG108 cells (Evans & von Zastrow, 1990; von Zastrow & Evans, 1990). The binding change results in a >2000-fold decrease in apparent affinity for all opioid peptides tested, with no detectable changes in alkaloid ligand binding (Fig. 3-2). Opioid agonists can therefore induce an intriguing state of the delta-opioid receptor that is effectively "blind" to opioid peptides, yet still can bind opiate alkaloids. The effect can be blocked by co-administration of opiate antagonists and does not occur with treatment of agonist at 4°C. The affinity change has an extremely quick onset (effects are seen after only 5 minutes following etorphine treatment) and

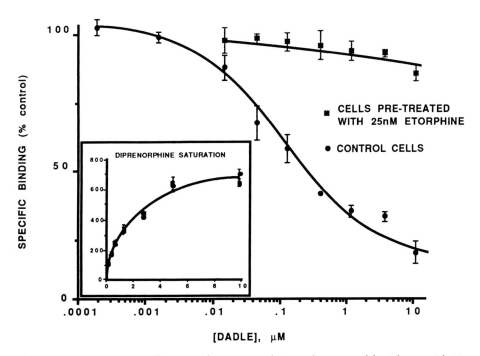

Figure 3-2.   NG108-15 cells were either untreated (control) or treated for 2 hours with 25 nM etorphine at 37°C in culture media. After treatment, the cells were cooled to 4°C, harvested, and washed extensively, and intact cell binding was analyzed using ^{3}H diprenorphine as the receptor probe (Law et al., 1983). All steps subsequent to harvesting and including binding were conducted between 0 and 4°C. Specific binding was determined by counts displacable by the addition of 400 nM diprenorphine. The insert represents diprenorphine saturation curves for treated (*circles*) and untreated cells (*squares*), the X axis representing the ^{3}H diprenorphine concentration (nM) and the Y axis the concentration of ^{3}H diprenorphine (fmoles) specifically bound per mg protein. The experiments demonstrate that etorphine pretreatment of NG108-15 cells can induce a dramatic change in interaction of DADLE with receptors labeled with ^{3}H diprenorphine without a change in ^{3}H diprenorphine binding. This study was in collaboration with Dr. Mark von Zastrow.

occurs below the measured K_d of etorphine for the delta opioid receptor yet comparable to the K_i for cyclase inhibition. These results show that opioid peptides and opiate alkaloids may interact differently with receptors and suggest that alkaloid ligands may elude a regulatory desensitization process. This observation does have an intuitive rationale if one assumes that cellular tolerance mechanisms evolved to respond to the major exogenous ligands—the opioid peptides—and not to exogenous alkaloids, such as etorphine.

Additional experiments relating to the peptide-selective affinity change have revealed that morphine does not induce the effect. Furthermore, morphine can antagonize the ability of other agonists (e.g., DADLE and etorphine) to induce this cellular adaptation. Moreover, morphine was found to block the peptide-selective binding change without inhibiting opioid-stimulated receptor downregulation. It would therefore seem that these two agonist-induced cellular adaptations have differing pharmacologies, and they may have separate molecular triggers.

It is becoming very clear that a series of cellular adaptive processes are associated with opioid and opiate tolerance. The delta receptor clone we have recently isolated will no doubt prove to be as invaluable for studying these adaptations as they have been in analogous neurotransmitter/receptor fields.

THE QUESTION OF DIVERSITY

The potential for diversity within the vertebrate opioid system is vast. Figure 3-3 outlines various aspects of the system to highlight how regulation at certain points may lead to diversity. There are three opioid precursors to ligands, namely proopiomelanocortin (pOMC), proenkephalin (pENK), and pro-

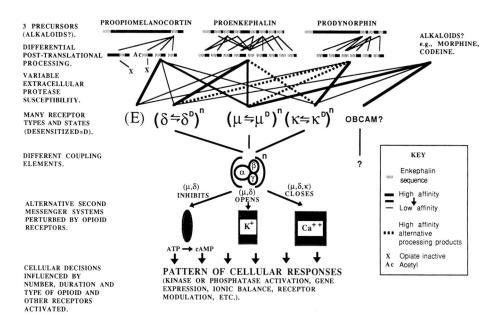

Figure 3-3. Diversity within the endogenous opioid system.

dynorphin (pDYN). Highly specific proteolytic processing is an absolute requirement for activation of all three of these opioid precursors. Differential processing can result in a wide variety of opioid peptides with very different extracellular stabilities, different receptor on-rates, and different affinities for the various opioid receptors (Akil et al., 1984; Evans et al., 1988; Hollt; 1986). The high affinity kappa and mu ligand BAM18 if processed to met enkephalin now becomes a high affinity delta ligand with low affinity for the kappa sites. Perhaps the most illustrative example of the power of differential processing is found in the pOMC system. The pOMC-derived peptide beta-endorphin 1-31 is found as the predominant endorphin form in the human adrenal and rat arcuate nucleus and is a highly potent analgesic. Removal of the C-terminal 4 amino acids forms beta-endorphin 1-27, the major form found in midbrain (Zakarian & Smyth, 1979), which has only 1% of the analgesic activity of beta-endorphin 1-31. Furthermore, beta-endorphin 1-27 has been reported to be capable of antagonizing the activity of beta-endorphin 1-31 (Suh et al., 1988). In the intermediate lobe of the rat pituitary the beta-endorphin-containing molecules are 90% α-N-acetylated, a modification that totally obliterates opioid effects (Smyth et al., 1979).

It has been commonly assumed that each precursor is biologically designed for a specific subtype of receptor, i.e., prodynorphin for kappa, proenkephalin for delta and mu, etc. However, the distribution of endogenous opioids and receptors does not support this hypothesis (Herkenham, 1987; Kuhar, 1985), and it should be remembered that all endogenous opioid peptides are agonists (or possibly partial agonists) for all major receptor subtypes, with the important caveat that receptor affinities are very different.

Pertinent to the theme of this chapter is the ability of the cell to express a specific precursor (or combination of precursors) and to process the precursor(s) to target a specific mosaic of opioid receptors. When might this ability be important? It has been demonstrated that neuronal cells express different combinations of opioid receptor types on the cell surface (Werz & Macdonald, 1982). These neurons may have inputs from a considerable number of other neurons—some expressing pENK, some pDYN, and possibly co-localized with a series of other neurotransmitters or neuroregulators. One mechanism that target cells could employ to discriminate inputs would be recognition of patterns of receptors activated, i.e., ratios of delta to mu or muscarinic to kappa, etc. To achieve such an "input signature," diversity of neurotransmitter receptor systems is a critical feature. The demands of intricate neuronal communication utilizing these neurotransmitter mosaics would go a long way in explaining the confusing and subtle pharmacological differences in the activity of different opioid ligands.

There is one problem with the notion of a neurotransmitter signature mechanism for input differentiation—the fact that many of the receptors converge with respect to second-messenger systems. As indicated earlier, all the opioid receptor types can inhibit calcium influx, and both the mu and delta receptors can couple to potassium channels and adenylate cyclase via inhibitory G-proteins. Although many different receptor ligands can exhibit the same changes in ion channels and levels of cyclic nucleotides, this feature does not necessarily translate to the cell responding identically. The diversity of

G-proteins that have recently been discovered and cloned provides a mechanism by which subtle changes in coupling to effector systems may alter cellular decisions. It is probable that receptor activation will trigger a series of complex molecular cascades that will depend on the G-proteins to which the receptors are coupled, the stability of the activated receptor-effector complex, the membrane microenvironment of the receptor complexes, and the phosphorylation state of surrounding effector proteins. Thus, although there seem to be no differences electrophysiologically between the actions of mu and delta agonists, their activation may have completely different results on some critical cellular systems.

This type of second-messenger complexity has been observed in PC12 cells (Hershman, 1989) in which the same second-messenger systems and early response genes are activated by both mitogens and growth factors. The cells thus respond very differently—either dividing in the case of mitogens or differentiating in the case of growth factors—when apparently the same intracellular machinery is set in motion. It seems therefore that cellular decisions are not made merely on the basis of single second-messenger activation; the situation is considerably more subtle and complex.

Returning to the question of why such diversity exists in the endogenous opioid system, the answer that I find most appealing is that neuronal communication demands diversity to enable differentiation of inputs. The common associations of opiates (e.g., analgesia) have perhaps led to oversimplification of the endogenous opioid system. It is apparent from the study of neurotransmitters that it is difficult to assign them a "behavioral function"; transmitters are used to communicate information in the brain, and different areas may have behaviorally opposing things to say using the same transmitters.

The opioid field now awaits the cloning of the receptor types and subtypes so that the receptor classifications can be clarified and studies of receptor regulation can begin at the molecular level. The endogenous opioid system, with its depth of pharmacological data, multiplicity of receptors and ligands, and relevance to medical issues, has been the promising focus of much neurobiological research, and it is indeed frustrating that cloning of these receptors has proven to be so problematic.

ACKNOWLEDGMENTS

I would like to thank Cathey Heron for her help in the preparation of this manuscript and Dr. Nigel Maidment for his critique. The original studies presented in this chapter were done in collaboration with Dr. Mark von Zastrow and Dr. Jacques Maddaluno and funded by NIDA grant #DA-05010. We would also like to acknowledge the support of the W.M. Keck Foundation.

Note
1. Since the original submission of this chapter, two groups have independently isolated clones for a delta opioid receptor (Evans et al. (1992). *Science, 258,* 1952-1955; Kieffer et al. (1992). *Proc. Natl. Acad. Sci. USA 89,* 12048-12052). Identification of other opioid receptors will undoubtedly soon follow.

REFERENCES

Akil, H., Watson, S., Young, E., Lewis, M., Khachaturian, H., & Walker, J. (1984). Endogenous opioids biology and function. *Annu. Rev. Neurosci., 7*, 223-255.

Blume, A.J., Lichtshtein, D., & Boone, G. (1979). Coupling of opiate receptors to adenylate cyclase: Requirement for Na+ and GTP. *Proc. Natl. Acad. Sci. USA, 76*(11), 5626-5630.

Bochet, P., Icard-Liepkalns, C., Pasquini, F., & Garbay-Jaureguiberry, C. (1988). Photoaffinity labeling of opioid delta receptors with an iodinated azido ligand: [125I][D Thr2,pN3Phe4,Leu5]enkephalyl-Thr6. *Mol. Pharmacol., 34*(4), 436-443.

Brady, L.S., Herkenham, M., Long, J.B., & Rothman, R.B. (1989). Chronic morphine increases mu-opiate receptor binding in rat brain: A quantitative autoradiographic study. *Brain Res., 477*(1-2), 382-386.

Brog, J.S., & Beinfeld, M.C. (1990). Inhibition of carbachol-induced inositol phosphate accumulation by phencyclidine, phencyclidine-like ligands and sigma agonists involves blockade of the muscarinic cholinergic receptor: A novel dioxadrol-preferring interaction. *J. Pharmacol. Exp. Ther., 254*(3), 952-956.

Collier, H.O.J., & Roy, A.C. (1973). Morphine-like drugs inhibit the stimulation by E prostaglandins of cyclic AMP formation by rat brain homogenate. *Nature, 248*, 24-27.

Erspamer, V., Melchiorri, P., Falconieri-Erspamer, G., Negri, L., Corsi, R., Severini, C., Barra, D., Simmaco, M., & Kreil, G. (1989). Deltorphins: a family of naturally occurring peptides with high affinity and selectivity for delta opioid binding sites. *Proc. Natl. Acad. Sci. USA, 86*(13), 5188-92.

Evans, C.J., & von Zastrow M. (1990). A state of the delta opioid receptor that is "blind" to opioid peptides yet retains high affinity for opiate alkaloids. In J.M. van Ree, et al. (Eds.), *New leads in opioid research* (pp. 159-161). Amsterdam: Excerpta Medica.

Evans, C.J., Erdelyi, E., & Barchas, J.D. (1985). Opioid peptides in the adrenal pituitary axis. *Psychopharm. Bull., 21*(3), 466-471.

Evans, C.J., Fredrickson, R., & Hammond, D. (1988). Processing of endogenous opioid precursors. In G.W. Pasternak (Ed.), *The opiate receptors* (pp. 23-71). Clifton, NJ: Humana Press.

Evans, C.J., Keith, D.E.Jr., Morrison, H., Magendzo, K., & Edwards, R.H. (1992). Cloning of a delta opioid receptor by Functional Expression. *Science* (1).

Gilbert, P.E., & Martin, W.R. (1976). The effects of morphine and nalorphine-like drugs in the nondependent, morphine-dependent and cyclazocine-dependent chronic spinal dog. *J. Pharmacol. Exp. Ther., 198*(1), 66-82, 1976.

Griffin, M.T., Law, P.Y., & Loh, H.H. (1985). Involvement of both inhibitory and stimulatory guanine-nucleotide binding proteins in the expression of adenylate-cyclase activity in NG108-15 cells. *J. Neurochem., 45*(5), 1585-1589.

Gross, R.A., Moises, H.C., Uhler, M.D., & Macdonald, R.L. (1990). Dynorphin A and cAMP-dependent protein kinase independently regulate neuronal calcium currents. *Proc. Natl. Acad. Sci. USA., 87*(18), 7025-7029.

Harada, H., Ueda, H., Katada, T., Ui, M., & Satoh, M. (1990). Phosphorylated mu-opioid receptor purified from rat brains lacks functional coupling with Gi1, a GTP-binding protein in reconstituted lipid vesicles. *Neurosci. Let., 113*(1), 47-49.

Herkenham, M. (1987). Mismatches between neurotransmitter and receptor localizations in brain: Observations and implications. *Neuroscience, 23*, 1-38.

Herschman, H.R. (1989). Extracellular signals, transcriptional responses and cellular specificity. *Trends Biochem. Sci., 14*, 455-458.

Hollt, V. (1986). Opioid peptide processing and receptor selectivity. *Annu. Rev. Pharmacol. Toxicol., 26,* 59-77.

Hurlbut, D.E., Evans, C.J., Barchas, J.D., & Leslie, F.M. (1987). Pharmacological properties of a proenkephalin A-derived opioid peptide: BAM 18. *Eur. J. Pharmacol., 138,* 359-366.

Knapp, R.J., Kazmierski, W., Hruby, V.J., & Yamamura, H.I. (1989). Structural characteristics of two highly selective opioid peptides. *Bioessays, 10*(2-3), 58-61.

Konkoy, C.S., & Childers, S.R. (1991). Relationship of kappa opioid receptor binding and inhibition of adenylate cyclase in guinea pig brain. *Soc. Neurosci. Abstr., 17*(1), 236.16, 593.

Koski, G., & Klee, W.A. (1987). Opiate inhibits cyclase by stimulating GTP hydrolysis. *Proc. Natl. Acad. Sci. USA, 78,* 4185-4189.

Kuhar, M.J. (1985). The mismatch problem in receptor mapping studies. *Trends Neurosci., 8,* 190-191.

Law, P.Y., Hom, D.S., & Loh, H.H. (1983). Opiate receptor down-regulation and desensitization in neuroblastoma X glioma NG108-15 hybrid cells are two separate cellular adaptation processes. *Mol. Pharmacol., 24,* 413-424.

Leslie, F. (1987). Methods used for the study of opioid receptors. *Pharmacol. Rev., 39,* 197-249.

Lord, J.A., Waterfield, A.A., Hughes, J., & Kosterlitz, H.W. (1977). Endogenous opioid peptides: Multiple agonists and receptors. *Nature, 267,* 495-499.

Maidment, N.T., Siddal, B., Rudolph, V.D., Erdelyi, E., & Evans, C.J. (1991). Postmortem changes in opioid peptide release in the rat brain monitored with microdialysis. *J. Neurochem., 56*(6), 1980-1984.

Mansour, A., Khachaturian, H., Lewis, M.E., Akil, H., & Watson, S.J. (1988). Anatomy of CNS opioid receptors. *Trends Neurosci., 11*(7), 308-314.

McKenzie, F.R., & Milligan, G. (1990). Delta-opioid-receptor-mediated inhibition of adenylate cyclase is transduced specifically by the guanine-nucleotide-binding protein Gi2. *Biochem. J., 267*(2), 391-398.

Morris, B.J., & Herz, A. (1989). Control of opiate receptor number in vivo: Simultaneous kappa-receptor down-regulation and mu-receptor up-regulation following chronic agonist/antagonist treatment. *Neuroscience, 29*(2), 433-442.

Nock, B., Giordano, A.L., Cicero, T.J., & O'Connor, L.H. (1990). Affinity of drugs and peptides for U-69,593-sensitive and -insensitive kappa opiate binding sites: The U-69,593-insensitive site appears to be the beta endorphin-specific epsilon receptor. *J. Pharmacol. Exp. Ther., 254*(2), 412-419.

North, A.R., Williams, J.T., Surprenant, A., & Christie, M.J. (1987). μ and ∂ receptors belong to a family of receptors that are coupled to potassium channels. *Proc. Natl. Acad. Sci. USA, 84,* 5487-5491.

O'Dowd, B.F., Lefkowitz, R.J., & Caron, M.G. (1989). Structure of the adrenergic and related receptors. *Annu. Rev. Neurosci., 12,* 67-83.

Paul, D., Bodnar, R.J., Gistrak, M.A., & Pasternak, G.W. (1989). Different mu receptor subtypes mediate spinal and supraspinal analgesia in mice. *Eur. J. Pharmacol., 168*(3), 307-314.

Ross, S.B. (1990). Is the sigma opiate receptor a proadifen-sensitive subform of cytochrome P-450? *Pharmacol. Toxicol., 67*(1), 93-94.

Schofield, P.R., McFarland, K.C., Hayflick, J.S., Wilcox, J.N., Cho, T.M., Roy, S., Lee, N.M., Loh, H.H., & Seeburg, P.H. (1989). Molecular characterization of a new immunoglobulin superfamily protein with potential roles in opioid binding and cell contact. *Embo J., 8*(2), 489-495.

Sharma, S.K., Klee, W.A., & Nirenberg, M. (1975). Dual regulation of adenylate cyclase accounts for narcotic dependence and tolerance. *Proc. Natl. Acad. Sci. USA, 72*(8), 3092-3096.

Sharma, S.K., Klee, W.A., & Nirenberg, M. (1977). Opiate-dependent modulation of adenylate cyclase. *Proc. Natl. Acad. Sci. USA, 74*(8), 3365-3369.

Smyth, D.G., Massey, D.E., Zakarian, S., & Finnie, M.D.A. (1979). Endorphins are stored in biologically active and inactive forms: Isolation of a-N-acetyl peptides. *Nature, 279*, 252-254.

Stevens, K.E., Leslie, F.M., Evans, C.J., Belluzzi, J.D., & Stein, L. (1988). Bam 18 analgesia, hyperalgesia and locomotor effects. *Neuropeptides, 12*(1), 21-27.

Suh, H.H., Tseng, L.F., & Li, C.H. (1988). Beta-endorphin-(1-27) antagonizes beta-endorphin- but not morphine-,D-Pen2-D-Pen5-enkephalin- and U50, 488H-induced analgesia in mice. *Neuropharmacology, 27*(9), 957-963.

Tao, P.L., Law, P.Y., & Loh, H.H. (1987). Decrease in delta and mu opioid receptor binding capacity in rat brain after chronic etorphine treatment. *J. Pharmacol. Exp. Ther., 240*(3), 809-816.

Tao, P.L., Chang, L.R., Law, P.Y., & Loh, H.H. (1988). Decrease in delta-opioid receptor density in rat brain after chronic:D-Ala2,D-Leu5:enkephalin treatment. *Brain Res., 462*(2), 313-320.

Taussig, R., Sanchez, S., Rifo, M., Golman, A.G., & Belardetti, F. (1992). Inhibition of the omega-conotoxin-sensitive calcium current by distinct G proteins. *Neuron 8*(4), 799-809.

Tempel, A., Gardner, E.L., & Zukin, R.S. (1985). Neurochemical and functional correlates of naltrexone-induced opiate receptor up-regulation. *J. Pharmacol. Exp. Ther., 232*(2), 439-444.

Tempel, A., Habas, J., Paredes, W., & Barr, G.A. (1988). Morphine-induced down-regulation of mu opioid receptors in neonatal rat brain. *Dev. Brain Res., 41*(1-2), 129-133.

Traynor, J. (1989). Subtypes of the kappa-opioid receptor: Fact or fiction? *Trends Pharmacol. Sci., 10*(2), 52-53.

Vaupel, D.B. (1983). Naloxone fails to antagonize the sigma effects of PCP and SKF10,047 in the dog. *Eur. J. Pharmacol., 92*, 269-274.

von Zastrow, M.A., & Evans, C.J. (1990). Morphine blocks the peptide-selective binding change without blocking receptor downregulation. In J.M. van Ree, et al. (Eds.), *New leads in opioid research* (pp. 101–103). Amsterdam: Excerpta Medica.

Wagner, J.J., Evans, C.J., & Chavkin, C. (1991). Focal stimulation of the mossy fibers releases endogenous dynorphins that bind K$_1$opioid receptors in guinea pig hippocampus. *J. Neurochem., 57*(1), 333–343.

Weber, E., Esch, F.S., Bohlen, P., Paterson, S., Corbett, A.D., McKnight, A.T., Kosterlitz, H.W., Barchas, J.D., & Evans, C.J. (1983). Metorphamide: Isolations, structure and biologic activity of a novel amidated opioid octapeptide from bovine brain. *Proc. Natl. Acad. Sci. USA, 80*, 7362-7366.

Werling, L.L., McMahon, P.N., & Cox, B.M. (1989a). Effects of pertussis toxin on opioid regulation of catecholamine release from rat and guinea pig brain slices. *Naunyn Schmiedebergs Arch Pharmacol., 339*(5), 509-513.

Werling, L.L., McMahon, P.N., & Cox, B.M. (1989b). Selective changes in mu opioid receptor properties induced by chronic morphine exposure. *Proc. Natl. Acad. Sci. USA, 86*(16), 6393-6397.

Werz, M.A., & Macdonald, R.L. (1982). Heterogeneous sensitivity of cultured dorsal root ganglion neurones to opioid peptides selective for mu- and delta-opiate receptors. *Nature, 299*, 730-733.

Wollemann, M. (1990). Recent developments in the research of opioid receptor subtype molecularcharacterization. *J. Neurochem., 54*(4), 1095-1101.

Xie, G.X., Miyajima, A., & Goldstein, A. (1992). Expression cloning of cDNA encoding a seven-helix receptor from human placenta with affinity for opioid ligands. *Proc. Natl. Acad. Sci. USA, 89*, 4124-4128.

Yang, H-Y.T., & Majane, E.A. (1989). FMRF-NH$_2$-like peptide. A putative antiopioid peptide in mammalian CNS. INRC Research Conference, Abstract #S-19.

Young, E.A., Walker, J.M., Houghten, R., & Akil, H. (1987). The degradation of dynorphin A in brain tissue in vivo and in vitro. *Peptides, 8*(4), 701-707.

Yu, V.C., Eiger, S., Duan, D.S., Lameh, J., & Sadee, W. (1990). Regulation of cyclic AMP by the mu-opioid receptor in human neuroblastomaSH-SY5Y cells. *J. Neurochem., 55*(4), 1390-1396.

Zakarian, S., & Smyth, D. (1979). Distribution of active and inactive forms of endorphins in rat pituitary and brain. *Proc. Natl. Acad. Sci. USA, 76*, 5927-5976.

Zukin, R.S., & Zukin, S.R. (1988). The sigma receptor. In G.W. Pasternack (Ed.), *The opiate receptors* (pp. 143-163). Clifton, NJ: Humana Press.

4

Second-Messenger and Protein Phosphorylation Mechanisms Underlying Opiate and Cocaine Addiction

ERIC J. NESTLER, XAVIER GUITART, AND DANA BEITNER-JOHNSON

The mechanism by which opiates induce tolerance and dependence in target neurons has been the subject of intensive investigation. The discovery of opiate receptors in the 1970s raised the possibility that opiate addiction might be mediated by alterations in these endogenous receptors. However, over a decade of research has failed to identify consistent changes in the number of opiate receptors or in their affinity for opiates ligands under conditions of opiate addiction (Johnson & Fleming, 1989; Loh et al., 1988; Redmond & Krystal, 1984). Changes in levels of endogenous opioid peptides also do not seem to explain prominent aspects of opiate tolerance, dependence, and withdrawal.

Similarly, the biochemical mechanisms underlying cocaine addiction remain obscure. The primary acute action of cocaine, acting as a drug of abuse, seems to be the inhibition of dopamine reuptake by dopaminergic nerve terminals. Acutely, cocaine thereby results in transient increases in dopaminergic neurotransmission. However, studies of the levels of the dopamine transporter protein itself or of various dopamine receptor subtypes have not reported consistent changes in cocaine-sensitive brain regions in response to chronic cocaine exposure (Clouet et al., 1988; Peris et al., 1990).

The failure to account for important aspects of opiate and cocaine addiction through regulation of neurotransmitters and receptors per se has shifted attention to postreceptor mechanisms. Thus, it is now known that opiate and dopamine receptors, as well as most other types of receptors present in brain, produce most of their physiological responses in target neurons through a

This work was supported by USPHS Grants DA05490, DA07359, 2 PO1 MH25642, and 5 P50 DA04060, by the VA-Yale Alcoholism Research Center, and by the Abraham Ribicoff Research Facilities of the Connecticut Mental Health Center, State of Connecticut Department of Mental Health.

complex cascade of intracellular messengers involving (1) G-proteins (Gilman, 1987) that couple the receptors to intracellular effector systems and (2) the intracellular effector systems themselves, which include second messengers, protein kinases, and phosphoproteins (Fig. 4-1) (Nestler & Greengard, 1984,

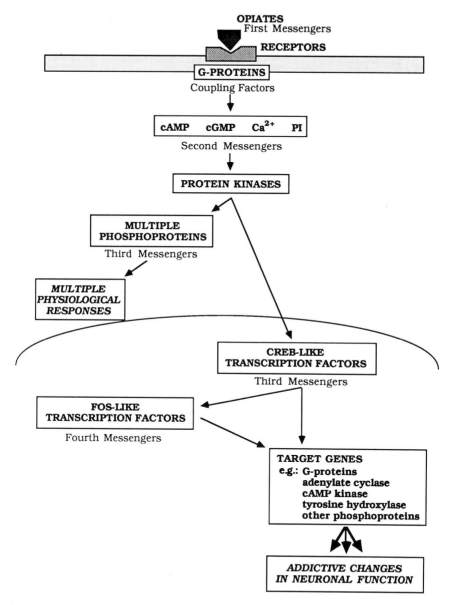

Figure 4-1.   Intracellular messenger pathways through which diverse extracellular signals produce multiple types of physiological responses, including the regulation of gene expression, in target neurons. The figure illustrates the likely central role played by these intracellular messengers in mediating the addictive actions of opiates and other drugs of abuse. Adapted from Hyman & Nestler, 1993.

1989). Regulation of these intracellular messenger pathways mediates the effects of the neurotransmitter-receptor systems on diverse aspects of neuronal function. Increasing evidence indicates that one role of these intracellular pathways is to mediate neurotransmitter regulation of gene expression in target neurons (Hyman & Nestler, 1993; Montminy et al., 1990), a process that would be expected to be particularly important for long-term changes in brain function, such as the changes associated with drug addiction.

Over the past several years, we have used the increasing knowledge of intracellular messenger pathways as an experimental framework within which to study possible postreceptor mechanisms of opiate and cocaine addiction. The studies have demonstrated that adaptations in G-proteins and the cyclic AMP second-messenger and protein phosphorylation system mediate important aspects of opiate and cocaine addiction in several drug-responsive brain regions. Interestingly, the results suggest that similar types of biochemical changes, occurring in these various brain regions, are involved in mediating both physical and psychological aspects of drug addiction.

INTRACELLULAR ACTIONS OF CHRONIC OPIATES IN THE LOCUS COERULEUS

The locus coeruleus (LC) has served as a useful model of opiate action. It is the largest noradrenergic nucleus in the brain and is located bilaterally on the floor of the fourth ventricle in the anterior pons (Foote et al., 1983). The LC is particularly well suited for biochemical and molecular investigations: It is a relatively homogeneous brain region, and it has been extensively characterized anatomically and electrophysiologically.

Acute Opiate Actions in the LC

The mechanism of acute opiate action in the LC, based on electrophysiological and biochemical studies, is shown schematically in Figure 4-2 (top). Opiates acutely inhibit LC neurons through the regulation of two types of ion channels: increased conductance of a voltage-dependent K^+ channel and decreased conductance of a slowly depolarizing Na^+ channel (Wang & Aghajanian, 1987). Regulation of both channels is mediated by pertussis toxin-sensitive G-proteins, i.e., G_i and G_o (Aghajanian & Wang, 1986; North et al., 1987), and the Na^+ channel is regulated by reduced neuronal levels of cyclic AMP (Aghajanian & Wang, 1987; Wang & Aghajanian, 1987). Biochemically, opiates acutely inhibit adenylate cyclase activity in the LC (Beitner et al., 1989; Duman et al., 1988), as seen in other brain regions (see Johnson & Fleming, 1989), and inhibit cyclic AMP-dependent protein phosphorylation (Guitart & Nestler, 1989). Such regulation of protein phosphorylation presumably mediates the effects of opiates on the Na^+ channel through the phosphorylation of the channel itself or some associated protein. In addition, opiate regulation of protein phosphorylation probably mediates the effects of opiates on many other aspects of LC neuronal function, even including some of the initial steps underlying longer-term changes associated with addiction.

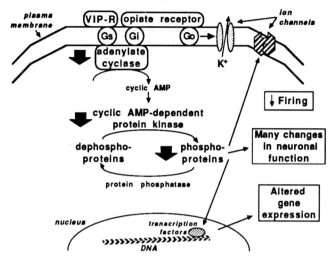

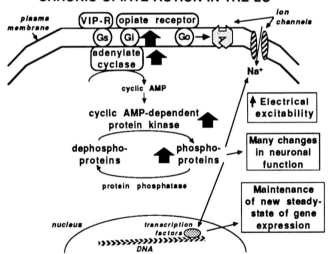

Figure 4-2. Mechanisms of acute and chronic opiate action in the locus coeruleus. From Nestler (1992).

Chronic Opiate Actions in the LC

LC neurons become tolerant to the acute inhibitory effects of opiates, as LC firing rates return toward normal levels during chronic opiate exposure (Agha-janian, 1978; Andrade et al., 1983; Christie et al., 1987). The neurons also become dependent on opiates, as their firing rates increase more than sixfold during opiate withdrawal precipitated in vivo by administration of opiate receptor antagonists (Aghajanian, 1978; Rasmussen et al., 1990). These chronic changes in LC neuronal excitability seem to play an important role in mediating aspects of physical opiate addiction—namely, physical dependence and physical abstinence syndromes—in several mammalian species (Rasmussen et al., 1990; Redmond & Krystal, 1984).

However, electrophysiological signs of tolerance, dependence, and withdrawal in the LC occur in the absence of detectable changes in opiate receptors[1] or opiate-regulated ion channels themselves, raising the possibility that intervening intracellular steps might be involved. Indeed, we have found that chronic treatment of rats with opiates results in a dramatic upregulation of the cyclic AMP system at every major step between receptor and physiological response (Fig. 4-2, bottom). Chronic opiates increase levels of $G_{i\alpha}$ and $G_{o\alpha}$ (without changes in other G-protein subunits), adenylate cyclase, cyclic AMP-dependent protein kinase, and a number of "MARPPs" (morphine- and cyclic AMP-regulated phosphoproteins) (Duman et al., 1988; Guitart & Nestler, 1989, 1990; Nestler & Tallman, 1988; Nestler et al., 1989). Among these MARPPs is tyrosine hydroxylase (Guitart et al., 1990), the rate-limiting enzyme in the biosynthesis of catecholamines. These various intracellular adaptations to chronic opiates are mediated via persistent activation of opiate receptors; the responses are blocked by concomitant treatment of rats with naltrexone, an opiate receptor antagonist, and are not produced by acute morphine. Moreover, the changes are not generalized responses exhibited by all brain regions in that they were not observed in several other brain regions studied originally, which included the frontal cortex, caudate/putamen, and dorsal raphe.

Evidence for a Functional Role of an Upregulated Cyclic AMP System in Opiate Addiction

The upregulated cyclic AMP system in the LC can be viewed as a homeostatic response to persistent opiate inhibition of the cells. According to this view, the upregulated cyclic AMP system, by increasing the intrinsic excitability of LC neurons, represents part of the biochemical mechanisms underlying opiate tolerance, dependence, and withdrawal exhibited by these neurons (Guitart et al., 1990; Nestler, 1992; Rasmussen et al., 1990). Thus, the concurrent presence of morphine and the upregulated cyclic AMP system in opiate-treated animals results in LC firing rates close to levels in control rats, i.e., tolerance. When the morphine is "withdrawn" abruptly by administration of naltrexone, the upregulated cyclic AMP system, unopposed by morphine, increases the activity of LC neurons, i.e., dependence and withdrawal. This model, which is similar to one proposed previously based on studies of cultured neuroblastoma × glioma cells (Sharma et al., 1975), is supported by several lines of evidence.

---

[1] It is important to note that the lack of consistent effects of chronic opiates on opiate receptors in the LC and elsewhere is based exclusively on ligand binding studies, since to date no opiate receptor has been cloned or purified. It may well prove to be true that a more complete analysis of opiate receptors will reveal changes in opiate receptors (e.g., altered expression, phosphorylation) associated with drug addiction.

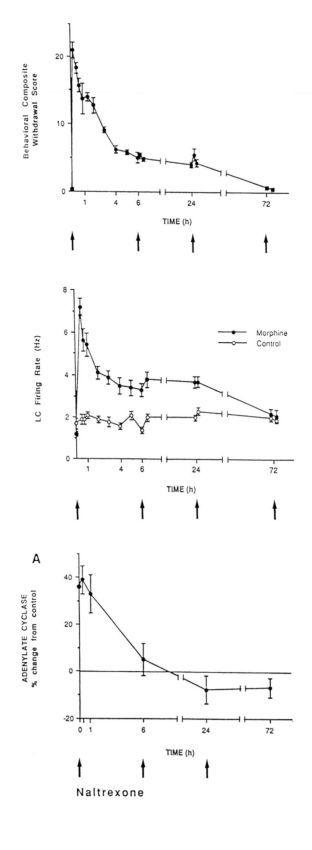

Behavioral Composite Withdrawal Score

TIME (h)

LC Firing Rate (Hz)

● Morphine
○ Control

TIME (h)

A

ADENYLATE CYCLASE % change from control

TIME (h)

Naltrexone

First, LC neurons from opiate-dependent animals exhibit spontaneous firing rates in vitro that are more than twofold higher than in LC neurons from control animals (Kogan et al., 1992). Since these recordings from LC neurons were performed in brain slices in which virtually all synaptic inputs to the LC are removed, the results demonstrate increased intrinsic excitability of the neurons in the opiate-dependent state. Second, LC neurons from opiate-dependent animals exhibit electrophysiological supersensitivity to cyclic AMP analogs, and to agents that increase neuronal cyclic AMP levels compared to neurons from control animals (Kogan et al., 1992). This supersensitivity is direct electrophysiological evidence for an upregulated cyclic AMP system in the LC during opiate dependence. Third, recovery of alterations in G-proteins, adenylate cyclase, and cyclic AMP-dependent protein kinase during opiate withdrawal in vivo parallels the time course by which LC firing rates and numerous behavioral signs and symptoms of withdrawal recover during the early phases of antagonist-precipitated withdrawal (Rasmussen et al., 1990), as illustrated in Figure 4-3. Finally, systemic administration of phosphodiesterase inhibitors, which increase cyclic AMP levels, produces a morphine-like withdrawal syndrome in normal rats (Collier et al., 1981) and potentiates opiate antagonist discrimination (Holtzman, 1989) and opiate abstinence behaviors (D. Marby, J.H. Krystal, and E.J. Nestler, unpublished observations) in opiate-dependent animals. These effects of systemic phosphodiesterase inhibitors could be mediated in part by upregulation of the cyclic AMP system seen in response to chronic morphine in the LC. Taken together, these results provide strong evidence to support the view that the opiate-induced upregulation of the cyclic AMP system represents one mechanism by which opiates produce addictive changes in LC neurons.

Molecular Mechanisms Underlying Opiate Upregulation of the Cyclic AMP System

One of the central questions raised by our studies concerns the precise molecular mechanisms by which chronic opiate administration leads to upregulation of the cyclic AMP system in the LC. Recent evidence indicates that many of the

---

Figure 4-3. Studies of the locus coeruleus during opiate withdrawal: behavioral, electrophysiological, and biochemical correlates. Note the striking parallel in the time course by which opiate abstinence behaviors (top) and increased LC firing rates (middle) recover during naltrexone-precipitated opiate withdrawal. Two phases are evident: an early, rapid phase during which withdrawal behaviors and LC firing rates recover by more than 50% over the first 6 hours of withdrawal and a slower phase during which the remaining recovery occurs after 72 hours of withdrawal. In addition, the time course by which increased levels of adenylate cyclase activity (bottom) recover during opiate withdrawal parallels the early phase of physiological and behavioral withdrawal. Similar results were seen with cyclic AMP-dependent protein kinase and G-proteins. The results provide correlative evidence for a role of these intracellular messengers in mediating changes in LC neuronal activity during early opiate withdrawal. From Rasmussen et al. (1990).

intracellular adaptations occur at the protein and messenger RNA level. Chronic morphine increases levels of immunoreactivity of $G_{i\alpha}$, $G_{o\alpha}$, cyclic AMP-dependent protein kinase regulatory subunit (type II) and catalytic subunit, and tyrosine hydroxylase in the LC by immunoblotting and increases mRNA levels of $G_{i\alpha}$, cyclic AMP-dependent protein kinase catalytic subunit, and tyrosine hydroxylase by Northern blotting and/or in situ hybridization (Guitart et al., 1990; Nestler, 1990; M.D. Hayward, J.A. Clark, R.Z. Terwilliger, & E.J. Nestler, unpublished observations). These findings raise the possibility that opiate regulation of the G-protein/cyclic AMP system is mediated, at least in part, by changes in gene expression.

Neurotransmitter regulation of gene expression is now known to occur via second-messenger-dependent phosphorylation and/or induction of a class of proteins referred to as transcription factors—proteins that bind to specific DNA sequences (termed response elements) in the promoter regions of genes and thereby increase or decrease the rate at which those genes are transcribed (Hyman & Nestler, 1993; Montminy et al., 1990). Two general types of mechanisms seem to be involved (see Fig. 4-1). In the first, protein kinases, activated in response to a first- and second-messenger stimulus, phosphorylate and activate transcription factors that are already present in the cell. CREB proteins (cyclic AMP response element binding proteins) function in this manner. CREB proteins consist of a family of related transcription factors that mediate many of the effects of cyclic AMP, and of those neurotransmitters that act through cyclic AMP, on gene expression. Alternatively, protein kinases, through the phosphorylation and activation of CREB or a CREB-like protein, would stimulate the expression of a family of transcription factor genes referred to as immediate early genes, e.g., c-fos, c-jun, zif268. The newly synthesized immediate early gene products would return to the nucleus where they would regulate the expression of other target genes. Figure 4-1 illustrates the potential role played by these mechanisms in mediating addictive actions of opiates in the nervous system.

We have recently initiated a series of studies to identify the specific transcription factors through which opiates might regulate the expression of G-proteins and the cyclic AMP system in the LC. Our initial studies focused on c-fos and other immediate early genes because of the relative ease with which these transcription factors can be studied. We have found that, acutely, opiates decrease levels of c-fos expression in the LC and that such decreased expression persists with chronic opiate administration (Hayward et al., 1990). In contrast, c-fos expression is induced several-fold during naltrexone-precipitated opiate withdrawal. Similar regulation of c-jun was observed. These studies indicate that decreased levels of c-fos (and related transcription factors) might play a role in triggering and in maintaining some of the intracellular adaptations to chronic morphine and that increased levels of the transcription factors might be involved in the recovery of these adaptations during withdrawal. Current studies are aimed at testing this possibility directly, as well as identifying other classes of transcription factors, most notably CREB proteins (see Guitart et al., 1992a), that might be involved in mediating the effects of opiates on LC gene expression.

A General Role for Adaptations in G-proteins and the Cyclic AMP System in Opiate Addiction

Our progress in identifying molecular mediators of chronic opiate action in the LC led us to examine whether similar mechanisms are involved in opiate action in other regions of the CNS. Indeed, there are increasing indications that an upregulated cyclic AMP system may mediate aspects of opiate addiction in several regions of the CNS. Chronic opiates have been shown to increase adenylate cyclase activity in dorsal root ganglion/spinal cord explants (DRG/SC) (Makman et al., 1988), and more recent experiments have demonstrated a concomitant increase in cyclic AMP-dependent protein kinase as well (Terwilliger et al., 1991). Similar changes in the cyclic AMP system have also been found recently in the nucleus accumbens, amygdala, and thalamus (Terwilliger et al., 1991). An upregulated cyclic AMP system may therefore be a common mechanism by which a number of opiate-sensitive neurons adapt to chronic morphine. Such increases in adenylate cyclase and cyclic AMP-dependent protein kinase could contribute to aspects of opiate tolerance, dependence, and withdrawal in these neuronal cell types as outlined above for the LC. These possibilities need to be studied directly in electrophysiological investigations.

Chronic opiates have also been shown to regulate $G_{i\alpha}$ and $G_{o\alpha}$ in most of the opiate-responsive regions of the CNS mentioned above, although different effects are seen in the different regions. Chronic opiates increase the levels of these G-protein subunits in the amygdala, as in the LC (Terwilliger et al., 1991), but decrease levels of $G_{i\alpha}$ in DRG/SC (Attali & Vogel, 1989) and nucleus accumbens (Terwilliger et al., 1991). Such differential regulation of G-proteins may determine whether chronic exposure to opiates induces heterologous or homologous desensitization in specific target neurons (Terwilliger et al., 1991). Thus, in addition to inducing desensitization to opiates (i.e., tolerance) in all of these regions, chronic opiates also induce desensitization to other similarly acting agonists, such as $alpha_2$-adrenergic agonists, in the DRG/SC. Such heterologous desensitization could be accounted for by the reduced levels of $G_{i\alpha}$ (together with the upregulated cyclic AMP system) induced in the DRG/SC in response to chronic opiates. In contrast, opiates induce homologous desensitization in the LC. In this situation, tolerance to opiates could be mediated by the upregulated cyclic AMP system plus some postulated uncoupling of opiate receptors from G-proteins. Increased levels of $G_{i\alpha}$ and $G_{o\alpha}$ would enable normal responsiveness to $alpha_2$-adrenergic agonists acting against the upregulated cyclic AMP system. Clearly, further work is needed to test the validity of this hypothesis.

COMMON INTRACELLULAR ACTIONS OF CHRONIC OPIATES AND CHRONIC COCAINE IN BRAIN REWARD REGIONS

Regulation of G-proteins and the Cyclic AMP System in the Nucleus Accumbens

Most of the brain regions discussed above (e.g., LC, DRG-SC, and thalamus) are thought to play prominent roles in mediating physical opiate addiction, i.e., physical dependence and physical abstinence syndromes. In contrast, the nucleus accumbens (nACC), along with dopaminergic neurons originating in the ventral tegmental area (VTA), are thought to play a prominent role in psychological aspect of drug addiction; namely, drug reinforcement and craving (Bozarth & Wise, 1987; Koob & Bloom, 1988; Liebman & Cooper, 1989). Rats will self-administer opiates directly into the VTA and nACC, and develop opiate place preference after local opiate infusion into these brain regions. Furthermore, lesions of the nACC have been reported to attenuate opiate self-administration and place preference. Morphine regulation of the G-protein/cyclic AMP system in the nACC raised the possibility that these intracellular adaptations contribute to mechanisms of drug reward and craving mediated by this brain region.

This possibility was tested further by determining whether similar intracellular adaptations occur in the nACC in response to chronic cocaine, since the mesolimbic dopamine system has been postulated to play an important role in the reinforcing actions of this drug as well (Bozarth & Wise, 1987; Clouet et al., 1988; DiChiara & Imperato, 1988; Kalivas & Duffy, 1988; Koob & Bloom, 1988; Liebman & Cooper, 1989). As shown in Figure 4-4, we found that chronic cocaine produced very similar changes, compared to chronic morphine, in levels of $G_{i\alpha}$, adenylate cyclase, and cyclic AMP-dependent protein kinase in the nACC (Nestler et al., 1990; Terwilliger et al., 1991). Similar effects were not observed in several other brain regions studied. The effects of cocaine in the nACC were not seen after acute cocaine administration, indicating that these changes are a result of chronic exposure to the drug. Moreover, in contrast to morphine and cocaine, no changes in these intracellular messengers were observed in the nACC in response to chronic administration of several other classes of psychotropic drugs without prominent reinforcing properties: halo-

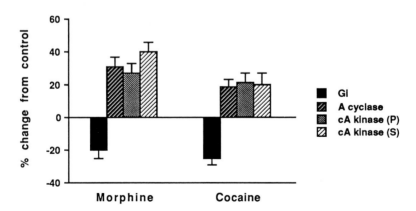

Figure 4-4. Common adaptations in G-proteins and the cyclic AMP system in the nACC in response to chronic morphine and chronic cocaine. Gi, immunoreactivity of Giα subunit; A cyclase, adenylate cyclase activity; cA kinase, cyclic AMP-dependent protein kinase activity in particulate (P) and soluble (S) fractions. Data represent means ± s.e.m. (N=8–14). All changes shown in the figure are statistically significant by χ^2 test. From Terwilliger et al. (1991).

peridol (an antipsychotic, dopamine receptor antagonist), imipramine and fluoxetine (antidepressants, monoamine reuptake blockers), and clonidine (an antihypertensive, alpha$_2$-adrenergic agonist).

These findings indicate that adaptations in G-proteins and the cyclic AMP system may represent common responses by nACC neurons to drugs of abuse and may underlie some of the functional changes in these neurons that mediate drug reward and craving. Adaptations observed in response to chronic cocaine can be understood within a functional context of the known electrophysiological effects of chronic cocaine on nACC neurons. Chronic cocaine has been shown to produce supersensitivity of nACC neurons to the inhibitory actions of D$_1$-dopaminergic agonists on these cell (Henry & White, 1991). This functional supersensitivity occurs in the absence of consistent changes in levels or affinity of D$_1$ receptors in this brain region (Clouet et al., 1988; Peris et al., 1990). As D$_1$ agonists are thought to exert their effects through cyclic AMP, the observed increase in adenylate cyclase and cyclic AMP-dependent protein kinase, together with the observed decrease in G$_{i\alpha}$ (without a change in G$_{s\alpha}$ or G$_\beta$), could account for the supersensitivity of nACC neurons demonstrated electrophysiologically. Based on our biochemical data, we would predict that chronic treatment of rats with morphine, at least under our treatment conditions, would result in similar alterations in the physiological sensitivity of these neurons, a possibility that needs to be studied directly.

Identification of Morphine- and Cocaine-Regulated Phosphoproteins in the VTA and nACC

In addition to regulation of G-proteins, adenylate cyclase, and cyclic AMP-dependent protein kinase, chronic morphine and cocaine also produce some similar changes in the next step in the cyclic AMP pathway; namely, in individual phosphoproteins. Chronic morphine and chronic cocaine treatments have been shown to regulate many of the same phosphoproteins in the VTA and NAc; we have designated these proteins as *morphine*- and *cocaine-regulated phosphoproteins* or "MCRPPs" (Beitner-Johnson & Nestler, 1991; Beitner-Johnson et al., 1992). The effects of chronic morphine on cyclic AMP-dependent protein phosphorylation in the VTA, as analyzed by back phosphorylation and two-dimensional gel electrophoretic procedures, are shown in Figure 4-5. Among the MCRPPs identified are some that have been shown previously to be regulated by chronic morphine in the LC (tyrosine hydroxylase and MCRPPs-71, 62, and 51), as well as several additional phosphoproteins (MCRPPs-165, 66, and 39). Interestingly, three of these phosphoproteins—tyrosine hydroxylase, MCRPP-165, and MCRPP-66—are regulated in the same way by both morphine and cocaine treatments. Drug regulation of the various MCRPPs was not seen in response to acute morphine or cocaine treatment, indicating the requirement for chronic drug administration. Drug regulation of these phosphoproteins also shows regional specificity in that most of the changes were not observed in the substantia nigra or caudate/putamen, components of the nigrostriatal dopamine system that are generally not implicated in drug reward mechanisms. The results support the view that regulation of these MCRPPs may

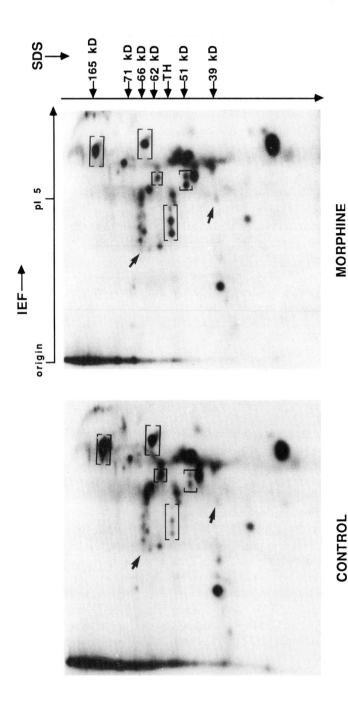

Figure 4-5. Autoradiograms showing the effect of chronic morphine on protein phosphorylation in the VTA. Extracts of VTA from control and morphine-treated rats were subjected to back phosphorylation with [γ-³²P]ATP and purified cyclic AMP-dependent protein kinase and to two-dimensional gel electrophoresis and autoradiography. The figure illustrates the positions of seven phosphoproteins regulated by chronic morphine. Proteins of 165, 66, and 39 kD, and tyrosine hydroxylase (TH) were also regulated by chronic cocaine and are designated MCRPPs. Proteins of 71 and 51 kD also seem to be regulated by chronic cocaine, but this has not yet been established with certainty. From Beitner-Johnson et al., 1992.

represent part of a common molecular basis for morphine and cocaine addiction mediated by dopaminergic brain reward regions.

Of particular interest is the similar regulation of tyrosine hydroxylase in the VTA in response to chronic morphine and chronic cocaine. Both drug treatments have been shown to increase levels of enzyme immunoreactivity in this brain region (Beitner-Johnson & Nestler, 1991). It is possible that such upregulation of the enzyme underlies a common functional change induced in VTA neurons by these two drugs of abuse. Tyrosine hydroxylase, as stated above, is the rate-limiting enzyme in catecholamine biosynthesis, and its expression in adrenal medulla, peripheral sympathetic neurons, and central catecholaminergic neurons appears to be induced by conditions that increase synaptic activation of the cells (Nestler & Greengard, 1984, 1989; Zigmond et al., 1989). An increase in tyrosine hydroxylase expression in the VTA in response to morphine or cocaine may therefore result from an elevated level of VTA neuronal activity. Indeed, such an increase has been reported to occur in response to chronic cocaine treatment: Henry et al. (1989) found a greater number of spontaneously active VTA neurons, with significantly higher firing rates, in cocaine-treated rats compared to controls. It is not known how VTA neurons respond electrophysiologically to chronic morphine treatment, but it is reasonable to hypothesize that chronic morphine (at least under our treatment conditions) may also increase the firing rate or intrinsic excitability of VTA neurons.

We have also observed an apparent dephosphorylation of tyrosine hydroxylase, without a change in its total amount, in the nACC in response to both chronic morphine and chronic cocaine. As cyclic AMP-dependent protein kinase and other protein kinases are known to phosphorylate and activate tyrosine hydroxylase (Nestler & Greengard, 1989; Zigmond et al., 1989), dephosphorylation of the enzyme would suggest reduced catalytic activity in response to chronic morphine and cocaine.

The explanation for the presence of less active tyrosine hydroxylase in dopaminergic nerve terminals in the nACC and of more total enzyme in cell bodies in the VTA is unknown, but the findings are consistent with the view that dopaminergic neurotransmission subserves different functional roles in these two brain regions. In the VTA, where dopamine is known to act upon inhibitory D_2 autoreceptors and possibly on nondopaminergic nerve terminals as well (Bayer & Pickel, 1990; Roth et al., 1987), increased levels of tyrosine hydroxylase could reflect increased local dopaminergic tone, consistent with increased VTA firing rates that occur with chronic cocaine treatment as mentioned above (Henry et al., 1989). In the nACC, where dopamine has distinct physiological and biochemical actions on multiple subtypes of receptors localized both pre- and postsynaptically (Bunney et al., 1987; Wachtel et al., 1989), lower tyrosine hydroxylase activity may reflect decreased dopamine synthesis. This is supported by the recent report that chronic cocaine treatment decreases dopamine synthesis in the nACC as measured by in vivo microdialysis (Brock et al., 1990). Moreover, D_1-dopamine receptor supersensitivity seen electrophysiologically in the nACC in response to chronic cocaine (Henry & White, 1991) could reflect a compensatory response to decreased dopamine synthesis.

These observations are in contrast to the reported ability of chronic co-caine treatment to increase the amount of dopamine released in the nACC in response to a subsequent challenge of cocaine (Pettit et al., 1990). The various data, however, can be reconciled by the following scheme. Chronic cocaine use results in decreased basal levels of dopaminergic neurotransmission in the nACC, which are reflected by decreased levels of dopamine synthesis. These decreased levels might be expected to result in D_1 receptor supersensitivity (as described above) and an increase in readily releasable pools of dopamine (Ng et al., 1990). Then, in response to a subsequent acute dose of cocaine, more dopamine is released, which acts on supersensitive postsynaptic cells, resulting in a temporary synergistic enhancement in dopaminergic neurotransmission. Clearly, further studies are needed to test the validity of these and alternative hypotheses. Nevertheless, the data suggest that chronic morphine and chronic cocaine use produces similar changes in dopaminergic function in both the VTA and nACC, but by distinct mechanisms in these two brain regions.

Three of the other MCRPPs, MCRPP-165, 66, and 62, are highly enriched in the VTA, and have been shown recently to be neurofilament proteins (Beit-ner-Johnson et al., 1992). Morphine- and cocaine-induced decreases in the in vitro phosphorylation of neurofilaments (see Figure 5) are associated, in most cases, with equivalent decreases in the total amounts of these proteins in the VTA. As neurofilaments are major determinants of neuronal morphology and are associated with axonal caliber and transport, morphine and cocaine regula-tion of these proteins would suggest that chronic exposure to the drugs reflects prominent structural and functional changes in VTA dopamine neurons possi-bly associated with the drug-addicted state (Beitner-Johnson et al., 1992; Nestler, 1992).

Different Levels of MCRPPs in the VTA and nACC of Lewis and Fischer Rats

Genetic factors are generally thought to contribute to individual differences in susceptibility to drug addiction in both animals and people, although the spe-cific factors involved remain unknown. One model system for such differences are Lewis and Fischer 344 rats, inbred strains that show dramatically different levels of self-administration of several types of drugs of abuse. Lewis rats self-administer opiates, cocaine, and alcohol at much higher rates than Fischer rats (George & Goldberg, 1989; Suzuki et al., 1988) and develop greater degrees of conditioned place preference to opiates and cocaine (Guitart et al., 1992b). To identify possible factors that contribute to the different levels of drug prefer-ence exhibited by these strains, we studied cyclic AMP-dependent protein phosphorylation in dopaminergic brain reward regions. Prominent differences were found between the two rat strains in levels of five MCRPPs—tyrosine hydroxylase and 165, 66, 62, and 51—in the VTA and nACC (Beitner-Johnson et al., 1991).

The strain differences in tyrosine hydroxylase phosphorylation are associ-ated with different levels of enzyme immunoreactivity. The VTA of drug-naive Lewis rats was found to contain ~45% higher levels of tyrosine hydroxylase immunoreactivity and the nACC contained ~45% lower enzyme levels compared to those brain areas in Fischer rats. In contrast, no differences in tyrosine hydroxylase phosphorylation or immunoreactivity were seen in the substantia nigra or caudate/putamen (Beitner-Johnson et al., 1991).

The different pattern of tyrosine hydroxylase levels in the VTA and nACC of drug-naive Lewis versus Fischer rats resembles the influence of chronic morphine and cocaine on the enzyme in these brain reward regions. Higher levels of enzyme are seen in the VTA both in the drug-treated state and in Lewis rats. Moreover, lower levels of enzyme activity seem to occur in the nACC, with lower levels of enzyme activity achieved in the drug-treated state through decreases in enzyme phosphorylation (i.e., decreased catalytic activity) and with lower total levels of the enzyme in Lewis rats. The observation of higher enzyme levels in the VTA, but lower levels in the nACC, further supports the view expressed above that dopaminergic neurotransmission within these two brain regions subserves different functional roles. The results are consistent with the view that the drug-preferring (drug-addicted) state is associated with higher enzyme levels in the VTA, but lower enzyme levels in the nACC.

Similarly, the strain differences in levels of MCRPPs-165, 66, and 62, now known to be neurofilament proteins, are also due to differences in the total amounts of these proteins in the VTA of Lewis versus Fischer rats (Guitart et al., 1992b). As with tyrosine hydroxylase, the levels of neurofilaments in the VTA of Lewis (compared to Fischer) rats resembles the influence of chronic morphine and chronic cocaine on these proteins in Sprague-Dawley rats.

The genetic basis for the strain differences in levels of tyrosine hydroxylase and the other MCRPPs could conceivably reside in mutations in the genes for these phosphoproteins themselves or in alterations of other gene(s) that code for proteins that then regulate the five phosphoproteins in a concerted fashion. That several phosphoproteins show differences in Lewis versus Fischer rats and the observation of coordinated regulation of the same proteins in response to morphine or cocaine treatment would appear to support the latter alternative.

Role of the MCRPPs in Drug Addiction

Several lines of evidence, presented above, support the possibility that the MCRPPs play an important role in mediating drug reinforcement and craving. First, chronic morphine and chronic cocaine regulate the same series of phosphoproteins in the VTA and nACC. Such regulation is specific, in most cases, to these brain reward regions, which are known to play a prominent role in drug reinforcement. Second, one of the drug-regulated phosphoproteins is tyrosine hydroxylase, and increasing evidence supports a central role of dopaminergic neurotransmission in the VTA-nACC pathway in mediating aspects of drug reward. Third, several of the other drug-regulated phosphoproteins—the neurofilaments MCRPPs-165, 66, and 62—are highly enriched in the VTA. Fourth, five of the drug-regulated phosphoproteins are present at markedly different levels in the VTA and nACC of drug-naive Fischer and Lewis rats, two inbred rat strains that show significantly different levels of self-administration of several types of drug abuse. Taken together, the results are consistent with the possibility that these phosphoproteins mediate not only aspects of opiate and cocaine reinforcement but also contribute to individual differences in vulnerability to drug addiction.

CONCLUSIONS AND PERSPECTIVES FOR FUTURE RESEARCH

The studies described in this chapter support the view that, through the investigation of intracellular messenger pathways, it will be possible to learn a great deal about the biochemical and molecular mechanisms by which drugs of abuse induce changes in brain function that underlie addiction. Studies of the LC have provided the clearest indication to date of the specific biochemical mechanisms involved in opiate addiction. Adaptations in G-proteins and the cyclic AMP second-messenger and protein phosphorylation system have been shown to play an important role in mediating opiate tolerance, dependence, and withdrawal in this cell type. There are indications that similar mechanisms may be involved in a number of other opiate-responsive neurons. Among these other neurons are those in the nACC, which has been implicated in drug reward mechanisms. Our results thereby suggest that adaptations in G-proteins and the cyclic AMP system may be a common response by many types of neurons to chronic opiates, with such adaptations mediating both *physical* and *psychological* aspects of drug addiction depending on the neuronal cell type involved. The findings emphasize that the distinction between physical and psychological addiction is arbitrary; both are due to changes in brain function mediated by biochemical adaptations in specific neuronal cell types that lead to alterations in the functional state of these neurons.

Of particular interest are our findings that chronic morphine and chronic cocaine exert many of the same effects on G-proteins and the cyclic AMP second-messenger and protein phosphorylation system, specifically in the nACC and VTA, whereas other classes of psychotropic drugs, which are not reinforcing, have no significant effect on these intracellular messenger pathways. The results raise the interesting possibility that common biochemical changes mediate aspects of morphine and cocaine reinforcement and craving. It will be interesting in future studies to characterize the effects of other types of drugs of abuse on these same intracellular pathways. For example, the nACC and VTA have been implicated in mediating the rewarding properties of many types of drugs of abuse, including ethanol, amphetamine, nicotine, and tetrahydrocannabinol (Chen et al., 1990; Di Chiara and Imperato, 1988; Koob & Bloom, 1988; Lieberman & Cooper, 1989), and it will be important to study the chronic actions of these drugs on G-proteins and the cyclic AMP system in these dopaminergic brain reward regions.

The studies also identify a number of other avenues for future research. It will be critical to determine the identity of the various MARPPs and MCRPPs found in our investigations. Given the paramount role played by protein phosphorylation in virtually all aspects of neuronal function (Nestler & Greengard, 1984, 1989), the study of drug-regulated phosphoproteins offers an open-ended approach with which to identify the types of proteins, and therefore the types of neuronal processes, altered under states of drug addiction. We are also utilizing subtraction hybridization as an additional open-ended method of identifying drug-regulated proteins. Subtraction hybridization enables the isolation of specific mRNAs enriched in one tissue sample compared to another. Preliminary results involving the identification of mRNAs regulated by chronic cocaine in the nACC support the feasibility and great potential value of this novel approach (Sevarino et al., 1990).

It will also be important to identify the precise molecular pathways through which chronic opiate and chronic cocaine treatments produce alterations in intracellular messenger pathways. Given the preliminary evidence that such alterations are mediated, at least in part, at the level of gene expression, opiate and cocaine regulation of transcription factors would seem to represent the ultimate mechanism by which addictive changes are induced in the brain (see Fig. 4-1). Studies are needed therefore to characterize the effects of acute and chronic drug treatment on specific types of transcription factors in opiate- and cocaine-responsive brain regions. Eventually, transfection studies can be used to provide direct evidence for a causal role of a particular transcription factor in mediating changes in brain function associated with addiction.

One of the major advantages of the LC, as discussed above, is the relative ease with which it has been possible to relate biochemical and molecular phenomena to electrophysiological changes known to reflect opiate tolerance, dependence, and withdrawal. In contrast, our relative lack of knowledge of the influence of chronic opiates and cocaine on VTA and nACC neurons has made it less straightforward to assess the functional significance of adaptations in G-proteins and the cyclic AMP system in these other brain regions. Clearly, studies that attempt to correlate biochemical and electrophysiological regulation of these cells are needed. Eventually, the role played by specific biochemical changes in a given brain region in mediating aspects of drug addiction can be tested in transgenic animal models. For example, induction of a change associated with chronic morphine and cocaine treatment in brain reward regions of a transgenic animal should mimic the effects of the drug on reinforcement and craving, whereas blockade of the change should attentuate drug action. This raises the possibility of identifying genetic factors that contribute to an individual's vulnerability for drug addiction. Our preliminary findings in Lewis and Fischer rats indicate that studies of intracellular messenger pathways will help reveal some of these genetic factors. It is intriguing that some of the proteins involved in these genetic factors may be the same as those regulated pharmacologically under conditions of drug abuse and addiction.

These studies of the biochemical and molecular basis of drug addiction have many potential implications. A better understanding of the mechanisms underlying drug addiction will lead to the development of pharmacological agents that prevent or reverse the actions of the drugs on specific target neurons. Such drugs could be used not only to treat physical abstinence syndromes but also to reduce the craving for abused substances. Such latter actions by pharmacological agents would represent a revolutionary step in our battle against drug addiction. Moreover, identification of some of the genetic factors that predispose individuals to drug abuse would greatly advance our understanding of drug addiction, as well as eventually its treatment and prevention.

REFERENCES

Aghajanian, G.K. (1978). Tolerance of locus coeruleus neurons to morphine and suppression of withdrawal response by clonidine. *Nature, 267,* 186-188.

Aghajanian, G.K., & Wang, Y.Y. (1986). Pertussis toxin blocks the outward currents evoked by opiate and α_2-agonists in locus coeruleus neurons. *Brain Res., 371,* 390-394.

Aghajanian, G.K., & Wang, Y.Y. (1987). Common alpha-2 and opiate effector mechanisms in the locus coeruleus: Intracellular studies in brain slices. *Neuropharmacology, 26,* 789-800.

Andrade, R., VanderMaelen, C.P., & Aghajanian, G.K. (1983). Morphine tolerance and dependence in the locus coeruleus: Single cell studies in brain slices. *Eur. J. Pharmacol., 91,* 161-169.

Attali, B., & Vogel, Z. (1989). Long-term opiate exposure leads to reduction of the αi-1 subunit of GTP-binding proteins. *J. Neurochem., 53,* 1636-1639.

Bayer, V.E., & Pickel, V.M. (1990). Ultrastructural localization of tyrosine hydroxylase in the rat ventral tegmental area: Relationship between immunolabeling density and neuronal associations. *J. Neurosci., 10,* 2996-3013.

Beitner, D.B., Duman, R.S., & Nestler, E.J. (1989). A novel action of morphine in the rat locus coeruleus: Persistent decrease in adenylate cyclase. *Mol. Pharmacol., 35,* 559-564.

Beitner-Johnson, D., & Nestler, E.J. (1991). Morphine and cocaine exert common chronic actions on tyrosine hydroxylase in dopaminergic brain reward regions. *J. Neurochem., 57,* 344-347.

Beitner-Johnson, D., Guitart, X., & Nestler, E.J. (1991). Dopaminergic brain reward regions of Lewis and Fischer rats display different levels of tyrosine hydroxylase and other morphine- and cocaine-regulated phosphoproteins. *Brain Res., 561,* 146-149.

Beitner-Johnson, D., Guitart, X., & Nestler, E.J. (1992). Neurofilaments and mesolimbic dopamine system. Common regulation by chronic morphine and chronic cocaine in the rat ventral tegmental area. *J. Neurosci., 12,* 2165-2176.

Bozarth, M.A., & Wise, R.A. (1987). Involvement of the ventral tegmental dopamine system in opioid and psychomotor stumulant reinforcement. In L.S. Harris (Ed.), *Problems of drug dependence, 1985* (pp. 190-196). Washington, DC: US Government Printing Office.

Brock, J.W., Ng, J.P., & Justice Jr, J.B. (1990). Effect of chronic cocaine on dopamine synthesis in the nucleus accumbens as determined by microdialysis perfusion with NSD-1015. *Neurosci. Lett., 117,* 234-239.

Bunney, B.S., Sesack, S.R., & Silva, N.L. (1987). Midbrain dopaminergic systems: Neurophysiology and electrophysiological pharmacology. In H.Y. Meltzer (Ed.), *Psychopharmacology: The third generation of progress* (pp. 81-94). New York: Raven Press.

Chen, J., Paredes, W., Li, J., Smith, D., Lowinson, J., & Gardner, E.L. (1990). Δ^9-tetrahydrocannabinol produces naloxone-blockable enhancement of presynaptic basal dopamine efflux in nucleus accumbens of conscious, freely-moving rats as measured by intracerebral microdialysis. *Psychopharmacology, 102,* 156-162.

Christie, M.J., Williams, J.T., & North, R.A. (1987). Cellular mechanisms of opioid tolerance: Studies in single brain neurons. *Mol. Pharmacol., 32*, 633-638.

Clouet, D., Asghar, D., & Brown, R., eds (1988). Mechanisms of cocaine abuse and toxicity. *NIDA* Res. Monogr. 88.

Di Chiara, G., & Imperato, A. (1988). Drugs abused by humans preferentially increase synaptic dopamine concentrations in the mesolimbic system of freely moving rats. *Proc. Natl. Acad. Sci. USA., 85*, 5274-5278.

Collier, H.O.J., Cuthbert, N.J., Francis, D.L. (1981). Character and meaning of quasi-morphine withdrawal phenomena elicited by methylxanthines. *Fed. Proc., 40*, 1513-1518.

Duman, R.S., Tallman, J.F., & Nestler, E.J. (1988). Acute and chronic opiate-regulation of adenylate cyclase in brain: Specific effects in locus coeruleus. *J. Pharmacol. Exp. Ther., 246*, 1033-1039.

Foote, S.L., Bloom, F.E., & Aston-Jones, G. (1983). Nucleus locus coeruleus: New evidence of anatomical and physiological specificity. *Physiol. Rev., 63*, 844-914.

George, F.R., & Goldberg, S.R. (1989). Genetic approaches to the analysis of addiction processes. *Trends Pharmacol. Sci., 10*, 78-83.

Gilman, A.G. (1987). G-proteins: Transducers of receptor-generated signals. *Annu. Rev. Biochem., 56*, 615-650.

Guitart, X., & Nestler, E.J. (1989). Identification of morphine- and cyclic AMP-regulated phosphoproteins (MARPPs) in the locus coeruleus and other regions of the rat brain: Regulation by acute and chronic morphine. *J. Neurosci., 9*, 4371-4387.

Guitart, X., Nestler, E.J. (1990). Identification of MARPP-14-20, morphine- and cyclic AMP-regulated phosphoproteins of 14-20 kD, as myelin basic proteins: Evidence for their acute and chronic regulation by morphine in rat brain. *Brain Res., 516*, 57-65.

Guitart, X., Hayward, M., Nisenbaum, L.K., Beitner-Johnson, D.B., Haycock, J.W., & Nestler, E.J. (1990). Identification of MARPP-58, a morphine- and cyclic AMP-regulated phosphoprotein of 58 kDa, as tyrosine hydroxylase: Evidence for regulation of its expression by chronic morphine in the rat locus coeruleus. *J. Neurosci., 10*, 2649-2659.

Guitart, X., Thompson, M.A., Mirante, C.K., Greenberg, M.E., & Nestler, E.J. (1992a). Regulation of CREB phosphorylation by acute and chronic morphine in the rat locus coeruleus. *J. Neurochem., 58*, 1168-1171.

Guitart, X., Beitner-Johnson, D., Marby, D., Kosten, T.A., & Nestler, E.J. (1992b). Neurofilament proteins and the mesolimbic dopamine system: strain differences between Lewis and Fischer rats in basal levels of neurofilament proteins and in their regulation by chronic morphine. *Synapse,* in press.

Hayward, M.D., Duman, R.S., & Nestler, E.J. (1990). Induction of the c-fos proto-oncogene during opiate withdrawal in the locus coeruleus and other regions of rat brain. *Brain Res., 525*, 256-266.

Henry, D.J., & White, F.J. (1991). Repeated cocaine administration causes persistent enhancement of D1 dopamine receptor sensitivity within the rat nucleus accumbens. *J. Pharmacol. Exp. Ther., 258*, 882.

Henry, D.J., Greene, M.A., & White, F.J. (1989). Electrophysiological effects of cocaine in the mesoaccumbens dopamine system: Repeated administration. *J. Pharmacol. Exp. Ther., 251*, 833-839.

Holtzman, S.G. (1989). Phosphodiesterase inhibitors potentiate opiate-antagonist discrimination by morphine-dependent rats. *Pharmacol. Biochem. Behav., 33*, 875-879.

Hyman, S.E., & Nestler, E.J. (1993). *The molecular foundations of psychiatry.* Washington, DC: American Psychiatric Press.

Johnson, S.M., & Fleming, W.W. (1989). Mechanisms of cellular adaptive sensitivity changes: Applications to opioid tolerance and dependence. *Pharmacol. Rev., 41,* 435-488.

Kalivas, P.W., & Duffy, P. (1988). Effects of daily cocaine and morphine treatment on somatodendritic and terminal field dopamine release. *J. Neurochem., 50,* 1498-1504.

Kogan, J.H., Nestler, E.J., & Aghajanian, G.K. (1992). Elevated basal firing rates and enhanced responses to 8-Br-cAMP in locus coeruleus neurons in brain slices from opiate-dependent rats. *Eur. J. Pharmacol., 211,* 47-53.

Koob, G.F., & Bloom, F.E. (1988). Cellular and molecular mechanisms of drug dependence. *Science, 242,* 715-723.

Liebman, J.M., & Cooper, S.J. (1989). *Neuropharmacological basis of reward.* New York: Oxford Press.

Loh, H.H., Tao, P.L., & Smith, A.P. (1988). Invited review: Role of receptor regulation in opioid tolerance mechanisms. *Synapse, 2,* 457-462.

Makman, M.H., Dvorkin, B., & Crain, S.M. (1988). Modulation of adenylate cyclase activity of mouse spinal cord-ganglion explants by opioids, serotonin and pertussis toxin. *Brain Res., 445,* 303-313.

Montminy, M.R., Gonzalez, G.A., & Yamamoto, K.K. (1990). Regulation of cAMP-inducible genes by CREB. *Trends Neurosci., 13,* 184-188.

Nestler, E.J. (1990). Adaptive changes in signal transduction systems: Molecular mechanisms of opiate addiction in the rat locus coeruleus. *Progr. Cell Res., 1,* 73-88.

Nestler, E.J. (1992). Molecular mechanisms of drug addiction. *J. Neurosci., 12,* 2439-2450.

Nestler, E.J., & Greengard, P. (1984). *Protein phosphorylation in the nervous system.* New York: John Wiley and Sons.

Nestler, E.J., & Greengard, P. (1989). Protein phosphorylation and the regulation of neuronal function. In G.J. Siegel, B. Agranoff, R.W. Albers, & P. Molinoff (Eds.), Basic neurochemistry: Molecular, cellular, and medical aspects, 4th ed (pp. 373-378). New York: Raven Press.

Nestler, E.J., & Tallman, J.F. (1988). Chronic morphine treatment increases cyclic-AMP-dependent protein kinase activity in the rat locus coeruleus. *Mol. Pharmacol., 33,* 127-132.

Nestler, E.J., Erdos, J.J., Terwilliger, R., Duman, R.S., & Tallman, J.F. (1989). Regulation of G-proteins by chronic morphine treatment in the rat locus coeruleus. *Brain Res., 476,* 230-239.

Nestler, E.J., Terwilliger, R.Z., Walker, J.R., Sevarino, K.A., and Duman, R.S. (1990). Chronic cocaine treatment decreases levels of the G protein subunits $G_{i\alpha}$ and $G_{o\alpha}$ in discrete regions of rat brain. *J. Neurochem., 55,* 1079-1082.

Ng, J., Hubert, G.W., & Justice Jr, J.B. (1990). Increased stimulated release and uptake of dopamine in nucleus accumbens after repeated cocaine administration as measured by in vivo voltammetry. *J. Neurochem.* (in press).

North, R.A., Williams, J.T., Suprenant, A., & Christie, M.J. (1987). Mu and delta receptors belong to a family of receptors that are coupled to potassium channels. *Proc. Natl. Acad. Sci. USA., 84,* 5487-5491.

Ottiger, H.-P., Battenberg, E.F., Tsou, A.-P., Bloom, F.E., & Sutcliffe, J.G. (1990). 1B1075: A brain- and pituitary-specific mRNA that encodes a novel chromogranin/secretogranin-like component of intracellular vesicles. *J. Neurosci., 10,* 3135-3147.

Peris, J., Boyson, S.J., Cass, W.A., Curella, P., Dwoskin, L.P., Larson, G., Lin, L.H., Yasuda, R.P., & Zahniser, N.R. (1990). Persistence of neurochemical changes in dopamine systems after repeated cocaine administration. *J. Pharmacol. Exp. Ther., 253,* 38-44.

Pettit, H.O., Pan, H., Parsons, L.H., & Justice Jr, J.B. (1990). Extracellular concentrations of cocaine and dopamine are enhanced during chronic cocaine administration. *J. Neurochem., 55,* 798-804.

Rasmussen, K., Beitner-Johnson, D.B., Krystal, J.H., Aghajanian, G.K., & Nestler, E.J. (1990). Opiate withdrawal and the rat locus coeruleus: Behavioral, electrophysiological, and biochemical correlates. *J. Neurosci., 10,* 2308-2317.

Redmond, D.E., Jr, & Krystal, J.H. (1984). Multiple mechanisms of withdrawal from opioid drugs. *Annu. Rev. Neurosci., 7,* 443-478.

Roth, R.H., Wolf, M.E., & Deutch, A.Y. (1987). Neurochemistry of midbrain dopamine systems. In H.Y. Meltzer (Ed.), *Psychopharmacology: The third generation of progress.* (pp. 81-94). New York: Raven Press.

Sevarino, K.A., Walker, J.R., Duman, R.S., & Nestler, E.J. (1990). Identification of cocaine-regulated proteins in rat nucleus accumbens by subtraction hybridization. *Soc. Neurosci. Abst., 16,* 745.

Sharma, S.K., Klee, W.A., & Nirenberg, M. (1975). Dual regulation of adenylate cyclase accounts for narcotic dependence and tolerance. *Proc. Natl. Acad. Sci. USA, 72,* 3092-3096.

Suzuki, T., George, F.R., & Meisch, R.A. (1988). Differential establishment and maintenance of oral ethanol reinforced behavior in Lewis and Fischer 344 inbred rat strains. *J. Pharmacol. Exp. Ther., 245,* 164-170.

Terwilliger, R.Z., Beitner-Johnson, D., Sevarino, K.A., Crain, S.M., & Nestler, E.J. (1991). A general role for adaptations in G-proteins and the cyclic AMP system in mediating the chronic actions of morphine and cocaine on neuronal function. *Brain Res., 548,* 100-110.

Wachtel, S.R., Hu, X.-T., Galloway, M.P., & White, F.J. (1989). D1 dopamine receptor stimulation enables the postsynaptic, but not autoreceptor, effects of D2 dopamine agonist in nigrostriatal and mesoaccumbens dopamine systems. *Synapse, 4,* 327-346.

Wang, Y.Y., & Aghajanian, G.K. (1990). Excitation of locus coeruleus neurons by vasoactive intestinal peptide: Role of cAMP and protein kinase A. *J. Neurosci., 10,* 3335-3343.

Zigmond, R.E., Schwarzschild, M.A., & Rittenhouse, A.R. (1989). Acute regulation of tyrosine hydroxylase by nerve activity and by neurotransmitters via phosphorylation. *Annu. Rev. Neurosci., 12,* 415-461.

5

A Cocaine Receptor: Properties and Significance

MICHAEL J. KUHAR, F. IVY CARROLL, JOHN BOJA,
ROBERT LEW, URSULA SCHEFFEL, SAKIRE PÖĞÜN,
RABI SIMANTOV, AND ROXANNE VAUGHAN

To understand the mechanism of action of a drug, it is necessary to identify the molecular site where the drug interacts to produce its initial physiological effects. These studies are usually carried out by using biochemical binding techniques, an approach that has been very successful over the past 20 years (Yamamura et al., 1990). Studies of binding proteins for cocaine began about 10 years ago. Reith et al. (1980) identified a cocaine binding site in rat brain that proved to be the serotonin transporter. Soon after, Kennedy and Hanbauer (1983) identified a different cocaine binding site in rat striatal tissue, and this was the dopamine transporter. A variety of different ligands, in addition to [^{3}H]cocaine, have been used to study the dopamine transporter (Anderson, 1987; Dubocovich & Zahniser, 1985; Janowsky et al., 1986; Javitch et al., 1984; Madras et al., 1989a; Ritz et al., 1990; Schoemaker et al., 1985). The fact that cocaine binding sites include two transporters was not surprising since it had been known for many years that cocaine inhibits monoamine uptake at nerve terminals (see Krueger, 1990 for references). Transporters are thought to play a role in terminating the action of a neurotransmitter and are uniquely localized to specific neurons (Kuhar, 1973). Other cocaine binding sites have been identified in the brain and periphery as well (Calligaro & Eldefrawi, 1987).

The relevant question for drug abuse is, of course, which of these cocaine binding sites is related to the addictive properties of cocaine. Cocaine has many actions; it produces local anesthesia, increases locomotor activity, reduces appetite, increases heart rate and blood pressure, causes euphoria, and is a powerful reinforcer. Thus, it is important to associate the various binding sites or potential receptors with the various physiological effects of cocaine.

Because drug self-administration in animals is thought to be an excellent model of the reinforcing properties of cocaine (Griffiths et al., 1980), it has been used as a tool to help identify the cocaine receptor related to addiction. Ritz et al. (1987) showed that the rank order of potencies of a variety of cocaine-like drugs at the dopamine transporter could be correlated to the rank order of potency of the same compounds in monkey drug self-administration (Fig. 5-1). Because the cocaine binding sites associated with the dopamine transporter had the same pharmacological properties as the monkey model for drug self-administration, it was proposed that the dopamine transporter (or the cocaine binding site at the dopamine transporter) was the cocaine receptor that somehow ultimately causes its reinforcing properties. Similar data were presented by Bergman et al. (1989).

The identification of the cocaine binding site at the dopamine transporter as a cocaine receptor related to drug addiction has led to the "dopamine hypothesis" of cocaine-reinforcing properties. The dopamine hypothesis states that the reinforcing properties of cocaine are due to the binding of cocaine at the dopamine transporter, which results in inhibition of dopamine reuptake and potentiation of dopaminergic transmission in the mesolimbic pathway. A variety of lesion experiments involving specific neuronal tracts indicate that the mesolimbic dopaminergic system is the critical system for reinforcement (see Bozarth, 1989 for references). A very large number of experiments support the involvement of dopamine with the dependence-producing properties of cocaine. For example, PET scanning studies have shown that the time course of occupancy of the dopamine transporter by cocaine is similar to the time course of production of subjective effects by cocaine (Fowler et al., 1989). Also, many studies have shown that chronic administration of cocaine causes regulatory changes in levels of dopamine receptors in brain (for example, Goeders & Kuhar, 1986; Peris et al., 1990).

These results have focused attention on the dopamine transporter and cocaine's interactions with it. The following sections summarize many of the

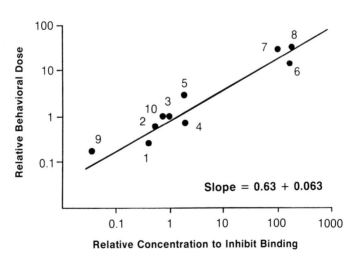

Figure 5-1.   Relation between the relative behavioral doses of cocaine and related compounds in self-administration studies and their relative inhibitory concentrations for 3H-mazindol binding at the dopamine transporter. Each point represents data for a cocaine analog as shown in Ritz et al., 1987.

recent findings about cocaine and the dopamine transporter and shed light on the molecular nature of the transporter.

STRUCTURE ACTIVITY STUDIES

A variety of studies involving cocaine analogs have been carried out to shed some light on the conformation of the binding site for cocaine (Fig. 5-2) at the dopamine transporter. These studies have examined the inhibitory potency of the various analogs in biochemical binding studies. After examining more than 70 cocaine analogs, it is now possible to make several generalizations about the binding site for cocaine.

First, the cocaine binding site at the dopamine transporter is both enantiomeric and stereoselective. The seven possible stereoisomers of (−)-cocaine including (+)-cocaine were synthesized and were found to inhibit the binding of ^{3}H-WIN 35,428, with potencies ranging from 1/600th to about 1/60th of that of (−)-cocaine (Carroll et al., 1991).

Removal of the N-methyl group of cocaine to give norcocaine resulted in only a small reduction in affinity. In contrast, the addition of a second N-methyl group to cocaine to give the methiodide, as well as the acetylation and benzylation of norcocaine to give N-nor-N-acetylcocaine and N-nor-N-benzylcocaine, respectively, yielded compounds with very low or no affinity for the transporter.

When various substituents were made at the C2 carbon of the tropane ring, conversion of the carbomethoxy group to a hydroxymethyl ($-CH_2OH$), carboxyl ($-CO_2H$), or N-methylcarboxamide ($-CO_2NHCH_3$) resulted in inactive compounds. However, if the methyl group of the ester is changed to a longer straight chain, branched chain, or alkyl phenyl group $[(CH_2)_xC_6H_5]$, the binding potency is not greatly affected. Changes in the substituent at the C3 carbon produced quite interesting results. Removal of the benzoyl group to give ecgonine methyl ester resulted in complete loss of affinity for the transporter. Even the addition of substituents to the phenyl ring of cocaine caused a reduction in binding to the dopamine transporter; however, when the ester group was removed and the phenyl group attached directly to the tropane ring, a more potent compound was produced. If the phenyl group possessed p-methyl or p-halo substituent, highly potent compounds were produced (Boja et al., 1990). Also, where tested, the binding potency of these compounds at the transporter paralleled their behavioral potency (Ritz et al., 1987).

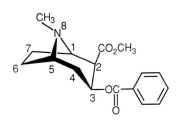

Figure 5-2. Structure of (−)cocaine.

CHARACTERIZATION OF THE TRANSPORTER PROTEIN

Several binding ligands are useful in studying the dopamine transporter (for references, see Ritz et al., 1990; Madras et al., 1989a and b). One of these ligands, [^{125}I]DEEP, was developed as an irreversible photoaffinity label (Grigoriadis et al., 1989). After labeling the transporter with this radioactive probe, it was possible to estimate the molecular weight of the transporter protein using SDS-page gels. Depending on assay conditions and standards used, the molecular weight seems to be between 58,000 and 80,000 daltons (Berger et al., 1990; Grigoriadis et al., 1989; Sallee et al., 1989).

Initially, it was observed that the [^{125}I]DEEP-transporter complex bound to wheat germ agglutinin columns and was eluted with N-acetylglucosamine Grigoriadis et al., 1989). These findings suggested that the transporter was a glycoprotein that contained sialic acid residues. Accordingly, after photoaffinity labeling the transporter in membrane fragments, the membranes were treated with a variety of enzymes that cleaved various sugar moeties from them. In these experiments, treatment with neuraminidase caused a decrease in the apparent molecular weight of the DEEP-transporter complex, whereas treatment with mannosidase did not; these data suggest that the transporter contains sialic acid residues, but not mannose. Furthermore, the carbohydrate appears to be attached to the protein through a nitrogen link since treatment with N-glycanase causes a similar loss in apparent molecular weight (Lew et al., 1991a; Sallee et al., 1989). These findings suggest that the dopamine transporter is a N-linked glycoprotein containing sialic acids. The significance of the carbohydrate side chain is presently unknown. Neither is it known whether the side chain is required for binding of ligands to the transporter or for the functioning of the dopamine transporter.

HETEROGENEITY OF TRANSPORTERS: THE DOPAMINE TRANSPORTER FROM THE STRIATUM IS DIFFERENT IN APPARENT MOLECULAR WEIGHT FROM THE TRANSPORTER IN THE NUCLEUS ACCUMBENS

When comparing the [^{125}I]DEEP-transporter complex from different brain regions of the rat, it was found that the transporter complex from the nucleus accumbens and from the olfactory tubercle seemed to have a slightly larger molecular weight than that from the striatum (Lew et al., 1991a and b). This slight difference occurred in every experiment and was statistically significant. Accordingly, it seems that the apparent molecular weight of the transporter from the nucleus accumbens is slightly larger than that from the striatum (Fig. 5-3).

This observation may be important in that, as mentioned above, the mesolimbic system seems to be the most relevant dopaminergic system in relation to the reinforcing properties of psychostimulants. If so, then the transporter in the mesolimbic neurons will be most relevant to the action of psychotropic drugs. Since the molecular weight of the transporter from mesolimbic neurons seems to be a little different, it may be that the transporter functions somewhat differ-

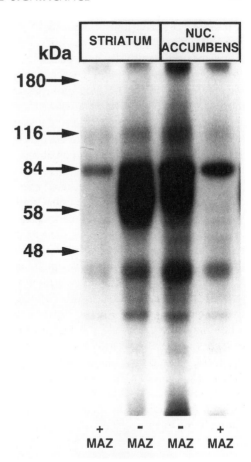

Figure 5-3. ^{125}I-DEEP-transporter complex in nucleus accumbens has a higher molecular weight than that in striatum. Membranes from striatum and nucleus accumbens were photoaffinity labeled, solubilized with SDS sample buffer, and underwent electrophoresis on a 10% acrylamide gel. The first and third lanes show total levels (tot) of ^{125}I-DEEP incorporation, and the third and fourth lanes show nonspecific incorporation defined by inclusion of mazindol (Maz). The transporter proteins had apparent molecular weights of 72400 d and 76800 d under these conditions. (From Lew et al., 1991, with permission.)

ently or that cocaine interacts with these transporters in a slightly different way. Thus, all transporters may not interact in the same way with drugs and may have different functions, and the mesolimbic transporters may be in need of greater study. Most experiments on dopamine transporters have involved those from the nigro striatal pathway since striatal tissue is readily available in large quantities.

IN VIVO LABELING OF DOPAMINE TRANSPORTERS: POTENTIAL FOR IMAGING

Various ligands have been used to label dopamine transporters in vivo (Aquilonius et al., 1987; Fowler et al., 1989; Kilbourne, 1988; Kuhar et al., 1990; Leenders et al., 1988). Unfortunately, most of these ligands have somewhat low ratios of specific to nonspecific binding. For example, both ^{3}H-nomifensine and ^{3}H-cocaine localize to dopamine transporters after in vivo administration, but only about 30–40% of the radioactivity in the brain region is "specific" binding (Fowler et al., 1989; Kuhar et al., 1990). Thus, it was quite interesting when we observed that some cocaine analogs, such as ³H-WIN 35,065-2 and ³H-WIN 35,428, bound to dopamine transporters in the mouse in vivo with much higher specific to nonspecific binding ratios (Fig. 5-4) (Scheffel et al., 1989, 1991). Studies of in vivo binding have some advantages over in vitro binding in which the binding environment and tissue preparation are artificial compared to the in vivo situation.

Because of the availability of this mouse model in which it is possible to label cocaine receptors in vivo very efficiently, we decided to study the rate of entry of various psychostimulant drugs into brain. This is an interesting problem because it has been suggested that the rate of occupancy of receptors by various drugs is important in determining the effects of drugs. For example, with reinforcing drugs, it has been suggested that abuse liability is greater for those drugs that enter the brain and occupy receptors more rapidly (Sellers et al., 1989). Using the in vivo labeling mouse model, we were able to quantify the relative rate of occupancy of cocaine receptor in mouse striatum after injection of cocaine, mazindol, or GBR 12909 (Fig. 5-5).

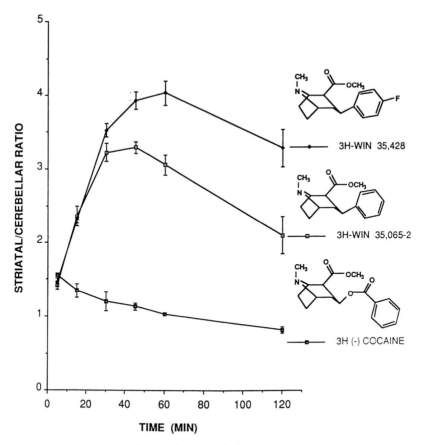

Figure 5-4. Time course of striatal to cerebellar ratios for ³H-WIN 35,065-2 and ³H-(−)cocaine. Data are expressed as ± SEM, n = 4. The structures of the compounds are shown next to their respective data. (From Scheffel et al., 1989, with permission.)

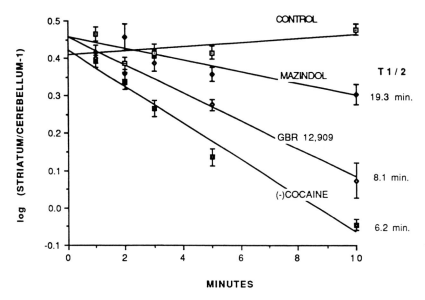

Figure 5-5. Half-time of clearance of [³H]WIN 34,428 from the corpus striatum as a result of competition by various dopamine uptake site blockers. The logs of the ratios of specific to nonspecific binding in the corpus striatum (C. Striatum/Cerebellum −1) are plotted versus time after injection of the drugs. Data represent means ± S.E.M. (n=4−10). Cocaine enters the brain and occupies receptors more rapidly than mazindol as indicated by the finding that the half-life of [³H]WIN 35,428 is shorter in the presence of cocaine than in the presence of mazindol. (Adapted from Pöğün et al., 1991.)

These studies were carried out in the following way. ³H-WIN 35,428 was injected into the tail veins of mice, and 30 minutes later, a time at which maximum labeling has occurred, various drugs were again injected into the tail vein. The quantity of drug injected was about the same amount required to displace in vivo binding of ³H-WIN 35,428 under equilibrium conditions. Under these experimental conditions, it was observed that cocaine displaced ³H-WIN 35,428 binding from striatal cocaine receptors more rapidly than mazindol. These data indicate that cocaine enters the brain and occupies cocaine receptors much more rapidly than mazindol. This finding correlates to the observation that mazindol has a lower abuse liability than cocaine. Thus, the availability of this in vivo mouse model allows us to examine this question directly and in a quantifiable manner.

CONCLUSIONS AND PERSPECTIVES FOR FUTURE RESEARCH

The goal of using a molecular approach to the cocaine receptor is to identify exactly how cocaine exerts its effects. The dopamine hypothesis suggests that cocaine produces its reinforcing effects by initially blocking dopamine reuptake and thereby potentiating dopaminergic transmission. One research issue is to find out precisely how cocaine blocks reuptake. Does it simply block the channel that dopamine moves through, or is a different mechanism used? By knowing exactly how cocaine blocks transport, would it be possible to rationally design a cocaine antagonist—that is, a compound that would block the action of cocaine but that would not block dopamine uptake? Such a compound could have important clinical applications. The structure-activity work and protein research are directed toward understanding the nature of the transporter and the nature of the interaction of cocaine with this transporter.

Future research will shed additional light on these questions. For example, the recent cloning of a cDNA for the GABA transporter (Guastella et al., 1990) makes it clear that we will be able to clone a cDNA for the dopamine transporter protein in the near future. This will provide a more detailed knowledge of the nature of the transporter and allow us to carry out a number of interesting experiments aimed at elucidating the interaction of cocaine with this transporter.

Yet another area of interesting research is the imaging of the cocaine receptor. Although it is difficult to cause changes in densities of cocaine receptors by cocaine administration, recent studies suggest that some changes in transporter density may occur. Thus, the ability to measure transporters in vivo in living human subjects will provide another piece of the puzzle of what cocaine is doing in the living human brain.

REFERENCES

Anderson, P.H. (1987). Biochemical and pharmacological characterization of [^{3}H]GBR 12395 binding in vitro to rat striatal membranes: Labeling of the dopamine uptake complex. *J. Neurochem.*, *48*, 1887-1896.

Aquilonius, S.M., Bergstrom, K., Eckernas, S.A., Hartvig, P., Leenders, K.L., Lundquist, H., Antoni, G., Gee, A., Rimoand, A., Uhlin, J., & Langstrom, B. (1987). In vivo evaluation of striatal dopamine reuptake sites using 11C-nomifensine and positron emission tomography. *Acta Neurol. Scand.*, *76*, 283-287.

Berger, P., Martenson, R., Laing, P., Thurcauf, A., De Costa, B., Rice, K.C., & Paul, S.M. (1990). Photoaffinity labeling of the dopamine reuptake carrier protein using a novel high affinity azido-derivative of GBR-12935. *Soc. Neurosci. Abst.*, *16*, 13.

Bergman, J., Madras, B.K., Johnson, S.E., & Spealman, R.D. (1989). Effects of cocaine and related drugs in nonhuman primates. III. Self-administration by squirrel monkeys. *J. Pharmacol. Exp. Ther.*, *251*, 150-155.

Boja, J.W., Ivy Carroll, F., Rahman, M.A., Philip, A., Lewin, A.H., & Kuhar, M.J. (1990). New, potent cocaine analogs: Ligand binding and transport studies in rat striatum. *Eur. J. Pharmacol.*, *184*, 329-332.

Bozarth, M.A. (1989). New perspectives on cocaine addiction: Recent findings from animal research. *Can. J. Physiol. Pharmacol.*, *67*, 1158-1167.

Calligaro, D.O., & Eldefrawi, M.E. (1987). Central and peripheral cocaine receptors. *J. Pharm. Exp. Pharmacol.*, *243*, 61-67.

Calligaro, D.O., & Eldefrawi, M.E. (1988). High affinity stereospecific binding of [^{3}H] cocaine in striatum and its relationship to the dopamine transporter. *Membrane Biochem.*, *7*, 87-106.

Carroll, F.I., Lewin, A.H., Abraham, P., Parhana, K., Boja, J.W., & Kuhar, M.J.

(1991). Synthesis and ligand binding of cocaine isomers at the cocaine receptor. *J. Med. Chem., 34*, 883-886.

Dubocovich, M.L., & Zahniser, N.R. (1985). Binding characteristics of the dopamine uptake inhibitor [³H]nomifensine to striatal membranes. *Biochem. Pharmacol., 34*, 1137-1144.

Fowler, J.S., Volkow, N.D., Wolf, A.P., Dewey, S.L., Schlyer, D.J., MacGregor, R.R., Hitzemann, R., Logan, J., Bendriem, B., Gatley, S.J., & Christman, D. (1989). Mapping cocaine binding sites in human and baboon brain in vivo. *Synapse, 4*, 371-377.

Goeders, N.E., & Kuhar, M.J. (1987). Chronic cocaine administration induces opposite changes in dopamine receptors in the striatum and nucleus accumbens. *Alcohol Drug Res., 7*, 207-216.

Griffiths, R.R., Bigelow, G.E., & Henningfield, J.E. (1980). Similarities in animal and human drug-taking behavior. In N.K. Mellow, (Ed.), *Advances in substance abuse* (Vol. 1, pp. 1-90). Greenwich, CT: JAI Press.

Grigoriadis, D.E., Wilson, A.A., Lew, R., Sharkey, J.S., & Kuhar, M.J. (1989). Dopamine transporter sites selectively labeled by a novel photoaffinity probe: ¹²⁵I-DEEP. *J. Neurosci., 9*, 2664-2670.

Guastella, J., Nelson, N., Nelson, H., Czyzyk, L., Keynan, S., Miedel, M.C., Davidson, N., Lester, H.A., & Kanner, B.I. (1990). Cloning and expression of a rat brain GABA transporter. *Science, 249*, 1303-1306.

Janowsky, A., Berger, P., Vocci, F., Labarca, R., Skolnick, P., & Paul, S.M., (1986). Characterization of sodium-dependent [³H]GBR-1935 binding in brain: A radioligand for selective labelling of the dopamine transport complex. *J. Neurochem., 46*, 1272-1276.

Javitch, J.A., Blaustein, R.O., & Snyder, S.H. (1984). [³H] Mazindol binding associated with neuronal dopamine and norepinephrine uptake sites. *Mol. Pharmacol., 26*, 35-44.

Kennedy, L.T., & Hanbauer, I. (1983). Sodium-sensitive cocaine binding to rat striatal membrane: Possible relationship to dopamine uptake sites. *J. Neurochem., 41*, 172-178.

Kilbourne, M.R. (1988). In vivo binding of [¹⁸F]GBR 13119 to the brain dopamine uptake system. *Life Sci., 42*, 1347-1353.

Kuhar, M.J. (1973). Neurotransmitter uptake: A tool in identifying neurotransmitter-specific pathways. *Life Sci., 13*, 1623-1634.

Kuhar, M.J., Sanchez-Roa, P.M., Wong, D.F., Dannals, R.F., Grigoriadis, D.E., Lew, R., & Milberger, M. (1990). Dopamine transporter: Biochemistry, pharmacology and imaging. *Eur. Neurol., 30*(Suppl.), 15-20.

Krueger, B.K. (1990). Kinetics and block of dopamine uptake in synaptosomes from rat caudate nucleus. *J. Neurochem., 55*, 260-267.

Leenders, K.L., Aquilonius, S.M., Bergstrom, K., Bjurling, P., Crossman, A.R., Eckernas, S.A., Gee, A.G., Hartvig, P., Lundqvist, H., Langstrom, B., Rimland, A., & Tedroff, J. (1988). Unilateral MPTP lesion in a rhesus monkey: Effects on the striatal dopaminergic system measured in vivo with PET using various novel tracers. *Brain Res., 445*, 61-67.

Lew, R., Grigoriadis, D., Wilson, A., Boja, J.W., Simantov, R., & Kuhar, M.J. (1991). Dopamine transporter: Deglycosylation with exo- and endoglycosidases. *Brain Res., 539*, 239-246.

Madras, B.K., Spealman, R.D., Fahey, M.A., Neumeyer, J.L., Saha, J.K., & Milius, R.A. (1989a). Cocaine receptors labeled by [³H]-2β-carbomethoxy-3β-(4-fluorophenyl)tropane. *Mol. Pharmacol., 36*, 518-524.

Madras, B.K., Fahey, M.A., Bergman, J., Canfield, D.R., & Spealman, R.D. (1989b). Effects of cocaine and related drugs in nonhuman primates. I. [^{3}H]Cocaine binding in caudateputamen. *J. Pharmacol. Exp. Ther., 251,* 131-141.

Peris, J., Boyson, S.J., Cass, W.A., Curella, P., Dworkin, L.P., Larson, G., Lin, L., Yasuda, R.P., & Zahniser, N.R. (1990). Persistence of neurochemical changes in dopamine systems after repeated cocaine administration. *J. Pharmacol. Exp. Ther., 253,* 38-44.

Reith, M.E.A., Shershen, H., & Lajtha, A. (1980). Saturable (^{3}H)cocaine binding in central nervous system in mouse. *Life Sci., 27,* 1055-1062.

Ritz, M.C., Lamb, R.J., Goldberg, S.R., & Kuhar, M.J. (1987). Cocaine receptors on dopamine transporters are related to self-administration of cocaine. *Science, 237,* 1219-1223.

Ritz, M.C., Boja, J.W., Grigoriadis, D.E., Zaczek, R., Carroll, F.I., Lewin, A.H., & Kuhar, M.J. (1990). [^{3}H]WIN 35065-2: A ligand for cocaine receptors in striatum. *J. Neurochem., 55,* 1556-1562.

Sallee, F.R., Fogel, E.L., Schwartz, E., Choi, S.M., Curran, D.P., & Niznik, H.B. (1989). Photoaffinity labeling of the mammalian dopamine transporter. *FEBS Lett., 256,* 219-224.

Scheffel, U., Boja, J.W., & Kuhar, M.J. (1989). Cocaine receptors: In vivo labeling with ^{3}H-(−)cocaine, ^{3}H-WIN 35,065-2 and ^{3}H-35,428. *Synapse, 4,* 390-392.

Scheffel, U., Pogun, S., Stathis, M., Boja, J.W., & Kuhar, M.J. (1991). In vivo labeling of cocaine binding sites on dopamine transporters with [^{3}H] WIN 35,428. *J. Pharmacol. Exp. Ther., 257(3),* 954-958.

Schoemaker, H., Pimoule, C., Arbilla, S., Scatton, B., Javoy-Agid, F., & Langer, S.Z. (1985). Sodium dependent [^{3}H]cocaine binding associated with dopamine uptake sites in the rat striatum and human putamen decrease after dopaminergic denervation and in Parkinson's disease. *Nauyn-Schmiederberg's Arch. Pharmacol., 329,* 227-235.

Sellers, E.M., Busto, M., & Kaplan, H.L. (1989). Pharmacokinetic and pharmacodynamic drug interactions: Implications for abuse liability testing. In M.W. Fischman & N.K. Mello (Eds.), *Testing for abuse liability of Drugs in humans. NIDA Res. Monogr., 92,* 287.

Yamamura, H.I., Enna, S.J., & Kuhar, M.J. (1990). *Methods in neurotransmitter receptor analysis.* New York: Raven Press.

6

Pharmacological Diversity of Nicotine Receptors

JAMES W. PATRICK AND CHARLES W. LUETJE

The primary addicting effects of nicotine presumably occur as a result of the interaction of nicotine with specific nicotine binding sites. Molecules that are candidates for the binding site(s) associated with nicotine's addictive action include the nicotinic acetylcholine receptors. Recent research suggests that these potential binding sites are structurally and functionally diverse (for review, see Luetje et al., 1990a).

We owe most of our insights into the nicotinic acetylcholine receptors to studies of the receptor found on the postsynaptic membrane of the neuromuscular junction. This muscle-type nicotinic acetylcholine receptor is composed of four different polypeptide chains—alpha, beta, gamma or epsilon, and delta—in the stochiometry $\alpha_2\beta\gamma\delta$ or $\alpha_2\beta\varepsilon\delta$ (for review, see Popot & Changeux, 1984). The receptors present before innervation differ from those found after innervation, most notably by the substitution of the epsilon for the gamma subunit in the adult innervated form (Gu & Hall, 1988; Methfessel & Sakmann, 1986). The arrangement of the polypeptide chains in the multimeric receptor molecule has been deduced from low-angle diffraction studies (Kistler & Stroud, 1982; Toyashima & Unwin, 1988), and various distributions of individual polypeptide chains across the membrane, based on deduced amino acid sequences and biochemical studies, have been proposed (for review, see Stroud & Finer-Moore, 1985). The alpha subunit is known to carry the agonist binding site and is labeled by affinity labeling reagents that react with a pair of contiguous cysteine residues at positions homologous to positions 192 and 193 in the *Torpedo* alpha subunit (Kao et al., 1984). Activation of this muscle type of nicotinic acetylcholine is blocked by the elapid alpha-neurotoxins, including alpha-bungarotoxin. This receptor is activated by nicotine, but only at relatively high concentrations (Chang et al., 1987). Few, if any, of the addictive effects of nicotine seem to be mediated by the nicotinic acetylcholine receptors found at the neuromuscular junction.

The receptors that mediate nicotinic cholinergic transmission between neurons differ pharmacologically and structurally from those found at the neuromuscular junction. In particular, the neuronal nicotinic acetylcholine receptors seem to be composed of just two, as opposed to four, different types of subunits. cDNA clones, isolated from brain-derived cDNA libraries, have defined two different classes of subunits that participate in the formation of neuronal nicotinic acetylcholine receptors. All the neuronal nicotinic acetylcholine receptor subunit sequences that contain contiguous cysteine residues at positions homologous to 192 and 193 in the *Torpedo* sequence are classified as alpha subunits. All sequences lacking these cysteine residues have been called non-alpha (Nef et al., 1988) or beta (Deneris et al., 1987) subunits. At this time there are eight published alpha subunits, one derived from muscle (called α1) and seven from brain—α2 (Nef et al., 1988; Wada et al., 1988); α3 (Boulter et al., 1986; Nef et al., 1988), α4 (Goldman et al., 1987; Nef et al., 1988), α5 (Boulter et al., 1990; Couturier et al., 1990b), α6 (Lamar et al., 1990), α7 (Couturier et al., 1990a; Schoepfer et al., 1990), and α8 (Schoepfer et al., 1990) cDNA libraries. There are four published beta subunits, one (β1) derived from muscle and three—β2 (Deneris et al., 1987; Nef et al., 1988), β3 (Deneris et al., 1988), and β4 (Boulter et al., 1990; Couturier et al., 1990b; Duvoisin et al., 1989)—derived from brain cDNA libraries.

Although the amino acid sequences of these subunits are very similar and the proteins clearly have common structural domains, not all have been shown to participate in the formation of functional ligand gated ion channels. Injection of *Xenopus* oocytes with RNA encoding either the β2 or β4 subunit, in pairwise combination with RNA encoding either α2, α3, or α4, results in the formation of a nicotine gated ion channel. It is clear, therefore, that both alpha and beta subunits contribute to the formation of the nicotine gated ion channel (Boulter et al., 1987). What is not clear is the nature of the contributions that these subunits make to the functional receptor. We assume that both subunits become part of the receptor, as opposed to acting catalytically in its formation, and that the oocyte contributes nothing more to the receptor than the machinery for its synthesis. Immunoprecipitation of detergent extracts of whole rat brain with antireceptor antibody yields both alpha and beta subunits (Whiting & Lindstrom 1986, 1987), suggesting that both subunits are components of the receptor. We do not know, however, the number of subunits in the mature receptor, the ratio of alpha subunits to beta subunits, whether this ratio is a constant, or whether other subunits contribute to the receptor in vivo. We do know that these two subunit types can combine in the oocyte in a minimum of six different ways to make six different neuronal nicotinic acetylcholine receptors. Subunit α7 is an interesting exception to the requirement for pairwise expression of alpha and beta subunits to form functional nicotine gated ion channels. Injection of *Xenopus* oocytes with RNA encoding the α7 subunit results in the formation of a homo-oligomeric nicotine gated ion channel (Couturier et al., 1990a).

The genes encoding each of these structurally different proteins are expressed in overlapping but unique subsets of neuronal structures (Fig. 6-1; Wada et al., 1989). In situ hybridization shows a pattern of β2 gene expression that is consistent with the idea that this subunit is common to different receptor subtypes. Thus, a signal for β2 was found in most regions of the brain. In contrast, alpha subunits show a unique but somewhat overlapping pattern of gene expression. Alpha3 subunits are strongly expressed in layer IV of isocortex, in entorhinal cortex, medial habenula, in certain thalamic nuclei of the anterior and ventral group, in medial and dorsolateral geniculate, in supramamillary nucleus, and lateral hypothalamus. Brainstem structures, such as the locus coeruleus, trigeminal ganglion, area postrema, and specific motor nuclei, are also labeled with high intensity. Alpha4-1 and alpha4-2 mRNAs, likely corresponding to different spliced products of the alpha4 gene, show to date the most extensive distribution of nicotinic agonist-binding subunit transcripts in the rat brain. Most regions examined contained weak to strong levels of expression of this gene. Regions particularly rich in alpha4 were the medial habenula, anterior and lateral thalamus, medial and dorsolateral geniculate nucleus, layer III and V of isocortex, certain hypothalamic and somatosensory brainstem nuclei, parasubiculum and subiculum, septum, substantia nigra pars compacta, ventral tegmental area, and interpeduncular nucleus. The only strong hybridization signal expression of the alpha2 gene was the interpeduncular nucleus, but low to moderate levels of expression were detected in many other parts of the brain. The alpha5 gene, coding for a protein of unknown function, has a pattern of expression distinct from the other alpha subunit genes (Wada et al., 1990). No hybridization was observed in septum, thalamus, hypothalamus, or cerebellum, but relatively high expression was found in the subiculum, presubiculum, and parasubiculum; in substantia nigra pars compacta; ventral tegmental area; and the interpeduncular nucleus. Moderate signals were detected in deep layers of the isocortex, in contrast to the band of high-density labeling observed in layers III to V when using probes for other alpha subunit genes. High levels of alpha6 mRNA expression were detected in the medial habenula, substantia nigra, ventral tegmental area, and the locus coeruleus (Lamar et al., 1990). Moderate expression was also detected in the reticular nucleus of the thalamus, the supramamillary nucleus, and the medial mamillary nucleus of the hypothalamus.

There are interesting exceptions to the general rule of co-localization of $\beta2$ and known alpha subunits. In some regions, such as the subfornical organ, the supraoptic and arcuate nucleus, the hippocampus, and in a subpopulation of cerebellar Purkinje cells, the $\beta2$ gene was expressed, but expression of alpha genes was not detected, suggesting that some neuronal alpha subunits remain to be discovered. The inverse situation has been observed in layer III-IV of the cerebral cortex and in the inner plexiform layer of the olfactory tubercle, where the signal for $\beta2$ does not correlate with the observed density of alpha3 and alpha4. These results suggest the existence of receptor complexes composed of alpha3 or alpha4 associated with as yet uknown subunits. $\beta3$ subunit transcription has been observed in a small subset of alpha4 rich regions; namely, the reticular nucleus of the thalamus, medial habenula, ventral tegmental area, and mesencephalic nucleus of the trigeminal nerve (Deneris et al., 1988). Only medial habenula neurons seem to transcribe mRNA coding for beta4 subunit at a detectable level (Boulter et al., 1990; Duvoisin et al., 1989). The distribution of the three known neuronal beta subunits overlaps that of alpha subunits, indicating the existence of specific regional receptor combinations with ex-

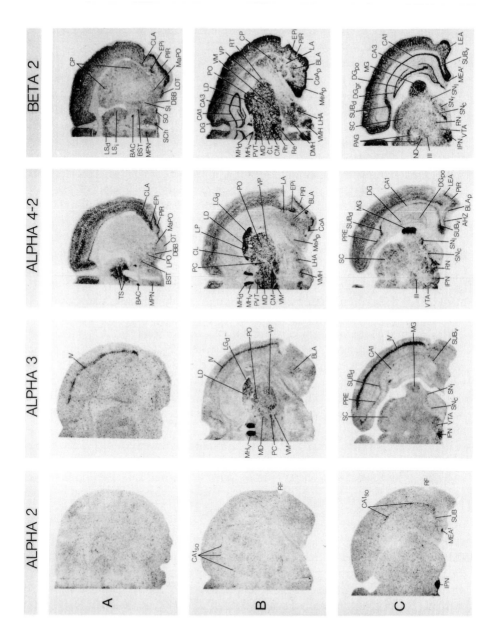

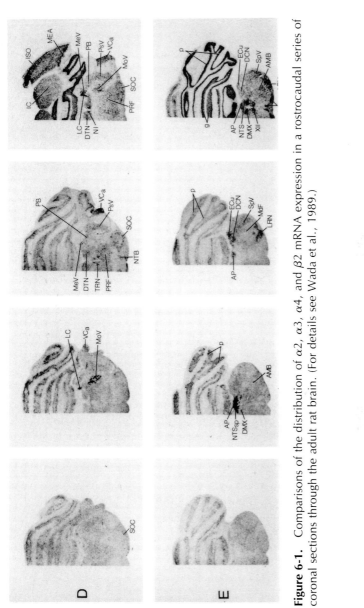

Figure 6-1. Comparisons of the distribution of α2, α3, α4, and β2 mRNA expression in a rostrocaudal series of coronal sections through the adult rat brain. (For details see Wada et al., 1989.)

pected different functional properties. Despite the large amount of anatomical data collected, the resolution of this technique does not allow differentiation in regions where more than one alpha subunit is expressed between co-expression in the same neurons and expression in mixed subpopulations of neurons.

The diversity of structure and distribution seen with these subunits is also found in the pharmacological properties of nicotinic receptors expressed in the nervous system and of those produced by the expression of various combinations of subunits in *Xenopus* oocytes. The earliest demonstration of functional nicotinic receptors and of their involvement in neurotransmission in the CNS was made in the Renshaw cell recurrent collateral synapse (Curtis & Ryall, 1966; Eccles et al., 1954). Since then, functional nicotinic receptors have been shown to be present throughout the CNS (for review, see Luetje et al., 1990a). In fact, there seem to be multiple pharmacologically distinct subtypes of nicotinic receptor in the CNS. The receptor examined by Vidal and Changeux (1989) in a rat prefrontal cortex slice preparation, which was antagonized by dihydro-beta-erythroidine (DHBE) and neuronal bungarotoxin but not mecamylamine, hexamethonium, or d-tubocurarine, is clearly different from the receptor studied by Mulle and Changeux (1990) in acutely dissociated rat medial habenular neurons, which was blocked by DHBE, mecamylamine, hexamethonium, and d-tubocurarine, but was insensitive to neuronal bungarotoxin. Both of these receptors seem to differ from the receptor on cultured rat retinal ganglion neurons shown by Lipton et al. (1987) to be antagonized by d-tubocurarine, DHBE, mecamylamine, hexamethonium, and neuronal bungarotoxin. The work of Garza et al. (1987a and b) also suggests multiple forms of nicotinic receptors in the rat cerebellum. Multiple biophysically distinct subtypes of neuronal nAChRs have also been shown to be present in the nervous system (for review, see Steinbach & Ifune, 1989), and the expression of different functional subtypes is developmentally regulated (Moss et al., 1989; Schuetze and Role, 1987).

Experiments examining the functional properties of various subunit combinations expressed in *Xenopus* oocytes suggest differential subunit association as a mechanism by which receptor diversity is generated in the nervous system. Single-channel analysis of pairwise subunit combinations reveals that each functional combination possesses unique characteristics (Papke et al., 1989). There is a similar diversity in the sensitivity of different subunit combinations to nicotinic neurotoxins and antagonists. Sensitivity to neuronal bungarotoxin, for example, is particularly diverse, with the $\alpha3\beta2$ subunit combination being very sensitive (extensive blockade occurring at a concentration of 10 nm), the $\alpha4\beta2$ subunit combination being much less sensitive (substantial blockade occurring only at a concentration of 1 μm), and the $\alpha2\beta2$ apparently insensitive to neuronal bungarotoxin blockade (Luetje & Patrick, 1989; Luetje et al., 1990b; Wada et al., 1988). Interestingly, in contrast to $\alpha3\beta2$, the $\alpha3\beta4$ subunit combination seems to be insensitive to neuronal bungarotoxin (Duvoisin et al., 1989; Luetje & Patrick, 1991). The homo-oligomeric $\alpha7$ receptor is blocked by alpha-bungarotoxin but not neuronal bungarotoxin (Couturier et al., 1990). The effect of DHBE on different subunit combinations is also diverse, with the $\alpha4\beta2$ subunit combination being most sensitive (IC_{50} = 4 nm) and the $\alpha3\beta2$ subunit combination being least sensitive ($IC_{50} = 127$ nm) to blockade by this antagonist (Luetje & Patrick, 1989).

The six neuronal nAChR α/β subunit combinations that can be formed with the $\alpha2$, $\alpha3$, $\alpha4$, $\beta2$ and $\beta4$ subunits also differ in their sensitivities to a panel of four nicotinic agonists (Fig. 6-2). A profile of the responses of these six nicotinic receptor subtypes is shown in Figure 6-3. Rapid, extensive desensitization of nAChRs makes the maximal response an unreliable standard with which to normalize data (Luetje & Patrick, 1991). For this reason, we constructed partial dose-response curves normalizing all data relative to the response to 1 μm acetylcholine.

Structural homology with the alpha subunit of muscle and *Torpedo* nAChRs suggests that the alpha subunits of neuronal nAChRs contain the agonist binding site. For this reason, they would be expected to contribute to the pharmacological character of neuronal nAChRs. Results presented in Figure 6-3 confirm this expectation. Oocytes expressing the $\alpha2\beta2$ subunit combination show greater sensitivity to nicotine (closed circles) than to acetylcholine (open circles) (Fig. 6-3A). In contrast, oocytes expressing the $\alpha3\beta2$ subunit combination are much less sensitive to nicotine than to acetylcholine (Fig. 6-3C). Oocytes expressing the $\alpha4\beta2$ subunit combination show equal sensitivity to both agonists (Fig. 6-3E). Clearly then, since each of these receptors includes the same beta subunit ($\beta2$), the different alpha subunits contribute to the differences in sensitivity to nicotine and acetylcholine.

A contribution by the alpha subunit to the pharmacological character of neuronal nAChRs is not surprising, given the probable location of the agonist binding site on it. However, the results presented in Figure 6-3 show that the beta subunit also contributes to the pharmacological character of neuronal nAChRs. Receptors that include the $\beta2$ subunit ($\alpha2\beta2$, $\alpha3\beta2$, and $\alpha4\beta2$) are almost completely unresponsive to cytisine (triangles; Fig. 6-3A, C, E). In contrast, receptors that contain the $\beta4$ subunit ($\alpha2\beta4$, $\alpha3\beta4$, and $\alpha4\beta4$) are more sensitive to cytisine than to any other agonist tested (Fig. 6-3B, D, F).

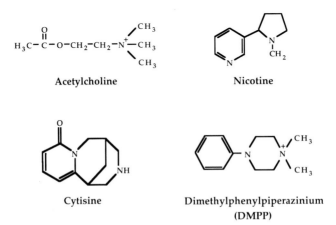

Acetylcholine

Nicotine

Cytisine

Dimethylphenylpiperazinium
(DMPP)

Figure 6-2. Structures of nicotinic agonists.

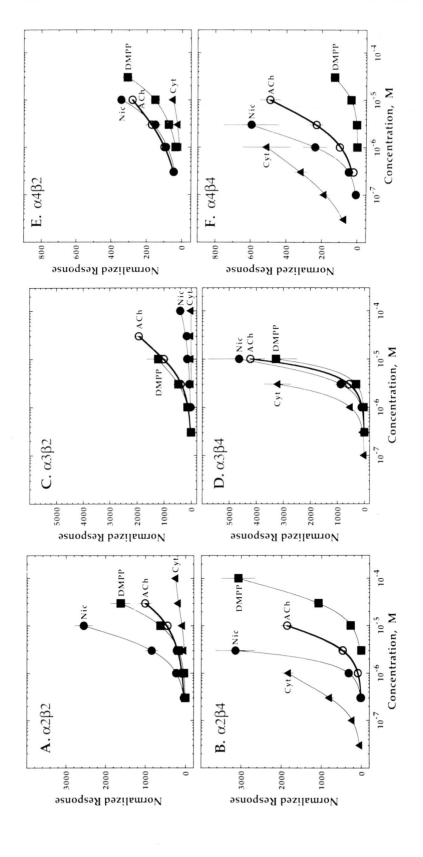

Thus, differences in sensitivity to cytisine seem not to be a function of which presumed agonist binding subunit ($\alpha2$, $\alpha3$, or $\alpha4$) is present, but rather of the particular beta subunit ($\beta2$ or $\beta4$) present in the receptor.

Use of DMPP (squares) also reveals a combination by the beta subunit to the pharmacological character of neuronal nAChRs. Receptors containing $\alpha3$ with either $\beta2$ or $\beta4$ are equally sensitive to acetylcholine and DMPP (Fig. 6-3C, D). Although the $\alpha2\beta2$ subtype was also equally sensitive to both acetylcholine and DMPP (Fig. 6-3A), the $\alpha2\beta4$ subtype was about fivefold more sensitive to acetylcholine than to DMPP (Fig. 6-3B). Receptors containing $\alpha4$ with either $\beta2$ or $\beta4$ were more sensitive to acetylcholine than to DMPP. However, the respective differences in sensitivity were about threefold for $\alpha4\beta2$ and approximately 20-fold for $\alpha4\beta4$ (Fig. 6-3E, F). The differences between the $\alpha2\beta2$ and $\alpha2\beta4$ subtypes, and between the $\alpha4\beta2$ and $\alpha4\beta4$ subtypes, demonstrate the importance of the beta subunit in determining the relative sensitivity to DMPP and acetylcholine.

It is important to note that the pharmacological properties of the receptors produced in the oocyte reflect those of the receptor produced by its cell of origin. The BC3H1 cell line produces a muscle-type nicotinic receptor (Patrick et al., 1977), and cDNA clones encoding this receptor have been isolated. The pharmacological properties of the receptor determined in the BC3H1 cell line are known (Sine & Steinbach, 1986, 1987), and the pharmacological properties of the receptor generated in the oocyte using clones encoding this receptor are very similar to those determined in situ (Luetje & Patrick, 1991). The accuracy of our observations might also be affected by differences in the degree of expression of different RNA transcripts, perhaps resulting in artificial variation of subunit stoichiometry. This difference in expression might then be more important in accounting for the pharmacological differences we have characterized than differences in subunit combination. We have ruled out this possibility by using multiple lots of both RNA and oocytes and by showing that varying the ratio of alpha to beta RNA injected into the oocytes does not alter the pharmacological properties of the expressed receptors (Luetje & Patrick, 1991).

Figure 6-3. Each neuronal nAChR subunit combination has unique pharmacological properties. Agonist-induced current responses of oocytes expressing $\alpha2\beta2$ (**A**), $\alpha2\beta4$ (**B**), $\alpha3\beta2$ (**C**), $\alpha3\beta4$ (**D**), $\alpha4\beta2$ (**E**), and $\alpha4\beta4$ (**F**) were measured under two electrode voltage clamps at a holding potential of -70 mV. Currents were elicited by bath application of various concentrations of acetylcholine (*open circles*), nicotine (*closed circles*), cytisine (*triangles*), and DMPP (*squares*). Responses are presented after normalization to the response of the same oocyte to 1 μm acetylcholine (response to 1 μm acetylcholine = 100). Each point represents the mean $\pm$ SD of the responses of three to eight separate oocytes. These results were obtained using two to three different lots of RNA and oocytes from two to six different donors. Data were fit by a nonlinear least squares program using the equation: current = maximum current/$[1 + (EC_{50}/[agonist])^n]$, where n and EC_{50} represent the Hill coefficient and the agonist concentration producing half-maximal response, respectively.

Figure 6-3 shows several examples of diversity among neuronal nAChRs composed of different combinations of subunits. This diversity cannot be explained only as a result of the particular alpha subunit present in a particular subunit combination. It is clear that the particular beta subunit present also contributes to the pharmacological character of the receptor. This can be appreciated most fully by considering the $\alpha3\beta2$ subunit combination in detail. The $\alpha3\beta2$ receptor differs from the other five subunit combinations examined by its relative insensitivity to nicotine. Furthermore, Figure 6-4 suggests that the $\alpha3\beta2$ subunit combination is much less sensitive to nicotine than to acetylcholine because of its low affinity for nicotine. The response of $\alpha3\beta2$ to nicotine differs from the responses of other $\beta2$-containing receptors ($\alpha2\beta2$ and $\alpha4\beta2$). The nicotine sensitivity of $\alpha3\beta2$ also differs from that of the other $\alpha3$-containing receptor ($\alpha3\beta4$). Thus, receptors are more sensitive to nicotine when they are formed by the $\beta2$ subunit and a different α subunit ($\alpha2$ or $\alpha4$) or when they are formed by the $\alpha3$ subunit and a different β subunit ($\beta4$) than when $\alpha3$ and $\beta2$ form a receptor together. This is strong evidence that both alpha and beta subunits contribute to the pharmacological character of neuronal nAChRs.

Figure 6-3 suggests nicotine and cytisine as good probes of the structure-function relationships of neuronal nAChRs. Nicotine is a weak agonist on $\alpha3\beta2$, but a potent agonist on $\alpha2\beta2$ and $\alpha4\beta2$, providing insight into the func-

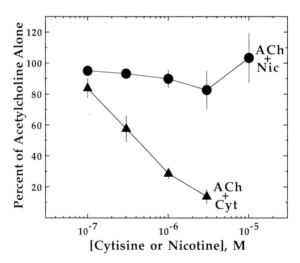

Figure 6-4. Low concentrations of cytisine, but not nicotine, block the response of $\alpha3\beta2$ expressing oocytes to acetylcholine. Agonist-induced current responses of $\alpha3\beta2$ expressing oocytes were measured under two electrode voltage clamps at a holding potential of -70 mV. Current responses were elicited by bath application of 3 μm acetylcholine in the absence and presence of various concentrations of nicotine (*circles*) or cytisine (*triangles*). Responses to acetylcholine in the presence of nicotine or cytisine are presented as a percent of the response to acetylcholine alone. Each point represents the mean ± SD of the responses of three to four separate oocytes.

tional contribution of the alpha subunits. Cytisine is a weak agonist on $\beta2$-containing receptors, but becomes a potent agonist by inclusion of the $\beta4$ subunit, rather than the $\beta2$ subunit. There are several explanations for these observations. Weak responses may simply reflect a low affinity of receptor for agonist. Alternatively, the receptor might have a high affinity for agonist, but the response is blocked through some subsequent effect of the agonist. Another possibility is that cytisine or nicotine might be partial agonists, in which case occupation of the agonist-binding site would not result as efficiently in open ion channels (Colquhoun et al., 1987). To determine which of these possibilities best explains our observations with nicotine and cytisine, we compared the response of $\alpha3\beta2$-expressing oocytes to 3 μm acetylcholine in the absence and presence of various concentrations of nicotine or cytisine (Fig. 6-4). If the weak responses to nicotine or cytisine were due to the low affinity of the receptor for these agonists, then the presence of nicotine or cytisine would have little effect on the response to acetylcholine. If the weak responses were due to partial agonism or to a secondary blocking effect of nicotine or cytisine, then the acetylcholine response would be blocked when acetylcholine is applied in the presence of a sufficiently high concentration of nicotine or cytisine.

The response to 3 μm acetylcholine was not significantly affected by co-application of nicotine (closed circles) at concentrations ranging from 100 nm to 10 μm (Fig. 6-4). This finding suggests that the weak response of $\alpha3\beta2$-expressing oocytes to nicotine is a result of a low affinity of this subunit combination for nicotine. In contrast, co-application of cytisine (closed triangles) results in dramatic inhibition of the response to 3 μm acetylcholine, with an IC_{50} for cytisine of approximately 400 nm. This finding suggests that the weak responses of $\beta2$-containing receptors to cytisine result from a blocking effect of cytisine secondary to its role as an agonist, or from cytisine being a partial agonist. Possible mechanisms that might account for a blocking effect of cytisine include open channel block (Sine & Steinbach, 1984) or an effect of cytisine at an allosteric modulatory site (Changeux et al., 1987). Experiments in which a constant concentration of cytisine showed an increasing ability to block acetylcholine-induced responses as the acetylcholine concentration was increased suggest that cytisine has a preference for the open form of the channel and may therefore be an open channel blocker (Luetje & Patrick, 1991).

Nicotine clearly activates receptors composed of these various alpha and beta subunits and does so with varying efficiency, depending upon which of the various subunits are present. It seems likely that the addictive properties of nicotine may involve only a subset of nicotinic receptors in the CNS and that identification of the particular subset will be important in understanding nicotine addiction. The pharmacological experiments described here may provide a means of identifying particular receptor subtypes in the brain. Likewise, the discovery of novel or unexpected pharmacological profiles of nicotinic receptors in the brain may suggest that we have not yet identified all the members of this gene family, that other untested subunit combinations exist in vivo, or that modifications, perhaps through cytoplasmic mechanisms, alter the properties of these receptors in the brain.

REFERENCES

Boulter, J., Evans, K., Goldman, D., Martin, G., Treco, D., Heinemann, S., & Patrick, J. (1986). Isolation of a cDNA clone coding for a possible neural nicotinic acetylcholine receptor alpha-subunit. *Nature, 319,* 368-374.

Boulter, J., Connolly, J., Deneris, E., Goldman, D., Heinemann, S., & Patrick, J. (1987). Functional expression of two neuronal nicotinic acetylcholine receptors from cDNA clones identifies a gene family. *Proc. Natl. Acad. Sci. USA., 84,* 7763-7767.

Boulter, J., O'Shea-Greenfield, A., Duvoisin, R., Connolly, J., Wada, E., Jensen, A., Ballivet, M., Gardner, P.D., Deneris, E., McKinnon, D., Heinemann, S., & Patrick, J. (1990). Alpha3, alpha5 and beta4: Three members of the rat neuronal nicotinic acetylcholine receptor-related gene family form a gene cluster. *J. Biol. Chem., 265,* 4472-4482.

Chang, C.C., Jou, M.J., Hong, S.J., & Chiou, L.C. (1987). Pre- and postsynaptic effects of nicotine on the mouse phrenic nerve-diaphragm preparation. *Proc. Natl. Sci. Counc. Repub. China, 11,* 148-154.

Changeux, J.-P., Giraudat, J., & Dennis, M. (1987). The nicotinic acetylcholine receptor: Molecular architecture of a ligand-regulated ion channel. *Trends Pharmacol. Sci., 8,* 459-465.

Colquhoun, D., Ogden, D.C., & Mathie, A. (1987). Nicotinic acetylcholine receptors of nerve and muscle: Functional aspects. *Trends Pharmacol. Sci., 8,* 465-472.

Couturier, S., Bertrand, D., Matter, J.M., Hernandez, M.C., Bertrand, S., Millar, N., Valera, S., Barkas, T., & Ballivet, M. (1990a). A neuronal nicotinic acetylcholine receptor subunit ($\alpha7$) is developmentally regulated and forms a homo-oligomeric channel blocked by a-BTX. *Neuron, 5,* 847-856.

Couturier, S., Erekman, L., Valera, S., Rungger, D., Bertrand, S., Boulter, J., Ballivet, M., & Bertrand, D. (1990b). $\alpha5$, $\alpha3$, and Non-$\alpha3$, three clustered avian genes encoding neuronal nicotinic acetylcholine receptor-related subunits. *J. Biol. Chem., 265,* 17560-17567.

Curtis, D.R., & Ryall, R.W. (1966). The acetylcholine receptors of Renshaw cells. *Exp. Brain Res., 2,* 66-80.

Deneris, E.S., Connolly, J., Bouler, J., Patrick, J., & Heinemann, S. (1987). Identification of a gene that encodes a non-alpha subunit of neuronal nicotinic acetylcholine receptors. *Neuron, 1,* 45-54.

Deneris, E.S., Boulter, J., Swanson, L., Patrick, J., & Heinemann, S. (1988). β-3, a new member of the nicotinic acetylcholine receptor gene family is expressed in the brain. *Biol. Chem., 264,* 6268-6272.

Duvoisin, R.M., Deneris, E.S., Boulter, J., Patrick, J., & Heinemann S. (1989). The functional diversity of the neuronal nicotinic acetylcholine receptors is increased by a novel subunit: $\beta4$. *Neuron, 3,* 487-496.

Eccles, J.C., Fatt, P., & Koketsu, K. (1954). Cholinergic and inhibitory synapses in a pathway from motor-axon collaterals to motoneurones. *J. Physiol., 126,* 524-562.

Garza, R. de la, Bickford-Wimer, P.C., Hoffer, B.J., & Freedman, R. (1987a). Heterogeneity of nicotine actions in the rat cerebellum: An in vivo electrophysiologic study. *Pharmacol. Exp. Ther., 240,* 689-695.

Garza, R. de la, McGuire, T.J., Freedman, R., & Hoffer, B.J. (1987b). Selective antagonism of nicotine actions in the rat cerebellum with α-bungarotoxin. *Neuroscience, 23,* 887-891.

Goldman, D., Deneris, E., Luyten, W., Kohchar, A., Patrick, J., & Heinemann, S.

(1987). Members of a nicotinic acetylcholine receptor gene family are expressed in different regions of the mammalian central nervous system. *Cell, 48,* 965-973.

Gu, Y., & Hall, Z.W. (1988). Immunological evidence for a change in subunits of the acetylcholine receptor in developing and denervated rat muscle. *Neuron, 1,* 117-125.

Kao, P.N., Dwork, A.J., Kaldany, R.J., Silver, M.L., Wideman, J., Stein, S., & Karlin, A. (1984). Identification of two alpha-subunit half-cystines specifically labeled by an affinity reagent for the acetylcholine binding site. *J. Biol. Chem., 259,* 1162-1165.

Kistler, J., & Stroud, R.M. (1982). Crystalline arrays of membrane-bound acetylcholine receptor. *Proc. Natl. Acad. Sci. USA, 78,* 3678-3682.

Lamar, E., Miller, K., & Patrick, J. (1990). Amplification of genomic sequences identifies a new gene, alpha 6, in the nicotinic acetylcholine receptor gene family. *Soc. Neurosci. Abst., 16,* 681.

Lipton, S.A., Aizenman, E., & Loring, R.H. (1987). Neural nicotinic acetylcholine responses in solitary mammalian retinal ganglion cells. *Pflugers Arch., 410,* 37-43.

Luetje, C.W., & Patrick, J.W. (1989). Members of the neuronal nicotinic acetylcholine receptor family display distinct pharmacological and toxicological properties. *Soc. Neurosci. Abst., 15,* 677.

Luetje, C.W., & Patrick, J. (1991). Both α- and β-subunits contribute to the agonist sensitivity of neuronal nicotinic acetylcholine receptors. *J. Neurosci.* (in press).

Luetje, C.W., Patrick, J., & Séguéla, P. (1990a). Nicotine receptors in the mammalian brain. *FASEB J., 4,* 2753-2760.

Luetje, C.W., Wada, K., Rogers, S., Abramson, S.N., Tsuji, K., Heinemann, S., & Patrick, J. (1990b). Neurotoxins distinguish between different neuronal nicotinic acetylcholine receptor subunit combinations. *J. Neurochem., 55,* 632-640.

Methfessel, C., & Sakmann, B. (1986). Molecular distinction between fetal and adult forms of muscle acetylcholine receptor. *Nature, 321,* 406-411.

Moss, B.L., Schuetze, S.M., & Role, L.W. (1989). Functional properties and developmental regulation of nicotinic acetylcholine receptors on embryonic chicken sympathetic neurons. *Neuron, 3,* 597-607.

Mulle, C., & Changeux, J.P. (1990). A novel type of nicotinic receptor in the rat central nervous system characterized by patch-clamp techniques. *J. Neurosci., 10,* 169-175.

Nef, P., Oneyser, C., Alliod, C., Couturier, S., & Ballivet, M. (1988). Genes expressed in the brain define three distinct neuronal nicotinic acetylcholine receptors. *Embo J., 7,* 595-601.

Papke, R.L., Boulter, J., Patrick, J., & Heinemann, S. (1989). Single-channel currents of rat neuronal nicotinic acetylcholine receptors expressed in *Xenopus* oocytes. *Neuron, 3,* 589-596.

Patrick, J., McMillan, J., Wolfson, H., & Chin-O'Brien, J. (1977). Acetylcholine receptor metabolism in a non-fusing muscle cell line. *J. Biol. Chem., 252,* 2143.

Popot, J.L., & Changeux, J.P. (1984). Nicotinic receptor of acetylcholine structure of an oligomeric integral membrane protein. *Physiol. Rev. USA, 64,* 1162-1239.

Schoepfer, R., Conroy, W.G., Whiting, P., Gore, M., & Lindstrom, J. (1990). Brain α-bungarotoxin binding protein cDNAs and MAbs reveal subtypes of this branch of the ligand-gated ion channel gene superfamily. *Neuron, 5,* 35-48.

Schuetze, S.M., & Role, L.W. (1987). Developmental regulation of nicotinic acetylcholine receptors. *Annu. Rev. Neurosci., 10,* 403-457.

Sine, S.M., & Steinbach, J.H. (1984). Agonists block currents through acetylcholine receptor channels. *Biophys. J., 46,* 277-284.

Sine, S.M., & Steinbach, J.H. (1986). Activation of acetylcholine receptors on clonal mammalian BC3H-1 cells by low concentrations of agonist. *J. Physiol., 373,* 129-162.

Sine, S.M., & Steinbach, J.H. (1987). Activation of acetylcholine receptors on clonal mammalian BC3H-1 cells by high concentrations of agonist. *J. Physiol., 385,* 325-359.

Steinbach, J.H., & Ifune, C. (1989). How many kinds of nicotinic acetylcholine receptor are there? *Trends Neurosci., 12,* 3-6.

Stroud, R.M., & Finer-Moore, J. (1985). Acetylcholine receptor structure, function and evolution. *Annu. Rev. Cell Biol., 1,* 369-401.

Surgeon General. (1988). *The health consequences of smoking; nicotine addiction. A report of the Surgeon General* (U.S. Department of Health and Human Services). Washington, DC: U.S. Government Printing Office.

Toyashima, C., & Unwin, N. (1988). Ion channel of acetylcholine receptor reconstructed from images of post-synaptic membranes. *Nature, 336,* 247-250.

Vidal, C., & Changeux, J.-P. (1989). Pharmacological profile of nicotinic acetylcholine receptors in the rat prefrontal cortex: An electrophysiological study in a slice preparation. *Neuroscience, 29,* 261-270.

Wada, K., Ballivet, M., Boulter, J., Connolly, J., Wada, E., Deneris, E.S., Swanson, L.W., Heinemann, S., & Patrick, J. (1988). Functional expression of a new pharmacological subtype of brain nicotinic acetylcholine receptor. *Science, 240,* 330-334.

Wada, E., Wada, K., Boulter, J., Deneris, E., Heinemann, S., Patrick, J., & Swanson, L.W. (1989). Distribution of alpha2, alpha3, alpha4, and beta2 neuronal nicotinic receptor subunit mRNAs in the central nervous system: A hybridization histochemical study in the rat. *J. Comp. Neurol., 284,* 314-335.

Wada, E., McKinnon, D., Heinemann, S., Patrick, J., & Swanson, L.W. (1990). The distribution of mRNA encoded by a new member of the neuronal nicotinic acetylcholine receptor gene family (α5) in the rat central nervous system. *Brain Res., 526,* 45-53.

Whiting, P.J., & Lindstrom, J.M. (1986). Purification and characterization of a nicotinic acetylcholine receptor from chick brain. *Biochemistry, 25,* 2082-2093.

Whiting, P., & Lindstrom, J. (1987). Affinity labeling of neuronal acetylcholine receptors localizes acetylcholine-binding sites to the beta-subunits. *FEBS Lett., 213,* 55-60.

7

The THC Receptor and Its Implications

LISA A. MATSUDA, STEPHEN J. LOLAIT,
MICHAEL J. BROWNSTEIN, AND TOM I. BONNER

The term "cannabinoid" is a chemical classification for a group of C_{21} compounds typical of the plant *Cannabis sativa* (marijuana) and its carboxylic acids, analogs, and transformation products (Mechoulam, 1973). Since the identification of Δ9-tetrahydrocannabinol (Δ9-THC) as the major psychoactive substance in marijuana (Gaoni & Mechoulam, 1964), much effort has been devoted to the study of marijuana and its cannabinoid components. For many years, however, progress in elucidating the mechanisms responsible for cannabinoid-induced effects in animals and humans was difficult. This difficulty can be attributed to the very hydrophobic properties of these substances that, in many instances, complicated not only the execution of studies but also the interpretation of the findings (Dewey, 1986; Pertwee, 1988). In addition, both in animals and in humans, these compounds elicit a wide range of complex effects (for reviews, see Dewey, 1986; Pertwee, 1988), and consequently, there have been many conflicting results (for reviews, see Martin, 1986; Pertwee, 1988). Although early studies did not conclusively define the mechanism(s) responsible for cannabinoid-induced effects, the development of novel cannabinoid analogs and tests to evaluate the psychoactive component of cannabinoid activity laid important groundwork for our current understanding of cannabinoids and marijuana (for review, see Razdan, 1986).

A specific receptor that interacts with cannabinoids has been characterized at the biochemical, pharmacological, and most recently the anatomical and molecular levels. Although the existence of such a receptor was first suggested by behavioral responses of animals treated with individual enantiomers of cannabinoid compounds (Dewey et al., 1984), the pioneering work conducted by Howlett and colleagues (1990a) defined the receptor-mediated responses of both neural cell lines and brain tissue in vitro to cannabinoid compounds. Their studies demonstrated that cannabinoids interact with a specific receptor to inhibit the activity of adenylate cyclase in a reversible, stereoselective, dose-dependent, and pertussis toxin-sensitive manner. This response is also most readily observed in cells treated with cannabinoids capable of producing psychoactive effects (Howlett, 1987; Howlett et al., 1988, 1990b). Although several laboratories helped establish the existence and define the nature of this receptor by describing the structure-activity relationships of numerous cannabinoids and synthetic analogs, a series of nonclassical cannabinoids designed by Johnson and Melvin (1986) greatly accelerated progress in characterizing a cannabinoid receptor. A radiolabeled ligand of high specific activity and high affinity for the cannabinoid receptor enabled researchers to define the binding properties of this site (Devane et al., 1988) and to localize the receptor in brain (Bidaut-Russell et al., 1990; Herkenham et al., 1990). This ligand (^{3}H-CP 55940) will undoubtedly be used to define further the nature of the receptor and the substances with which it interacts. More recently, the cloning of the complementary DNA (cDNA) that encodes this receptor conclusively established the existence of this protein and gave important information about its molecular nature (Matsuda et al., 1990). Determining the physiological significance of this receptor and realizing the potential therapeutic benefits of compounds that interact with it are the challenges that researchers must now address.

THE CLONED RECEPTOR

As described by Matsuda et al. (1990), the cannabinoid receptor clone was obtained by using a strategy designed to clone novel receptor proteins belonging to a family of functionally and structurally related receptors, and *not* a strategy designed to obtain the cannabinoid receptor specifically. The receptor family of interest was the G-protein-coupled receptors—integral membrane proteins that interact with guanine-nucleotide binding proteins (G-proteins) to initiate various cellular responses, such as the stimulation or inhibition of adenylate cyclase, stimulation of phospholipase C, etc. To date, the G-protein-coupled receptors with known amino acid sequences include biogenic amine, neuropeptide, phospholipid, glycoprotein-hormone, and amino acid receptors. Structurally, each of these receptors comprises a single polypeptide molecule, within which are seven hydrophobic domains. Figure 7-1 illustrates the amount of amino acid sequence identity between several G-protein-coupled receptors in the region corresponding to their respective second hydrophobic domains. At the time this project was initiated, this region seemed to be the most conserved among known receptor sequences; therefore, a 56-base oligonucleotide probe designed to recognize nucleic acid sequences corresponding to the majority of the second hydrophobic domain was used to screen a cDNA library (Bonner et al., 1987; Matsuda et al., 1990). This probe was based on the sequence of the bovine substance K receptor sequence that, at the time, was the only neuropeptide G-protein-coupled receptor cloned.

A cDNA clone (SKR6) was isolated and analyzed using hybridization conditions that allow the oligonucleotide probe to associate with similar yet different sequences in the library (rat cerebral cortex). This 5.7 kilobase cDNA contained a long open reading frame that would encode a 473 amino acid protein (minimum molecular weight of 53850 daltons). Present within the sequence were a number of the highly conserved amino acids found in other G-protein-coupled receptors, seven hydrophobic domains, and three potential

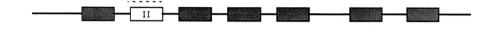

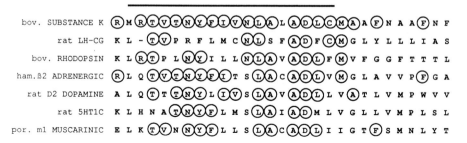

```
bov. SUBSTANCE K    R M R T V T N Y F L V N L A L A D L C M A A F N A A F N F
      rat LH-CG     K L - T V P R F L M C N L S F A D F C M G L Y L L L I A S
   bov. RHODOPSIN   K L R T P L N Y I L L N L A V A D L F M V F G G F T T T L
ham. ß2 ADRENERGIC  R L Q T V T N Y F I T S L A C A D L V M G L A V V P F G A
 rat D2 DOPAMINE    A L Q T T N Y L I V S L A V A D L L V A T L V M P W V V
     rat 5HT1C      K L H N A T N Y F L M S L A I A D M L V G L L V M P L S L
por. m1 MUSCARINIC  E L K T V N N Y F L L S L A C A D L I I G T F S M N L Y T
```

Figure 7-1. Amino acid sequence identity from the second hydrophobic domain of various G-protein-coupled receptors. The polypeptide structure of G-protein-coupled receptors is shown above the sequences. The boxes represent the characteristic seven hydrophobic domains. Circled residues in the LH-CG (leutinizing hormone-chorianogonadotropin), rhodopsin, beta-adrenergic, dopaminergic, serotonergic, and muscarinic receptor sequences are identical to the corresponding residues in the substance K receptor sequence. The dotted line above these sequences indicates the region of corresponding nucleic acid sequences that the 56-base oligonucleotide probe was designed to recognize.

glycosylation sites (Matsuda et al., 1990). Although the predicted amino acid sequence of the protein indicated that this clone was a member of this receptor family, it was not similar enough to any other known sequence to be able to predict the identity of the ligand for this receptor.

The critical finding that suggested the cannabinoids as candidate ligands for the SKR6 receptor clone was the cell line-specific expression of the SKR6 mRNA as determined by Northern blot analysis. Previous studies indicate that two neural cell lines, N18TG-2 and NG108-15, express G-protein-coupled cannabinoid receptors and that the C6 glial cell line, among others, does not (Howlett et al., 1986). This cell-specific expression pattern of receptors was consistent with that for the SKR6 mRNA (Matsuda et al., 1990) and provided a strong impetus to test cannabinoids on cell lines expressing the SKR6 cDNA. Further evidence that supported the testing of cannabinoids as ligands for the SKR6 clone came from comparisons of the localization patterns of the SKR6 mRNA and the cannabinoid receptor in rat brain. Although mismatches between in situ hybridization signals and autoradiographic ligand-binding images are to be expected in the CNS (receptors can be detected in terminal projection areas that are often quite distant from cell bodies, whereas mRNA is usually detectable only in the immediate vicinity of the cell body), the localization pattern of SKR6 mRNA showed notable similarity with that of cannabinoid binding. Both receptors and message were readily detected in cerebral cortex, hippocampus, caudate putamen, and cerebellum (Fig. 7-2). Consequently, various cannabinoids were tested for their ability to inhibit cAMP accumulation in CHO-K1 cells stably expressing the SKR6 cDNA.

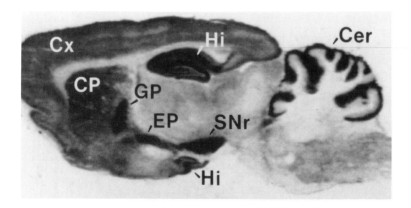

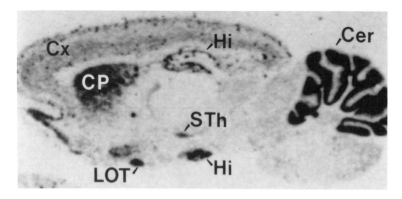

Figure 7-2. Sagittal sections through adult rat brain showing localization of cannabinoid receptors and SKR6 mRNA. **Top,** Autoradiographic image of receptors localized with ³H-CP 55940 binding. (Used with permission, Herkenham et al., 1990 and 1991.) **Bottom,** Localization of the SKR6 mRNA as determined using in situ hybridization histochemistry with the ³⁵S-SKR6-1 probe (Matsuda et al., 1990). Specifically bound ligand and hybridizing probe appear as dark images in both autoradiograms. Cer, cerebellum; CP, caudate putamen; Cx, cerebral cortex; EP, entopeduncular nucleus; GP, globus pallidus; Hi, hippocampus; LOT, lateral olfactory tract; SNr, substantia nigra reticulata; STh subthalamic nucleus.

As shown in Figure 7-3, the major psychoactive cannabinoid found in marijuana, Δ9-THC, and the synthetic cannabinoid, CP 55940, inhibit cAMP accumulation in SKR6-transfected cells. This effect is stereoselective and is not observed in nontransfected CHO cells (not shown) nor in cells transfected with other cloned G-protein-coupled receptors (Matsuda et al., 1990). As was previously observed with N18TG-2 cells (Howlett, 1987), cannabinoids considered to be psychoactive (Δ9-THC, 11-OH Δ9-THC, nabilone, and Δ8-THC) have more potent actions on SKR6-transfected cells than do those with little or no psychoactivity—cannabinol, cannabidiol (Matsuda et al., 1990). Furthermore, the cannabinoid-induced effects seen in SKR6-transfected cells are completely prevented in cells cultured with pertussis toxin (PTX) (Fig. 7-3).

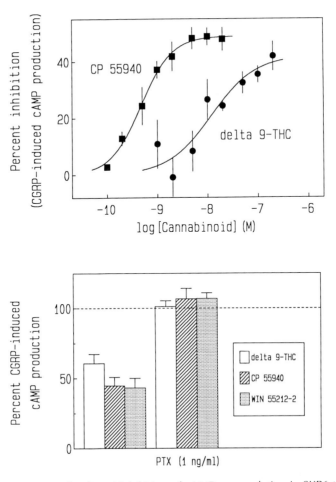

Figure 7-3. Cannabinoid-induced inhibition of cAMP accumulation in SKR6-transfected CHO-K1 cells. **Top,** Concentration-dependent inhibition of stimulated cAMP accumulation. Points are averaged values ± S.E.M. from three experiments, each of which was performed in triplicate. A stably expressing clonal cell line was established as described (Matsuda et al., 1990). Intact cells, in suspension, were incubated (37°C, 5 minutes) with various concentrations of cannabinoids and 250 nm calcitonin-gene related peptide (CGRP) to stimulate cAMP production. The average (± S.E.M.) CGRP-induced increase of cAMP (determined by RIA) was 44.9 ± 1.6 pmol/10^6 cells/5 min. **Bottom,** Effect of PTX on cannabinoid-induced inhibition of cAMP accumulation. Bars represent the averaged results from three to four experiments (performed in triplicate) of cAMP produced as a percentage of the CGRP-induced response (100%, dashed horizontal line). Cells were treated with CGRP (250 nm) ± Δ9-THC (100 nm), CP 55940 (5 nm), or WIN 55212-2 (100 nm) as described for data shown in top. Average CGRP-induced cAMP production was 52.3 (pmol/10^6 cells/5 min) and ranged from 28.8 to 64.8 (pmol/10^6 cells/5 min) in control cells. Average CGRP-induced cAMP production was 50.6 (pmol/10^6 cells/5 min) in cells pretreated with PTX (1 ng/ml, 18-20 hours before the experiment) and ranged from 22.7 to 83.2 (pmol/10^6 cells/5 min). Δ9-THC was obtained from the National Institute of Drug Abuse; CP 55940 and WIN 55212-2 were donated by Pfizer Research, Corp. and Sterling Drug, Inc., respectively.

Although the SKR6 receptor clone functions similarly to the cannabinoid receptor found in neural cell lines and rat brain, the biochemical characterization of cannabinoid-induced effects in cultured cells cannot directly confirm mechanisms for cannabinoid-induced psychoactivity or other subjective effects, such as euphoria. Several laboratories have used drug discrimination studies and other behavioral tests in laboratory animals to estimate the cannabimimetic properties of various compounds (Razdan, 1986). Although these studies use indirect measures, their results quite accurately predict a compound's psychoactive potential. These studies use various laboratory animals in addition to rodents, including pigeons, monkeys, and dogs. Using oligonucleotide probes specific for the SKR6 mRNA (or the human mRNA), a single hybridizing signal was observed on a Northern blot containing cerebellar RNAs from human, common marmoset, pig, and dog tissues (Fig. 7-4). These data indicate that the corresponding SKR6-receptor gene is active in other species that are typically used in whole-animal determinations of cannabinoid activity.

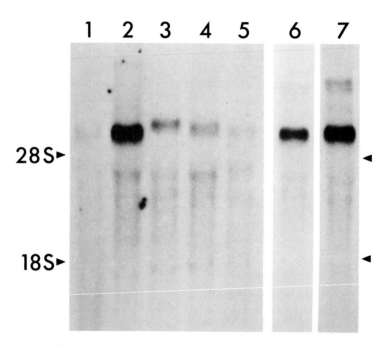

Figure 7-4. Northern blot analysis of cerebellar RNA prepared from various mammalian species. SKR6 message (ca. 6 kb) is visible in each lane of total RNA (10 μg) from human (lane 1), common marmoset (lane 2), pig (lane 3), dog (lane 4), and rat (lanes 5,6,7) cerebellar tissue. RNAs in lanes 6 and 7 were hybridized to ^{32}P-tailed SKR6-1 and SKR6-2 probes, respectively (Matsuda et al., 1990). RNAs in lanes 1 through 5 were hybridized to two similar probes (human probes, HC-1 and HC-2), which were designed to hybridize to the corresponding sequences in the human gene (data not shown). RNAs shown as lanes 1 through 5 were run on a 1% agarose/formaldehyde gel, RNAs shown as lanes 6 and 7 were run on a 1.2% agarose/formaldehyde gel. Positions of 18s and 28s RNA are indicated by arrows.

These data are consistent with the presence of cannabinoid receptors in such species as determined by ^{3}H-CP 55940 binding (Herkenham et al., 1990).

The human cannabinoid receptor has also been cloned (Gérard et al., 1991). The amino acid sequence of the human receptor exhibits more than 97% identity with that of the rat receptor and, when expressed in CHO cells, the human receptor also mediates a cannabinoid-induced reduction in cAMP production. The cloned human receptor has also been expressed in COS-7 and mouse L cells and its ligand-binding properties determined using ^{3}H-CP 55940 (Gérard et al., 1991; Felder et al., in press). As determined in these studies, the ligand specificity of this receptor is consistent with its involvement in the psychoactive effects that typically occur during marijuana intoxication. The gene for the human receptor has been genetically linked to chromosome 6 (Hoehe et al., 1991). Physically mapping the cannabinoid receptor gene using a biotinylated cosmid probe and in situ hybridization on metaphase chromosomes has confirmed these findings and further localized this gene to 6q14-q15 (Hoehe et al., 1991).

IMPLICATIONS

Although the characterization of the SKR6-receptor clone as a G-protein-coupled cannabinoid receptor confirms previous findings of a cannabinoid receptor in brain and neural cell lines, the sequence information and potential for various manipulations of the receptor through recombinant DNA technology will enable researchers to define more thoroughly the actions of cannabimimetic compounds and their receptor. The sequence information will enable researchers to verify and localize potential post-translational modifications of the receptor (glycosylation, phosphorylation, acylation) and to determine what significance these modifications have on receptor structure and function. Similarly, specific domains of the protein, as well as individual amino acid residues, can be studied to determine their potential role(s) in receptor-ligand binding and/or receptor-G-protein coupling. These types of studies will add to our growing understanding of receptor biochemistry and should facilitate future design and development of cannabimimetic compounds.

The anatomical characterization of the cannabinoid receptor has been initiated with the autoradiographic mapping of ^{3}H-CP 55940 binding in brain (Herkenham et al., 1991). Subsequently, the neurons in which the cannabinoid receptor gene is active have been localized by in situ hybridization histochemical methods (Mailleux & Vanderhaeghen, 1992; Matsuda et al., in press). Future studies that utilize immunohistochemical techniques and antibodies specific for the receptor will increase our understanding of the detailed circuitry of these neurons and interactions and their interactions with other neural systems. Moreover, researchers will be able to examine the regulation of this gene and the involvement of this receptor in various aspects of brain function (ontogeny, learning and memory processes, sensory perception, etc.) or dysfunction and disease by using the histochemical methods in conjunction with other techniques.

The identity of its endogenous ligand is one of the most important unknowns associated with this receptor. A similar scenario of a receptor and its unknown ligand eventually led to the isolation and characterization of the endogenous opiates (enkephalins, dynorphins, endorphins) and has resulted in research efforts that have contributed substantially to numerous aspects of biology, physiology, and pharmacology. The notably high abundance of the cannabinoid receptor in the CNS (Herkenham et al., 1990) suggests that the ligand for this receptor has a unique, important role in brain function.

The nature of this endogenous "cannabinoid" is, at present, unknown. As shown in Figure 7-5, Δ9-THC and CP 55940 have similar chemical features, including a phenolic ring and a long hydrocarbon chain at the same position relative to the phenolic hydroxyl group. Although the endogenous ligand may have structural features similar to Δ9-THC or CP 55940, a structurally dissimilar series of synthetic compounds were recently reported to interact with a cannabinoid receptor. These compounds, termed aminoalkylindoles, bind to a cannabinoid receptor, and inhibit adenylate cyclase activity and electrically stimulated contractions of smooth muscles in vitro (Pacheco et al., 1991; D'Ambra et al., 1992). One of these aminoalkylindoles, WIN 55212-2, also inhibits cAMP production in SKR6-transfected cells in a pertussis toxin-sensitive manner (Fig. 7-3). Although it is tempting to speculate on the chemical nature of the endogenous ligand based on the structures of various agonists, the lack of similarity between the structure of WIN 55212-2 (Fig. 7-5) and the Δ9-THC/CP 55940-type of structure suggests that predicting the nature of the endogenous ligand will be difficult. However, the deduced amino acid sequence of the cloned receptor may indicate what this substance is likely not to be. An aspartic acid residue found in the third hydrophobic domain in monoaminergic G-protein-coupled receptors (histaminergic, dopaminergic, serotonergic, muscarinic, and adrenergic) is absent from the SKR6 sequence. This residue seems to interact with the cationic amino group found in catecholaminergic neuro-

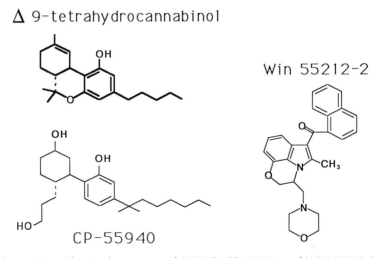

Figure 7-5. Chemical structures of Δ9THC, CP 55940, and WIN 55212-2.

transmitters (Strader et al., 1988). Therefore, its absence from the canna receptor suggests that the endogenous "cannabinoid" is chemically diss to these monoamines. In addition to deducing the chemical characteristics of the ligand itself, the search for this substance will be greatly facilitated by the use of receptor-specific antagonists or cell lines expressing the cloned receptor. Indeed, a transfected cell line together with its untransfected parent cell line can serve as an important tool for determining a cannabinoid receptor-specific response.

Cannabinoid-induced euphoria, sensory alterations, and calming effects have popularized the use of marijuana and hashish throughout history. Although these effects are themselves worthy of investigation, the more beneficial therapeutic effects of cannabinoids have compelled researchers to characterize fully the actions of these compounds and to define their mechanisms. Because of the ability of these compounds to block pain perception, dilate bronchial passages, and decrease intraocular pressure, cannabinoids could provide therapeutic relief to a potentially large number of individuals (Lemberger, 1980). One of the most exciting implications of the characterization of the cannabinoid receptor is therefore the possibility for developing new therapeutically useful compounds (both receptor agonists and antagonists).

The wide range of effects that are associated with cannabinoid use may well result from mechanisms not involving its particular receptor. Until a substantial amount of research has been completed, non-receptor-mediated mechanisms and receptors other than the cloned cannabinoid receptor (SKR6) should not be overlooked as potential mechanisms for cannabinoid-induced effects. Based on the example of other G-protein-coupled receptors, it is quite possible that one or more additional subtypes of cannabinoid receptors exist. Indeed, some indication of the involvement of multiple receptors is found when individual cannabinoid compounds are examined in a series of behavioral tests and physiological measures that reflect cannabinoid activity (Compton et al., 1990). The effectiveness of some cannabimimetic compounds differs between specific tests, which may implicate more than a single mechanism of action for the observed effects. However, such factors as metabolic processing and distributional properties that are often unique to individual compounds do not allow for simple and conclusive interpretations of the findings obtained from whole-animal studies. If there are additional cannabinoid receptor genes, our analysis of genomic blots indicates that they are not closely enough related to the SKR6 clone to expect that they will be identified easily.

The identification and characterization of receptor subtypes or other mechanisms that specifically mediate some cannabinoid responses will increase the likelihood of developing therapeutic agents that would benefit a large number of patients. To date, the mood-altering or psychoactive effects of commercially available cannabinoids greatly limit their usefulness. The nausea and vomiting associated with cancer chemotherapy are currently the only symptoms for which the use of cannabinoids is indicated. A number of nonclassical cannabinoids have been identified as potentially useful analgesic agents (Johnson & Melvin, 1986); however, the side effects of these compounds have precluded their approval for therapeutic use. Therefore, a cannabinoid-receptor subtype or specific mechanism that does not produce psychoactive effects needs to be found, or alternatively, reformulation of existing psychoactive cannabinoids will be necessary to counteract the undesirable components of their actions or reduce their access to the CNS.

Although marijuana is one of the oldest and most widespread drugs of abuse in the world, cannabinoids are relatively nontoxic and have not been considered to have serious addictive potential. However, tolerance (for reviews, see Dewey, 1986; Hollister, 1986) and sensitization (Weil et al., 1968) do occur in humans exposed to marijuana. Since cannabinoid-induced tolerance has also been observed in cultured neuroblastoma cells (Dill & Howlett, 1988), basic cellular mechanisms that result in drug tolerance may be analogous to those occurring with other substances that are capable of producing severe physical dependence. With regard to reward mechanisms, however, a recent report indicates that systemically administered Δ9-THC increases dopamine release in the medial prefrontal cortex of rats (Chen et al., 1990). Increases in dopaminergic activity in this and other regions have also been observed in rats treated with phencyclidine (Deutch et al., 1987). In studies in which drugs are self administered intracranially, rats will deliver cocaine to this area of the brain directly (Goeders & Smith, 1983). Although these data may suggest that marijuana and cannabinoids may act at key neuroanatomical sites for reward or drug-induced reinforcement in a manner similar to that observed with other controlled substances (Koob & Goeders, 1989), it is not clear whether cannabinoid receptors are directly involved. Interestingly, cannabinoid-induced effects on dopamine reuptake in synaptosomes have also been reported (Hershkowitz & Szechtman, 1979; Poddar & Dewey, 1980). Clearly, more research addressing marijuana's actions on reward-specific neuronal circuits is indicated. Similarly, the cannabinoid-induced effects of analgesia and altered sensory perception are reminiscent of some opiate- and hallucinogen-induced actions. Therefore, further investigations of cannabinoids, their receptor(s), and other drugs of abuse will ultimately add to our understanding of the physiology of these effects as well.

REFERENCES

Bidaut-Russell, M., Devane, W.A., & Howlett, A.C. (1990). Cannabinoid receptors and modulation of cyclic AMP accumulation in the rat brain. *J. Neurochem., 55,* 21-26.

Bonner, T.I., Buckley, N.J., Young, A.C., & Brann, M.R. (1987). Identification of a family of muscarinic acetylcholine receptor genes. *Science, 237,* 527-532.

Chen, J., Paredes, W., Lowinson, J.H., & Gardner, E.L. (1990). Δ9-Tetrahydrocannabinol enhances presynaptic dopamine efflux in medial prefrontal cortex. *Eur. J. Pharmacol., 190,* 259-262.

Compton, D.R., Little, P.J., Martin, B.R., Gilman, J.W., Saha, J.K., Jorapur, V.S., Sard, H.P., & Razdan, R.K. (1990). Synthesis and pharmacological evaluation of amino, azido, and nitrogen mustard analogues of 10-substituted cannabidiol and 11- or 12-substituted Δ8-tetrahydrocannabinol. *J. Med. Chem., 33,* 1437-1443.

D'Ambra, T.E., Estep, K.G., Bell, M.R., Eissenstat, M.A., Josef, K.A., Ward, S.J.,

Haycock, D.A., Baizman, E.R., Casiano, F.M., Beglin, N.C., Chippari, S.M., Grego, J.D., Kullnig, R.K., & Daley, G.T. (1992). Conformationally restrained analogues of praradoline: Nanomolar potent enantioselective (Aminoalkyl) indole agonists of the cannabinoid receptor. *J. Med. Chem., 35,* 124-135.

Deutch, A.Y., Tam, S-Y., Freeman, A.S., Bowers, M.B., Jr., & Roth, R.H. (1987). Mesolimbic and mesocortical dopamine activation induced by phencyclidine: Contrasting pattern to striatal response. *Eur. J. Pharmacol., 134,* 257-264.

Devane, W.A., Dysarz, F.A., III, Johnson, M.R., Melvin, L.S., & Howlett, A.C. (1988). Determination and characterization of a cannabinoid receptor in rat brain. *Mol. Pharmacol., 34,* 605-613.

Dewey, W.L. (1986). Cannabinoid pharmacology. *Pharmacol. Rev., 38,* 151-178.

Dewey, W.L., Martin, B.R., & May, E.L. (1984). Cannabinoid stereoisomers: Pharmacological effects. In D.F. Smith (Ed.), *CRC handbook of stereoisomers: Drugs in psychopharmacology,* (pp. 317–326). Boca Raton, FL: CRC Press.

Dill, J.A., & Howlett, A.C. (1988). Regulation of adenylate cyclase by chronic exposure to cannabimimetic drugs. *J. Pharmacol. Exp. Ther., 244,* 1157-1163.

Felder, C.C., Veluz, J.S., Williams, H.L., Briley, E.M., & Matsuda, L.A. (in press). Cannabinoid agonists stimulate both receptor- and nonreceptor-mediated signal transduction pathways in cells transfected with and expressing cannabinoid receptor clones. *Mol. Pharmacol.*

Gaoni, Y., & Mechoulam, R. (1964). Isolation, structure, and partial synthesis of an active constituent of hashish. *J. Am. Chem. Soc., 86,* 1646-1647.

Gérard, C.M., Mollereau, C., Vassart, G., & Parmentier, M. (1991). Molecular cloning of a human cannabinoid receptor which is also expressed in testis. *Biochem. J., 279,* 129-134.

Goeders, N.E., & Smith, J.E. (1983). Cortical dopaminergic involvement in cocaine reinforcement. *Science, 221,* 773-775.

Herkenham, M., Lynn, A.B., Little, M.D., Johnson, M.R., Melvin, L.S., deCosta, B.R., & Rice, K.C. (1990). Cannabinoid receptor localization in brain. *Proc. Natl. Acad. Sci. USA., 87,* 1932-1936.

Herkenham, M., Lynn, A.B., Johnson, M.R., Melvin, L.S., deCosta, B.R., Rice, K.C. (1991). Characterization and localization of cannabinoid receptors in rat brain: A quantitative in vitro autoradiographic study. *J. Neurosci., 11,* 563-583.

Hershkowitz, M., & Szechtman, H. (1979). Pretreatment with Δ1-tetrahydrocannabinol and psychoactive drugs: Effects on uptake of biogenic amines and on behavior. *Eur. J. Pharmacol., 59,* 267-276.

Hoehe, M.R., Caenazzo, L., Martinez, M.M., Hsieh, W.-T., Modi, W.S., Gershon, E.S., & Bonner, T.I. (1991). Genetic and physical mapping of the human cannabinoid receptor gene to chromosome 6q14-q15. *New Biologist, 3,* 880-885.

Hollister, L.E. (1986). Health aspects of cannabis. *Pharmacol. Rev., 38,* 1-20.

Howlett, A.C. (1987). Cannabinoid inhibition of adenylate cyclase: Relative activity of constituents and metabolites of marihuana. *Neuropharmacology, 26,* 507-512.

Howlett, A.C., Qualy, J.M., & Khachatrian, L.L. (1986). Involvement of G_i in the inhibition of adenylate cyclase by cannabimimetic drugs. *Mol. Pharmacol., 29,* 307-313.

Howlett, A.C., Johnson, M.R., Melvin, L.S., & Milne, G.M. (1988). Nonclassical cannabinoid analgetics inhibit adenylate cyclase: Development of a cannabinoid receptor model. *Mol. Pharmacol., 33,* 297-302.

Howlett, A.C., Bidaut-Russell, M., Devane, W.A., Melvin, L.S., Johnson, M.R., & Herkenham, M. (1990a). The cannabinoid receptor: Biochemical, anatomical and behavioral characterization. *Trends Neurosci., 13,* 420-423.

Howlett, A.C., Champion, T.M., Wilken, G.H., & Mechoulam, R. (1990b). Stereo-chemical effects of 11-OH-Δ8-tetrahydrocannabinol-dimethylheptyl to inhibit adenylate cyclase and bind to the cannabinoid receptor. *Neuropharmacology,* *29,* 161-165.

Johnson, M.R., & Melvin, L.S. (1986). The discovery of nonclassical cannabinoid analgetics. In R. Mechoulam (Ed.), *Cannabinoids as therapeutic agents* (pp. 121-145). Boca Raton, FL: CRC Press.

Koob, G.F., & Goeders, N.E. (1989). Neuroanatomical substrates of drug self-administration. In J.M. Liebman & S.J. Cooper (Eds.), *The neuropharmacological basis of reward* (pp. 214–263). New York: Oxford University Press.

Lemberger, L. (1980). Potential therapeutic usefulness of marijuana. *Annu. Rev. Pharmacol. Toxicol., 20,* 151-172.

Mailleux, P., & Vanderháeghen, J.-T. (1992). Distribution of neuronal cannabinoid receptor in the adult rat brain: A comparative receptor binding radioautography and in situ hybridization histochemistry. *Neurosci., 48,* 655-668.

Martin, B.R. (1986). Cellular effects of cannabinoids. *Pharmacol. Rev., 38,* 45-74.

Matsuda, L.A., Lolait, S.J., Brownstein, M.J., Young, A.C., & Bonner, T.I. (1990). Structure of a cannabinoid receptor and functional expression of the cloned cDNA. *Nature, 346,* 561-564.

Matsuda, L.A., Bonner, T.I., & Lolait, S.J. (in press). Localization of cannabinoid receptor mRNA in rat brain. *J. Comp. Neurol.*

Mechoulam, R. (1973). Cannabinoid chemistry. In R. Mechoulam (Ed.), *Marijuana: Chemistry, pharmacology, metabolism, and clinical effects* (pp. 1-99). New York: Academic Press.

Pacheco, M., Childers, S.R., Arnold, R., Casiano, F., & Ward, S.J. (1991). Amino-alkylindoles: Actions on specific G-protein-linked receptors. *J. Pharmacol. Exp. Ther., 257,* 170-183.

Pertwee, R.G. (1988). The central neuropharmacology of psychotropic cannabinoids. *Pharmacol. Ther., 36,* 189-261.

Poddar, M.K., & Dewey, W.L. (1980). Effects of cannabinoids on catecholamine uptake and release in hypothalamic and striatal synaptosomes. *J. Pharmacol. Exp. Ther., 214,* 63-67.

Razdan, R.K. (1986). Structure-activity relationships in cannabinoids. *Pharmacol. Rev., 38,* 75-149.

Strader, C.D., Sigal, I.S., Candelore, M.R., Rands, E., Hill, W.S., & Dixon, R.A.F. (1988). Conserved aspartic acid residues 79 and 113 of the β-adrenergic receptor have different roles in receptor function. *J. Biol. Chem., 263,* 10267-10271.

Weil, A.T., Zinberg, N.E., & Nelsen, J.M. (1968). Clinical and psychological effects of marihuana in man. *Science, 162,* 1234-1242.

8

Mechanisms of Action of the Steroid Receptor Superfamily of Gene Regulatory Proteins

BERT W. O'MALLEY

Over the past two decades, a great deal of evidence has accumulated to support the hypothesis that steroid hormones act at the level of nuclear DNA to regulate gene expression (Gorski et al., 1968; Jensen et al., 1968; O'Malley & Means 1974; O'Malley et al., 1979). The earliest studies were qualitative and involved experiments that showed that steroid hormones (1) caused the accumulation of new species of hybridizable RNAs that did not exist before stimulation, (2) caused stimulation of synthesis of new specific proteins, (3) caused a corresponding increase in the cellular levels of specific mRNAs, and (4) stimulated the rate of transcription of certain nuclear genes (O'Malley et al., 1969). By the early 1970s, the primary pathway for steroid hormone action was defined as follows: steroid → (steroid-receptor) → (steroid-receptor-DNA) → mRNA → functional response (Fig. 8-1; O'Malley et al., 1979). Steroid enters cells by passive diffusion and allosterically activates receptors in either the cytoplasm or nucleus. The activated receptor binds usually at the 5'-flanking region of target genes and stimulates transcription and protein synthesis. Precursor mRNAs are synthesized, processed, and translated to produce new proteins.

The first receptors were subsequently purified to near homogeneity and characterized as to size, charge, etc. Antibodies were developed, structural domains were postulated by proteolytic analyses, and assay of sex steroid receptors became commonplace in the diagnosis and determination of therapy for breast cancer. Investigators isolated specific target genes for steroid hormones, defined their structure, and proved that cis-acting regulator sequences were located nearby to such genes, usually in the 5'-flanking sequences (Payvar et al., 1983). When such sequences—termed steroid response elements (SREs)—are occupied by receptors, these genes come under hormonal control.

Molecular biologists became interested in these receptors for steroid hormones as they came to realize that they were the most intensively studied and

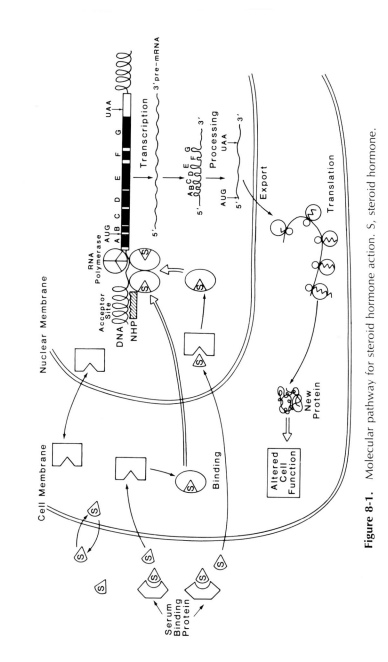

Figure 8-1. Molecular pathway for steroid hormone action. S, steroid hormone.

highly purified transactivation factors for the control of eucaryotic transcription and that they were the specific activators of an emerging and fascinating genetic cis-element, the enhancer. In the past 5 years, a great deal more has been learned about the structure-function relationships of steroid receptors and the mechanisms by which they interact with DNA. Biochemical studies conducted in the late 1970s suggested that steroid receptors, thyroid receptors, and receptors for vitamin D and vitamin A belonged to a family of gene-regulatory proteins. Furthermore, it was thought that these proteins were organized into domains that contained the functions of (1) specific and high-affinity ligand binding, (2) specific DNA binding, and (3) "transcriptional modulation." Molecular cloning of the receptors confirmed the "superfamily" concept. A schematic representation of the major members of this family is shown in Figure 8-2. Molecular cloning and sequence analyses not only substantiated the existence of domains but also showed that they could be rearranged as independent cassettes within their own molecules or as hybrid molecules with other regulatory peptides (Evans, 1988).

Perhaps the most intensively studied domain has been that responsible for DNA binding. This domain has been shown to be a cysteine-rich region that is capable of binding zinc in a manner that creates two peptide projections, which are referred to as "zinc fingers." These zinc fingers promote the interactions of receptors with target enhancers and clearly mark each as a member of this

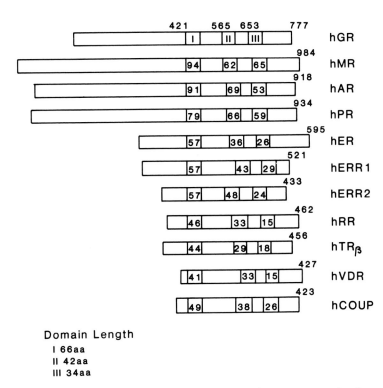

Domain Length
I 66aa
II 42aa
III 34aa

Figure 8-2. Sequence homology of the steroid receptor superfamily.

evolutionary conserved family. Each zinc finger is important for high-affinity binding to target DNA sequences, although some experiments indicate that the first (N-terminal) finger plays a greater role in specific sequence recognition. A surprising observation has been that certain oncogenes, such as v-erb A, are members of this receptor gene family. The avian erythroblastosis virus seems to have captured the cellular gene coding for thyroid receptor, as this retrovirus uses this mutated molecule for its own oncogenic purposes.

One of the most fascinating observations to emerge from the cloning of cDNAs for steroid receptors is the unexpected large size of the steroid receptor superfamily of related genes. After elucidation of the receptors for the more traditional members of this family (glucocorticoids, mineralocorticoids, sex steroids, thyroid hormone, vitamin D_3, and retinoic acid), a large number of cloned receptoroids have been discovered. These molecules can be considered to be "orphan receptors" in search of a function and a ligand. Since they were cloned by cDNA cross-hybridization screening using cDNA probes, we have little clue as to their cellular physiology. A function is implicit, however, since they are expressed in cells as fully processed cytoplasmic mRNAs. The first report of two such molecules was by the Evans laboratory; they were termed ERR-1 (estrogen-receptor related) and ERR-2 (Giguere et al., 1988). Their function remains unknown to date. More receptor sequences have since been published. They can be recognized easily by their homology in the DNA binding region and their conservation of type I zinc fingers. More than 20 additional related molecules may have been cloned; several of these molecules have been cloned from *Drosophila* (Mlodzik, 1990). Until recently, all of these putative receptors were without designated functions.

A recent discovery in our laboratory has stimulated my conceptual appreciation of these orphan receptors. We have been involved in the purification and cloning of a transcription factor called COUP-TF (*c*hicken *o*valbumin *u*pstream *p*romoter-*t*ranscription *f*actor). As suggested by its name, it is a high-affinity and specific DNA binding protein, which interacts as a dimer with the distal promoter sequence of the ovalbumin gene and promotes initiation of transcription of this gene by RNA polymerase (Wang et al., 1987). COUP-TF is thought to activate a number of other genes, including the mammalian insulin gene (Hwung et al., 1988), apolipoprotein genes (VLDL; Wijnholds et al., 1988), and the gene coding for proopiomelanocortin.

When COUP-TF was cloned and its amino acid sequence was derived, we were surprised to find that it was an authentic member of the steroid receptor superfamily (Wang et al. 1987). The assignment of COUP-TF to the steroid receptor superfamily of proteins has several implications. For the first time, it designated promoter regulatory proteins as a legitimate subtype in this family. The family had been thought previously to include only enhancer regulatory proteins. Second, it provides information that is useful for understanding the evolution of this family of regulators. Third, it raises the question whether COUP-TF, and other promoter activators for that matter, may be ligand-activated gene regulators. This latter query remains to be answered experimentally. Deductive reasoning should permit us to conclude that if one of these orphan receptors now has been found to have a function, then in time, others will follow suit.

Although direct evidence for regulation of these molecules by ligands does not exist, the conservation of amino acids in the ligand-binding region of authentic receptors with those present in the orphan receptors supports that hypothesis. A recent study has shown that the *Drosophila* analog of human COUP-TF, which is called seven-up and regulates retinal cell differentiation, contains a 93% identity with the human protein in the C-terminal region (Mlodzik, 1990). This observation suggests strong conservation of function and implies ligand regulation for both molecules.

The sequences of the target enhancers referred to as steroids response elements (SREs) and regulated by steroid hormones have been described for most members of this family to date (Evans 1988; Jantzen et al., 1987; Payvar et al., 1983; Renkawitz et al., 1984). Consensus regulatory sequences for genes responsive to glucocorticoid and progesterone (GRE/PRE), estrogen (ERE), thyroid hormone (TRE), and COUP-TF (COUP, RIPE) are shown in Figure 8-3. There are 15 base-pair consensus sequences, composed of two half-sites of six base-pairs arranged in a dyad axis of symmetry (inverted repeats) around a few central base-pairs of random composition. The SREs for various receptors share similarities in sequence; in fact, the identical sequence allows activation by glucocorticoid, progesterone, and androgen receptors. One copy of such an SRE is sufficient usually to bring a promoter under moderate hormonal control, and two copies often provide a synergistic response to the cognate hormone.

The precise mechanism of interaction of receptors with their target SREs has come under close scrutiny of late (Fig. 8-4). After cytoplasmic synthesis, many steroid receptors form transient complexes with heat shock proteins,

GRE/PRE	G G T A C A (with T T under first two G's, C under A)	N3	T G T T C T (C under second T)
ERE	– G G T C A (T under second G)	N3	T G A C C –
TRE	A G A T C A	N1	G G A C G T
COUP	G T G T C A	N1	A G G T C A
RIPE	A G T C C A	N1	G G G T C A
Consensus	– G – – C A	N1–3	– G – T C – (C under T)

Figure 8-3. Consensus sequences for steroid response elements GRE/PRE, glucocorticoid/progesterone/response element; ERE, estrogen response element; TRE, thyroid hormone response element; COUP, chicken ovalbumin upstream promoter; RIPE, rat insulin promoter element.

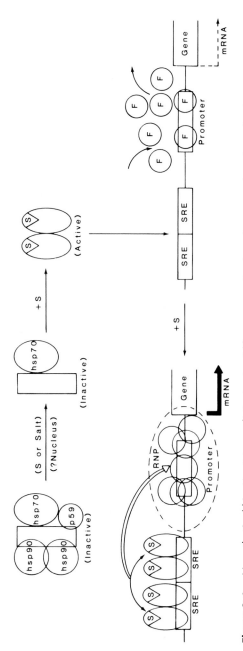

Figure 8-4. Hypothetical kinetics intermediates in steroid hormone activation of receptor. hsp, heat shock protein; s, steroid hormone; SRE, steroid response element; F, transcription factors; RNP, RNA polymerase.

such as hsp90, hsp70, etc. Certain extracts of receptors for glucocorticoid, progesterone, and estrogen are prepared from cells in vitro as such aggregates. In cells, this interaction may promote proper folding and stability of the molecule; in complex with heat shock proteins, receptors cannot bind to DNA. When a receptor is complexed with a heat shock protein, hormone binding drives in vitro dissociation of the complex. The exact meaning of this putative association of receptors with heat shock proteins is unclear at present. In any event, the hormone causes dissociation of all heat shock proteins (Fig. 8-4). The hormone then directs an allosteric change in the receptor, followed by a covalent modification that completes hormone-mediated ''activation'' of the molecule.

Recent evidence shows that glucocorticoid, progesterone, and estrogen receptors bind to their SREs as dimers, one molecule to each half-site. This interaction seems to be cooperative, at least for glucocorticoid and progesterone receptors, and is shown schematically in Figure 8-4. In this manner, receptor dimers bind with greater affinity and stability to their SREs than do monomers (Tsai et al., 1988). In addition, interactions between receptor dimers at separate SREs allow a higher order cooperative interaction, which stabilizes the two dimers into a tetrameric structure with a 100-fold greater affinity for its SRE sequences than does a single dimer (Tsai et al., 1989). Such protein-protein interactions may occur among homologous receptor complexes, heterologous receptor complexes, or receptor-promoter/TATA complexes. These interactions are thought to stabilize transcription factors at the promoters of target genes, thereby inducing a high degree of initiation of transcription (Fig. 8-4). Receptors appear to enhance transcription by stabilizing general transcription factors (e.g., TFIID, IIA, IIB, IIE/F RNA polymerase, etc.) at the TATA box directly (O'Malley, 1990). Alternatively, stabilization may be ''referred'' through interaction of receptors first with proteins bound to upstream promoters, e.g., COUP, NF-1, etc. (Klein-Hitpass et al., 1990). Incompatible complexes or proteins that disrupt such interactions should promote negative control by decreasing the chance that RNA polymerase will initiate transcription at a gene. Protein-protein interaction is the currently popular hypothesis for the formation of stable transcription complexes at regulated genes. However, a great deal more needs to be known about chromatin structure in regions of genetic control. Recent experiments suggest that specific phasing of nucleosomes around select SREs may allow recognition by receptors. Some studies indicate that hormonal stimulation may result in structural arrangements of nucleosomes that promote transcriptional changes at target genes.

The definitive role of ligand in receptor activation remains still a bit of a mystery. Certainly, receptors are inactive in cells in the absence of hormone. Hormone administration in vivo results in formation of a bound protein complex at SREs of hormone-regulated genes, as evidenced by in vivo footprint analyses. Crude receptor extracts of cells bind DNA poorly until they undergo a temperature- and salt-aided ''activation'' that is driven by hormone (Bagchi et al., 1990). As a first step, activation is promoted by disaggregation of receptors from heat shock and/or other proteins. Antihormones promote such disaggregation, but do not activate target genes, indicating an additional level of ligand-induced allosteric control. Recent evidence implicates a second step in which some allosterically altered form of receptor becomes a suitable substrate for a protein kinase and is activated by phosphorylation.

The role of steroid receptors has been defined now for genetic diseases of hormone resistance. Receptor defects have been shown to be the cause of testicular feminization, vitamin D resistant rickets, and hypercortisolism without Cushing's syndrome. Our recent familial studies have proven that vitamin D resistance can result from a single amino acid mutation at the tip of either "zinc finger" of the DNA binding domain of its receptor (Hughes et al., 1988) or from single amino acid mutations in the carboxy terminus of the protein (Lubahn et al., 1989). These observations are important in proving that mutations in human steroid receptors or in a transcription factor can cause a human genetic disease. Many recent reports show that genetic mutations in the androgen receptor are a frequent cause of the androgen insensitivity syndrome, commonly called testicular feminization (Lubahn et al., 1989).

Recently, we have made a series of exciting observations that may enhance our understanding of steroid receptor action in such organs as the brain. For the past 20 years, it has been accepted dogma that steroid receptors can be activated only by their specific cognate ligands. Surprisingly, we observed that certain receptors, such as the progesterone receptor and perhaps the estrogen, thyroid, and vitamin D receptors as well, can be activated to turn on target genes by 8-bromo-cyclic AMP. Although this observation is largely pharmacological, the principle has been established that activation of protein phosphokinase pathways can convert an inactive progesterone receptor to its activated state in the absence of its specific ligand. This heretical concept is supported by similar activation of these receptors by okadaic acid, a potent inhibitor of phosphatases 1 and 2A, which also enhances accumulation of phosphate residues on proteins.

Our observations led us to consider whether the binding to membrane receptors of certain physiological stimuli, such as those that emanate from chemical regulators (hormones, neurotransmitters, interleukins, etc.), could result in activation of target genes of the steroid superfamily. Using cloned receptors and target genes transfected into host cells, we tested a large series of compounds. We found that the neurotransmitter dopamine activates selected members of this receptor family, notably classic receptors, such as those for progesterone and vitamin D, as well as "orphan receptors," such as COUP-TF.

These results have several important implications. We can now state that pathway cross-talk can occur between membrane receptor and intracellular receptor pathways, a phenomenon not known to occur previously. We suggest that the steroid activation pathway is redundant in eucaryotes and can be modulated by selected perturbations in intracellular phosphorylation. Finally, we can now describe a logical hypothesis explaining how CNS neurotransmitters can reach the neuronal genome—perhaps the mechanism by which long-term effects, such as learning, memory, and drug addiction, are modulated.

Studies of the molecular mechanisms of steroid hormone action have had an immense impact on the field of endocrinology, advancing it as a legitimate discipline wherein technologies inherent to biochemistry, molecular biology, biophysics, pharmacology, and immunology can be unified toward the study of cellular physiology and regulatory biology. Since the CNS is replete with classical and orphan receptors, there seems little doubt that this family will be shown to play important roles in normal neurophysiology and drug addiction. Much excitement has already arisen, but the near future holds promise for a greater understanding of fertility, early embryonic development, genetic disease, stress, eating and nutritional disorders, addictions, emotional and depressive disorders, cancers, and aging through research in this field. Our results to date should facilitate not only the discovery of a series of new hormones and pathways but also the rational design and synthesis of new agonists and antagonists for therapy of certain of the above-mentioned disorders.

REFERENCES

Bagchi, M.K., Tsai, S.Y., Tsai, M.-J., & O'Malley, B.W. (1990). Progesterone-dependent cell free transcription: Identification of a functional intermediate in receptor activation. *Nature, 345,* 547.

Evans, R.M. (1988). The steroid and thyroid hormone receptor superfamily. *Science, 240,* 889-895.

Giguere, V., Yang, N., Segui, P., & Evans, R. (1988). Identification of a new class of steroid hormone receptors. *Nature, 331,* 91-94.

Gorski, J., Toft, D., Shyamala, G., Smith, D., & Notides, A. (1968). Hormone receptors: Studies on the interaction of estrogen with the uterus. *Rec. Prog. Horm. Res., 24,* 45-80.

Hughes, M.R., Malloy, P.J., Kieback, D.G., et al. (1988). Point mutations in the human vitamin D receptor gene cause hypocalcemic rickets. *Science, 242,* 1702-1705.

Hwung, Y.P., Crowe, D.T., Wang, L.H., Tsai, S.Y., & Tsai, M.-J. (1988). The COUP transcription factor binds to an upstream promoter element of the rat insulin II gene. *Mol. Cell. Biol., 8,* 2070-2077.

Jantzen, H.-M., Strahle, U., Glass, B., et al. (1987). Cooperativity of glucocorticoid response elements located far upstream of the tyrosine amino transferase gene. *Cell, 49,* 29-38.

Jensen, E.V., Suzuki, T., Kawashima, T., et al. (1968). *Proc. Natl. Acad. Sci. USA., 59,* 632-638.

Klein-Hitpass, L., Tsai, S.Y., Weigel, N.L., et al. (1990). Native progesterone receptor stimulates cell-free transcription by enhancing formation of a stable preinitiation complex. *Cell, 60,* 247.

Lubahn, D.B., Brown, T.R., Simental, J.A., Higgs, H.N., Migeon, C.J., Wilson, E.M., & French, F.S. (1989). Sequence of the intron/exon junctions of the coding region of the human androgen receptor gene and identification of a point mutation causing complete androgen insensitivity. *Proc. Natl. Acad. Sci. USA., 86,* 9534-9538.

Mlodzik, M., Hiromi, Y., Weber, U., Goodman, C.S., & Rubin, G.M. (1990). The Drosophila seven-up gene, a member of the steroid receptor gene superfamily, controls photoreceptor cell fates. *Cell, 60,* 211-224.

O'Malley, B.W. (1990). The steroid receptor superfamily: More excitement predicted for the future. *Mol. Endocrinol., 4,* 363-369.

O'Malley, B.W., & Means, A.R. (1974). Female steroid hormones and target cell nuclei. *Science, 183,* 610-620.

O'Malley, B.W., McGuire, W.L., Kohler, P.O., & Korenman, S.G. (1969). Studies on the mechanism of steroid hormone regulation of synthesis of specific proteins. *Rec. Prog. Hormone Res., 25,* 105.

O'Malley, B.W., Roop, D.R., Lai, E.C., et al. (1979). The ovalbumin gene: Organization, structure, transcription and regulation. *Rec. Prog. Horm. Res., 35,* 1-46.

Payvar, F., DeFranco, D., Firestone, G.L., et al. (1983). Sequence-specific binding of glucocorticoid receptor to MTV DNA at sites within and upstream of the transcribed region. *Cell, 35,* 381-392.

Renkawitz, R., Schutz, G., Von der Ahe, D., & Beato, M. (1984). Sequences in the promoter region of the chicken lysozyme gene required for steroid regulation and receptor binding. *Cell, 37,* 503-510.

Tsai, S.Y., Carlstedt-Duke, J., Weigel, N.L., et al. (1988). Molecular interactions of steroid hormone receptor with its enhancer element: Evidence for receptor dimer formation. *Cell, 55,* 361-369.

Tsai, S.Y., Tsai, M.-J., & O'Malley, B.W. (1989). Cooperative binding of hormone receptors contributes to transcriptional synergism at steroid response elements. *Cell, 57,* 43-448.

Wang, L.H., Tsai, S.Y., Sagami, I., & O'Malley, B.W. (1987). Purification and characterization of COUP transcription factor from HeLa cells. *J. Biol. Chem., 262,* 16080.

Wijnholds, J., Philipsen, S., & Geert, A.B. (1988). Steroid-dependent interaction of transcription factors with the inducible promoter of the chicken apo-VLDL II gene in vivo. In *UCLA Symposium on Molecular and Cellular Biology* (p. 235). New York: Alan R. Liss.

II
NEURAL SYSTEMS

One of the most rapidly moving areas of research on substance abuse has dealt with fundamental neuronal mechanisms, whether in individual cells or in groups of cells and their interactions. This section demonstrates some of those processes as they apply to several different forms of drug abuse.

Opiates, as described by Trujillo and his colleagues, affect brain systems involved in reward. They have an impact on a number of neuronal groups and also on the electrophysiology of specific neurons, as noted by North. The preparations that are used for these investigations can be quite varied. Dunwiddie and Brodie have used brain slice preparations to study the cellular processes involved in the action of cocaine. The interactions of cocaine with dopaminergic and serotonergic neuronal systems are examined by White and Bunney. Some mechanisms such as long-term potentiation are of enormous importance in the nervous system, as noted by Malenka, but their relation to behavioral and drug effects have been only sparingly investigated.

Newly discovered systems are particularly interesting as their roles in cognition and behavior are not yet understood. Herkenham examines the cannabinoid receptor system as it relates to motor and behavioral processes. Interactions between systems are elucidated in studies of the effects of cannabinoids and nicotine on brain neurons, as described by Deadwyler and associates.

9

Drug Reward and Brain Circuitry: Recent Advances and Future Directions

KEITH A. TRUJILLO, JAMES P. HERMAN,
MARTIN K.-H. SCHÄFER, ALFRED MANSOUR,
JAMES H. MEADOR-WOODRUFF, STANLEY J. WATSON, AND
HUDA AKIL

It is readily apparent that social, cultural, and psychological factors contribute to drug abuse. However, it is also becoming increasingly apparent that biological factors play a very important role in the self-administration of drugs. The purpose of this chapter is to examine the current state of knowledge regarding biological substrates of drug-seeking behavior and to speculate on how emerging techniques may be helpful in the further elucidation of these substrates.

We will begin by exploring how the psychological concepts of positive and negative reinforcement help us understand the ability of drugs to motivate behavior. Next we will discuss the current state of knowledge regarding the neuroanatomy and neurochemistry of the positive reinforcing actions of drugs of abuse, paying particular attention to the opiates and psychomotor stimulants. Then we will examine in some detail the tools and techniques that have been used in the past to analyze the neurochemistry and neuroanatomy of drug-seeking behavior and those that may be helpful in the future, with a particular focus on recent advances in molecular and cellular biology. Due to space restrictions, our exploration of these areas is somewhat limited in scope. For more detailed discussions of these various facets of drug abuse research, the reader is referred to several excellent sources (Bozarth, 1987; Engel et al., 1987; Goldberg & Stolerman, 1986; Goldstein, 1989; Kalivas & Nemeroff, 1988; Liebman & Cooper, 1989; Smith & Lane, 1983; White & Franklin, 1989).

REINFORCEMENT AND DRUG SELF-ADMINISTRATION

It is well established that drugs can powerfully influence behavior. Of particular relevance to the present discussion are the abilities of certain drugs to serve as

This work was supported by NIDA Grant DA02265, the Theophile Raphael Research Fund, and the Lucille P. Markey Charitable Trust.

motivational influences on behavior. The effects of a drug such as heroin or cocaine can be so potent as to become the primary motivational force in an individual's life. In the terminology of operant psychology (Skinner, 1938), these drugs influence behavior by acting as reinforcers of behavior.

According to operant psychology, behavior is controlled by its consequences. A consequence that increases the likelihood of a behavior occurring again in the future is called a *reinforcer,* whether it is a positive or a negative stimulus. In the case of drug abuse, the relevant stimulus is the drug (or more precisely the subjective effects that the drug produces after administration), and the behavior of interest is the self-administration of that drug. Two types of reinforcers are recognized by operant psychologists: positive reinforcers and negative reinforcers. A *positive reinforcer* is a stimulus that upon *presentation* produces an increase in behavior. Positive reinforcers are typically associated with positive affect (or mood) and are often referred to as rewards (in the following discussion the terms "positive reinforcement" and "reward" are used interchangeably). A well-known example of positive reinforcement is the presentation of a food pellet to a laboratory rat when the rat presses a lever. The positive reinforcer in this case is the food pellet. The rat will repeatedly press the lever to obtain the food. A *negative reinforcer* is a stimulus that upon *omission* produces an increase in behavior. Negative reinforcers are typically associated with negative affect. An example of negative reinforcement is the omission of an electric shock to a laboratory rat when the rat presses a lever. The negative reinforcer in this case is the electric shock. The rat will repeatedly press the lever to stop the shock. Note that in both examples of positive and negative reinforcement the rat is pressing the lever; however, in the first case the rat is working to obtain a positive stimulus, whereas in the second case the rat is working to stop a negative stimulus. (Negative reinforcement needs to be distinguished from *punishment,* which is also typically associated with negative affect. In contrast to negative reinforcement, however, the effect of punishment is to decrease behavior. An example of punishment is the presentation of an electric shock to a laboratory rat when the rat presses a lever. The rat will cease pressing the lever in order to avoid the shock. Although the stimulus may be the same as that in negative reinforcement, the presentation is different, resulting in a decrease rather than an increase in the behavior of interest).

Positive reinforcement and negative reinforcement have each been used as explanations for the self-administration of drugs. For many years, researchers focused on drug dependence, and in particular the negative reinforcing properties of the withdrawal syndrome to explain drug use. This focus stemmed primarily from the observation that chronic administration of opiates results in physical dependence on these drugs. If chronic drug administration is stopped abruptly, the individual shows many signs and symptoms of physiological disturbance and reports profound dysphoria and desire for further administration. This disturbance is called a *withdrawal* or *abstinence syndrome,* and an individual who undergoes withdrawal when drug administration is stopped is said to be *physically dependent.* According to researchers who focus on physical dependence, the withdrawal syndrome serves as a powerful negative reinforcer of drug self-administration; drug use is reinforced by the ability of further administration to suppress withdrawal. More recently, it has been recognized that drugs of abuse have very potent positive reinforcing actions—that individuals will self-administer drugs in the absence of physical dependence, primarily for their hedonic or pleasurable qualities. This observation has led many researchers in recent years to focus on the positive reinforcing effects of drugs as an explanation for self-administration. Although researchers have alternately chosen to focus on either positive or negative reinforcement in their theories of drug self-administration, these two concepts are not mutually exclusive. Although positive reinforcement may be the primary motivating factor for the initiation of drug use, before the development of physical dependence, both positive reinforcement and negative reinforcement will motivate the physically dependent user to self-administer.

OPIOID AND DOPAMINERGIC MECHANISMS IN POSITIVE REINFORCEMENT

It is striking how few drug classes are represented in the list of compounds that are self-administered by humans or experimental animals. The fact that so few drug classes are self-administered gives important clues as to why drugs are abused. We now recognize that it is the ability of these drugs to interact with specific brain systems that gives them their positive reinforcing actions. Two of the most readily self-administered and most widely studied classes of drugs are the opiates and the psychomotor stimulants. Opiates are drugs, such as heroin, morphine, and codeine, that are extracted from the opium poppy *Papaver somniferum,* as well as synthetic and semisynthetic analogs of these drugs. These drugs produce their marked effects, including analgesia and a sense of well-being, by interacting with brain opioid receptors. Psychomotor stimulants are drugs such as amphetamine or cocaine that elicit arousal and excitation by acting on brain catecholamine systems. Humans have long reported that these two classes of drugs produce pleasurable sensations, and recent research on both animals and humans has revealed that they can act as positive reinforcers. Evidence from a variety of sources indicates that the brain systems upon which these drugs act may normally mediate the positive reinforcing actions of natural reinforcers, such as food, water, and social interactions. In other words, opiates and psychomotor stimulants produce positive reinforcement by bypassing sensory systems and directly activating the brain systems normally involved in reward function. Although other neurotransmitter systems may be involved in reward, endogenous opioids and catecholamines have each been shown to play an important role in the positive reinforcing actions of drugs and other stimuli.

Neurobiology of Opiate Actions

Opiates act on the brain by mimicking the effects of endogenous opioid peptides at opioid receptors. There are currently three recognized "families" of endogenous opioid peptides, each of which is encoded for by a specific gene: the proenkephalin family, the proopiomelanocortin family, and the prodynorphin family (Akil et al., 1984). The proenkephalin gene produces methionine-enkephalin, leucine-enkephalin, and several extended forms of these peptides. The proopiomelanocortin gene codes for the 31 amino acid opioid peptide beta-endorphin and the nonopioid melanocyte-stimulating hormones (MSH) and adrenocorticotropin (ACTH). The prodynorphin gene produces dynorphin A peptides, dynorphin B peptides, and neo-endorphin peptides. Opioid peptides, when released from neurons in the brain, produce effects by binding to cell-surface opioid receptors, of which there are three primary types—mu receptors, delta receptors, and kappa receptors (Akil et al., 1984), each of which probably has multiple subtypes. The fact that there are three opioid peptide families and three opioid receptor types is coincidental— there is no direct pharmacological or anatomical correspondence between a particular opioid peptide family and opioid receptor. Although some of the peptides of a given family may have a pharmacological preference for one receptor type over another, this should be viewed as a *selectivity,* rather than a *specificity* of action. The pharmacological consequence of this lack of specificity is that each known opioid peptide, if exogenously administered at a high enough dose, has the ability to activate each of the three known classes of opioid receptors. In regard to physiological function, the actions at a particular opioid synapse will be determined both by which peptides are released and by which receptors are located in that synapse.

When administered to a human or an animal, opiates interact with opioid receptors throughout the brain, spinal cord, and periphery, thereby producing the varied opiate effects. For example, after administration of an opiate to a subject, activation of opioid receptors in the gut is primarily responsible for the constipating effects of the drug; activation of opioid receptors in brainstem nuclei is responsible for respiratory depression and vomiting; activation of opiate receptors in spinal cord and brain pain pathways is responsible for analgesia; and as discussed below, activation of opiate receptors at several brain sites within a well-defined circuit is responsible for positive reinforcement. Because of their different anatomical localization and different cellular effects, each of the three opioid receptor types is differentially involved in the various opiate actions. Psychopharmacological studies have revealed that injection of mu or delta receptor agonists is rewarding, and it is therefore mu and delta receptors that are most likely responsible for the positive reinforcing actions of opiates. In contrast, injection of kappa receptor agonists is aversive (Herz & Shippenberg, 1989); kappa receptors may therefore be involved in negative reinforcement or punishment.

Neurobiology of Psychomotor Stimulants

Psychomotor stimulants have several actions on dopamine, norepinephrine, and serotonin neurons, which together result in an increase in synaptic levels of these monoamines. As discussed elsewhere in this book, cocaine prevents reuptake of the monoamines by binding to the uptake sites for these neurotransmitters, thereby producing increased concentrations of synaptic dopamine, norepinephrine, and serotonin. Amphetamine and its analogs prevent reuptake of the monoamines (via mechanisms different than cocaine), increase release, and inhibit the metabolic enzyme monoamine oxidase, thereby increasing synaptic concentrations of these neurotransmitters. Although the psychomotor stimulants have profound actions on neurons containing each of the three monoamines, it is the release of dopamine from nerve terminals at forebrain sites, and the consequent binding of this neurotransmitter to dopamine receptors, that is believed to be responsible for the reinforcing properties of these drugs.

Although pharmacological analyses have distinguished only two types of dopamine receptors, D_1 and D_2, recent molecular genetic studies have thus far identified at least five types: D_1, D_2, D_3, D_4, and D_5 (Bunzow et al., 1988; Dearry et al., 1990; Sokoloff et al., 1990; Sunahara et al., 1990, 1991; Van Tol et al., 1991; Zhou et al., 1990). D_3 and D_4 receptors are structurally and pharmacologically similar to D_2, whereas D_5 is similar to D_1. Psychopharmacological studies have yielded conflicting results as to which dopamine receptor type is responsible for the positive reinforcing actions of psychomotor stimulants. Although some studies suggest that the D_1 receptor is responsible, others suggest that the D_2 is the critical receptor (the D_3, D_4, and D_5 receptors have yet to be studied in this context). However, since co-activation of D_1 and D_2 receptors has been found to be important in several behavioral and physiological effects of dopamine (Walters et al., 1987), it is possible that co-activation of two or more dopamine receptor types is necessary for proper expression of psychomotor stimulant reward.

BRAIN CIRCUITRY OF OPIATE AND PSYCHOMOTOR STIMULANT REWARD

Numerous psychopharmacological studies have examined the brain sites involved in opioid and psychomotor stimulant reward. There are several techniques available for determining such sites. Investigators may examine whether animals will self-administer the drug in question into a particular brain site or whether injections into that site will produce conditioned reinforcement. Alternatively, they may inject an antagonist into a specific brain site to determine whether the antagonist will disrupt the reinforcing properties of peripherally administered drug. In a similar manner, researchers may lesion a specific brain site and determine whether the lesion will disrupt the rewarding effects of a drug. Such psychopharmacological studies are consistent in demonstrating that the positive reinforcing actions of amphetamine and its analogs are mediated by dopamine activation in the nucleus accumbens (nACC). There is, however, debate over the primary locus for the rewarding actions of cocaine. Some evidence suggests that the nACC is the primary site of action, whereas other studies suggest that the medial prefrontal cortex (MPC) is most important. Interestingly, each of these brain regions is a primary terminal area for dopamine neurons originating in the ventral tegmental area (VTA).

Like the psychomotor stimulants, opiates can produce positive reinforcement by actions in the nACC. However, in addition to the nACC, opiates are also rewarding when injected into the ventral tegmental area (VTA), the lateral hypothalamus (LH), and the hippocampus (Corrigal & Linseman, 1988; Stein & Belluzzi, 1989; Watson et al., 1989). Activation of opioid receptors in the region of the VTA causes release of dopamine in VTA terminal regions, such as the nACC. Evidence suggests that this dopamine release mediates the rewarding actions of intra-VTA injections of opiates. In contrast, the positive reinforcing actions of opiates injected directly into the nACC seem to be independent of dopamine and are more likely due to direct actions on postsynaptic neurons in this nucleus. The positive reinforcing actions of opiates in the LH and hippocampus may also be independent of dopamine. In summary, although future studies may show that other brain sites play a role in the positive reinforcing actions of opiates and psychomotor stimulants, the available evidence thus far suggests that the MPC, the nACC, the LH, the VTA, and the hippocampus are important sites of action for these effects.

One might ask whether these five brain sites are independently involved in drug reinforcement or whether some factor links them in this role. In fact, examination of the neuroanatomical relationships reveals that these brain sites are closely linked not only functionally but also anatomically—important monosynaptic pathways connect each of these nuclei (Fallon & Loughlin, 1987). As noted above, VTA dopamine neurons send dense projections to the nACC and the MPC. These dopamine neurons also project to the LH. In addition, the MPC, the LH, and the hippocampus provide strong inputs to the nACC, the nACC and the MPC project to the VTA, and the nACC sends projections to the LH. These nuclei therefore seem to be linked in a functional and anatomical circuit, which has been called the "limbic-motor reinforcement circuit" (Watson et al., 1989). The "limbic" aspect of this nomenclature derives from the fact that these nuclei are traditionally identified as part of the limbic circuitry of the brain and are involved in motivation and emotion. The "motor" aspect derives from the fact that a major output from the circuit as a whole is to motor systems via outputs from the nACC, which is itself involved in locomotor activation (see below). Finally, the "reinforcement" denotation arises from the demonstrated role that these nuclei have in the positive reinforcing actions of drugs and other rewarding stimuli (Fig. 9-1).

Although each of the five nuclei in the limbic-motor reinforcement circuit seems to be involved in drug reward, the nACC may play a central role in this circuitry. The nACC receives strong inputs from each of the other four nuclei and sends outputs to the VTA and the LH. In addition, it receives inputs from several important limbic regions, including limbic cortex, amygdala, and limbic thalamus (Fig. 9-2). In contrast, input from traditional sensory and motor systems and from the neocortex and striatum is limited. The output of the nACC involves both limbic and motor systems. For instance, outputs of this nucleus include the VTA, preoptic area, bed nucleus of the stria terminalis, and lateral hypothalamus, components of the limbic system; and the ventral pallidum, entopeduncular nucleus, and substantia nigra pars reticulata, regions implicated in motor function (Fig. 9-3). The motor projections of the nACC may serve as an important output pathway for the limbic-motor reinforcement circuit. The outputs to the ventral pallidum and the pedunculopontine tegmentum,

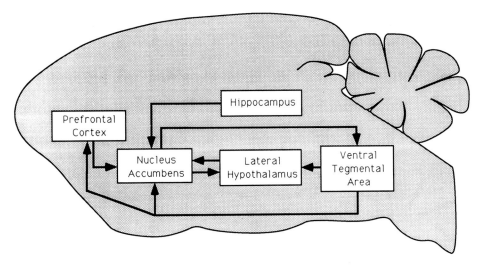

Figure 9-1. A saggital section from a rat brain illustrating the principal nuclei of the limbic-motor reinforcement circuit.

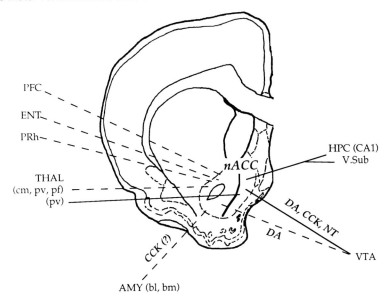

Figure 9-2. Connectivity of the nucleus accumbens (nACC): afferents. Direct connections are illustrated by lines. The neurotransmitter/neuropeptide(s) utilized, if known, are designated along the lines. Among the cell groups providing the richest innervation of the VTA are dopamine (DA)/cholecystokinin (CCK)/neurotensin (NT) neurons of the ventral tegmental area (VTA) and neurons of the ventral subiculum and ventral hippocampus (CA1), which are believed to use the excitatory amino acid glutamate as a neurotransmitter. There is a particularly heavy aggregation of both VTA and hippocampal afferents in the medial nACC—the "shell" region (*solid lines*). The lateral nACC ("core") receives afferents from limbic cortex (entorhinal, medial prefrontal, and perirhinal), some midline thalamic nuclei, and the basomedial and basolateral amygdala (dashed lines). Some of the latter projections contain the neuropeptide CCK.

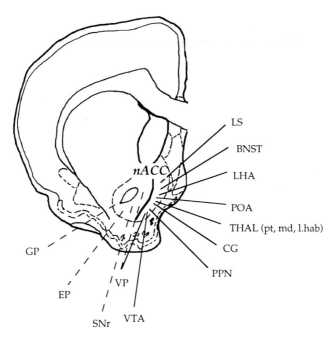

Figure 9-3. Connectivity of the nucleus accumbens (nACC): efferents. Direct connections are illustrated by lines. Note that there seems to be some differentiation among projectional fields, which loosely obeys the medial-lateral (or shell-core) distinction. Neurons localized to the medial nACC project to sites associated with limbic function (*solid lines*), include the ned nucleus of the stria terminalis (BNST), preoptic area (POA), lateral hypothalamic area (LHA), and VTA, as well as the ventral pallidum (VP) and pedunculopontine nucleus (PPN). Neurons located within the lateral nACC, on the other hand, are more likely to project to regions associated with extrapyramidal motor function (dotted lines), include the substantia nigra pars reticulata (SNr), entopeduncular nucleus (EP), and the VP.

in particular, seem to be very important in the rewarding and locomotor stimulant actions of opiates and psychomotor stimulants (Bechara & van der Kooy, 1989; Koob & Bloom, 1988).

Because of the central location of the nACC between limbic inputs and motor outputs, this nucleus has been called a limbic-motor interface, where emotions are translated into behavioral actions (Mogenson et al., 1980). It appears that limbic inputs to the nACC may be gated or amplified in this nucleus, thereby gaining access to motor output pathways for expression as behavioral actions. Dopamine and opioids may serve as the "gates" or "amplifiers," biasing the inputs and allowing them access to the motor systems (Fibiger & Phillips, 1986; Mogenson et al., 1980; Simon & Le Moal, 1988; Watson et al., 1989). In this respect, it is quite interesting that the nACC is not only important in the rewarding properties of both opiates and psychomotor stimulants but is also the site where these drugs produce locomotor stimulation. Both opiates and psychomotor stimulants produce locomotor stimulation in laboratory rats, in addition to positive reinforcement. Psychopharmacological studies have demonstrated that this stimulation is mediated by the nACC for both classes of drugs. The nACC may therefore be responsible for the well-described association between positive reinforcement and locomotor behavior (Glickman & Schiff, 1967; Watson et al., 1989; Wise & Bozarth, 1987). Interestingly, the nACC may play an important role in the positive reinforcing actions not only of opiates and psychomotor stimulants but also of other self-administered drugs (Clarke, 1990; Di Chiara & Imperato, 1988; Koob & Bloom, 1988; Spyraki et al., 1988). Because of the central role of the nACC in the positive reinforcing properties of opiates, psychomotor stimulants, and perhaps other drugs, we now examine in some detail the chemical neuroanatomy of this nucleus as it relates to drug reward, focusing in particular on opioid and dopaminergic elements of the nucleus.

Opioid Peptide and Dopamine Systems in the Nucleus Accumbens

Dopamine innervation of the nACC arises from neurons in the VTA (A10 cell region). Dopamine fibers can be seen throughout the nACC, with a particularly dense innervation of the medial zone, also known as the shell (Heimer et al., 1991). The dopamine projection to the nACC parallels the projections to the dorsal striatum by the substantia nigra pars compacta (A9) and to some extent may be topographically continuous with it (Fallon & Loughlin, 1987). However, in contrast to the nigrostriatal system, the VTA contains a substantial population of neurons in which the neuropeptides cholecystokinin (CCK) and/ or neurotensin (NT) are co-localized with dopamine. Neurons co-localizing CCK or NT with dopamine have a characteristic distribution within the medial or shell portion of the nACC. The presence of CCK and NT in VTA dopamine neurons projecting to the nACC indicates that these peptides are in a position to play a role in dopamine-mediated reward, a suggestion supported by recent psychopharmacological studies.

The nACC is rich in proenkephalin and prodynorphin peptides, containing numerous cell bodies and dense aggregations of fibers and terminals. Interestingly, like dopamine, CCK, and NT, enkephalin and dynorphin fibers are heaviest in the medial or shell portion of the nucleus (Fig. 9-4). This medial zone of the nucleus accumbens also receives a minor innervation from beta-endorphin-containing neurons originating in the arcuate nucleus of the hypothalamus. Therefore, all three opioid peptide families are present in the nACC, with cell bodies and fibers localized in the immediate proximity of ascending dopamine projections from the VTA (many of which contain CCK or NT), as well as limbic afferents from the hippocampus.

Receptor autoradiographic studies have localized D_1 and D_2 dopamine receptors and mu, delta, and kappa opioid receptors in the nACC. D_1 and D_2 receptors are densely distributed throughout the nACC (Fig. 9-5). Strikingly, the three opioid receptor types are found in greatest density in the medial accumbens, overlapping the heavy localization of opioid peptide-containing terminals and cell bodies in this subregion. Throughout the rest of the nACC, delta receptors are located diffusely, whereas mu receptors appear in patches, as is characteristic of the striatum (Fig. 9-6).

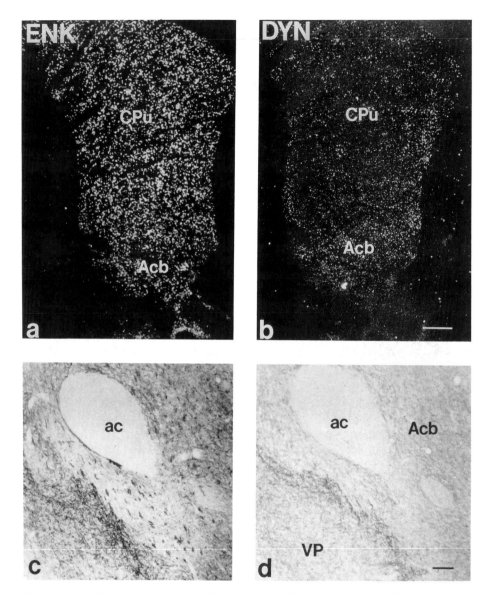

Figure 9-4. Histological sections illustrating localization of enkephalin (ENK) and dynorphin mRNA (**A,B**) and peptide (**C,D**) in the nucleus accumbens of the rat. **A,B,** In situ hybridization of sagittal sections of rat striatum with a 35S-UTP-labeled ENK cRNA probe (**A**) and a DYN cRNA probe (**B**). Note the high abundance and uniform distribution of ENK mRNA-containing cells in the nucleus accumbens (Acb) and caudate-putamen (CPu). DYN mRNA-producing cells, in contrast, are predominantly localized in the nucleus accumbens. **C,D,** Immunohistochemical localization of ENK and DYN peptide-containing fibers in coronal sections of caudal nucleus accumbens in the rat. Note the heavy ENK fiber staining throughout this region (**C**), and the concentration of both peptides in the ventrome-dial portion of this nucleus (**C,D**). Heavy staining for both ENK and DYN is seen in the ventral pallidum (VP) at this level. ac, anterior commissure. Magnification bars: **A,B** = 1 mm, **C,D** = 100 μm.

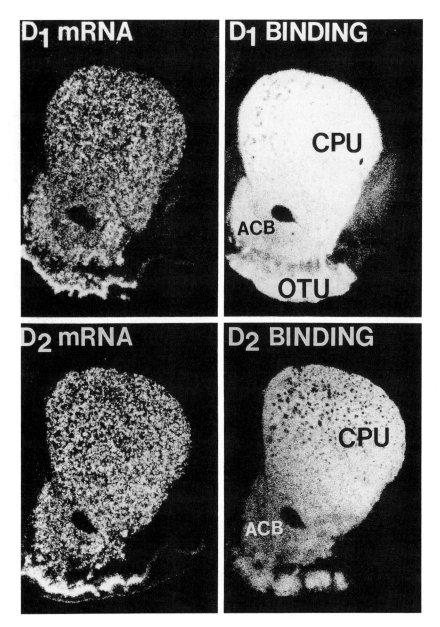

Figure 9-5. Dopamine D_1 and D_2 receptor mRNA (*left*) and binding (*right*) in coronal sections through the nucleus accumbens (ACB) of the rat. Caudate-putamen (CPU) and olfactory tubercle (OTU) are also shown. D_1 and D_2 mRNAs were visualized with [^{35}S]-labeled cnRNA probes generated to transmembrane regions III-VI of the rat D_1 receptor (bp 383-843), and a Sac I-Bgl II fragment of the rat D_2 receptor. In situ hybridization was performed using procedures previously described elsewhere (Meador-Woodruff et al., 1989). D_1 and D_2 receptor binding images were generated with the selective D_1 antagonist [^{3}H]-SCH23390 (in the presence of 1 μm ketanserin), and the D_2 antagonist [^{3}H]-raclopride, using standard autoradiographic procedures (Mansour et al., 1990).

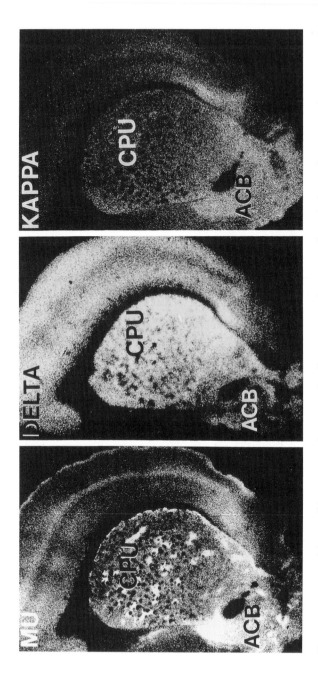

Figure 9-6. Mu, delta, and kappa opioid receptor binding in coronal sections through the nucleus accumbens (ACB) of the rat. Caudate-putamen (CPU) and olfactory tubercle (OTU) are also shown. Mu and delta receptors were labeled with the selective ligands [³H]-DAGO (Tyr-D-Ala-Gly-MePhe-Gly-ol) and [³H]-DPDPE (D-Pen², D-Pen⁵-enkephalin), respectively, whereas kappa receptors were labeled with [³H]-bremazocine in the presence of a 300-fold excess of unlabeled DAGO and DPDPE (Mansour et al., 1987). Each ligand selectively occupied approximately 75% of each opioid receptor type.

The presence of all three opioid receptors in relatively high abundance within the nACC indicates the potential for opioid neuromodulation in this region, in accordance with the psychopharmacological data. Unfortunately, the relatively unclear relationship between the three peptide systems and the three opioid receptor subtypes noted above, and the close proximity of all three peptide families and all three receptors in the nACC, makes identification of the specific role of individual peptide systems in nACC-mediated reinforcement processes quite difficult. It is therefore unknown whether enkephalin, dynorphin, or beta-endorphin neurons or perhaps all three are involved in nACC reinforcement processes. Further research identifying the specific neurons and circuits involved in reward will help determine the individual contributions of these peptide systems.

In summary, the chemical neuroanatomy of the nACC strongly supports the conclusions of psychopharmacological studies that opioid neuromodulation and dopamine neurotransmission are important in this nucleus. Of particular interest is the dense concentration of limbic inputs, opioid cell bodies and fibers, and dopamine terminals in the medial, shell region of the nACC. Whether this zone of potentially rich interactions plays a special role in opioid and dopaminergic mechanisms of positive reinforcement remains to be determined.

Although much is known about the input and output circuitry of the nACC, as well as the localization of opioid and dopamine systems in this nucleus, there is still much to be learned about the circuitry of positive reinforcing actions of opiates and psychomotor stimulants. Which tools and techniques will allow us to identify the specific neurons and circuits affected by a rewarding stimulus, whether that stimulus is a drug, a food pellet, or a sexual encounter? Which methods will help us understand how these neurons and circuits respond to the stimulus and how that reponse is involved in positive reinforcement? Below, we explore some of the technologies that have been useful in the past, as well as some that may be useful in the future, for answering these questions. However, it is important first to describe some of the difficulties involved in studying the brain substrates of drug reward.

To study the brain mechanisms involved in the negative reinforcing actions of drugs, researchers typically produce physical dependence in an animal by chronic administration of a drug and then examine the changes in the brain caused by either the chronic treatment or by withdrawal from the chronic treatment. Changes in the brain produced in such experiments can be quite robust. This strategy has therefore been very fruitful in suggesting neural systems that might be involved in physical dependence and withdrawal, and thus in the negative reinforcing actions of drugs. For example, recent studies have found changes in opioid peptides and opioid peptide mRNA after chronic treatment with drugs of abuse (Bronstein et al., 1990; Mochetti et al., 1989; Trujillo & Akil, 1990; Uhl et al., 1988), suggesting that alterations in endogenous opioid systems may be important in the negative reinforcing actions of drug withdrawal. In contrast, the study of cellular and molecular events involved in the positive reinforcing actions of drugs is particularly difficult for neuroscientists.

Since positive reinforcement occurs in the absence of chronic administration and is a discrete, time-limited event, researchers studying the brain mechanisms involved in the positive reinforcing actions of drugs must examine the brain after a single, acute injection of a drug. Effects of such treatment can be quite small and difficult to detect. Therefore, new techniques must be developed or old techniques must be adapted to allow researchers to better understand the brain substrates of positive reinforcement.

TOOLS AND TECHNIQUES FOR ANALYZING NEUROANATOMY AND CIRCUITRY

Techniques from several disciplines have contributed significantly to the identification of the neural systems and circuits involved in drug reward. Psychopharmacological studies, in particular, have been critical in determining the neurochemicals and the brain nuclei that mediate the positive reinforcing properties of drugs (Bozarth, 1987). As discussed above, these studies have revealed that endogenous opioid and dopamine systems within the limbic-motor reinforcement circuit, most notably the nACC, are important mediators of drug reward. Although this knowledge helps us understand the brain substrates of positive reinforcement and drug abuse at a relatively gross level, it is important to explore these systems at more refined levels of analysis. In particular, researchers would like to identify not only the nuclei involved in the positive reinforcing actions of drugs but also the specific neurons within these nuclei, the neurochemicals within these neurons, and the inputs and outputs of the neurons.

Histofluorescence, immunocytochemistry, and receptor autoradiography have long (at least by neuroscience research standards) been the mainstays of research into the neurochemical anatomy of the brain. Histofluorescent techniques have enabled the identification and visualization of specific monoamine neurons, whereas immunocytochemistry has made it possible to identify and visualize peptidergic neurons (Björklund & Hökfelt, 1983; Fig. 9-4). In a similar manner, autoradiography has been used to localize specific receptors (Björklund & Hökfelt, 1983; Figs. 9-5 and 9-6). The combination of these techniques with tract tracing has proven to be a powerful methodology for analyzing specific neurochemical circuits within the brain. Thus, these techniques have revealed much of what is currently known about the chemical neuroanatomy of the brain.

More recently, molecular biological techniques have expanded our ability to explore the neurochemistry and neuroanatomy of specific brain systems. The genes encoding many neurotransmitter precursors, biosynthetic enzymes, and receptors have been identified, and techniques have been developed for detecting their messenger RNA (mRNA) within specific brain regions. To date, there are several important molecular biological tools available for the study of brain substrates of drug reward. The mRNAs coding for the precursors of each of the three endogenous opioid peptide families have been cloned, as well as the mRNAs that code for the dopamine biosynthetic enzymes, tyrosine hydroxylase and dopa decarboxylase. In addition, the mRNAs coding for at least five dopamine receptors have been cloned, and the genes coding for the opioid receptors, although as yet unidentified, are the focus of intensive research. Thus, the tools for identifying endogenous opioid- and dopamine-*producing* cells (see Fig. 9-4), as well as those for identifying dopamine-*receptive* cells (see Fig. 9-5) are already in use, and the tools for identifying opioid-*receptive* cells may soon be available (1). Of particular interest is the ability to identify dopamine- and opioid-receptive neurons and their inputs and outputs, since these neurons should represent the first stage of integration for the positive reinforcing actions of psychomotor stimulants and opioids, and should point to the critical output pathways in the brain that mediate drug reward. Studies designed to localize dopamine- and opioid-receptor mRNA in the limbic-motor reinforcement circuit will therefore provide important data regarding the circuitry of drug reinforcement.

A valuable technique for the identification and localization of mRNA is in situ hybridization. This technique allows one to identify the cells that express a given gene, whether the gene is coding for a neuropeptide precursor, a biosynthetic enzyme, or a neurotransmitter receptor. Briefly, in situ hybridization involves incubation of tissue sections with radioactive- or enzymatic-labeled DNA or RNA probes complementary to the coding strand of the mRNA of interest. The probes base-pair specifically with the appropriate mRNA in the tissue, leaving a signal in the cells that synthesize that mRNA, thus allowing specific anatomical localization of this message. In addition, since expression of a given gene product is often reflected in levels of mRNA for that gene, this technique has also proven useful for the analysis of biosynthetic activity. However, changes in mRNA may not be relevant in an acute process, such as positive reinforcement, since reinforcement may influence a cell without affecting gene transcription. Moreover, even if changes in mRNA do occur, because they must emerge over an already existing pool to become detectable, there may be a considerable delay between gene transcriptional events and the ability to detect any changes in mRNA. Therefore, analysis of the regulation of neurotransmitter or receptor mRNA by in situ hybridization may be of limited value in the study of drug reward.

However, the use of in situ hybridization for localization of specific mRNAs, in combination with other techniques such as tract tracing, may prove to be quite valuable in the study of the circuitry of positive reinforcing actions of drugs. Using such strategies, Gerfen and co-workers (1990) recently found different neuropeptide expression, different projection targets, and different dopaminergic regulation of D_1- and D_2-receptive neurons in the dorsal striatum. Their study helps demonstrate the utility of combinations of molecular and neuroanatomical techniques in elucidating the neurochemical circuitry of the brain. Moreover, if the relationships observed by Gerfen et al. (1990) in the dorsal striatum are found to be similar in the nACC (or ventral striatum), the results may have important consequences regarding the circuitry of drug reward.

TOOLS AND TECHNIQUES FOR EXAMINING CHANGES IN NEURONAL ACTIVITY

A second approach to identifying the neurons involved in the reinforcing effects of drugs of abuse is to look for evidence of cell activation or inhibition in selected brain regions after treatment with the drug of interest. The most widely used neuroanatomical technique for studying cell activity has been the quantitative autoradiographic 2-deoxyglucose (2-DG) method (Björklund & Hökfelt, 1983). This method takes advantage of the fact that, in brain tissue, glucose utilization is an excellent marker of functional activity. By using a radioactively labeled, nonmetabolized analog of glucose, 2-deoxyglucose, one can measure rates of glucose utilization, and therefore functional activity, in specific brain regions at a discrete point in time. This technique has been useful in identifying changes in metabolic activity in the brain after a variety of experimental manipulations. Importantly, changes in functional activity have been observed in the limbic-motor reinforcement circuit after treatment with heroin, amphetamine, or cocaine (Porrino & Kornetsky, 1988; Trusk & Stein, 1988). However, since the 2-DG technique measures all changes produced by a drug, both direct and indirect and both specific and nonspecific, one cannot assume that the changes observed after treatment with a particular drug are specifically related to its reinforcing properties. Nonetheless, examination of the changes in functional activity produced in brain regions known to be involved in positive reinforcement may help identify the subregions, neurons, and circuits important in this action. Similar autoradiographic techniques have been used to study changes in second-messenger activation (Olds et al., 1989) and could be quite useful in identifying specific subsets of neurons activated or inhibited during drug-induced reward, i.e., those neurons that utilize a given second-messenger system.

The recent identification of transacting factors (sometimes called proto-oncogenes) has provided another tool for the study of short-term activation of neurons. Numerous transacting factors have already been identified, including c-fos, c-jun, CREB, c-myc, ras, and several others. These factors, which are activated by a variety of different processes that influence cellular activity, play an important role in the regulation of gene transcription. Because of their position in the biochemical cascade of cellular events—between second-messenger events and gene transcription—they have been called "third messengers." The most extensively studied of these factors, the proto-oncogene c-fos, has been demonstrated to exhibit a rapid (less than 15 minutes for c-fos mRNA; 1-4 hours for c-fos protein) and transient (less than 1 hour for c-fos mRNA) induction in response to experimental manipulation (Sagar et al., 1988). This induction is apparently indicative of a metabolically active neuron, in that increases in c-fos mRNA and protein occur in neurons known to be undergoing active depolarization or secretion (Sagar et al., 1988). As discussed above for 2-DG, the mapping of the induction of c-fos or other transacting factors after administration of a drug of interest can help identify the neurons and circuits involved in the actions of that drug. Initial studies on drugs of abuse have revealed interesting changes in the limbic-motor reinforcement circuit after treatment with amphetamine or cocaine (Graybiel et al., 1990). However, like 2-DG, induction of transacting factors is a relatively nonspecific signal. Therefore, induction of these factors in a given neuron by a drug does not necessarily indicate that the cell is involved in the rewarding actions of the drug—it merely indicates that the neuron has been activated. On the other hand, like second-messenger autoradiography, activation of transacting factors will identify specific subsets of neurons that are affected by the drug treatment, i.e., only neurons that use the particular transacting factor in their cellular machinery.

Although the above techniques, including 2-DG, second-messenger autoradiography, and transcription factor labeling, are relatively nonspecific indicators of cellular activity, by combining these techniques with other methods, such as in situ hybridization, one may be able to study changes produced by an experimental manipulation in specific neurons of interest, such as those synthesizing endogenous opioids or dopamine, or those synthesizing receptors for these neurotransmitters. Recent studies in the brain have demonstrated the elegance of such double-labeling methodology, in which induction of c-fos has been reported in opioid peptide neurons after a painful stimulus (Weihe et al., 1990).

Although the specificity of the above techniques may be helped by the use of double-labeling, it would be of considerable interest to use a more direct technique for assessing drug-induced changes in neurochemically identified neurons. However, most of the techniques currently available are unable to assess *both* acute cellular changes *and* neurochemistry. As discussed above, although 2-DG, second-messenger autoradiography, and transacting factor assays can measure acute cellular activity, they cannot identify the neurotransmitters or receptors produced by the neuron. In contrast, although in situ hybridization can identify the neurotransmitters and receptors of a particular neuron, it cannot easily assess acute cellular activity. In an attempt to establish relationships between cellular activation and gene expression in defined anatomical circuits, methods have been developed for the detection and quantitation of heteronuclear RNA (hnRNA) (Fremeau et al., 1986, 1989). Heteronuclear RNA for a given gene represents the primary transcripts and spliced transcripts of that gene, i.e., hnRNA is the first class of RNA to appear after transcription. With the splicing of introns in the nucleus, the hnRNA matures to mRNA and is transported to the cytoplasm. Heteronuclear RNA species are detected by intron probes that recognize sequences specific for unprocessed RNAs (Fig. 9-7). Given that splicing of introns occurs rapidly within the nucleus and that spliced introns are degraded rapidly, the lifetime of a given hnRNA species is generally quite short, and as such, it exists within the nucleus at quite low copy numbers at any given time (Lewin, 1990). If gene transcription is stimulated, hnRNA levels increase rapidly, generating a signal proportional to the extent of transcriptional activation of a given cell. Conversely, cessation of transcriptional stimulation should rapidly decrease detectable hnRNA levels. The timing of cellular events and the small existing pools of hnRNA render intronic in situ hybridization a potentially valuable tool for

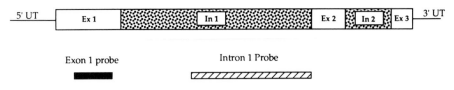

Figure 9-7. Structural organization of a "prototypical" gene, possessing three exons and two introns. Exons are represented in mature mRNA, whereas introns are spliced out in the cell nucleus and thus are present only in nuclear hnRNA form. The bars beneath exon 1 (exon 1 probe) and intron 1 (intron 1 probe) illustrate points where exon (mRNA) and intron (hnRNA) probes may be effectively designed. For exon probes, it is desirable to generate probes against a region of the protein-coding domain that is free of sequences that are highly homologous to sequences present in other genes, e.g., transmembrane-spanning domains of membrane receptors, DNA binding domains of steroid receptors. For intron probes, the sequence utilized should be contained wholly within the intron and should be free of repetitive DNA sequences. 5'-UT, 5' untranslated domain; 3'-UT, 3' untranslated domain.

accurate assessment of the relationship between onset of a stimulus of inter-rest, such as drug administration, and activation of genes responsive to that stimulus.

Application of this method to the study of dynamic CNS processes is still in its infancy. In our laboratory, we have begun to characterize the intronic in situ method by utilizing endocrine (POMC) and neuronal (vasopressin) model systems. As can be seen in Figure 9-8, proopiomelanocortin hnRNA can be reliably localized to intermediate and anterior lobe cells of the pituitary gland. Utilizing a nonradioactive in situ protocol, localization of the signal generated by the intron probe can be localized to the nucleus of POMC cells. In contrast, exon probe labeling is densest in the cell cytoplasm, in accordance with the predominantly extranuclear localization of mature mRNA. Initial regulatory studies performed in our laboratory demonstrate the utility of intronic in situ hybridization as a tool for examining rapid changes in neuronal gene expression in response to experimental manipulation. Using a traditional stimulus for magnocellular vasopressin neurons (e.g., acute salt loading), we can detect changes in vasopressin hnRNA levels (two- to threefold) within 30 minutes of an injection of 2M saline. In contrast, mRNA levels are not significantly altered until 2 hours after an acute salt load, further demonstrating that acute changes in gene transcription are difficult to detect at the level of mature message. The ability to detect rapid changes in gene activation (operationally defined as a change in hnRNA) in response to an appropriate stimulus, coupled with an obvious delay in the ability to detect such changes in gene expression as changes in mRNA levels, points to the importance of the intronic in situ hybridization technique as a means of assessing conditions promoting rapid activation in neuronal systems.

The potential for intronic in situ hybridization as a tool for the study of neuronal regulatory processes is great. However, several caveats should be acknowledged. First, to date, intronic in situ hybridization has been applied to

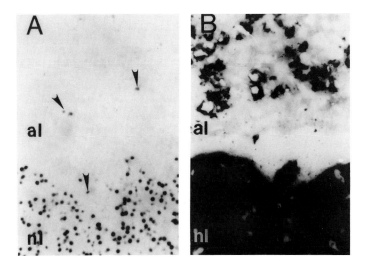

Figure 9-8. Photomicrographs showing hybridization with digoxigenin-labeled proopiomelanocortin intron A (**A**) and exon III (**B**) probes in the anterior (al) and neurointermediate (nl) lobes of the rat pituitary gland. Note the punctate appearance of POMC intron A in the anterior and neurointermediate lobes (**A**), consistent with its localization to the cell nucleus. The exon probe, in contrast, primarily labels the cell cytoplasm (**B**), consistent with the abundance of mRNA in this cell compartment. Note the greater density of labeling utilizing the exon probe. From Schäfer et al. (1990) with permission of the publisher.

systems containing considerable resting pools of mRNA (vasopressin, POMC), which may reflect high resting rates of gene transcription. When this method is applied to molecules that are present in small quantities, there may be relatively difficult detection problems. Second, many genes contain multiple introns, which are almost certainly spliced at different rates (Lewin, 1990). Thus, depending on the intron selected for probing, one may hybridize to a more or less stable form of hnRNA. If known (and if possible), it is ideal to work with the most rapidly spliced intron. This form constitutes the shortest-lived nuclear transcript and thus provides a better estimate of actual transcription rate. Third, it is important to carefully consider the potential for alternative splicing when using this method. Many genes have multiple mRNA forms resulting from multiple intron splicing schemes. In other words, what is an intron in one cell may be part of an exon in another. Therefore, it is important to carefully localize all intron signals to nerve cell nuclei to ensure that one is actually assessing hnRNA, rather than or in addition to mRNA.

The technique of intronic in situ hybridization, if found to be as useful as it promises, will allow researchers to characterize the activation of specific genes, in specific neurons, along particular anatomical circuits, in relatively rapid time frames. The ability to visualize rapid, specific, cellular changes in this manner will bring the field of chemical neuroanatomy into the realm of acute events. This method could therefore prove to be quite useful in analyzing the brain circuitry of discrete events, such as positive reinforcement.

SUMMARY AND CONCLUSIONS

In this chapter, we discussed the importance of positive reinforcement in the self-administration of drugs of abuse and described the limbic-motor reinforcement circuit—a brain circuit that seems to be critically involved in rewarding effects of opiates and psychomotor stimulants. This circuitry may also be important in the rewarding effects of other drugs of abuse, as well as other positive reinforcing stimuli, such as food, water, and social interactions. The ventral tegmental area, nucleus accumbens, hypothalamus, prefrontal cortex, and hippocampus are the primary components of this circuit, with the nucleus accumbens playing a particularly central role. Opiates act on this circuit by binding to opioid receptors, mimicking the endogenous opioid peptides, whereas psychomotor stimulants act by facilitating dopaminergic neurotransmission. Opiates and psychomotor stimulants may produce their reinforcing actions in the nucleus accumbens and perhaps in other components of this circuit by serving a "gating" or "amplifying" function, increasing the ability of reward-related stimuli to gain access to motor output pathways.

Our focus on positive reinforcement is not meant to suggest that it is the only factor or even the most critical factor in drug abuse by humans. Indeed, many factors contribute to the compulsive use of drugs by an individual. It will be important to understand each of these factors both individually and collectively before we can understand fully the phenomenon of drug abuse. Yet, since positive reinforcement is an important factor common to drugs of abuse, and is readily observable and quantifiable both in experimental animals and humans, the study of drug reward has proven to be an important area of research in the study of drug abuse.

Although psychopharmacological studies have permitted the gross identification of neurotransmitters and brain nuclei important in the rewarding properties of drugs, these studies have not had the resolution necessary for elucidating the "microanatomy" and "microcircuitry" of drug reward; they have thus far been unable to identify the specific reward-responsive neurons in the brain and their critical inputs and outputs. The behavioral pharmacologists have, however, provided an excellent foundation on which to proceed in the study of the brain systems involved in drug abuse. As stated by Koob and Bloom (1988), "It is time for the cellular and molecular analyses to exploit the spoils of these studies of behavior to identify the potentially critical cell types, locations, and molecular mechanisms for reinforcing effects of dependent drugs." In this chapter we attempted to identify some of the tools and techniques that have proven useful and some that may be useful in the future for identifying the specific neural circuitry of drug reinforcement. Methodologies that combine measures of cellular activity and/or neurochemistry with tract-tracing are of particular value in this area. Intronic in situ hybridization seems to be an especially promising technique for identifying the cells and circuits involved in drug reward, as well as other behaviors and functions.

An important issue that we did not address in this chapter is the potential role of individual differences in neuroanatomy and neurochemistry in the compulsive use of drugs. It is evident from reports on humans, and is becoming increasingly evident in animal studies, that some individuals are more inclined to self-administer drugs than others. Is the neuroanatomy or the neurochemistry of these individuals different from those who are not predisposed to self-administer? Recent studies have demonstrated that the behavioral response to amphetamine or to stress is quite different in animals that self-administer amphetamine from those that do not (Deminiere et al., 1989), suggesting that the brain systems mediating these effects may also be different. Will we someday have the ability to identify individuals who are at risk for drug abuse? By gaining a more complete understanding of the neurochemistry and neuroanatomy of the reinforcing actions of drugs of abuse, we may be able not only to answer these questions but also to more adequately prevent and treat the compulsive use of drugs.

ACKNOWLEDGMENTS

We would like to thank Dr. J.L. Olds for helpful comments and Drs. L. Fox and R. Alpert for their valuable perspective.

Note
1. Since the original submission of this chapter, two groups have independently isolated clones for a delta opioid receptor (Evans et al. (1992). *Science, 258,* 1952-1955; Kieffer et al. (1992). *Proc. Natl. Acad. Sci. USA 89,* 12048-12052). Identification of other opioid receptors will undoubtedly soon follow.

REFERENCES

Akil, H., Watson, S.J., Young, E., Lewis, M.E., Khachaturian, H., & Walker, J.M. (1984). Endogenous opioids: Biology and function. *Annu. Rev. Neurosci., 7,* 233-255.

Bechara, A., & van der Kooy, D. (1989). The tegmental pedunculopontine nucleus: A brain-stem output of the limbic system critical for the conditioned place preferences produced by morphine and amphetamine. *J. Neurosci., 9,* 3400-3409.

Björklund, A., & Hökfelt, T. (Eds.). (1983). *Methods in chemical neuroanatomy.* New York: Elsevier.

Bozarth, M.A. (Ed.). (1987). *Methods of assessing the reinforcing properties of abused drugs.* New York: Springer-Verlag.

Bronstein, D.M., Przewlocki, R., & Akil, H. (1990). Effects of morphine treatment on pro-opiomelanocortin systems in rat brain. *Brain Res., 519,* 102-111.

Bunzow, J.R., Van Tol, H.H.M., Grandy, D.K., Albert, P., Salon, J., Christie, M., Machida, C.A., Neve, K.A., & Civelli, O. (1988). Cloning and expression of a rat D_2 dopamine receptor cDNA. *Nature, 336,* 783-787.

Clarke, P.B.S. (1990). Mesolimbic dopamine activation—the key to nicotine reinforcement? In G. Bock & J. Marsh (Eds.), *The biology of nicotine dependence* (pp. 153-168). New York: Wiley.

Corrigal, W.A., & Linseman, M.A. (1988). Conditioned place preference produced by intra-hippocampal morphine. *Pharmacol. Biochem. Behav., 30,* 787-789.

Dearry, A., Gingrich, J.A., Falardeau, P., Fremeau, R.T., Bates, M.D., & Caron, M.G. (1990). Molecular cloning and expression of the gene for a human D_1 dopamine receptor. *Nature, 347,* 72-76.

Deminiere, J.M., Piazza, P.V., Le Moal, M., & Simon, H. (1989). Experimental approach to individual vulnerability to psychostimulant addiction. *Neurosci. Biobehav. Rev., 13,* 141-148.

Di Chiara, G., & Imperato, A. (1988). Drugs abused by humans preferentially increase synaptic dopamine concentrations in the mesolimbic system of freely moving rats. *Proc. Natl. Acad. Sci. USA, 85,* 5274-5278.

Engel, J., Oreland, L., Ingvar, D.H., Pernow, B., Rössner, S., & Pellborn, L.A. (Eds.). (1987). *Brain reward systems and abuse.* New York: Raven Press.

Fallon, J.H., & Loughlin, S.E. (1987). Monoamine innervation of cerebral cortex and a theory of the role of monoamines in cerebral cortex and basal ganglia. In E.G. Jones & A. Peters (Eds.), *Cerebral cortex* (pp. 41-127). New York: Plenum.

Fibiger, H.C., & Phillips, A.G. (1986). Reward, motivation, cognition: Psychobiology of mesotelencephalic dopamine systems. In V. B. Mouncastle, F.E. Bloom, & S.R. Geiger (Eds.), *Handbook of physiology: The nervous system IV* (pp. 647-675). Bethesda, MD: American Physiological Society.

Fremeau, R.T., Lundblad, J.R., Pritchett, D.B., Wilcox, J.N., & Roberts, J.L. (1986). Regulation of pro-opiomelanocortin gene transcription in individual cell nuclei. *Science, 234,* 1265-1269.

Fremeau, R.T., Autelitano, D.J., Blum, M., Wilcox, J., & Roberts, J.L. (1989). Intervening sequence-specific in situ hybridization: Detection of the pro-opiomelanocortin gene primary transcript in individual neurons. *Mol. Brain Res., 6,* 197-201.

Gerfen, C.R., Engber, T.M., Mahan, L.C., Susel, Z., Chase, T.N., Monsma, F.J., & Sibley, D.R. (1990). D_1 and D_2 dopamine receptor-regulated gene expression of striatonigral and striatopallidal neurons. *Science, 250,* 1429-1432.

Glickman, S.E., & Schiff, B.B. (1967). A biological theory of reinforcement. *Psychol. Rev., 74,* 81-109.

Goldberg, S.R., & Stolerman, I.P. (Eds.). (1986). *Behavioral analysis of drug dependence.* Orlando, FL: Academic Press.

Goldstein, A. (Ed.). (1989). *Molecular and cellular aspects of the drug addictions.* New York: Springer-Verlag.

Graybiel, A.M., Moratalla, R., & Robertson, H.A. (1990). Amphetamine and cocaine induce drug-specific activation of the c-fos gene in striosome-matrix compartments and limbic subdivisions of the striatum. *Proc. Natl. Acad. Sci. USA, 87,* 6912-6916.

Heimer, L., Zahm, D.S., Churchill, L., Kalivas, P.W., & Wohltman, C. (1991). Specificity in the projection patterns of accumbal core and shell in the rat. *Neuroscience, 41,* 89-125.

Herz, A., & Shippenberg, T.S. (1989). Neurochemical aspects of addiction: Opioids and other drugs of abuse. In A. Goldstein (Ed.), *Molecular and cellular aspects of the drug addictions* (pp. 111-141). New York: Springer-Verlag.

Kalivas, P.W., & Nemeroff, C.B. (Eds.). (1988). *The mesocorticolimbic dopamine system.* New York: New York Academy of Sciences.

Koob, G.F., & Bloom, F.E. (1988). Cellular and molecular mechanisms of drug dependence. *Science, 242,* 715-723.

Lewin, B. (1990). *Genes IV.* New York: Oxford.

Liebman, J.M., & Cooper, S.J. (Eds.). (1989). *The neuropharmacological basis of reward.* New York: Oxford University Press.

Mansour, A., Khachaturian, H., Lewis, M.E., Akil, H., & Watson, S.J. (1987). Autoradiographic differentiation of mu, delta and kappa opioid receptors in the rat forebrain and midbrain. *J. Neurosci., 7,* 2445-2464.

Mansour, A., Meador-Woodruff, J.H., Bunzow, J.R., Civelli, O., Akil, H., & Watson,

S.J. (1990). Localization of D_2 receptor mRNA and D_1 and D_2 receptor binding in the rat brain and pituitary: An in situ hybridization-receptor autoradiographic analysis. *J. Neurosci., 10,* 2587-2600.

Meador-Woodruff, J.H., Mansour, A., Bunzow, J.R., Van Tol, H.H.M., Watson, S.J., & Civelli, O. (1989). Distribution of D_2 dopamine receptor mRNA in rat brain. *Proc. Natl. Acad. Sci. USA, 86,* 7625-7628.

Mochetti, I., Ritter, A., & Costa, E. (1989). Down-regulation of pro-opiomelanocortin synthesis and beta-endorphin utilization in hypothalamus of morphine-tolerant rats. *J. Mol. Neurosci., 1,* 33-38.

Mogenson, G.J., Jones, D.L., & Yim, C.Y. (1980). From motivation to action: Functional interface between the limbic system and the motor system. *Prog. Neurobiol., 14,* 69-97.

Olds, J.L., Anderson, M.L., McPhie, D.L., Staten, L.D., & Alkon, D.L. (1989). Imaging of memory-specific changes in the distribution of protein kinase C in the hippocampus. *Science, 245,* 866-869.

Porrino, L.J., & Kornetsky, C. (1988). The effects of cocaine on local cerebral metabolic activity. In D. Clouet, K. Asghar, & R. Brown (Eds.), *Mechanisms of cocaine abuse and toxicity: NIDA research monograph 88* (pp. 92-106). Rockville, MD: National Institute on Drug Abuse.

Sagar, S.M., Sharp, F.R., & Curran, T. (1988). Expression of c-fos protein in brain: Metabolic mapping at the cellular level. *Science, 240,* 1328-1331.

Schäfer, M.K.-H., Herman, J.P., & Watson, S.J. (1990). Rapid detection of POMC heteronuclear RNA in individual pituitary cells by in situ hybridization. In J.M. van Ree, A.H. Mulder, V.M. Wiegant, & T.B. van Wimersma Griedanus (Eds.), *New leads in opioid research* (pp. 307-309). New York: Elsevier Science.

Simon, H., & Le Moal, M. (1988). Mesencephalic dopamine neurons: Role in the general economy of the brain. *Ann. N.Y. Acad. Sci., 537,* 235-253.

Skinner, B.F. (1938). *The behavior of organisms: An experimental analysis.* New York: Appleton.

Smith, J.E., & Lane, J.D. (Eds.). (1983). *The neurobiology of opiate reward processes.* New York: Elsevier.

Sokoloff, P., Giros, B., Martres, M.-P., Bouthenet, M.-L., & Schwartz, J.-C. (1990). Molecular cloning and characterization of a novel dopamine receptor (D_3) as a target for neuroleptics. *Nature, 347,* 146-151.

Spyraki, C., Nomikos, G.G., Galanopoulou, P., & Daïfotis, Z. (1988). Drug-induced place preferences in rats with 5,7-dihydroxytryptamine lesions of the nucleus accumbens. *Behav. Brain Res., 29,* 127-134.

Stein, L., & Belluzzi, J.D. (1989). Cellular investigations of behavioral reinforcement. *Neurosci. Biobehav. Rev., 13,* 69-80.

Sunahara, R.K., Niznik, H.B., Weiner, D.M., Stormann, T.M., Brann, M.R., Kennedy, J.L., Gelernter, J.E., Rozmahel, R., Yang, Y., Israel, Y., Seeman, P., & O'Dowd, B.F. (1990). Human dopamine D_1 receptor encoded by an intronless gene on chromosome 5. *Nature, 347,* 80-83.

Sunahara, R.K., Guan, H.-C., O'Dowd, B.F., Seeman, P., Laurier, L.G., Ng, G., George, S.R., Torchia, J., Van Tol, H.H.M., & Niznik, H. (1991). Cloning of the gene for a human dopamine D_5 receptor with higher affinity for dopamine than D_1. *Nature, 350,* 614-619.

Trujillo, K. A., & Akil, H. (1990). Pharmacological regulation of striatal prodynorphin peptides. *Prog. Clin. Biol. Res., 328,* 223-226.

Trusk, T.C., & Stein, E.A. (1988). Effects of heroin and cocaine on brain activity in rats using [1-^{14}C]octanoate as a fast functional tracer. *Brain Res., 438,* 61-66.

Uhl, G.R., Ryan, J.P., & Schwartz, J.P. (1988). Morphine alters preproenkephalin gene expression. *Brain Res., 458,* 391-397.

Van Tol, H.H.M., Bunzow, J.R., Guan, H.-C., Sunahara, R.K., Seeman, P., Niznik, H.B., & Civelli, O. (1991). Cloning of the gene for a human dopamine D_4 receptor with high affinity for the antipsychotic clozapine. *Nature, 350,* 610-614.

Walters, J.R., Bergstrom, D.A., Carlson, J.H., Chase, T.N., & Braun, A.R. (1987). D_1 dopamine receptor activation required for postsynaptic expression of D_2 agonist effects. *Science, 236,* 719-722.

Watson, S.J., Trujillo, K.A., Herman, J.P., & Akil, H. (1989). Neuroanatomical and neurochemical substrates of drug-seeking behavior: Overview and future directions. In A. Goldstein (Ed.), *Molecular and cellular aspects of the drug addictions* (pp. 29-91). New York: Springer-Verlag.

Weihe, E., Iadarola, M.J., Nohr, D., Müller, S., Millan, M.J., Yanaihara, N., Stein, C., & Herz, A. (1990). Sustained expression and colocalization of proenkephalin and prodynorphin opioids and c-fos protein in dorsal horn neurons revealed in arthritic rats. In J.M. van Ree, A.H. Mulder, V.M. Wiegant, & T.B. van Wimersma Greidanus (Eds.), *New leads in opioid research* (pp. 92-94). New York: Elsevier Science.

White, N.M., & Franklin, K.B.J. (Eds.). (1989). Special issue: The neural basis of reward and reinforcement. *Neurosci. Biobehav. Rev., 13,* 59-186.

Wise, R.A., & Bozarth, M.A. (1987). A psychomotor stimulant theory of addiction. *Psychol. Rev., 94,* 469-492.

Zhou, Q.-Y., Grandy, D.K., Thambi, L, Kushner, J.A., Van Tol, H.H.M., Cone, R., Pribnow, D., Salon, J., Bunzow, J.R., & Civelli, O. (1990). Cloning and expression of human and rat D_1 dopamine receptors. *Nature, 347,* 76-80.

10

Cellular Basis of Opioid Action

R.A. NORTH

Whether opioids are administered in a therapeutic or a drug abuse environment, they ultimately exert their effects on cells by binding to receptors in the surface membrane of cells. Three main types of receptor have been distinguished on nerve cells—mu, delta, and kappa; these differ in their distribution throughout the nervous system and among species (Mansour et al., 1988). It is generally thought that the most widely abused opioids, such as morphine, act fairly selectively at mu receptors.

MOLECULAR CONCERNS

The structure of the receptors is not known, but there is considerable indirect evidence that they belong to a family of cell surface receptors that couple to and activate guanosine 5′-triphosphate-binding proteins (G-proteins). Other members of the receptor family include receptors for noradrenaline (α_2), 5-hydroxytryptamine (5-HT$_{1A}$), dopamine (D$_2$), acetylcholine (muscarinic M$_2$), adenosine (A$_1$), gamma-aminobutyric acid (GABA$_B$), and somatostatin (North, 1989a and b). The activated G-protein serves as a local intracellular messenger; the three best known molecular targets for the G-protein-activated by the opioids are potassium channels (opened), calcium channels (closed), and adenylyl cyclase (inhibited).

These molecular targets are membrane proteins situated relatively close to the receptors themselves. When a patch of membrane is isolated at the tip of a glass micropipette, opioids preserve their ability to open potassium channels within the membrane patch (Miyake et al., 1989). Thus, other cytoplasmic constituents are not required for the activated receptor to open the potassium channel, although as mentioned above, a G-protein couples the receptor to the channel. It is generally thought, although not explicitly shown, that the coupling from opioid receptors to calcium channels and adenylyl cyclase is organized similarly (Fig. 10-1).

This work was supported by grants from the U.S. Department of Health and Human Services (DAO3160, DAO3161, and MH40416).

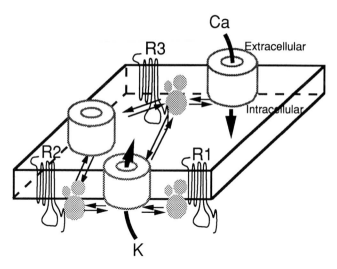

Figure 10-1. How activation of several membrane receptors might open the same potassium channel. R1, R2, and R3 represent distinct receptors, one of which would be an opioid receptor. The hatched symbols represent trimeric G-proteins (same or different). Three ion channels are depicted, including a potassium-selective channel (opened by receptor activation) and a voltage-dependent calcium-selective channel (closed by receptor activation).

Individual nerve cells usually express on their surface more than one member of this family of receptors. Even an excised patch of membrane in which only one potassium channel is active can have, for example, opioid, noradrenaline, and somatostatin receptors. Activation of any of these receptors by the appropriate agonists causes an increased opening of the potassium channel (Shen et al., 1990). This convergence of transmitter action onto a single ion channel is thought to account for similarities often observed in the overall pharmacological profile of action of the members of this receptor family. For example, somatostatin analogs, baclofen, and α_2 receptor agonists all have analgesic actions at the spinal level. The therapeutic use of clonidine to treat some symptoms of opiate withdrawal probably reflects the fact that the neurons responsible for the symptoms (preganglionic sympathetic for the most part) express both α_2 and mu receptors.

CELLULAR ACTIONS

When opioids open potassium channels, neuron firing is inhibited. Potassium ions leave the neuron, increasing the intracellular negativity (hyperpolarization). The hyperpolarization directly affects other membrane channels that are sensitive to membrane voltage. Spontaneously firing neurons, such as the noradrenaline cells of the locus ceruleus, slow their rate of firing. Cells excited by synaptic inputs, such as neurons in the dorsal horn of the spinal cord responding to painful stimulation, fire less vigorously. Because this inhibition of firing by opioids acting at mu receptors is widespread throughout the mammalian nervous system (Duggan & North, 1984; North, 1992) it is generally thought to be the action that accounts for most of the immediate behavioral effects of acutely administered opioid drugs. A similar effect has been shown to result from activation of delta receptors (North, 1992).

The effects of reducing current through the closing of voltage-dependent calcium channels are less well understood because many cellular mechanisms depend on calcium entry; these mechanisms include electrical signaling, exocytosis, and gene regulation. The inhibition of calcium entry, which has been described for mu, delta, and kappa receptors, has been studied in nerve cell bodies (North, 1992), but it is often suggested that a similar action occurring at nerve terminals would result in less transmitter being released. The ability of opioids to reduce transmitter release from a variety of mammalian nerves, which could be a possible mechanism (North & Williams, 1983), is well known. Such a reduction in transmitter release could account for the selective block of some pathways (for example, those involved in pain transmission) while sparing others.

The consequences to the cell of the inhibition of adenylyl cyclase are also manifold. The resulting reduction in levels of cyclic adenosine $3',5'$-monophosphate should reduce the activity of protein kinase A, which would change the phosphorylation state of many proteins, as well as reduce transcription of several genes. These effects of adenylyl cyclase inhibition (Guitart et al., 1989; see Chapter 4) seem to be unrelated to the ability of opioids to open potassium channels and close calcium channels, and they might contribute to some of the changes in sensitivity to opioids that occur with long-term use.

SYSTEMIC CONSIDERATIONS

The overall effect on behavior of the administration of opioids depends primarily on two factors: which neurons actually have the opioid receptors on their surface (and are therefore inhibited) and how different sets of neurons are connected together synaptically. One behavior that has been studied extensively relates to the rewarding effects of opioids.

Dopamine-containing neurons of the midbrain are important for the reinforcing actions of drugs of abuse (Fibiger & Philips, 1986; Liebman & Cooper, 1989). Animals will work to obtain opioids that are applied into the dopamine cell body region of the ventral tegmental area (Koob & Bloom, 1988; Wise & Bozarth, 1987; see Chapter 22). It is proposed that the reinforcing effect of opioids results from an excitation of dopamine cells, with an increased release in the nucleus accumbens (Di Chiara & Imperato, 1988).

It is not obvious how the primary cellular actions discussed above—opening potassium channels, closing calcium channels, and inhibiting adenylyl cyclase—result in an excitation of neurons. In fact, mu receptors are not present on the midbrain dopamine-containing cells (Dilts & Kalivas, 1989); instead, they are present on a group of GABA-containing interneurons interspersed

to accumbens

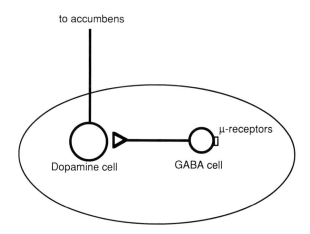

Figure 10-2. How dopamine cells of the ventral tegmental area are excited by disinhibition. Within the ventral tegmental area are dopamine-containing cells, which project to limbic targets such as the nucleus accumbens and GABA-containing cells. Release of GABA from the latter cells inhibits firing of dopamine cells. Mu-opioid receptors are on the GABA-containing cells. Activation of these receptors by opioids results in inhibition of firing of GABA cells, less GABA release, and excitation of the dopamine cells.

among the dopamine-containing cells. Electrophysiological studies show that potassium channels in these interneurons are opened by opioids, resulting in hyperpolarization and reduced frequency of firing (Johnson & North, 1990). Under normal circumstances, these interneurons release the inhibitory transmitter GABA onto the nearby dopamine cells. When hyperpolarized by opioids, they fire less frequently, and therefore release less GABA onto the dopamine cells; the dopamine cells thus fire more rapidly (Fig. 10-2). Neurons in other regions of the brain have also been shown to be excited by opioids by such an indirect mechanism—the removal of ongoing inhibition, which is termed disinhibition. These neurons include the pyramidal cells of the hippocampus and perhaps a group of descending 5-HT containing neurons that are involved in the control of pain input to the spinal cord.

CONCLUSIONS

The acute cellular actions of opioids result from inhibition of the firing of nerve cells by a molecular mechanism fundamentally similar to that used by several other neurotransmitters. The particular profile of actions observed in a given species depends on which cells express the receptors. The positive reinforcing action of the opioids seems to result from an excitation of mesolimbic dopamine-containing neurons, occurring secondarily through inhibition of local inhibitory interneurons.

REFERENCES

Di Chiari, G., & Imperato, A. (1988). Drugs abused by humans preferentially increase synaptic dopamine concentrations in the mesolimbic system of freely moving rats. *Proc. Natl. Acad. Sci. U.S.A., 85,* 5274-5278.

Dilts, R.P., & Kalivas, P.W. (1989). Autoradiographic localization of μ-opioid and neurotensin receptors within the mesolimbic dopamine system. *Brain Res., 488,* 311-327.

Duggan, A.W., & North, R.A. (1984). Electrophysiology of opioids. *Pharmacol. Rev., 35,* 219-281.

Fibiger, H.C., & Phillips, A.G. (1986). Reward, motivation, cognition: Psychobiology of mesotelencephalic dopamine systems. In *Handbook of Physiology:* Sect. 1, Vol. IV (pp. 647-676). Bethesda, MD: American Physiological Society.

Guitart, X., & Nestler, E.J. (1989). Identification of morphine- and cyclic AMP-regulated phosphoproteins (MARPPs) in the locus coeruleus and other regions of rat brain: Regulation by acute and chronic morphine. *J. Neurosci., 9,* 4371-4387.

Johnson, S.W., & North, R.A. (1990). Electrophysiological effects of opioids on neurons in the ventral tegmental area. *Soc. Neurosci. Abst., 16,* 1027.

Koob, G.F., & Bloom, F.E. (1988). Cellular and molecular mechanisms of drug dependence. *Science, 242,* 715-723.

Liebman, J.M., & Cooper, S.J. (1989). *The neuropharmacological basis of reward.* New York: Oxford University Press.

Mansour, A., Khachaturian, H., Lewis, M.E., Akil, H., & Watson, S.J. (1988). Anatomy of CNS opioid receptors. *Trends Neurosci., 11,* 308-314.

Miyake, M., Christie, M.J., & North, R.A. (1989). Single potassium channels opened by opioids in rat locus coeruleus neurons. *Proc. Natl. Acad. Sci. U.S.A., 86,* 3419-3422.

North, R.A. (1989a). Neurotransmitters and their receptors: From the clone to the clinic. *Sem. Neurosci., 1,* 81-90.

North, R.A. (1989b). Drug receptors and the inhibition of nerve cells. *Br. J. Pharmacol., 98,* 13-28.

North, R.A. (1992). Opioid actions on membrane ion channels. In A. Herz, E. Simon, H. Akil (Eds.), *Handbook on experimental pharmacology.* Berlin: Springer-Verlag.

North, R.A., & Williams, J.T. (1983). How do opiates inhibit transmitter release? *Trends Neurosci., 6,* 337-339.

Shen, K.-Z., Surprenant, A., & North, R.A. (1990). Somatostatin, opioids and α_2 receptor agonists increase activity of potassium channels and decrease activity of calcium channels in excised membrane patches. *Soc. Neurosci. Abst., 16,* 361.

Wise, R.A., & Bozarth, M.A. (1987). A psychomotor stimulant theory of addiction. *Psychol. Rev., 94,* 469-492.

11

Cellular Mechanisms of Cocaine Action: Effects in Brain Slice Preparations

THOMAS V. DUNWIDDIE AND MARK S. BRODIE

Although effective pharmacological strategies for limiting or terminating self-administration of cocaine are beginning to be developed (see Chapters 27–29), by and large these strategies do not seem to have significantly reduced cocaine consumption. Further refining pharmacological strategies for limiting substance abuse requires a better understanding of the effects of drugs such as cocaine at the cellular level. If we can link specific pharmacological properties of cocaine and its cellular actions in discrete brain regions to its reinforcing effects, then there is a possibility that we can selectively inhibit drug self-administration by disrupting the mechanisms underlying the response.

There are at least four distinct pharmacological actions of cocaine that could result in reinforcing effects. Cocaine blocks the transport of monoamines by interacting with the high-affinity dopamine (DA), norepinephrine (NE), and serotonin (5-HT) uptake mechanisms, and in addition, it is also an effective local anesthetic agent. Behavioral and biochemical studies have identified which potential mechanisms of action are most important from the drug reinforcement standpoint. The multiple regression analysis carried out by Kuhar's group (Ritz & Kuhar, 1989; Ritz et al., 1987), which is probably the most systematic attempt to address this issue, has done much to clarify the role played by the dopamine transporter in pharmacological reward. These studies have suggested that, *within the group of cocaine and structurally related compounds,* the ability to inhibit or bind to the DA transporter is most closely linked to reinforcement, whereas inhibition of the NE transporter seems to be unrelated and inhibition of the 5-HT transporter is, if anything, negatively related to reinforcement.

The multiple actions of cocaine make it difficult to predict what its effects should be within any given brain region, since they depend on the distribution within that region of monoamine transporters and receptors. Electrophysiologi-

This work was supported by grants from the National Institute on Drug Abuse (DA 02702) and the Veterans Administration Medical Research Service.

cal studies can be used to link the cellular actions of such drugs as cocaine to altered patterns of overall activity. Although 10 years ago we knew virtually nothing about the electrophysiological actions of cocaine on the nervous system, within the past 5 years numerous studies have helped define the specific actions of cocaine in reward-relevant brain structures. Although linking specific electrophysiological actions to reward per se is a difficult task, these types of studies nevertheless are beginning to bridge the gap between the known cellular actions of cocaine and the psychological constructs of reward or reinforcement.

Two basic types of electrophysiological studies have contributed significantly to our understanding of the pharmacological effects of cocaine. First, the recent development of techniques for maintaining slices of brain tissue in a physiologically viable state has permitted quantitative pharmacological studies of cocaine's effects, which have contributed markedly to our understanding of the cellular mechanisms by which cocaine exerts its effects. Because the region being studied is isolated in the slice preparation, the indirect effects of cocaine mediated via other brain regions, or even more indirectly by changes in heart rate, blood pressure, etc., are completely eliminated. In addition, intracellular recording and voltage clamping of neurons are feasible in brain slices and can provide much more specific information about the ways in which cocaine can alter neuronal activity. Finally, a variety of experimental parameters can be altered in a brain slice preparation that cannot be varied in vivo (e.g., temperature, ion concentrations, etc.), and such drugs as tetrodotoxin can be used that would be difficult to use in the intact animal.

Nevertheless, although we have gained much by this "divide and conquer" approach to the electrophysiological effects of cocaine, these studies do not provide sufficient information to enable us to predict what cocaine will do in an intact, freely moving animal. In some instances the activity of these brain regions is different in the slice and in vivo, and in any case much of the synaptic circuitry upon which cocaine probably acts is disrupted. For this reason, in vivo studies of the effects of cocaine in intact animals are just as important to our overall understanding of cocaine's actions as are the in vitro experiments, and in some cases they have provided results that would not have been predicted based solely upon the brain slice experiments. In particular, in vivo studies permit more direct comparisons between administration of pharmacologically reinforcing amounts of cocaine and physiological responses. In addition, both direct and indirect responses to cocaine can occur, and through appropriately designed experiments it is possible to determine to what extent each type of effect contributes to the overall action of the drug.

This chapter is not intended to serve as a comprehensive review of all of the electrophysiological studies of the effects of cocaine; rather we discuss in detail the results of in vitro studies that focus on the cellular bases for cocaine responses and attempt to determine whether there are general principles of cocaine action that can provide insights into the behavioral effects of this drug. The effects of cocaine in intact animals have been discussed in several recent reviews (Lakoski & Cunningham, 1988; Pitts & Marwah, 1988; White, 1990; see Chapter 12), some of which also deal with more specific aspects of cocaine's action (e.g., cocaine sensitization) that are not discussed in this chapter.

EFFECTS OF COCAINE IN MONOAMINE TARGET REGIONS

Hippocampus

Interactions of Cocaine with Exogenous NE
When we began to characterize the effects of cocaine in the hippocampal formation several years ago, virtually nothing was known about the electrophysiological effects of cocaine on the central nervous system, with the exception of a few EEG studies indicating that cocaine, like other local anesthetics, could increase the propensity of the hippocampus to show epileptiform activity (Lesse, 1980; Lesse & Collins, 1980; Lesse & Harper, 1985). In particular, no studies implicated inhibition of neurotransmitter uptake in any of the physiological actions of cocaine.

In our initial studies, we characterized the effects of superfused cocaine on the electrical activity of hippocampal brain slices. We observed that cocaine, as well as other NE uptake inhibitors, such as desipramine, imipramine, and phencyclidine (PCP), could potentiate the ability of NE to modulate evoked potentials in the CA1 region of the hippocampus, whereas equivalent concentrations of procaine and lidocaine had no such effect (Dunwiddie & Alford, 1987; Yasuda et al., 1984). Under normal conditions, the threshold for responses to bath superfusion with NE is approximately 5 μM, but in the presence of cocaine, the sensitivity to NE is increased approximately tenfold. The concentrations of cocaine that produced this effect are one to two orders of magnitude lower than those that elicited local anesthetic actions in the hippocampus (Fig. 11-1). The concentrations required to potentiate NE responses (threshold 300 nM, peak effect at 1 μM) are in the range that elicit pharmacological reward, whereas the conditions that elicit local anesthetic effects are in the range in which cocaine toxicity might be expected. This finding clearly does not establish whether the interactions between cocaine and NE relate to reinforcement, but it does suggest that self-administered concentrations of cocaine are sufficient to interact with noradrenergic systems.

Interactions of Cocaine with Endogenous NE
The preceding experiments demonstrated that cocaine could potentiate the actions of exogenous NE superfused over the brain slice. However, this effect is in many respects a nonphysiological response that probably bears little relation to the way in which neurotransmitter is normally released in the slice. For this reason, we recently characterized the interaction of cocaine and other uptake inhibitors with endogenously released NE. To do so, we used electrochemical rather than electrophysiological approaches to study endogenous NE. Under normal conditions, we and others have observed that there does not seem to be any tonic noradrenergic "tone" in the slice preparation, in that noradrenergic antagonists have no effect upon background activity. Further-

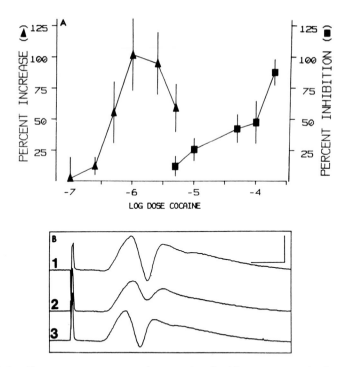

Figure 11-1. Dose-response curves for cocaine in hippocampus. **A,** Dose-response curves for the potentiating effects of cocaine on responses to 0.5 μM NE (*triangles* and *left axis*) and the local anesthetic effects of cocaine on the population spike amplitude (*squares*). Values shown are mean +/− SEM (N = 3-7 per point). **B,** Local anesthetic action of cocaine on the evoked population spike response (the downward-going spike on the positive waveform) from a single hippocampal slice. Each record is the average of three to four individual responses. The top record (1) was obtained during the predrug period, the middle trace (2) during superfusion with 50 μM cocaine, and the bottom trace (3) represents the population spike response after washout of cocaine. Calibration bars are 2 mV and 2 ms.

more, cocaine does not elicit noradrenergic responses in the absence of exogenous NE. This finding is perhaps not unexpected, since the NE terminals in the slice have been completely removed from their cell bodies of origin. However, even electrical stimulation in regions that contain noradrenergic fibers fails to elicit any kind of response mediated by noradrenergic receptors. The *only* condition under which we have been able to elicit such responses is when slices are superfused with indirectly acting noradrenergic agonists, such as tyramine (Mueller et al., 1982); the findings that noradrenergic nerve terminals still can take up NE and that they contain sufficient NE to elicit a postsynaptic response when released by tyramine suggest that the nerve terminals are viable, but that they are difficult to stimulate electrophysiologically.

For these reasons, we have used 35-μ carbon fiber electrochemical electrodes to measure the basal and K⁺-stimulated release of NE in hippocampal brain slices (Su et al., 1990). We observed that pretreatment of hippocampal slices with 10 to 50 μM cocaine markedly potentiates the amplitude of the increase in extracellular NE after K^+ superfusion. Cocaine pretreatment alone has no effect on the electrochemical baseline responses. In addition, cocaine does not seem to have any effect on the rate of recovery to baseline after the superfusion with K^+-containing buffer, suggesting that at least under these conditions, extracellular NE is being cleared by some process other than high-affinity uptake.

Local Anesthetic Actions in the Hippocampus

To gain a better understanding of other potential mechanisms through which cocaine might act, we also studied in greater detail its local anesthetic effects, which appear at somewhat higher concentrations (Yasuda et al., 1984; see Fig. 11-1). The threshold for direct inhibitory effects on synaptically evoked population spike responses is approximately 10 μM, and the EC_{50} values for different fiber populations range from approximately 50-125 μM. Because one of the symptoms of cocaine overdose is seizures and because other local anesthetics have proconvulsant effects as well, we determined whether the local anesthetic action of cocaine produced electrophysiological changes that would be consistent with a proconvulsant action. One proposed explanation for local anesthetic-induced excitatory effects is that they might interfere somewhat selectively with GABAergic inhibition. To examine this hypothesis, we stimulated excitatory and inhibitory pathways in the hippocampus and determined whether cocaine had a selective action on evoked inhibitory post-synaptic potentials (IPSPs). Although cocaine in rather high concentrations does reduce synaptic inhibition, it is at least as effective in blocking excitatory synaptic events (Dunwiddie et al., 1988). As another test, we determined the effects of cocaine on penicillin-induced interictal spiking, which has been used as an in vitro model for epilepsy (Dunwiddie, 1980; Mueller & Dunwiddie, 1983). However, cocaine invariably inhibits the rate of interictal spiking, regardless of the concentration tested (range: 5-100 μM; Dunwiddie et al., 1988).

Nucleus Accumbens

The nucleus accumbens (nACC), which receives significant 5-HT and DA innervation, was the site of another electrophysiological investigation of the effects of cocaine on a brain slice preparation by Uchimura and North (1990). The pharmacology in this nucleus is somewhat more complex, because it contains D_1, D_2, and 5-HT receptors that all mediate different responses. As with the hippocampal brain slice experiments, cocaine by itself does not have any indirect agonist properties at any of these receptors; superfusion with cocaine alone does not depolarize or hyperpolarize nACC neurons. Yet, cocaine *does* potentiate responses to exogenous DA and 5-HT, independently of the nature of the postsynaptic response. However, the concentrations of cocaine that were effective in this respect depend upon the neurotransmitter that was involved. The threshold concentration of cocaine for the potentiation of both D_1 and D_2 responses is approximately 1 μM, and the maximal effect is approximately a 40-times leftward shift in the dose-response curve for DA at 30 μM cocaine. The effects of 5-HT are potentiated to a significantly greater extent; the threshold of cocaine action is approximately 300 nM, and the maximal effect is an almost 120-times shift in the 5-HT dose-response curve.

Nucleus Prepositus Hypoglossi

The nucleus prepositus hypoglossi (PH) is a large brainstem nucleus that receives a dense 5-HT innervation from the raphe nuclei (Steinbusch, 1981), and electrical stimulation can evoke an IPSP in neurons within that area that is mediated by 5-HT (Bobker & Williams, 1991). As was found in the other monoaminergic target regions, cocaine (100 nM-10 μM) by itself has no direct effect on PH neurons that could be attributed to actions on serotonergic receptors. However, cocaine does potentiate responses to endogenous 5-HT released by stimulation of putative serotonergic synapses. The most pronounced effect is a change in the duration of the IPSP; the amplitude of the IPSP is also increased by cocaine concentrations below 1 μM, whereas at higher concentrations, the amplitude declines. Other 5-HT uptake inhibitors share these actions of cocaine, whereas local anesthetic drugs do not (Bobker & Williams, 1991). The concentration-response curve for 5-HT is shifted to the left by 10 μM cocaine, whereas the sensitivity to 8OH-DPAT, a 5-HT$_{1A}$ agonist that is *not* a substrate for uptake, is unaffected by cocaine (Bobker & Williams, 1991).

EFFECTS OF COCAINE IN MONOAMINE-CONTAINING REGIONS

Many of the initial studies of the effects of cocaine in intact animals focused on its action on monoamine-containing nuclei in the brain. The results of these studies have been remarkably consistent, both across laboratories and brain regions. In every region that has been examined to date, cocaine inhibits the rate of spontaneous firing of neurons, and it seems to do so by potentiating the effects of DA, NE, or 5-HT on autoreceptors. In the locus coeruleus, cocaine inhibits spontaneous firing, and this action is antagonized by the α_2 receptor antagonist piperoxane (Pitts & Marwah, 1986a, 1987a). Similarly, inhibition of dopamine-containing ventral tegmental area (VTA) and substantia nigra (SN) neurons is antagonized by haloperidol and sulpiride, which block dopamine D$_2$ autoreceptors (Einhorn et al., 1988; Pitts & Marwah, 1987b). Finally, in the dorsal raphe nucleus (DRN), cocaine inhibits firing, and this effect can be antagonized by spiperone, which blocks 5-HT1$_A$ autoreceptors (Cunningham & Lakoski, 1984). Subsequent in vitro examinations of the effects of cocaine in these brain regions have generally supported the results of the extracellular experiments and have provided additional information about its cellular mechanisms of action.

Locus Coeruleus

In the slice preparation, locus coeruleus (LC) neurons fire spontaneously, albeit at a somewhat more regular rate than is observed in intact animals (Egan et al., 1983). As in the intact animal, this spontaneous firing is inhibited by cocaine, and these types of inhibitory responses are antagonized by idazoxan (Surprenant & Williams, 1987), implicating α_2 adrenergic autoinhibitory receptors in this response. Similar effects are observed with other uptake blockers (e.g., desmethylimipramine) as well. The inhibition of the firing of LC neurons is accompanied by a hyperpolarization of the resting membrane potential, and in cells that are voltage-clamped at -60 mV, cocaine elicits an outward current ranging from 20-120 pA. Although the potassium-mediated outward current response to cocaine cannot be distinguished physiologically from the responses to α_2 adrenergic agonists, the maximal current elicited by cocaine is approximately 15-20% of the maximum current produced by NE. Thus, unlike the situation with noradrenergic target regions, such as the hippocampus, cocaine has direct effects on the LC that seem to be mediated through the potentiation of the effects of endogenous NE.

As might be expected, cocaine also potentiates the outward current or membrane hyperpolarization induced by exogenous NE (Surprenant & Williams, 1987); dose-response curves for NE are shifted to the left by 15-118 times. The half-maximal effect of cocaine is observed with a concentration of 4 μM cocaine, and the threshold is well below 1 μM. Finally, the IPSPs evoked by focal stimulation in the vicinity of the LC are significantly potentiated by cocaine superfusion (Fig. 11-2). Both the amplitude and the duration of the IPSP are markedly affected.

Dorsal Raphe

A picture very similar to that seen in the LC has emerged from experiments examining the effects of cocaine on dorsal raphe neurons. In slice preparations that are spontaneously active, cocaine inhibits spontaneous firing with an EC_{50} of 2.4 μM (Black & Lakoski, 1990). In nonspontaneously firing cells, cocaine induces a hyperpolarization that is similar in most respects to the response to 5-HT itself, with an EC_{50} of approximately 4 μM (Pan & Williams, 1989). Spiperone, a $5-HT_{1A}$ receptor antagonist, completely blocks the hyperpolarization induced by cocaine. What is unique about this response is that it does not depend upon the spontaneous firing of 5-HT neurons, implying that the source of the 5-HT with which the cocaine interacts must be a non-impulse-dependent pool of neurotransmitter (Pan & Williams, 1989). The observation that the cocaine-induced hyperpolarization is unaffected in animals that were pretreated with reserpine, which inhibits the vesicular storage of 5-HT, underscores this point as well.

As would be expected for an agent that blocks the high-affinity 5-HT uptake pump, cocaine shifts the 5-HT concentration response curve to the left (Pan & Williams, 1989). In addition, the duration of the putative serotonergic component of synaptic responses to focal stimulation in the area of the dorsal raphe is also markedly increased by cocaine. The maximum increase in the IPSP duration is about eightfold, with an EC_{50} of 1.5 μM. As in the PH, lower concentrations of cocaine generally increases the amplitude of the IPSP, whereas at higher concentrations the amplitude is depressed to less than control values.

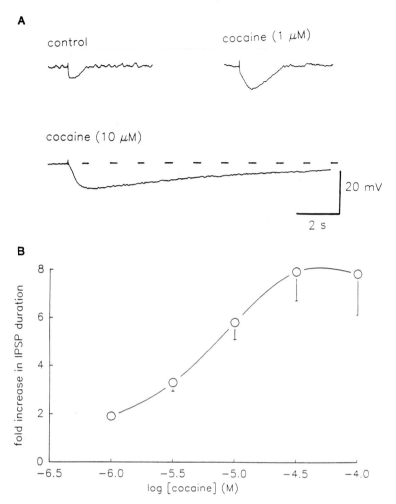

Figure 11-2. Prolongation of LC IPSPs by cocaine. Voltage recordings of IPSPs induced by local stimulation in a single locus coeruleus neuron are shown with and without superfusion with cocaine **A,** IPSPs were evoked by a single supramaximal electrical stimulation pulse. Both the amplitude and the duration of the IPSP were increased by cocaine, although the duration was increased to a considerably larger extent. **B,** Dose-response relation for the effect of cocaine on the duration of the IPSP. (From Dunwiddie et al., 1991, with permission; data from Surprenant & Williams, 1987).

Ventral Tegmental Region/Substantia Nigra

Studies of the effects of cocaine on the DA-containing cells of the VTA or SN have yielded conclusions paralleling those derived from dorsal raphe and LC studies. By itself, cocaine inhibits the slow spontaneous firing of VTA and SN neurons in brain slices (Brodie & Dunwiddie, 1990; Lacey et al., 1990). Moreover, this effect is completely antagonized by the D_2 receptor antagonist sulpiride (Fig. 11-3) and is potentiated by cholecystokinin$_{1-8}$ (CCK$_{1-8}$; Fig.

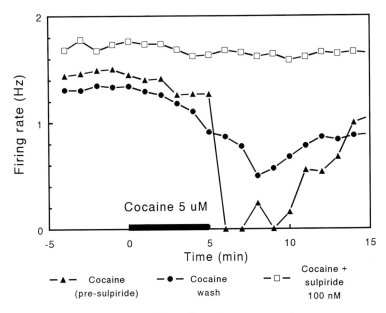

Figure 11-3. Electrophysiological effects of cocaine on a ventral tegmental area neuron in vitro. Spontaneous activity was recorded extracellularly from a single VTA neuron in an in vitro slice preparation, which was identified as a putative DA-containing neuron on the basis of its characteristic spike shape, duration, and sensitivity to inhibition by DA (Brodie & Dunwiddie, 1987). Each point represents the mean firing rate integrated over 1-minute intervals, and each line denotes a single cocaine trial before (*triangles*), during (*squares*), and after (*circles*) superfusion with 100 nM sulpiride. Note that the basal rate of firing of this cell was increased somewhat by sulpiride infusion and that the cocaine effect was completely blocked. In such cells as these, which were quite sensitive to DA, cocaine by itself was able to elicit a marked inhibition of the firing rate.

11-4). We have previously shown that DA-mediated inhibition of VTA firing is antagonized by sulpiride and potentiated by CCK$_{1-8}$ (Brodie & Dunwiddie, 1987). Both these lines of evidence suggest that the inhibitory action of cocaine is mediated via the dopamine autoreceptors on these neurons. We have also demonstrated that the inhibitory effect of cocaine is maintained or potentiated when the slices are incubated in medium containing 0.25 mM calcium and 10 mM magnesium, which does not support calcium-dependent release of transmitter (Brodie & Dunwiddie, unpublished data). Furthermore, cocaine-induced hyperpolarizations are not affected when slices are incubated in tetrodotoxin, indicating that full amplitude action potentials are not necessary to support the release process (Lacey et al., 1990). These results suggest that the DA with which cocaine interacts in the slice is released in a non-calcium-dependent, non-sodium-spike-dependent fashion, most probably from the dendrites of the DA-containing cells themselves.

In addition to its direct effects, cocaine also potentiates the inhibitory responses of VTA neurons to superfusion with subthreshold concentrations of DA, but has no effect upon responses to apomorphine, which is not a substrate

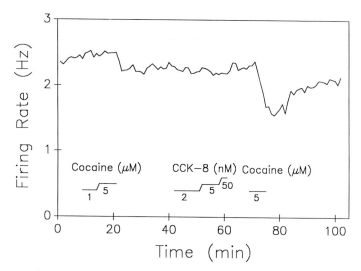

Figure 11-4. Cholecystokinin$_{1-8}$ (CCK$_{1-8}$) potentiation of cocaine responses, which occurs in the absence of any measurable CCK$_{1-8}$-induced change in the spontaneous firing rate, and can be observed for long periods after CCK$_{1-8}$ superfusion. The duration and concentration of superfusion with drugs are illustrated by the bars at the bottom.

for reuptake (Fig. 11-5). This effect can be observed at concentrations as low as 100 nM (Brodie & Dunwiddie, 1990), but are much more pronounced at higher concentrations. Intracellular experiments (primarily on SN neurons) have demonstrated that the hyperpolarization or outward current induced by low con-

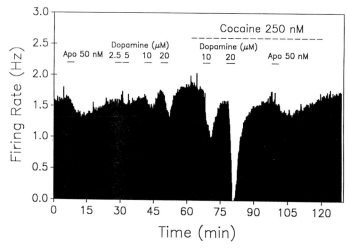

Figure 11-5. Potentiation of responses to DA by cocaine in VTA in vitro. Apomorphine (Apo), a DA agonist that is not a substrate for reuptake, and DA inhibited spontaneous firing of a putative DA-containing VTA neuron before cocaine superfusion. During concurrent superfusion with 250 nM cocaine, the responses to DA but not apomorphine were enhanced significantly.

centrations of DA is increased more than 200% in the presence of 10 μM cocaine, but the response to 100 μM DA is unaffected (Lacey et al., 1990). This lack of effect of cocaine on responses to high DA concentrations could reflect either a maximal response to DA itself or a saturation of the high-affinity uptake by DA, such that further inhibition by cocaine was not possible.

SUMMARY

This summary of cocaine's actions clearly establishes that cocaine can interact with a variety of neurotransmitter systems in the brain, and several conclusions can be drawn based upon the studies described above. In no region that has been studied do there seem to be direct monoaminergic agonistic effects in brain slices that are mediated by cocaine alone. Therefore, it seems safe to conclude that cocaine does not act as an indirect releasing agent, like amphetamine, but acts primarily to potentiate the effects of monoamines that have already been released by different kinds of stimuli. In the 5-HT system, this hypothesis has been confirmed directly by comparisons of cocaine and amphetamine in the nucleus prepositus hypoglossi (Bobker & Williams, 1991); it has been confirmed in the noradrenergic input to the hippocampus by comparing the effects of tyramine (Mueller et al., 1982) to those of cocaine (Yasuda et al., 1984).

A second major conclusion from these studies is that cocaine can significantly potentiate the effects of both exogenously and endogenously released monoamines. The potentiation of exogenous monoamines is perhaps not surprising, because exogenous neurotransmitter would have to traverse significant distances through the slice to reach synaptic sites, and hence uptake should play a major role in the inactivation of exogenous agonists. On a quantitative basis, the responses to endogenous transmitter seem to be potentiated to a somewhat lesser extent, perhaps because the close juxtaposition of release sites and neurotransmitter receptors gives uptake little chance to affect significantly the initial amplitude of the postsynaptic response. Nevertheless, some potentiation of the amplitude of monoamine responses is observed in every system that has been tested, particularly at lower doses. However, the most striking effect of cocaine on monoaminergic synaptic responses is a very marked prolongation of these postsynaptic potentials, which clearly suggests that reuptake plays a major role in the termination of the actions of these amines at their respective synapses. The only observation that might seem discordant with this conclusion is that, in hippocampus, the time course of the increase in extracellular NE evoked by K^+ is not significantly affected by cocaine. Although several reasons for this observation might be proposed, at least one possibility is that the extracellular NE that is measured by the electrochemical electrode is primarily NE that has already left the synapse (where most of the uptake sites are likely to be located) and thus is relatively free to diffuse in the extracellular space.

The primary observation that has been made both in vivo and in vitro on cocaine's effects on monoaminergic nuclei is that the spontaneous activity of neurons is reduced by the activation of autoreceptor-coupled K^+ channels and consequent hyperpolarizations. Interestingly enough, at least where it has been examined, this effect does not seem to depend on calcium-dependent, sodium-spike-dependent release of neurotransmitter; in addition, some (although not all) experiments suggest that these effects cannot be blocked by prior treatment with reserpine as well, which would deplete vesicular but not free cytoplasmic transmitter.

An important consideration, particularly in the context of behavioral studies, concerns the concentrations of cocaine at which it exerts its multiple actions. The approximate concentrations that can elicit significant electrophysiological actions are summarized in Figure 11-6. It is apparent that, within the various monoamine systems, cocaine is relatively equieffective in inhibiting uptake and altering electrophysiological activity. The most potent action of cocaine to date (significant effects at 100 nM) is the potentiation of the effects of exogenous DA in the VTA (Dunwiddie et al., 1991), but this apparently greater potency may reflect more the character of the electrophysiological response than an intrinsically higher activity of cocaine on this system. Nevertheless,

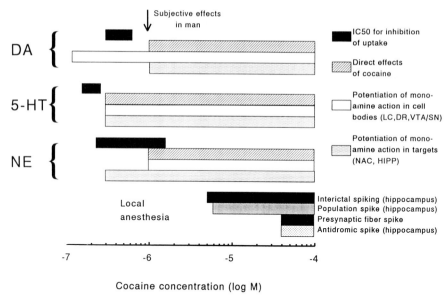

Figure 11-6. Pharmacologically effective concentrations of cocaine. Solid bars indicate the range of concentrations of cocaine that have been shown to inhibit high-affinity uptake or to displace radiolabeled ligands from binding to transporter sites (Hyttel, 1982; Ritz & Kuhar, 1989; Ritz et al., 1987). Diagonally hatched bars denote the concentrations of cocaine that were effective in reducing the spontaneous firing rates or hyperpolarizing monoaminergic neurons in brain slices, open bars indicate the effective concentrations for potentiating the effects of superfused exogenous monoamines in monoaminergic nuclei, and the shaded bars show the concentrations that potentiated monoaminergic effects in target regions. The bottom four bars indicate the effective concentrations of cocaine in eliciting local anesthetic effects in hippocampus (see Dunwiddie et al., 1988 for details).

this probably sets a kind of lower limit for the concentrations of cocaine that would be expected to have significant effects upon neural activity. At a concentration of 1 μM, which is in the range where most of the reinforcing effects of cocaine begin to appear, responses to DA, NE, and 5-HT are all affected significantly. Local anesthetic effects, however, do not begin to appear until the concentrations of cocaine are significantly higher, with threshold values between 5-10 μM for most types of responses. This finding certainly does not imply that local anesthetic actions are not functionally significant, and in fact animals can be trained to self-administer local anesthetic drugs, such as procaine (Ford & Balster, 1977). However, it does not seem likely that local anesthetic effects play a major role in pharmacological reinforcement, although their contributions to cocaine toxicity may be quite significant.

Finally, although cocaine may affect multiple brain systems in similar concentrations, its effects are not essentially equivalent. A good example is the different inhibitory effects of cocaine on the spontaneous activity of the monoamine-containing cells in the 5-HT and DA systems. In the serotonergic system both in vitro (Black & Lakoski, 1990) and in vivo (Cunningham & Lakoski, 1988; Pitts & Marwah, 1986b), cocaine completely inhibits the spontaneous firing of nearly all raphe neurons. In contrast, DA neurons in the VTA and SN are affected to a considerably lesser extent, and the mesocortical DA neurons in vivo show little if any sensitivity to cocaine (Brodie & Dunwiddie, 1990; Einhorn et al., 1988; Lacey et al., 1990; Pitts & Marwah, 1988). Thus, it might be predicted that the net effect of cocaine in serotonergic projection areas might be a decrease in 5-HT levels, since there will be no impulse-dependent 5-HT release with which cocaine can interact, whereas the net level of postsynaptic activation in DA projection areas might be an increase, based upon the facilitation of the actions of an only partially reduced DA release. Whether these generalizations are appropriate is unclear, although there is already a significant amount of information from electrophysiological, electrochemical, and in vivo microdialysis experiments that bear upon them. Nevertheless, it is clear that the net effects of cocaine action are quite complex and will have to be addressed not only through the in vitro types of studies but also through studies in intact (and perhaps optimally, cocaine self-administering) animals.

REFERENCES

Black, E.W., & Lakoski, J.M. (1990). In vitro electrophysiology of dorsal raphe serotonergic neurons in subchronic cocaine-treated rats: Development of tolerance to acute cocaine administration. *Mol. Cell. Neurosci., 1,* 84-91.

Bobker D.H., & Williams, J.J. (1991). Cocaine and amphetamine interact at 5-HT synapses through distinct mechanisms in guinea-pig prepositus hypogloss. *J. Neurosci. 11,* 2151-2156.

Brodie, M.S., & Dunwiddie, T.V. (1987). Cholecystokinin potentiates dopamine inhibition of mesencephalic dopamine neurons in vitro. *Brain Res., 425,* 106-113.

Brodie, M.S., & Dunwiddie, T.V. (1990). Cocaine effects in the ventral tegmental area:

Evidence for an indirect dopaminergic mechanism of action. *Naunyn-Schmiedeberg's Arch. Pharmacol., 342*, 660-665.

Cunningham, K.A., & Lakoski, J.M. (1988). Electrophysiological effects of cocaine and procaine on dorsal raphe serotonin neurons. *Eur. J. Pharmacol., 148*, 457-462.

Dunwiddie, T.V. (1980). Endogenously released adenosine regulates excitability in the in vitro hippocampus. *Epilepsia, 21*, 541-548.

Dunwiddie, T.V., & Alford, C. (1987). Electrophysiological actions of phencyclidine in hippocampal slices from the rat. *Neuropharmacology, 26*, 1267-1273.

Dunwiddie, T.V., Proctor, W.R., & Tyma, J. (1988). Local anaesthetic actions of cocaine: Effects on excitatory and inhibitory synaptic responses in the hippocampus in vitro. *Br. J. Pharmacol., 95*, 1117-1124.

Dunwiddie, T.V., Williams, J.T., Bobker, D.H., Pan, Z.Z., Gerhardt, G.A., & Brodie, M.S. (1991). In vitro approaches to characterizing the electrophysiological effects of cocaine upon the central nervous system. In J.M. Lakoski, M.P. Galloway & F.P. White (Eds.), *Cocaine: Pharmacology, physiology and clinical strategies*. Caldwell, NJ: Telford Press.

Egan, T.M., Henderson, G., North, R.A., & Williams, J.T. (1983). Noradrenaline-mediated synaptic inhibition in rat locus coeruleus neurones. *J. Physiol., 345*, 477-488.

Einhorn, L.C., Johansen, P.A., & White, F.J. (1988). Electrophysiological effects of cocaine in the mesoaccumbens dopamine system: Studies in the ventral tegmental area. *J. Neurosci., 8*, 100-112.

Ford, R.D., & Balster, R.L. (1977). Reinforcing properties of intravenous procaine in rhesus monkeys. *Pharmacol. Biochem. Behav., 6*, 289-296.

Hyttel, J. (1982). Citalopram-pharmacological profile of a specific serotonin uptake inhibitor with antidepressant activity. *Neuro-Psychopharmacol. Biol. Psychiat., 6*, 277-295.

Lacey, M.G., Mercuri, N.B., & North, R.A. (1990). Actions of cocaine on rat dopaminergic neurones in vitro. *Br. J. Pharmacol., 99*, 731-735.

Lakoski, J.M., & Cunningham, K.A. (1988). Cocaine interaction with central monoaminergic systems: Electrophysiological approaches. *Trends Pharmacol., 9*, 177-180.

Lesse, H. (1980). Prolonged effects of cocaine on hippocampal activity. *Comm. Psychopharmacol., 4*, 247-254.

Lesse, H., & Collins, J.P. (1980). Differential effects of cocaine on limbic excitability. *Pharmacol. Biochem. Behav., 13*, 695-703.

Lesse, H., & Harper, R.K. (1985). Frequency-related, bidirectional limbic responses to cocaine: Comparisons with amphetamine and lidocaine. *Brain Res., 335*, 21-31.

Mueller, A.L., & Dunwiddie, T.V. (1983). Anticonvulsant and proconvulsant actions of alpha- and beta-noradrenergic agonists on epileptiform activity in rat hippocampus in vitro. *Epilepsia, 24*, 57-64.

Mueller, A.L., Kirk, K.L., Hoffer, B.J., & Dunwiddie, T.V. (1982). Noradrenergic responses in rat hippocampus: Electrophysiological actions of direct- and indirect-acting sympathomimetics in the in vitro slice. *J. Pharmacol. Exp. Ther., 223*, 599-605.

Pan, Z.Z., & Williams, J.T. (1989). Differential actions of cocaine and amphetamine on dorsal raphe neurons in vitro. *J. Pharmacol. Exp. Ther., 251*, 56-62.

Pitts, D.K., & Marwah, J. (1986a). Effects of cocaine on the electrical activity of single noradrenergic neurons from locus coeruleus. *Life Sci., 38*, 1229-1234.

Pitts, D.K., & Marwah, J. (1986b). Electrophysiological effects of cocaine on central monoaminergic neurons. *Eur. J. Pharmacol., 131*, 95-98.

Pitts, D.K., & Marwah, J. (1987a). Cocaine inhibition of locus coeruleus neurons. *NIDA Res. Monogr., 76,* 334-340.

Pitts, D.K., & Marwah, J. (1987b). Cocaine modulation of central monoaminergic neurotransmission. *Pharmacol. Biochem. Behav., 26,* 453-461.

Pitts, D.K., & Marwah, J. (1988). Cocaine and central monoaminergic neurotransmission: A review of electrophysiological studies and comparison to amphetamine and antidepressants. *Life Sci., 42,* 949-968.

Ritz, M.C., & Kuhar, M.J. (1989). Relationship between self-administration of amphetamine and monoamine receptors in brain: Comparison with cocaine. *J. Pharmacol. Exp. Ther., 248,* 1010-1017.

Ritz, M.C., Lamb, R.J., Goldberg, S.R., & Kuhar, M.J. (1987). Cocaine receptors on dopamine transporters are related to self-administration of cocaine. *Science, 237,* 1219-1223.

Steinbusch, H. (1981). Distribution of serotonin-immunoreactivity on the central nervous system of the rat cell bodies and terminals. *Neuroscience, 6,* 557-618.

Su, M.T., Dunwiddie, T.V., & Gerhardt, G.A. (1990). Combined electrochemical and electrophysiological studies of monoamine overflow in rat hippocampal slice. *Brain Res., 518,* 149-158.

Surprenant, A., & Williams, J.T. (1987). Inhibitory synaptic potentials recorded from mammalian neurones prolonged by blockade of noradrenaline uptake. *J. Physiol., 382,* 87-103.

Uchimura, N., & North, R.A. (1990). Actions of cocaine on rat nucleus accumbens neurones in vitro. *Br. J. Pharmacol., 99,* 736-740.

White, F.J. (1990). Physiological basis for the rewarding effects of cocaine. *Behav. Pharmacol., 1,* 303-315.

Yasuda, R.P., Zahniser, N.R., & Dunwiddie, T.V. (1984). Electrophysiological effects of cocaine in the rat hippocampus in vitro. *Neurosci. Lett., 45,* 199-204.

12

Cocaine and Monoamine Neurons

FRANCIS J. WHITE AND BENJAMIN S. BUNNEY

In an attempt to unravel the complex neurobiological events that result in cocaine's powerful reinforcing properties, self-administration studies have directed attention toward the mesencephalic dopamine (DA) neurons (Wise & Rompré 1989). These cells innervate limbic-system-related areas of the ventral striatum, including the nucleus accumbens (nACC) and the medial prefrontal cortex (mPFC).

Lesion studies provide the main support for a role of the mesoaccumbens DA system in the rewarding effects of cocaine. Destruction of DA terminals within the nACC or A10 DA somata within the mesencephalic ventral tegmental area (VTA) by local administration of the selective catecholamine toxin 6-hydroxydopamine (6-OHDA) attenuates the rewarding effects of cocaine (Roberts & Koob, 1982; Roberts et al., 1980). Lesions of intrinsic neurons of the nACC, produced by the excitotoxin kainic acid, also disrupt cocaine self-administration (Zito et al., 1985), demonstrating that DA transmission to postsynaptic cells is an essential component of the reinforcement process.

By contrast, much of the evidence supporting a role for the mPFC DA system in cocaine reward has been obtained in studies using intracranial self-administration into the mPFC. Thus, rats will work for cocaine injections into the mPFC, but not the nACC (Goeders & Smith, 1983; Goeders et al., 1986). However, 6-OHDA lesions of DA terminals within the mPFC fail to disrupt cocaine self-administration once it has been established (Martin-Iverson et al., 1986). This finding has led to the suggestion that the mPFC DA system may be primarily responsible for the *initiation* of cocaine self-administration, whereas the mesoaccumbens DA system may *maintain* the behavior (Goeders et al., 1986).

Similar studies have begun to examine a possible role for serotonin (5-hydroxytryptamine, 5-HT) in cocaine self-administration. Some investigators argue that 5-HT systems play an opposing role to DA in psychomotor stimulant self-administration, so that decreasing 5-HT tone removes an aversive property and enhances self-administration (Loh & Roberts, 1990; Lyness et al., 1980). Selective lesions of the 5-HT system increase amphetamine self-administration (Leccese & Lyness, 1984; Lyness et al., 1980) and increase the number of responses (breaking point) that rats will make to obtain cocaine injections on a progressive ratio schedule of drug presentation (Loh & Roberts, 1990). In contrast, enhanced 5-HT function produced by precursor (1-tryptophan) loading or selective 5-HT uptake inhibitors diminishes cocaine self-administration (Carroll et al., 1990a,b). Others have agreed with the results of such manipulations on amphetamine self-administration, but have failed to see similar effects on cocaine self-administration (Porrino et al., 1989).

The neurochemical mechanism by which cocaine affects transmission in the CNS seems to involve primarily the inhibition of monoamine uptake. Because reuptake of released monoamines is the primary mechanism for terminating their synaptic actions, inhibition of this process enhances synaptic transmission. Radioligand binding studies have identified specific, saturable sites for cocaine located on both DA and 5-HT nerve endings in various brain areas, which seem to mark the uptake sites for these amines (Ritz & Kuhar, 1989; Ritz et al., 1987). The binding of cocaine and related agents to a site on the DA transporter labeled by [^{3}H]-mazindol is highly correlated with rewarding efficacy (Ritz et al., 1987). A significant *inverse* correlation between the affinities of amphetamine and related phenylethylamines for the 5-HT transporter (labeled by [^{3}H]paroxetine) and their reinforcing potency (Ritz & Kuhar, 1989) supports the possible aversive role of 5-HT in amphetamine self-administration. However, no such relationship exists for cocaine and related drugs (Ritz & Kuhar, 1989).

These behavioral and neurochemical studies indicate that the most relevant effect of cocaine on self-administration is enhanced DA transmission within the mesoaccumbens and mesocortical DA systems. The binding of cocaine to a site on the DA transporter (Ritz et al., 1987) results in diminished reuptake of the amine and in greatly enhanced synaptic levels, as recently confirmed by in vivo microdialysis studies (Bradberry & Roth, 1989; Hurd et al., 1989; Kalivas & Duffy, 1990; Moghaddam & Bunney, 1989; Nicolaysen et al., 1988). These findings raise an important question: What are the physiological effects of the enhanced synaptic DA levels induced by cocaine? This chapter analyzes how cocaine affects the activity of single DA neurons, as well as their target cells, and how such alterations in activity may result in overall changes in transmission from a systems perspective. Because of the postulated role for 5-HT in reward mechanisms, the electrophysiological actions of cocaine on 5-HT neuronal systems are also discussed.

Most of the studies reviewed in this chapter were conducted in anesthetized rats. This fact limits, to some extent, our ability to generalize the mechanisms elucidated to those operational in the awake behaving animal, particularly those engaging in self-administration of cocaine and other drugs of abuse. Almost all current knowledge regarding mesoaccumbens DA neurophysiology was acquired either from anesthetized rats in vivo or from brain slices in vitro. Mechanistic studies will continue to require these approaches because certain manipulations, such as local application of drugs, selective activation of relevant receptor populations, and alterations of transduction events, are difficult to achieve in awake animals. A thorough understanding of the mechanisms of action of cocaine will require the comprehensive use of the neuroscientists' complete armamentarium, with appreciation of both the strengths and weaknesses of each technique, as well as the interpretational restrictions imposed by the particular approach.

DOPAMINE NEURONS

Cocaine and Mesoaccumbens DA Neurons: In Vivo Studies

In chloral-hydrate-anesthetized rats, intravenously administered cocaine, like most other DA agonists, causes a dose-dependent inhibition of the activity of antidromically identified mesoaccumbens A10 DA neurons (Einhorn et al., 1988; White et al., 1987). Unlike amphetamine, apomorphine, and most other DA agonists, cocaine-induced inhibition is usually only partial (at sublethal doses) in that the maximal inhibition observed seldom exceeds 70% of the basal firing rate (Fig. 12-1). This partial inhibition is also observed after single bolus injections of cocaine (Einhorn et al., 1988; Pitts & Marwah, 1987). The duration of inhibition is quite short as most cells return to basal rates within 20-25 minutes (Einhorn et al., 1988).

Although cocaine inhibits the uptake not only of DA but also of 5-HT and NE, only the former action seems to be involved in its effects on mesoaccumbens DA neurons. Neither the selective 5-HT uptake inhibitor fluoxetine nor

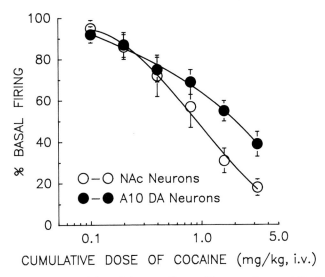

Figure 12-1. Comparison of the inhibitory effects of i.v. cocaine on A10 dopamine (DA) neurons in the rat ventral tegmental area and on neurons within the rat nucleus accumbens (nACC). Cocaine was administered to chloral-hydrate-anesthetized rats in a cumulative dose regimen in which each dose doubled the previous dose. Injections were separated by 60-90 seconds. Each point represents the mean ±SEM for 8 A10 DA cells and 12 nACC neurons. Asterisks represent the doses at which cocaine was more effective in inhibiting nACC neurons than A10 DA neurons (P < 0.01).

the selective noradrenergic uptake inhibitor desmethylimipramine alters the activity of A10 DA neurons (Einhorn et al., 1988). In contrast, other agents known to inhibit DA uptake, such as the catecholamine uptake inhibitor nomifensine and the selective DA uptake inhibitor GBR 12909, exhibit a potency and efficacy nearly identical to that of cocaine. The local anesthetic agents, procaine and lidocaine, which possess little to no psychomotor stimulant or rewarding properties, cause only a slight nonsignificant increase in the firing rates of A10 DA cells. Thus, the effects of cocaine on A10 DA neurons reflect its ability to inhibit the DA transporter and thereby increase the levels of DA available to interact with DA receptors. In support of this contention, the DA antagonist haloperidol reverses the inhibition of A10 DA neurons produced by cocaine, GBR 12909, and nomifensine (Einhorn et al., 1988). The possibility that cocaine acts directly on DA receptors is eliminated by studies indicating that reserpine pretreatment (5.0 mg/kg), which diminishes vesicular stores of DA, significantly attenuates the inhibitory effects of cocaine on A10 DA neurons. Thus, endogenous DA is required for cocaine to produce its inhibitory effects (Einhorn et al., 1988).

Experiments using microiontophoretic administration of cocaine indicate that cocaine inhibits DA neurons after local application. This finding suggests that cocaine might block dendritic uptake of DA in the VTA and thereby enhance the effects of endogenous DA at somatodendritic autoreceptors known to regulate DA neuronal activity (Aghajanian & Bunney, 1977; White & Wang, 1984b). The fact that simultaneous iontophoretic administration of cocaine with DA significantly enhances the inhibitory effects (increased efficacy and duration) of DA provides further support for this hypothesis. The inhibitory effects observed at currents of 20-40 nA seem to be mediated by DA autoreceptors since they are completely blocked by the D_2 receptor antagonist sulpiride. Because iontophoretic administration of cocaine alone produces only a 15-20% maximal inhibition of firing of mesoaccumbens DA neurons (Fig. 12–2), the effects of systemic cocaine on A10 neuronal activity may involve additional mechanisms.

Cocaine and Mesocortical DA Neurons: In Vivo Studies

In contrast to mesoaccumbens DA neurons, antidromically identified mesoprefrontal A10 DA neurons are largely insensitive to the rate-decreasing effects of cocaine. This finding is consistent with the view that these neurons may lack impulse-regulating autoreceptors (Chiodo et al., 1984), or may possess significantly fewer or less sensitive somatodendritic autoreceptors than either mesoaccumbens or nigrostriatal DA cells (White & Wang, 1984a).

Cocaine and Nigrostriatal DA Neurons: In Vivo Studies

Considerably less work has been published on the effects of cocaine on nigrostriatal DA neurons. However, there is evidence that cocaine exerts less pronounced and more variable effects on nigral A9 DA neurons than on VTA A10 DA neurons (Pitts & Marwah, 1987). At low doses (0.5 mg/kg i.v.), cocaine produces mild rate increases of A9 DA cells, but decreases of A10 unit activity.

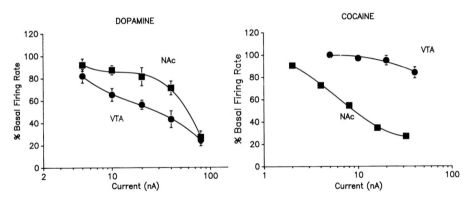

Figure 12-2. Comparison of the effects of both DA and cocaine, administered iontophoretically, on nucleus accumbens (nACC) neurons and A10 DA neurons in the rat ventral tegmental area (VTA). Both Type I and Type II neurons are included in the nACC data. Note that although DA is more potent on A10 DA neurons, cocaine is more potent on nACC neurons. Adapted from White (1990) with permission.

At higher doses, cocaine always inhibits VTA cells, whereas excitatory effects on nigral neurons are still occasionally observed. Finally, 40% of nigral DA neurons are unaffected by single bolus injections of 1.0 mg/kg cocaine (Pitts & Marwah, 1987).

Cocaine and DA Neurons: In Vitro Studies

Studies of cocaine effects on DA neurons using intracellular recordings from in vitro midbrain slice preparations indicate, as do the in vivo studies, that cocaine (1-10 μm) inhibits the spontaneous firing of both VTA and nigral DA neurons (Lacey et al., 1990). Unlike the in vivo situation, however, cocaine (10 μm) produces an 82% decrease in activity, and many neurons are completely inhibited. Since such complete inhibitions are not observed in the anesthetized rat in vivo, it seems unlikely that such concentrations of cocaine are achieved within the VTA after i.v. administration (up to 3.1 mg/kg). In fact, intraperitoneal doses of 30 mg/kg are required to achieve brain levels of 10 μm (Nicolaysen et al., 1988). Two i.v. doses of 1.5 mg/kg cocaine (90 minutes apart) result in approximately 1.5-2 μm concentrations in the rat striatum (Hurd et al., 1988). Thus, it is likely that the maximal dose of 3.1 mg/kg i.v. used by Einhorn et al. (1988) would have resulted in brain levels no greater than 3 μm, a concentration that causes an average inhibition of 45% during in vitro recordings.

The inhibition of DA neurons produced by cocaine is accompanied by small hyperpolarizations (3.4 mV at 10 μm) in cells held at -60 mV to prevent action potential discharge. The outward current elicited by cocaine in these voltage-clamped neurons is around 35 pA with applications of 5-10 minutes duration. Cocaine (10 μm) also enhances the effects of exogenous DA on inhibition of firing, hyperpolarization, and outward current. The D_2 antagonist sulpiride (up to 1 μm) rapidly and fully reverses the effects of cocaine, whereas tetrodotoxin (1 μm) does not (Lacey et al., 1990), indicating that the effects of cocaine are due to potentiation of the actions of DA, which is continuously released from DA neurons in the slice, at somatodendritic D_2 autoreceptors.

SEROTONIN NEURONS

Cocaine and 5-HT Neurons: In Vivo Studies

Cocaine effectively inhibits the activity of 5-HT-containing neurons within the rat dorsal raphe nucleus (DRN). Single bolus i.v. injections of cocaine inhibit DRN neurons in a dose-dependent manner (Pitts & Marwah, 1986). When administered in a cumulative dose paradigm, the ED_{50} is 0.66 mg/kg (Cunningham & Lakoski, 1988, 1990). This effect is stereoselective in that the behaviorally active isomer $(-)$-cocaine, but not the inactive isomers $(+)$-cocaine or $(+)$-pseudococaine, also inhibits DRN neurons.

Pharmacological analysis similar to that conducted on A10 DA neurons indicate that the effect of cocaine on DRN neurons is due to 5-HT uptake inhibition. Thus, similar inhibitory effects are produced by the selective 5-HT uptake inhibitor fluoxetine, but not by selective inhibition of DA or NE uptake. Although a lack of selective receptor antagonists for impulse-regulating somatodendritic $5-HT_{1A}$ receptors compromises this type of pharmacological study, the effect of cocaine has been reported to be reversed by the putative $5-HT_{1A}$ blocker spiperone on 7 of 11 neurons. Antagonists of several other receptors are ineffective in this regard (Cunningham & Lakoski, 1990). Finally, the effects of cocaine are significantly decreased by pretreating rats with the tryptophan hydroxylase inhibitor p-chlorophenylalanine, indicating a dependence on endogenous 5-HT (Cunningham & Lakoski, 1990).

Iontophoretic administration of cocaine inhibits the firing of DRN neurons in a current-dependent manner (Cunningham & Lakoski, 1988). In addition, low iontophoretic currents potentiate the effects of iontophoretically administered 5-HT. Taken together with the intravenous effects of cocaine, it is clear that cocaine is a much more effective inhibitor of 5-HT than of DA neurons (Pitts & Marwah, 1986).

Cocaine and 5-HT Neurons: In Vitro Studies

Studies of cocaine effects on DRN 5-HT neurons recorded intracellularly from a slice preparation reveal dose-dependent (0.3-100 nm) membrane hyperpolarizations that are completely antagonized by spiperone (Pan & Williams, 1989). The maximal effect is approximately a 15 mV hyperpolarization observed at 30 μm, with an EC_{50} of 4.2 μm. These findings again demonstrate a greater effectiveness of cocaine on 5-HT than on DA neurons. In addition to the direct hyperpolarization, cocaine also potentiates both the hyperpolarizing action of 5-HT and a 5-HT-mediated IPSP evoked by local stimulation. Importantly, these effects of cocaine are observed at very low, physiologically relevant concentrations (300 nm-3 μm). Reserpine treatment fails to reduce the hyperpolarizations produced by cocaine, suggesting that this effect is due to a potentiation of 5-HT released from newly synthesized, as opposed to vesicular, stores (Pan & Williams, 1989).

TARGET NEURONS OF DA AND 5-HT PROJECTIONS

Effects of Cocaine on nACC Neurons: In Vivo Studies

Intravenous cocaine suppresses the firing of nACC neurons (Fig. 12-1) in chloral-hydrate-anesthetized rats (White, 1990; White et al., 1987). The ability of cocaine to inhibit nACC neurons (ED_{50} = 0.67 ± 0.09 mg/kg) is similar to that for A10 DA cells (ED_{50} = 0.71 ± 0.03 mg/kg). However, cocaine is considerably more efficacious on nACC neurons than on mesoaccumbens A10 DA cells (Fig. 12-1). The inhibitory effects of cocaine on nACC neuronal activity can be reversed by both the nonselective (primarily D_2) DA antagonist haloperidol and the selective D_1 antagonist SCH 23390, although the D_1 receptor antagonist is both more potent and efficacious (White, 1990).

Iontophoretic administration of cocaine to nACC cells also inhibits neuronal firing (Qiao et al., 1990; White, 1990; White et al., 1987). In addition, low subinhibitory currents of cocaine potentiate the rate-suppressant effects of DA on nACC neurons. These inhibitory effects of cocaine are blocked by either D_1 (White et al., 1987) or D_2 selective antagonists (Qiao et al., 1990; White et al., 1987). As with intravenous administration, iontophoretic cocaine is significantly more effective in inhibiting nACC neurons than A10 DA neurons (Fig. 12-2). This finding is surprising in view of previous studies indicating that mesoaccumbens DA neurons are considerably more sensitive to DA than are nACC cells (White & Wang, 1986). This apparent discrepancy may be due to the fact that larger amounts of DA are released by nerve terminals than by dendrites (Bradberry & Roth, 1989; Kalivas et al., 1989). Accordingly, inhibition of the reuptake of synaptic DA within the nACC may have greater functional consequences than inhibiting the reuptake of DA within the VTA.

Interpreting the effects of cocaine on nACC neurons is complicated by the existence of at least two distinct subtypes of neurons, which are distinguishable on the basis of extracellular waveform (Skirboll & Bunney, 1979; White et al., 1987). The majority of nACC neurons seem to be Type I cells, which exhibit a negative/positive waveform, are seldom spontaneously active, and are typically inhibited by 5-HT (White et al., 1987). Type II neurons exhibit positive/negative waveforms, are more often spontaneously active, and often are excited by 5-HT. To study Type I neurons, iontophoretic administration of the excitatory amino acid glutamate is typically used to "drive" quiescent neurons. Cocaine is considerably more potent on Type I than Type II nACC cells, whereas DA is equipotent at inhibiting the two subtypes of nACC cells (Fig. 12-3). Direct comparisons revealed that cocaine is less potent than DA at inhibiting Type II nACC cells, but is more potent than DA on Type I nACC cells (White, 1990; White et al., 1987).

Based upon the differential effect of 5-HT on Type I and II nACC neurons, it seems likely that 5-HT mechanisms are related to the relatively greater effi-

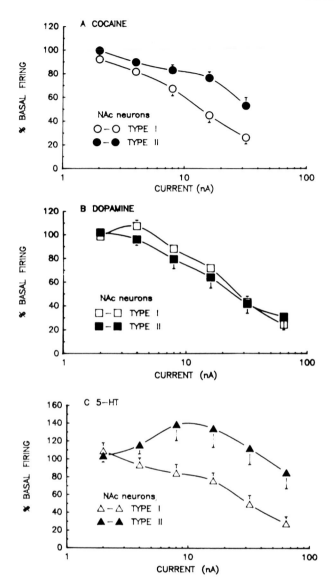

Figure 12-3. Comparison of the effects of cocaine (**A**), DA (**B**), and 5-HT (**C**) on the activity of Type I and Type II nucleus accumbens (nACC) neurons. These current-response curves demonstrate that cocaine (0.01 m) was more potent at inhibiting Type I than II nACC cells, whereas DA (0.01 m) was equally potent on the two subtypes. Serotonin (5-HT) inhibited Type I neurons, but excited most Type II neurons.

cacy of cocaine in inhibiting Type I nACC cells (Fig. 12-3). Because cocaine inhibits the reuptake of 5-HT, which, like DA, is inhibitory on Type I nACC neurons, enhanced activation of both DA and 5-HT receptors might result in potent inhibition of Type I nACC neurons. In contrast, because most Type II neurons are typically excited by iontophoretic 5-HT (Fig. 12-3), the ability of cocaine to block uptake of this amine would oppose the simultaneous inhibitory action of DA. Accordingly, the inhibitory effects of cocaine on Type I nACC neurons may reflect simultaneous potentiation of DA- and 5-HT-mediated inhibition, whereas the weaker inhibition of Type II neurons by cocaine may be due to competing inhibitory and excitatory influences of DA and 5-HT, respectively (White et al., 1987). Support for this hypothesis comes from findings indicating that combined administration of the selective DA uptake inhibitor GBR 12909 and the selective 5-HT uptake blocker fluoxetine is necessary to achieve the degree of inhibition of Type I nACC cells typically observed with cocaine (White et al., 1987; White, 1990).

Effects of Cocaine on nACC Neurons: In Vitro Studies

Uchimura and North (1990) recently reported that cocaine (10 μm) exerts no effect on the membrane potential of nACC cells, indicating that spontaneous release of DA or 5-HT is minimal in this preparation and that cocaine exerts no direct effect on nACC neurons. Dopamine produces both hyperpolarizations and depolarizations of nACC neurons in vitro, actions that seem to be mediated by D_1 and D_2 receptors, respectively (Uchimura & North, 1990). Cocaine potentiates each of these effects of DA as revealed by pretreatment with sulpiride to prevent D_2 receptor-mediated depolarizations or SCH 23390 to prevent D_1 receptor-mediated hyperpolarizations. The potentiation is approximately 20-fold for both effects when cocaine is administered at 10 μm. Cocaine (300 nm-10 μm) also potentiates 5-HT-induced depolarizations of nACC cells. At 10 μm, cocaine increases the potency of 5-HT by a factor of 100 (Uchimura & North, 1990). Thus, the 5-HT transporter seems much more sensitive to cocaine than the DA transporter in this nACC slice preparation.

Several aspects of Uchimura and North's report (1990) differ from the results obtained with in vivo extracellular recordings of nACC neurons combined with iontophoretic drug administration. First, whereas D_1 and D_2 receptor stimulation apparently produces opposite polarizations on nACC neurons in vitro, both of these receptors mediate inhibition of nACC neuronal activity in vivo (White & Wang, 1986). Second, D_1 and D_2 receptors function in a synergistic manner to control striatal neuronal activity in vivo (Clark & White, 1987), whereas they seem to function antagonistically in vitro. Reasons for these differences have not yet been elucidated, but it is likely that the presence of afferent activation in vivo may play an important role. Finally, inhibition of DA uptake seems to result in more effective alterations of nACC neurons in vivo, as compared to inhibition of 5-HT uptake, whereas the opposite appears to be true in vitro. Given the greater density of DA than 5-HT terminals within the nACC, it is possible that alterations of DA uptake result in greater functional consequences, even if the 5-HT transporter is more sensitive to cocaine than is its counterpart on DA terminals.

nACC-VTA Feedback Pathways and Cocaine Effects on DA Neurons

As described above, cocaine is more effective in inhibiting the firing of nACC neurons than of A10 DA cells in the VTA (White et al., 1987). When this finding is considered along with the observation that systemic cocaine is more effective in inhibiting A10 DA neurons than is iontophoretic cocaine, it seems likely that systemic cocaine inhibits DA firing by at least one other mechanism, in addition to enhanced autoreceptor stimulation by endogenous DA. One possibility is that the inhibition of DA neurons by systemic cocaine also involves an inhibitory nACC-VTA feedback pathway.

Although considerably less extensive than the striatonigral feedback pathway, a similar nACC-VTA pathway is known to exist (Walaas & Fonnum, 1980). Since the nACC-VTA long-loop is primarily an inhibitory GABAergic projection, it is likely that, as in the striatonigral feedback pathway (Grace & Bunney, 1985), the primary target of such afferents is an inhibitory neuron within the VTA that makes synaptic connections with A10 DA cells. Electrophysiological studies have suggested the existence of such non-DA inhibitory neurons, which are probably themselves GABAergic, within the VTA (Waszczak & Walters, 1980). Accordingly, the net effect of inhibiting nACC neurons might be a compensatory inhibition of A10 DA neurons through a GABA-GABA-DA feedback system, in which inhibition of the nACC GABA projection neurons would disinhibit the VTA GABA neurons and thereby inhibit the VTA DA neuron.

Einhorn et al. (1988) examined the possible role of a nACC-VTA negative feedback pathway in mediating the systemic effects of cocaine on A10 DA neurons. Both excitotoxin lesions of the nACC and acute hemitransections significantly attenuate the partial inhibitory effects of cocaine on A10 DA neurons (Einhorn et al., 1988). These results indicate that, by inhibiting DA and 5-HT uptake at nerve terminals within the nACC, cocaine causes a marked suppression of nACC neurons and activation of long-loop feedback pathways to the VTA.

Effects of Cocaine on mPFC Neurons

Preliminary studies within the mPFC have indicated that cocaine inhibits the firing of mPFC neurons within layers V and VI and that, as in the nACC, both DA and 5-HT mechanisms may be involved (White, 1990). Thus, iontophoretic cocaine partially inhibits DA-sensitive cells within the mPFC. When compared to the nACC, the effect of iontophoretic cocaine on mPFC cells is less pronounced. These findings correlate well with the recent results showing that cocaine causes larger increases in synaptic DA within the nACC than in the mPFC (Moghaddam & Bunney, 1989). Inhibitory effects of cocaine are also observed after i.v. injections. As in the nACC, a 5-HT mechanism may also play a role in cocaine's effects on mPFC cells since iontophretic cocaine potentiates the inhibitory effects of both DA and 5-HT.

ACUTE EFFECTS OF COCAINE ON DA AND 5-HT TRANSMISSION: A SYNTHESIS

Effects of Cocaine on Mesoaccumbens and Mesocortical DA Transmission

Given the electrophysiological effects of acute cocaine administration on single DA and 5-HT neuronal systems described above, is it possible to provide a coherent perspective from which to view the mechanisms responsible for co-caine-induced alterations in transmission through the mesoaccumbens and me-socortical DA pathways and their relation to important behavioral effects? The following synthesis attempts to do just that. It must first be noted that, although apparently contradictory, the cocaine-induced *decrease* of firing of mesoac-cumbens A10 DA is actually consistent with the hypothesis that reward mecha-nisms involve enhanced DA transmission because such decreases represent a compensatory, homeostatic response to enhanced DA neurotransmission within the primary target site of these cells, the nACC.

The poor compensatory inhibition of A10 DA neurons may be particularly important for the intensity of cocaine's rewarding efficacy. Cocaine is more effective in suppressing the firing of postsynaptic cells within the nACC than inhibiting the DA cells themselves, presumably due to an additive potentiation of DA and 5-HT effects on the postsynaptic cells. In fact, long-loop feedback inhibitory processes are required to compensate for increased postsynaptic inhibition after systemic cocaine administration. Even this combination of autoreceptor stimulation and feedback modulation is insufficient to suppress DA cell firing completely. Therefore, the net effect of systemic cocaine on the mesoaccumbens DA system is an initial increase in synaptic levels of DA within the nACC caused by blocking transport processes, followed by contin-ued impulse-dependent release of DA as a result of incomplete suppression of neuronal activity. Accordingly, cocaine causes considerable enhancement of mesoaccumbens DA neurotransmission because of the relatively poor com-pensatory response of DA cells and the resulting buildup of synaptic DA. Similarly, the lack of inhibition of mesocortical DA cells by i.v. cocaine sug-gests that enhanced DA transmission within the mesocortical DA system may be less well compensated by diminished impulse flow, presumably due to the relative paucity of somatodendritic autoreceptors on these neurons (Chiodo et al., 1984; White & Wang, 1984a). Given the clear role of nACC-VTA feedback processes in cocaine-induced suppression of mesoaccumbens DA cells, it also seems likely that the failure of cocaine to inhibit mesocortical DA neurons reflects differences between these DA pathways in regard to long-loop feed-back regulation.

Possible Role of 5-HT Systems

Cocaine is more potent and effective in inhibiting 5-HT neurons within the DRN than A10 DA neurons within the VTA (above). These findings may be attributable to the higher affinity of cocaine for the 5-HT, as compared to the DA, transporter (Ritz & Kuhar, 1989). Thus, when considering the overall effects of cocaine within the mesoaccumbens DA system, it seems that the influence on the DRN-nACC projection would be an initial increase in synaptic levels of 5-HT followed by a sharp and prolonged *decrease* in 5-HT release since activity in the DRN is completely suppressed and DRN cells do not recover from cocaine-induced inhibition for at least 1.5 hours (Cunningham & Laksoki, 1990). Thus, unlike DA transmission within the nACC, the initial increase in 5-HT transmission may be well compensated for by diminished impulse flow and release. Accordingly, the relative ratio of DA : 5-HT innervation may remain biased toward DA for an extended time after cocaine administration. Given the behavioral results indicating that heightened 5-HT activity might play an aversive role in the subjective effects of cocaine (Loh & Roberts, 1990), the increased ratio of DA to 5-HT transmission could be an important factor in the high efficacy of cocaine-induced reward processes.

EFFECTS OF REPEATED COCAINE ADMINISTRATION

VTA DA Cells

Because cocaine addiction is essentially chronic in nature, there have been numerous recent studies on the effects of repeated cocaine administration on monoaminergic transmission. One of the most pervasive behavioral consequences of repeated cocaine treatment is reverse tolerance or sensitization to its ability to enhance locomotion and cause stereotyped behaviors (Post & Weiss, 1988), both effects known to be mediated by midbrain DA systems.

Electrophysiological experiments have begun to determine the extent to which repeated cocaine administration alters the sensitivity of both somatodendritic DA autoreceptors on A10 DA neurons and of postsynaptic DA receptors located on target cells within the nACC (Henry et al., 1989). A10 DA neurons in animals treated repeatedly with cocaine (10 mg/kg i.p., twice daily) are significantly less sensitive to the inhibitory effects of i.v. apomorphine than those in control animals (Henry et al., 1989). A single administration of cocaine 12-24 hours before testing fails to produce this subsensitivity. Thus, repeated cocaine administration decreases the sensitivity of impulse-regulating somatodendritic D_2 autoreceptors on A10 DA cells by enhancing the degree of stimulation by the endogenous transmitter. Further evidence supporting this conclusion is provided by iontophoretic studies indicating that repeated cocaine administration reduces the responsiveness of A10 DA cells to DA, but not to GABA (Henry et al., 1989). Since GABA-B receptors and D_2 autoreceptors share the same K^+ conductance in midbrain DA neurons (Lacey et al., 1988), the locus of cocaine-induced desensitization would appear to be restricted to D_2 autoreceptors.

Because the basal activity of A10 DA cells is dependent on the density or sensitivity of A10 DA autoreceptors (White & Wang, 1984a), autoreceptor subsensitivity might be expected to increase the firing rate of spontaneously active A10 DA neurons and activate normally quiescent DA neurons. In fact, repeated cocaine administration increases both the number and the mean basal firing rate of spontaneously active A10 DA cells (Henry et al., 1989).

The subsensitivity of DA autoreceptors was observed to return to normal 4 to 8 days after the last injection of the cocaine treatment regimen (Ackerman & White, 1990). Thus, autoreceptor subsensitivity induced by repeated cocaine administration is not a persistent effect (Fig. 12-4). This finding raises questions about the relevance of this change to behavioral sensitization, which is known to be a long-lasting phenomenon.

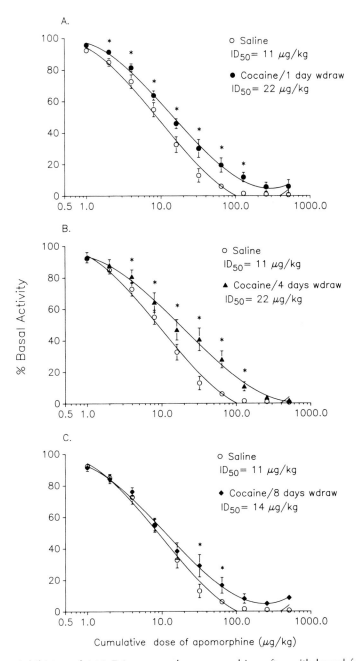

Figure 12-4. Inhibition of A10 DA neurons by apomorphine after withdrawal from re-peated cocaine treatment. The dose-response curve for apomorphine is shown for rats given 10 mg/kg cocaine or 1 ml/kg saline intraperitoneally twice daily for 14 days and tested 1 day (**A**), 4 days (**B**), or 8 days (**C**) after the last injection. The ID_{50} was calculated by linear regression analysis for individual cells, and statistical significance was determined by ANCOVA using basal firing rate as co-variate. A significant difference between points in the dose-response curve was determined by Dunnett's test. An asterisk indicates $P < 0.05$. (From Ackerman & White, 1990 with permission.)

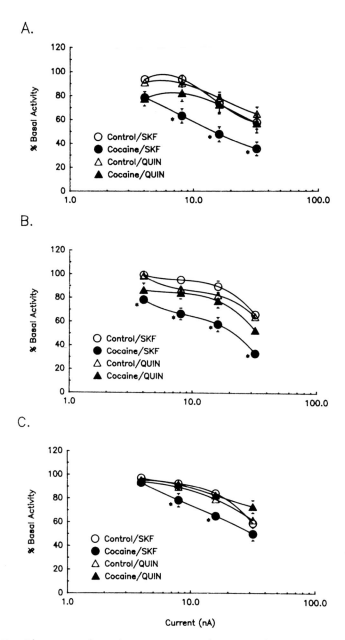

Figure 12-5. After repeated cocaine treatment, nucleus accumbens (nACC) neurons were supersensitive to the D_1 agonist SKF 38393 but not the D_2 agonist quinpirole (both administered at 0.01 m). In all three plots, rats had received either repeated cocaine (10 mg/kg i.p.) or saline for 14 days. **A,** Current-response curves illustrating the supersensitivity of nACC cells to iontophoretic administration of the D_1 agonist SKF 38393 12-24 hours after the last cocaine injection. After both a 1-week (**B**) and 1-month (**C**) withdrawal from cocaine treatment, nACC cells remained supersensitive to the effects of SKF 38393. Asterisks represent currents at which SKF 38393 was more effective in the rats that had received repeated cocaine administration.

DRN 5-HT Cells

Preliminary reports indicate that 5-HT neurons in the DRN are supersensitive to the inhibitory effects of both cocaine and the 5-HT$_{1A}$ agonist 8-OHDPAT after twice-daily injections of cocaine (15 mg/kg) for 7 days (Cunningham et al., 1992). Another study indicated that DRN neurons recorded with extracellular techniques from an in vitro slice preparation are subsensitive to the inhibitory effects of cocaine, with a shift in the EC$_{50}$ from 2.43 μm to 5.46 μm (Black & Lakoski, 1990). There was no observed tolerance to the effects of 5-HT, suggesting an alteration in the cocaine binding site as opposed to 5-HT autoreceptors. Further studies are needed to reconcile these discrepancies observed with in vivo and in vitro techniques.

nACC Neurons

In contrast to the effects of repeated cocaine treatment on VTA DA neurons, the responses of nACC neurons to iontophoretic cocaine are enhanced 1 day after the cessation of cocaine injections (Henry et al., 1989). nACC neurons also exhibit enhanced inhibitory responses to iontophoretic administration of 5-HT after repeated cocaine administration (Henry et al., 1989). Recently, Henry and White (1991) reported that these cells are significantly more sensitive to the inhibitory effects of the D$_1$ selective agonist SKF 38393 after 2 weeks of repeated cocaine injections. In contrast, the inhibitory effects of the selective D$_2$ agonist quinpirole are not altered (Fig. 12-5). Thus, the sensitization of nACC neurons to iontophoretic DA observed in the previous studies seems to be due primarily to enhanced sensitivity of the D$_1$ receptor.

Unlike D$_2$ autoreceptor subsensitivity, the supersensitivity of D$_1$ receptors within the nACC persists for 8 days after cocaine withdrawal (Fig. 12-5). In fact, supersensitive D$_1$ receptor-mediated responses are still evident after a 1-month withdrawal period. The sensitization of D$_1$ postsynaptic receptors within the nACC seems to be a relatively long-lasting adaptation produced by the repeated administration of cocaine and thus may be related to behavioral sensitization.

CHRONIC EFFECTS OF COCAINE ON DA AND 5-HT TRANSMISSION: SYNTHESIS

Repeated administration of cocaine to rats results in an enhancement of transmission through the mesoaccumbens neuronal system as compared to the first exposure to the drug. Electrophysiological studies have identified three components of this sensitized response. Each of these components may be essential for the development of behavioral sensitization accompanying repeated exposure to cocaine.

First, impulse-regulating somatodendritic autoreceptors on A10 DA cells within the VTA are rendered subsensitive by repeated cocaine administration. This adaptation results in an increase in the number of spontaneously active DA cells and their average basal firing rate. Although the autoreceptor subsensitivity does not seem to persist during withdrawal from the chronic treatment regimen, it seems likely that the resulting hyperactivity of DA cells may be an important initiating "trigger" for other, more permanent neuronal adjustments, including sensitization of D_1 receptors within the nACC. Thus, repeated administration of the selective D_1 agonist SKF 38393, as does cocaine, sensitizes striatal neurons to the inhibitory effects of D_1 agonists (White et al., 1990). However, unlike cocaine, the effect observed with SKF 38393 is not accompanied by an initial subsensitivity of DA autoreceptors and is very short-lived (<1 week).

Other results also support the notion that changes in VTA D_2 receptor sensitivity and the resulting increase in DA impulse flow might be necessary for behavioral sensitization. Repeated amphetamine injections into the VTA result in sensitized locomotor responses to systemic challenge with amphetamine, cocaine, and morphine (Kalivas & Weber, 1988; Vezina & Stewart, 1990). In contrast, repeated administration of amphetamine into the nACC does not produce behavioral sensitization (Dougherty & Ellinwood, 1981). Clearly, an essential component of sensitization occurs within the VTA and is probably related to alterations in impulse flow (Ackerman & White, 1990; Kalivas & Duffy, 1990).

The second electrophysiological component of repeated cocaine effects within the mesoaccumbens DA system is an enhanced sensitivity of D_1, but not D_2 receptors within the nACC. This finding may seem surprising in view of other studies indicating that similar treatments fail to increase D_1 receptor density within the nACC (Kleven et al., 1990; Peris et al., 1990). In fact, transient increases in nACC D_2 receptor density have been observed after such treatments (Goeders & Kuhar, 1987; Kleven et al., 1990; Peris et al., 1990). Taken together, these findings suggest that D_1 receptor supersensitivity may occur beyond the level of the recognition site.

Studies of D_1 receptor-activated transduction events have identified certain alterations that would be consistent with a supersensitivity of D_1 receptors. Nestler and colleagues have reported increased adenylate cyclase activity (forskolin-stimulated), augmented cAMP-dependent protein kinase activity, and reduced $G_{i\alpha}$ and $G_{o\alpha}$ levels in the nACC after repeated cocaine treatment regimens similar to that used in our experiments (Nestler et al., 1990; Terwilliger et al., 1991). Each of these changes could result in enhanced transmission through D_1 receptors.

The final electrophysiological component of repeated cocaine effects on mesoaccumbens DA transmission is actually an alteration in 5-HT action. Thus, increased 5-HT receptor-mediated inhibition, similar to that observed with DA, is observed after repeated cocaine administration. When combined with the subsensitivity of somatodendritic D_2 autoreceptors on A10 DA cells and their enhanced firing, the supersensitivity of nACC neurons to DA and 5-HT suggests that repeated exposure to cocaine produces a highly sensitized mesoaccumbens system. Thus, the unbalanced DA neurotransmission caused by acute cocaine administration is further magnified by repeated cocaine treatment. If DRN 5-HT neurons are supersensitive to cocaine after repeated administration, the altered DA : 5-HT ratio within the nACC might be further increased in favor of DA in sensitized animals because despite enhanced inhibitory effects of 5-HT within the nACC, the supersensitive response of DRN neurons to cocaine would diminish impulse-dependent 5-HT release.

The above account is not meant to overlook other possible mechanisms involved in sensitization. Clearly, repeated administration of cocaine results in a relatively persistent increase in DA release in response to subsequent challenge (Kalivas & Duffy, 1990; Peris et al., 1990). In addition, adaptations in the DA uptake processes (Izenwasser & Cox, 1990) and in nerve-terminal DA autoreceptor function (Peris et al., 1990; Yi & Johnson, 1990) may also play important roles. Finally, nondopaminergic systems projecting to the nACC may be altered to influence DA transmission indirectly (Post & Weiss, 1988). It is likely that behavioral sensitization results from a complex interplay among a number of neuronal adaptations, some of which may be necessary before others become manifest.

CONCLUSIONS AND FUTURE PERSPECTIVES

Cocaine exerts unique effects on mesoaccumbens and mesocortical DA systems. The highly efficacious inhibitory effects of cocaine on target neurons within the nACC and mPFC, combined with the relatively poor compensatory inhibition of the VTA DA neurons themselves, results in "unbalanced" transmission through these two reward-relevant DA systems. The mechanisms responsible for the greater efficacy of cocaine in inhibiting postsynaptic cells in these DA systems may be related to combined actions resulting from inhibition of both DA and 5-HT uptake. The potency and efficacy of cocaine as an inhibitor of 5-HT neurons within the DRN should result in better compensatory reductions in 5-HT activity than in the DA pathways. Thus, another result of cocaine administration may be an increase in the ratio of DA : 5-HT transmission within the nACC and mPFC.

Given the postulated roles of mesolimbic and mesocortical DA systems in mediating cocaine and other drug reinforcement, and of 5-HT systems as a possible aversive modulator of such processes, the interactions between DA and 5-HT within these pathways may be of considerable importance. Considerably more research is needed to further our understanding of the possible interactions between DA and 5-HT within reward relevant brain areas. The observation of additive inhibitory effects of these amines on most nACC cells, as well as opposing excitatory (5-HT) and inhibitory (DA) influences on others, is intriguing, but represents merely a first step in the identification of possible interactions. Heterologous regulation or modulation of release is clearly another possible site of DA/5-HT interaction.

The unbalanced nature of mesoaccumbens transmission is further magnified after repeated exposure to cocaine due to the subsensitivity of impulse-regulating A10 DA autoreceptors and the supersensitivity of D_1 receptors on nACC neurons. Although the autoreceptor subsensitivity seems to be an evanescent phenomenon, it may be necessary for more persistent alterations, including D_1 receptor supersensitivity. These changes, along with supersensitivity of 5-HT receptors and enhanced signal transduction mechanisms, are likely to participate in the behavioral sensitization to cocaine. The manner in which the neuronal alterations responsible for behavioral sensitization are related to cocaine craving and drug-seeking behavior in the cocaine addict is an important topic for further investigation.

Finally, it should again be appreciated that none of the studies reviewed in this chapter was conducted in freely moving animals. Thus, the conclusions reached herein must await appropriate testing in the intact, awake, behaving animal. Moreover, given the likelihood that the effects of cocaine will differ in rats that receive the drug in a response-contingent manner as opposed to experimenter discretion, the need for similar studies in animals that are actively self-administering the drug is paramount. Such experiments will be difficult because teasing out movement-related alterations in neuronal activity from those produced by drug administration will require precisely controlled experimental conditions. The neuronal mechanisms that we have implicated in this chapter were, by necessity, derived from experiments conducted in anesthetized rats or in brain slices. It is hoped that they will provide valuable heuristics for subsequent studies of cocaine effects in behaving animals.

ACKNOWLEDGMENTS

Many of the studies reviewed herein were made possible by USPHS Grants DA-04093 and MH-40832 (F.J.W.) and MH 28849 and DA 05119 (B.S.B.). The diligent efforts of Dr. Janice A. Ackerman, Dr. Leslie C. Einhorn, Douglas J. Henry, Dr. Xiu-Ti Hu, and Dr. Bita Moghaddam are gratefully acknowledged.

REFERENCES

Ackerman, J.A., & White, F.J. (1990). A10 somatodendritic dopamine autoreceptor sensitivity following withdrawal from repreated cocaine treatment. *Neurosci. Lett., 117*, 181-187.

Aghajanian, G.K., & Bunney, B.S. (1977). Dopamine "autoreceptors": Pharmacological characterization by microiontophoretic single cell recording studies. *Naunyn-Schmiedeberg's Arch. Pharmacol., 297*, 1-7.

Black, E.W., & Lakoski, J.M. (1990). In vitro electrophysiology of dorsal raphe serotonergic neurons in subchronic cocaine-treated rats: Development of tolerance to acute cocaine administration. *Mol. Cell. Neurosci., 1*, 84-91.

Bradberry, C.W., & Roth, R.H. (1989). Cocaine increases extracellular dopamine in rat nucleus accumbens and ventral tegmental area as shown by in vivo microdialysis. *Neurosci. Lett., 103*, 97-102.

Carroll, M.E., Lac, S.T., Asencio, M., & Kragh, R. (1990a). Fluoxetine reduces intravenous cocaine self-administration in rats. *Pharmacol. Biochem. Behav., 35*, 237-244.

Carroll, M.E., Lac, S.T., Asencio, M., & Kragh, R. (1990b). Intravenous cocaine self-administration is reduced by dietary 1-tryptophan. *Psychopharmacology, 100*, 293-300.

Chiodo, L.A., Bannon, M.J., Grace, A.A., Roth, R.H., & Bunney, B.S. (1984). Evidence for the absence of impulse-regulating somatodendritic and synthesis-modulating nerve terminal autoreceptors on subpopulations of mesocortical dopamine neurons. *Neuroscience, 12,* 1-16.

Clark, D., & White, F.J. (1987). Review: D1 dopamine receptor—the search for a function: A critical evaluation of the D1/D2 dopamine receptor classification and its functional implications. *Synapse, 1,* 347-388.

Cunningham, K.A., & Lakoski, J.M. (1988). Electrophysiological effects of cocaine and procaine on dorsal raphe serotonin neurons. *Eur. J. Pharmacol., 148,* 457-462.

Cunningham, K.A., & Lakoski, J.M. (1990). The interaction of cocaine with serotonin dorsal raphe neurons. Single-unit extracellular recording studies. *Neuropsychopharmacology, 3,* 41-50.

Cunningham, K.A., Paris, J.M., & Goeders, N.E. (1992). Chronic cocaine enhances serotonin autoregulation and serotonin uptake binding. *Synapse, 11,* 112-123.

Dougherty, Jr., G.G., & Ellinwood, Jr., E.E. (1981). Chronic amphetamine in nucleus accumbens: Lack of tolerance or reverse tolerance of locomotor activity. *Life Sci., 28,* 2295-2298.

Einhorn, L.C., Johansen, P.A., & White, F.J. (1988). Electrophysiological effects of cocaine in the mesoaccumbens dopamine system. *J. Neurosci., 8,* 100-112.

Goeders, N.E., & Kuhar, M.J. (1987). Chronic cocaine administration induces opposite changes in dopamine receptors in the striatum and nucleus accumbens. *Alcohol Drug Res., 7,* 207-216.

Goeders, N.E., & Smith, J.E. (1983). Cortical dopaminergic involvement in cocaine reinforcement. *Science, 221,* 773-775.

Goeders, N.E., Dworkin, S.I., & Smith, J.E. (1986). Neuropharmacological assessment of cocaine self-administration into the medial prefrontal cortex. *Pharmacol. Biochem. Behav., 24,* 1429-1440.

Grace, A.A., & Bunney, B.S. (1985). Opposing effects of striatonigral feedback pathways on midbrain dopamine cell activity. *Brain Res., 333,* 271-284.

Henry, D.J., & White, F.J. (1991). Repeated cocaine administration causes persistent enhancement of D1 dopamine receptor sensitivity within the rat nucleus accumbens. *J. Pharmacol. Exp. Ther., 258,* 882-890.

Henry, D.J., Greene, M.A., & White, F.J. (1989). Electrophysiological effects of cocaine in the mesoaccumbens dopamine system: Repeated administration. *J. Pharmacol. Exp. Ther., 251,* 833-839.

Hurd, Y.L., Kehr, J., & Ungerstedt, U. (1988). In vivo microdialysis as a technique to monitor drug transport: Correlation of extracellular cocaine levels and dopamine overflow in the rat brain. *J. Neurochem., 51,* 1314-1316.

Hurd, Y.L., Weiss, F., Koob, G.F., Anden, N.-E., & Ungerstedt, U. (1989). Cocaine reinforcement and extracellular dopamine overflow in rat nucleus accumbens. *Brain Res., 498,* 199-203.

Izenwasser, S., & Cox, B.M. (1990). Daily cocaine treatment produces a persistent reduction of [^{3}H]dopamine uptake in vitro in rat nucleus accumbens but not in striatum. *Brain Res., 531,* 338-341.

Kalivas, P.W., & Duffy, P. (1990). Effect of acute and daily cocaine treatment on extracellular dopamine in the nucleus accumbens. *Synapse, 5,* 48-58.

Kalivas, P.W., & Weber, (1988). Amphetamine injection into the ventral mesencephalon sensitizes rats to peripheral amphetamine and cocaine. *J. Pharmacol. Exp. Ther., 245,* 1095-1102.

Kalivas, P.W., Bourdelais, A., Abhold, R., & Abbott, L. (1989). Somatodendritic release of endogenous dopamine: In vivo dialysis in the A10 dopamine region. *Neurosci. Lett., 100,* 215-220.

Kleven, M.S., Perry, B.D., Woolverton, W.L., & Seiden, L.S. (1990). Effects of repeated injections of cocaine on D_1 and D_2 dopamine receptors in rat brain. *Brain Res., 532,* 265-270.

Lacey, M.G., Mercuri, N.B., & North, R.A. (1988). On the conductance increase activated by GABA-B and dopamine D2 receptors in rat substantia nigra neurones. *J. Physiol., 401,* 437-453.

Lacey, M.G., Mercuri, N.B., & North, R.A. (1990). Actions of cocaine on rat dopaminergic neurones in vitro. *Br. J. Pharmacol., 99,* 731-735.

Leccese, A.P., & Lyness, W.H. (1984). The effects of putative 5-hydroxytryptamine receptor active agents on *d*-amphetamine self-administration in controls and rats with 5,7-dihydroxytryptamine median forebrain bundle lesions. *Brain Res., 303,* 153-162.

Loh, E.A., & Roberts, D.C.S. (1990). Break-points on a progressive ration schedule reinforced by intravenous cocaine increase following depletion of forebrain serotonin. *Psychopharmacology, 101,* 262-266.

Lyness, W.H., Friedle, N.M., & Moore, K.E. (1980). Increased self-administration of *d*-amphetamine after destruction of 5-hydroxytryptaminergic nerves. *Pharmacol. Biochem. Behav., 12,* 937-941.

Martin-Iverson, M.T., Szostak, C., & Fibiger, H.C. (1986). 6-Hydroxydopamine lesions of the medial prefrontal cortex fail to influence intravenous self-administration of cocaine. *Psychopharmacology, 88,* 310-314.

Moghaddam, B., & Bunney, B.S. (1989). Differential effect of cocaine on extracellular dopamine levels in rat medial prefrontal cortex and nucleus accumbens: Comparison to amphetamine. *Synapse, 4,* 156-161.

Nicolaysen, L.C., Pan, H., & Justice, Jr., J.B. (1988). Extracellular cocaine and dopamine concentrations are linearly related in rat striatum. *Brain Res., 456,* 317-323.

Nestler, E.J., Terwilliger, R.Z., Walker, J.R., Sevarino, K.A., & Duman, R.S. (1990). Chronic cocaine treatment decreases levels of the G-protein subunits $G_{i\alpha}$ and $G_{o\alpha}$ in discrete regions of rat brain. *J. Neurochem., 55,* 1079-1082.

Pan, Z.Z., & Williams, J.T. (1989). Differential actions of cocaine and amphetamine on dorsal raphe neurons in vitro. *J. Pharmacol. Exp. Ther., 251,* 56-62.

Peris, J., Boyson, S.J., Cass, W.A., Curella, P., Dwoskin, L.P., Larson, G., Lin, L.-H., Yasuda, R.P., & Zahniser, N.R. (1990). Persistence of neurochemical changes in dopamine systems after repeated cocaine administration. *J. Pharmacol. Exp. Ther., 253,* 38-44.

Pitts, D.K., & Marwah, J. (1986). Electrophysiological effects of cocaine on central monoaminergic neurons. *Eur. J. Pharmacol., 131,* 95-98.

Pitts, D.K., & Marwah, J. (1987). Cocaine modulation of central monoaminergic neurotransmission. *Pharmacol. Biochem. Behav., 26,* 453-461.

Porrino, L.J., Ritz, M.C., Goodman, N.L., Sharpe, L.G., Kuhar, M.J., & Goldberg, S.R. (1989). Differential effects of the pharmacological manipulation of serotonin systems on cocaine and amphetamine self-administration in rats. *Life Sci., 45,* 1529-1535.

Post, R.M., & Weiss, S.R.B. (1988). Sensitization and kindling: Implications for the evolution of psychiatric symptomotology. In P.W. Kalivas & C.D. Barnes (Eds.), *Sensitization in the nervous system* (pp. 257-293) Caldwell, NJ: Telford Press.

Qiao, J.-T., Dougherty, P.M., Wiggins, R.C., & Dafny, N. (1990). Effects of microiontophoretic application of cocaine, alone and with receptor antagonists, upon the neurons of the medial prefrontal cortex, nucleus accumbens and caudate nucleus of rats. *Neuropharmacology, 29,* 379–385.

Ritz, M.C., & Kuhar, M.J. (1989). Relationship between self-administration of amphetamine and monoamine receptors in brain: Comparison with cocaine. *J. Pharmacol. Exp. Ther., 248,* 1010-1017.

Ritz, M.C., Lamb, R.J., Goldberg, S.R., & Kuhar, M.J. (1987). Cocaine receptors on dopamine transporters are related to self-administration. *Science, 237,* 1219-1223.

Roberts, D.C.S., & Koob, G.F. (1982). Disruption of cocaine self-administration following 6-hydroxydopamine lesions of the ventral tegmental area in rats. *Pharmacol. Biochem. Behav., 17,* 901-904.

Roberts, D.C.S., Koob, G.F., Klonoff, P., & Fibiger, H.C. (1980). Extinction and recovery of cocaine self-administration following 6-hydroxydopamine lesions of the nucleus accumbens. *Pharmacol. Biochem. Behav., 12,* 781-787.

Skirboll, L.R., & Bunney, B.S. (1979). The effects of acute and chronic haloperidol treatment on spontaneously firing neurons in the caudate nucleus of the rat. *Life Sci., 25,* 1419-1434.

Skirboll, L.R., Grace, A.A., & Bunney, B.S. (1979). Dopamine auto and postsynaptic receptors: Electrophysiological evidence for differential sensitivity to dopamine agonists. *Science, 206,* 80-83.

Terwilliger, R.Z., Beitner-Johnson, D., Sevarino, K.A., Crain, S.M., & Nestler, E.J. (1992). A general role for adaptations in G-proteins and the cyclic AMP system in mediating the chronic actions of morphine and cocaine on neuronal function. *Brain Res., 548,* 100-110.

Uchimura, N., & North, R.A. (1990). Actions of cocaine on rat nucleus accumbens neurons in vitro. *Br. J. Pharmacol., 99,* 736-740.

Vezina, P., & Stewart, J. (1990). Amphetamine administered to the ventral tegmenal area but not to the nucleus accumbens sensitizes rats to systemic morphine: Lack of conditioned effects. *Brain Res., 516,* 99-106.

Walaas, I., & Fonnum, F. (1980). Biochemical evidence for gamma-aminobutyrate-containing fibers from the nucleus accumbens to the substantia nigra and ventral tegmental area in the rat. *Neuroscience, 5,* 63-72.

Waszczak, B.L., & Walters, J.R. (1980). Intravenous GABA agonist administration stimulates firing of A10 dopaminergic neurons. *Eur. J. Pharmacol., 66,* 141-144.

White, F.J. (1990). The physiological basis of the rewarding effects of cocaine. *Behav. Pharmacol., 1,* 303-315.

White, F.J., & Wang, R.Y. (1984a). A10 dopamine neurons: Role of autoreceptors in determining firing rate and sensitivity to dopamine agonists. *Life Sci., 34,* 1161-1170.

White, F.J., & Wang, R.Y. (1984b). Pharmacological characterization of dopamine autoreceptors in rat ventral tegmental area: Microiontophoretic studies. *J. Pharmacol. Exp. Ther., 231,* 275-280.

White, F.J., & Wang, R.Y. (1986). Electrophysiological evidence for the existence of both D1 and D2 dopamine receptors in the rat nucleus accumbens. *J. Neurosci., 6,* 274-280.

White, F.J., Einhorn, L.C., Johansen, P.A., & Wachtel, S.R. (1987). Electrophysiological studies in the rat mesoaccumbens dopamine system: Focus on dopamine receptor subtypes, interactions, and the effects of cocaine. In L.A. Chiodo & A.S. Freeman (Eds.), *Neurophysiology of dopaminergic systems: Current status and clinical perspectives* (pp. 317-365). Detroit: Lakeshore Publishing Co.

White, F.J., Hu, X.-T., & Brooderson, R.J. (1990). Repeated stimulation of D1 dopamine receptors enhances the effects of DA agonists. *Eur. J. Pharmacol., 191,* 497-499.

Wise, R.A., & Rompre, P.-P. (1989). Brain dopamine and reward. *Annu. Rev. Psychol., 40,* 191-225.

Yi, S.-J., & Johnson, K.M. (1990). Chronic cocaine treatment impairs the regulation of synaptosomal ^{3}H-DA release by D_2 autoreceptors. *Pharmacol. Biochem. Behav., 36,* 457-461.

Zito, K.A., Roberts, D.C.S., & Vickers, G. (1985). Disruption of cocaine and heroin self-administration following kainic acid lesions of the nucleus accumbens. *Pharmacol. Biochem. Behav., 23,* 1029-1036.

13

Localization of Cannabinoid Receptors in Brain: Relationship to Motor and Reward Systems

MILES A. HERKENHAM

Marijuana (*Cannabis sativa*) is one of the oldest and most widely used drugs in the world, with a history of use dating back over 4000 years (Harris et al., 1977; Mechoulam, 1986). It was not until about 20 years ago that the principal psychoactive ingredient of the marihuana plant was isolated and found to be Δ^9-tetrahydrocannabinol (Δ^9-THC) (Gaoni & Mechoulam, 1964; Mechoulam, 1973; Mechoulam et al., 1970). Δ^9-THC and other natural and synthetic cannabinoids produce characteristic behavioral and cognitive effects (Dewey, 1986; Hollister, 1986), most of which can be attributed to actions on the central nervous system (Martin, 1986).

Until recently, very little was known about the cellular mechanisms through which cannabinoids act. The unique spectrum of cannabinoid effects and the stereoselectivity (enantioselectivity) of action of cannabinoid isomers in behavioral studies strongly suggested the existence of a specific cannabinoid receptor in brain, but early attempts to identify and characterize such a recognition site were not successful (see Devane et al., 1988; Herkenham, 1991; Herkenham et al., 1991b). (Enantioselectivity means that receptors will recognize a molecule in the correct three-dimensional conformation but not in a mirror-image form. This is a crucial criterion for identifying receptor-mediated drug actions.)

Without evidence that cannabinoids act through a specific receptor coupled to a functional effector system, researchers tended to study the effects of cannabinoids on membrane properties, membrane-bound enzymes, eicosanoid production, metabolism, and other neurotransmitter systems in vitro (Hilliard et al., 1985; Martin, 1986; Pertwee, 1988; Reichman et al., 1988). As noted by Howlett and colleagues (1990), most of the biochemical studies employed concentrations of Δ^9-THC that far exceeded those that might be found in brain tissue (for review, see Martin, 1986; Pertwee, 1988). In addition, the criterion of structure-activity relationship was not met—that is, the potencies of various

cannabinoids in the in vitro assays did not correlate with their relative potencies in eliciting characteristic behavioral effects (Howlett et al., 1990; Martin,
1986). Particularly damaging to the relevance of these in vitro studies was the
absence of enantioselectivity (Howlett et al., 1990).

Several groups have reported enantioselectivity of THC isomers in various
behavioral tests in vivo. Martin's group (1981) found that the potencies of (−)
and (+) forms of each of the cis and trans isomers of Δ^9-THC differ by 10- to
100-fold in producing static ataxia in dogs, depressing schedule-controlled responses in monkeys, and producing hypothermia and inhibiting spontaneous
activity in mice. Hollister et al. (1987) showed cannabinoid enantioselectivity in
human studies using indices of the subjective experience or "high." May's
group found enantioselectivity of a series of synthetic cannabinoids in tests of
motor depression and analgesia (Wilson & May, 1975; Wilson et al., 1976,
1979).

One of May's compounds, (−)-9-nor-9β-hydroxyhexahydrocannabinol
(β-HHC), was used as a lead compound by Johnson and Melvin (1986) for the
synthesis of a rather large series of structurally novel, classical and nonclassical cannabinoids for study of their potential use as analgesics (Fig. 13-1). The
synthetic cannabinoids share physicochemical properties with the natural cannabinoids and produce many behavioral and physiological effects characteristic
of Δ^9-THC, but are 5-1000 times more potent and show high enantioselectivity.

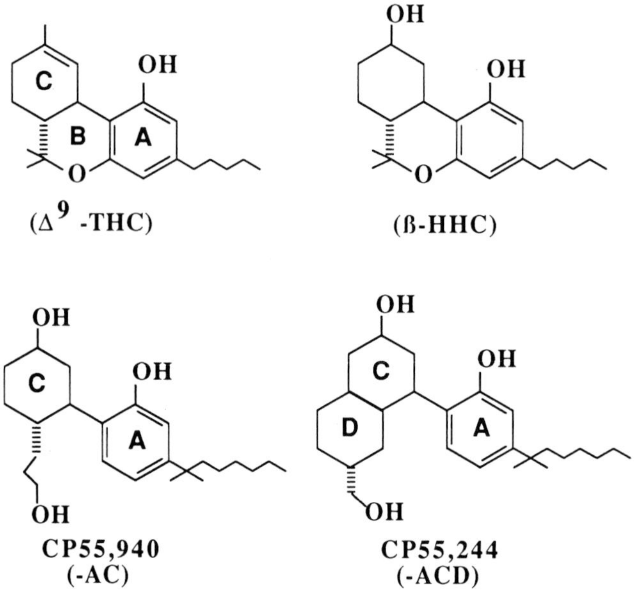

Figure 13-1. Chemical structures of Δ^9-THC and three synthetic cannabinoids. According to the nomenclature of Johnson and Melvin (1986), Δ^9-THC and 9-Nor-9β-hydroxy-
hexahydrocannabinol (β-HHC) are defined as members of the ABC-tricyclic cannabinoid
class. CP 55,940 is a hydroxypropyl analog of a 2-(3-hydroxycyclohexyl)phenol, defined
as an AC-bicyclic cannabinoid. CP 55,244 is an ACD-tricyclic cannabinoid with a rigidly
positioned hydroxypropyl moiety. (From Herkenham et al., 1991b, with permission.)

The availability of the nonclassical compounds revolutionized the study of the biochemical basis of cannabinoid activity. Howlett's group (1988) used them in neuroblastoma cell lines to show inhibition of adenylate cyclase activity. Such inhibition is enantioselective, and the pharmacological profile correlates well with that observed by Martin's group, which showed similar orders of potencies for the compounds in tests of mouse spontaneous activity, catalepsy, body temperature, and analgesia (Little et al., 1988).

One of the nonclassical compounds, CP 55,940, was tritiated and used by Howlett's group to identify and fully characterize a unique cannabinoid receptor in membranes from rat brain (Devane et al., 1988). The results from the centrifugation assay showed that [^{3}H]CP 55,940 receptor binding is saturable, has high affinity and enantioselectivity, and exhibits characteristics expected for a neuromodulator receptor associated with a guanine nucleotide regulatory (G) protein.

Recently, we characterized and validated the binding of [^{3}H]CP 55,940 in slide-mounted brain sections and described assay conditions to visualize autoradiographically the CNS distribution of cannabinoid receptors in a number of mammals, including humans (Herkenham et al., 1990). Autoradiography revealed a unique and conserved distribution; binding is most dense in outflow nuclei of the basal ganglia—the substantia nigra pars reticulata and globus pallidus—and in the hippocampus and cerebellum.

The discrete localization of dense receptors in the outflow nuclei of the basal ganglia suggests several important features of cannabinoid receptor distribution. Dense binding localized in the globus pallidus (GP), entopeduncular nucleus (EP), and substantia nigra pars reticulata (SNR) suggests an association of cannabinoid receptors with striatal efferent projections to these nuclei and therefore a role for cannabinoids in motor control. In addition, binding may be localized on mesostriatal dopaminergic neurons, which would implicate a role for cannabinoids in the direct control of dopamine release and therefore in brain reward mechanisms.

This chapter summarizes several key features of our cannabinoid receptor localization studies: (1) validation that the in vitro binding in brain sections is the same binding that mediates the effects of cannabinoids in vivo; (2) general features of brain distribution in several species, including human; and (3) neuronal localization of cannabinoid receptors to motor and/or limbic components of the basal ganglia, assessed by making selective chemical lesions of either the striatal GABAergic efferent or dopaminergic afferent pathways interconnecting the caudate-putamen (CP) and the substantia nigra.

RECEPTOR BINDING

The procedures for obtaining cryostat-cut slide-mounted brain sections have been described previously (Herkenham, 1991; Herkenham et al., 1990). The sections are incubated with [^{3}H]CP 55,940. For use in competition studies to characterize and validate binding, natural and synthetic cannabinoid ligands were obtained from the National Institute of Drug Abuse and Pfizer, Inc.

Names and stereochemical configurations of some of the cannabinoids are shown in Figure 13-1.

Autoradiography was performed on brain sections of rat, guinea pig, dog, rhesus monkey, and humans (dying of non-neurological disorders). Developed films were analyzed by a computer-based system for quantitative densitometry.

Both the D_1 and D_2 receptor assays were carried out as previously described (Richfield, 1990; Richfield & Herkenham, 1989; Richfield et al., 1986, 1987). The assay conditions had been optimized for selective labeling of each of the two dopamine receptor subtypes and for the dopamine uptake site. Subsequent film images of the radiolabeled ligand binding were analyzed as described above.

Selective neuronal lesions were made chemically, either by the placement of the neurotoxin ibotenate into the CP or of 6-hydroxydopamine (6-OHDA) into the medial forebrain bundle (MFB). These procedures resulted in either the destruction of striatal neurons and their projections to the pallidum and nigra (ibotenate) or of mesencephalic dopamine neurons and their projections to the striatum (6-OHDA) (Herkenham et al., 1991a).

A large series of cannabinoid and noncannabinoid drugs were assayed to test for competitive displacement of [^{3}H]CP 55,940 (Table 13-1). The competition curves and derived inhibition constants (Ki's) for the natural and synthetic cannabinoids provided a test for validation of binding. We found that highly significant ($P < 0.0001$) correlations exist between the Ki's and potencies of the drugs in tests of dog ataxia and human subjective experience, the two most reliable markers of cannabinoid activity (Dewey, 1986; Hollister, 1986). The Ki's also correlate very closely with relative potencies in tests of motor function (ataxia, hypokinesia, catalepsy), analgesia, and inhibition of contractions of guinea pig ileum and adenylate cyclase in neuroblastoma cell lines in vitro (Herkenham et al., 1990). Enantioselectivity is striking; the ($-$) and ($+$) forms of CP 55,244 differ by more than 10,000-fold in vitro, a separation predicted by the rigid structure of the molecule (Fig. 13-1) (Johnson & Melvin, 1986) and by potencies in vivo. Natural cannabinoids lacking psychoactive properties, such as cannabidiol, show extremely low potency at the receptor, and all tested noncannabinoid drugs had no potency (Table 13-1).

Autoradiography showed that in all species very dense binding is found in the globus pallidus, substantia nigra pars reticulata (SNR), and the molecular layers of the cerebellum and hippocampal dentate gyrus (Figs. 13-2 and 13-3). Dense binding is also found in the cerebral cortex, other parts of the hippocampal formation, and striatum. In rat, rhesus monkey, and human, the SNR contains the highest level of binding (Fig. 13-3). In dog, the cerebellar molecular layer is most dense (Fig. 13-2H). In guinea pig and dog, the hippocampal formation has selectively dense binding (Fig. 13-2E and F). Neocortex in all species has moderate binding across fields, with peaks in superficial and deep layers. Very low and homogeneous binding characterizes the thalamus and most of the brainstem, including all of the monoamine-containing cell groups; reticular formation; primary sensory, viscreomotor, and cranial motor nuclei; and the area postrema. The exceptions—hypothalamus, basal amygdala, central gray, nucleus of the solitary tract, and laminae I-III and X of the spinal cord—show slightly higher but still sparse binding (Figs. 13-2 and 13-3).

Table 13-1. Potencies of some cannabinoids in the section binding and other assays

Compound	Ki (nm)	Catalepsy/ataxia (mg/kg)	Mouse analgesia (mg/kg)	Cyclase Inh (nm)	Human "high" (mg)
CP 55,940 (−AC)	15 (Kd)	0.35	0.7	25	
CP 56,667 (+AC)	470	>10	>15	>5,000	
CP 55,244 (−ACD)	1.4	0.09	0.09	5	
CP 55,243 (+ACD)	18000	>10	>10	>10,000	
CP 50,556	14	1.5	0.4	100	0.5
CP 53,870	26000	>10	6.5	>5,000	
CP 54,939	14	0.05	0.7	7	
Nabilone	120	0.03		100	1
β-HHC	124	0.1	1.6		
α-HHC	2590	0.5	>50		
(−)Δ^9 THC	420	0.5	10	100	1
(+)Δ^9 THC	7700	>2.0	>100		
Δ^8 THC	498	0.5	8.8		2
11-OH-Δ^9 THC	210	0.05	1.9		1
TMA-Δ^8 THC	2300				
8β-OH-Δ^9 THC	4200				10
8α-OH-Δ^9 THC	8700				10
11-OH-Cannabinol	800				
Cannabinol	3200				>15
Cannabidiol	53000	Inactive	>100		>30
Cannabigerol	275000	>7			
9-COOH-11-nor-Δ^9 THC	75000	>40	10		
9-COOH-11-nor-Δ^8 THC	Inactive				

CP analogs were synthesized at Pfizer Central Research; their structures are given in Johnson and Melvin (1986). The first six analogs are enantiomeric pairs, as are α- and β-HHC and (−) and (+)Δ^9 THC. CP 50,556 is levonantradol; CP 53,870 is dextronantradol; CP 54,939 is desacetyl levonantradol; TMA-Δ^8 THC is trimethylammonium-Δ^8 THC. The last two compounds are Δ^9-THC metabolites. Ki's ± standard deviations are derived from binding surface analysis. Drugs that at 10 μm concentration show no inhibition of [^{3}H]CP 55,940 binding are amphetamine, beta-estradiol, cis-flupenthixol (dopamine receptor ligand), cocaine, corticosterone, cyclohexyladenosine, dexamethasone, etorphine (opiate receptor ligand), gamma-amino butyric acid (GABA), glutamate, leukotriene B$_4$ and D$_4$ (both at 1 μm), lysergic acid diethylamide (LSD), phencyclidine (PCP), prostaglandin E$_2$, Ro15-1788 (benzodiazepine receptor ligand), and thujone (the active ingredient of absinthe). Modified from Herkenham et al. (1990).

Quantitative autoradiography reveals very high numbers of receptors, exceeding 1 pmole/mg protein in densely labeled areas. Thus, cannabinoid receptor density is far in excess of densities of neuropeptide receptors and is similar to levels of cortical benzodiazepine (Zezula et al., 1988), striatal dopamine (Boyson et al., 1986; Richfield et al., 1986), and whole-brain glutamate receptors (Greenamyre et al., 1984).

The injection of ibotenate into the CP produced a large area of selective neuronal degeneration, in accordance with previous descriptions of toxicity in the dose range and location used (Köhler & Schwarcz, 1983). In the affected striatal territory, the losses on the lesion were the most profound for the dopamine D$_1$ receptors, showing a 96% reduction in binding at 4 weeks (Table 13-2). Cannabinoid and D$_2$ receptors were reduced by 78–80% in the affected territory, and the dopamine uptake site, which resides on afferent dopaminergic axons, was slightly reduced at 4 weeks (not shown).

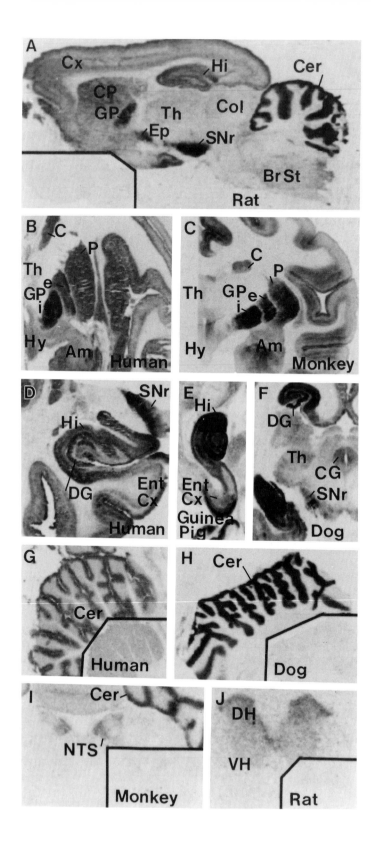

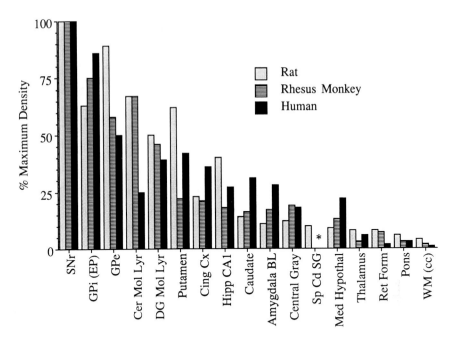

Figure 13-3. Relative densities of cannabinoid receptors across brain structures in rat, rhesus monkey, and human. Autoradiographic images were digitized by a solid-state camera and Macintosh II computer-based system for quantitative densitometry using Image™ software (Wayne Rasband, Research Services Branch, NIMH). Transmittance levels were converted to fmole/mg tissue using tritium standards and then normalized to the densest structure in each animal (SNr for all three). For every section incubated for total binding, an adjacent section was incubated in the presence of CP 55,244 to permit subtraction of nonspecific binding on a regional basis. Structure abbreviations not given in Figure 13-2 legend are Cing Cx, cingulate cortex; Hipp CA1, hippocampal field CA1; Med Hypothal, medial hypothalamus; Sp Cd SG, substantia gelatinosa of spinal cord (*only rat measured); Ret Form, reticular formation; WM (cc), white matter of corpus callosum. (From Herkenham et al., 1990, with permission.)

Figure 13-2. Autoradiography of 10 nm [³H]CP 55,940 binding in brain. Tritium-sensitive film exposed for 4 weeks, developed, and computer digitized. Images were photographed directly from the computer monitor. Gray levels represent relative levels of receptor densities. **A,** Sagittal section of rat brain. Coronal brain sections of human in **B, D,** and **G;** rhesus monkey in **C** and **I;** dog in **F** and **H;** and rat in **J.** Horizontal section of guinea pig brain in **E.** Insets show nonspecific binding in adjacent sections (miniaturized images are shown). Am, amygdala; Br St, brain stem; Cer, cerebellum; CG, central gray; C, caudate; Col, colliculi; CP, caudate-putamen; Cx, cerebral cortex; DG, dentate gyrus; DH, dorsal horn of spinal cord; Ent Cx, entorhinal cortex; Ep; entopeduncular nucleus (homolog of GPi); GP, globus pallidus (e, external; i, internal); Hi, hippocampus; Hy, hypothalamus; NTS, nucleus of solitary tract; P, putamen; SNR, substantia nigra pars reticulata; Th, thalamus; VH, ventral horn of spinal cord. (From Herkenham et al., 1990, with permission.)

Table 13-2. Effects of unilateral striatal ibotenate lesions at 4-weeks survival (n = 5)

Structure	Cannabinoid receptor	L % R	D_1 receptor	L % R	D_2 receptor	L % R
CP (L)	536 ± 37	20	69 ± 18	4	54 ± 25	18
(R)	2843 ± 849		1558 ± 111		299 ± 22	
GP (L)	719 ± 182	15	13 ± 6	12		
(R)	4763 ± 969		106 ± 28			
EP (L)	905 ± 340	22	57 ± 23	24		
(R)	4159 ± 834		240 ± 39			
SNR (L)	1023 ± 174	16	164 ± 16	13		
(R)	6421 ± 635		1254 ± 97			

Values are in fmole/mg protein and are the means and standard deviations of specific binding to approximately 50% of the total number (B_{max}) of receptors and 10% of uptake sites in each region, since ligand concentrations were near the K_d or below, in the case of [^{3}H]GBR-12935, for each drug. Corresponding locations on the control (R) side were outlined and measured. All left-right differences are significant at the $P < 0.005$ level of confidence except for the dopamine uptake site, which is significant at the $P < 0.05$ level (Student's paired t test). Data are from Herkenham et al. (1991a).

Both cannabinoid and D_1 dopamine receptors are lost in similar patterns (Fig. 13-4) and amounts (Table 13-2) in projection zones of lesioned striatal efferent neurons. In agreement with known medial-lateral topography of striatal projections (Altar & Hauser, 1987), receptor losses in both GP and SNR were greatest medially, with sparing of binding in lateral parts receiving projections from unlesioned parts of the lateral and posterior CP (Fig. 13-4). Reduction throughout the EP was evident for both D_1 and cannabinoid receptors. For cannabinoid receptor binding, losses in the labeled striatonigral pathway were also evident.

Following 6-OHDA lesions, Nissl-stained sections of the substantia nigra showed unilateral loss of neurons in the SNC (Fig. 13-4G). Autoradiography showed no change in cannabinoid receptor binding in either the striatum (Fig. 13-4D) or the nigra (Fig. 13-4E), whereas dopamine uptake sites were lost throughout the striatum and nigra on the lesioned side (Fig. 13-4F). Quantitative densitometry showed major losses of dopamine uptake sites in the CP, nucleus accumbens (nACC), and substantia nigra pars compacta (SNC), but no loss of cannabinoid receptors (Table 13-3).

Table 13-3. Effect of unilateral 6-OHDA lesions at 4-weeks survival (n = 4)

Structure	Cannabinoid receptor	L % R	Dopamine uptake site	L % R
CP (L)	4395 ± 266	99	62 ± 57	20
(R)	4422 ± 282		311 ± 60	
nACC (L)	2533 ± 384	102	38 ± 30	39
(R)	2491 ± 463		98 ± 13	
SNC (L)	1709 ± 320	95	1 ± 1	7
(R)	1807 ± 264		17 ± 7	

Values are in fmole/mg protein and are the means and standard deviations of specific binding to approximately 50% and 10% of the total number (B_{max}) of receptors and 10% of uptake sites in each region, respectively. Densitometric measures of CP, nACC, and SNC were each taken from the entire structure at the levels shown in Figure 13-3. Left-right cannabinoid receptor differences were not significant (Student's paired t test); dopamine uptake site left-right differences were significant in the CP ($P < 0.01$), nACC ($P = 0.05$), and SNC ($P < 0.03$). Data are from Herkenham et al. (1991a).

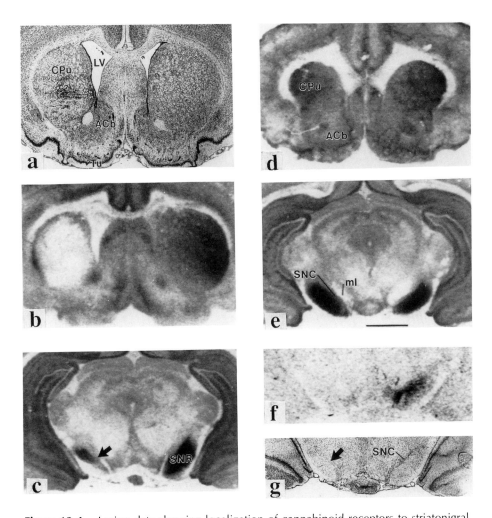

Figure 13-4. Lesion data showing localization of cannabinoid receptors to striatonigral neurons (**a-c**) and not to dopaminergic nigrostriatal neurons (**d-g**). As shown in **a-c**, a unilateral deposit of ibotenate was placed into the caudate-putamen (CPu). Nissl-stained section in (**a**) shows the area of selective neuronal loss and the enlarged lateral ventricle (LV). At 4-weeks survival, the losses of cannabinoid receptors in the CPu (**b**) and substantia nigra pars reticulata (SNR) (*arrow* in **c**) are shown autoradiographically. The losses are topographic; note sparing of laterally situated striatal neurons and their nigral projections. As shown in **d-g**, a unilateral lesion of the mesencephalic ascending dopamine system was made by depositing 6-OHDA into the medial forebrain bundle. At 4-weeks survival, degeneration of dopamine neurons in the substantia nigra pars compacta (SNC) is evident in the Nissl stain (*arrow* in **g**) and by the losses of dopamine uptake sites in the SNC (**f**), whereas cannabinoid receptor binding is unaffected in the striatum (**d**) and nigra (**e**). ACb, nucleus accumbens; ml, medial lemniscus; Tu, olfactory tubercle. Magnification bar measures 2 mm. (Modified from Herkenham et al., 1991a.)

DISCUSSION

Binding parameters depend on the assay used to characterize them. For this reason, optimization, kinetics, and validation must be done on slide-mounted brain sections of the type that will be used for autoradiographic visualization. In the case of cannabinoids, this requirement delivered an additional major dividend when it was discovered that the section assay, by its nature, obviates many of the technical problems associated with membrane binding. The section binding assay is easy to perform, does not require expensive equipment other than a cryostat, gives highly reproducible data, and shows high sensitivity to manipulations of binding conditions, such as the addition of guanine nucleotides (Herkenham et al., 1990). The assay circumvents technical problems inherent in membrane assays, such as adherence of ligand to glass, plastic surfaces, and to filters.

The structure-activity profile suggests that the receptor defined by the binding of [^{3}H]CP 55,940 is the same one that mediates many of the behavioral and pharmacological effects of cannabinoids (Table 13-1), including the subjective experience termed the human "high." All other tested psychoactive drugs, neurotransmitters, steroids, and eicosanoids at 10 μm concentrations fail to bind to this receptor. There is no compelling evidence for receptor subtypes from that analysis.

Autoradiography of cannabinoid receptors reveals a heterogeneous distribution pattern that conforms to cytoarchitectural and functional subdivisions in the brain. The distribution is unique—no other pattern of receptors is similar—and it is similar across several mammalian species, including human, suggesting that cannabinoid receptors are phylogenetically stable and conserved in evolution.

The locations of cannabinoid receptors help one understand cannabinoid pharmacology. Generally high densities in cerebral cortex (especially hippocampus), basal ganglia, and cerebellum implicate roles for cannabinoids in cognition and movement. Sparse densities in lower brainstem areas controlling cardiovascular and respiratory functions may explain why high doses of Δ^9-THC are not lethal.

The results of the 6-OHDA lesions indicate that cannabinoid receptors are not localized on mesencephalic dopamine neurons projecting to either the CP or the nACC. Systemically administered Δ^9-THC has been shown to elevate extracellular levels of dopamine in the CP (Ng Cheong Ton et al., 1988) and nACC (Chen et al., 1989). The mechanism of action seems to be indirect, as the effects are attenuated by naloxone (Chen et al., 1989). Nevertheless, it has been proposed that drugs that elevate dopamine levels in the striatum are those known to have abuse liability in humans (Di Chiara & Imperato, 1988; Kornetsky, 1985). In humans, cannabinoids can produce a feeling of euphoria as part of the subjective experience known as the marijuana "high," but dysphoria, dizziness, thought disturbances, and sleepiness are also reported (Dewey, 1986; Hollister, 1986; Johnson & Melvin, 1986). Animals generally do not self-administer Δ^9-THC (Harris et al., 1974; Leite & Carlini, 1974). Cannabinoids did not lower the threshold for electrical self-stimulation in one study

(Stark & Dews, 1980), although in another study they did (Gardner et al., 1988). However, apparently both this phenomenon and the enhancement of basal dopamine efflux from the nACC by Δ^9-THC are strain-specific, occurring only in the Lewis strain of rats (Gardner et al., 1989). Thus, the effects of cannabinoids on dopamine circuits thought to be common mediators of reward are indirect and differ from those of such drugs as cocaine and morphine, which interact directly with the dopamine neurons and produce craving and powerful drug-seeking behavior.

Accounts of cannabis use in humans stress a loosening of associations, fragmentation of thought, and confusion on attempting to remember recent occurrences (Hollister, 1986; Miller, 1984). These cognitive effects may be mediated by receptors in the cerebral cortex, especially the receptor-dense hippocampal cortex. The hippocampus "gates" information during memory consolidation and codes spatial and temporal relations among stimuli and responses (Douglas, 1967; Eichenbaum & Cohen, 1988). Δ^9-THC causes memory "intrusions" (Hooker & Jones, 1987), impairs temporal aspects of performance (Schulze et al., 1988), and suppresses hippocampal electrical activity (Campbell et al., 1986).

The localization of cannabinoid receptors in motor areas suggests therapeutic applications for movement disorders. Cannabinoids have been shown to be beneficial for some forms of dystonia, tremor, and spasticity (Clifford, 1983; Dewey, 1986; Hollister, 1986; Marsden, 1981; Meinck et al., 1989; Petro & Ellenberger, 1981). The lack of association of cannabinoid receptors with dopamine neurons indicates that cannabinoids do not directly affect dopamine release associated with reward and drug-seeking behavior. Further work may show the basis for its reported usefulness in controlling nausea and stimulating appetite in patients receiving chemotherapy for cancer or AIDS. Finally, the development of an antagonist could lead to additional therapeutic applications. The section binding assay can be used to screen the potencies of novel drugs and to identify cannabinoid receptor subtypes, which could lead to renewed interest in developing cannabinoid drugs without unwanted side effects.

REFERENCES

Altar, C.A., & Hauser, K. (1987). Topography of substantia nigra innervation by D_1 receptor containing striatal neurons. *Brain Res., 410,* 1-11.

Boyson, S.J., McGonigle, P., & Molinoff, P.B. (1986). Quantitative autoradiographic localization of the D_1 and D_2 subtypes of dopamine receptors in rat brain. *J. Neurosci., 6,* 3177-3188.

Campbell, K.A., Foster, T.C., Hampson, R.E., & Deadwyler, S.A. (1986). Effects of Δ^9-tetrahydrocannabinol on sensory-evoked discharges of granule cells in the dentate gyrus of behaving rats. *J. Pharmacol. Exp. Ther., 239,* 941-945.

Chen, J., Paredes, W., Li, J., Smith, D., & Gardner, E.L. (1989). In vivo brain microdialysis studies of Δ^9-tetrahydrocannabinol on presynaptic dopamine efflux in nucleus accumbens. *Soc. Neurosci. Abst., 15,* 1096.

Clifford, D.B. (1983). Tetrahydrocannabinol for tremor in multiple sclerosis. *Ann. Neurol., 13,* 669-671.

Devane, W.A., Dysarz, F.A.I., Johnson, M.R., Melvin, L.S., & Howlett, A.C. (1988). Determination and characterization of a cannabinoid receptor in rat brain. *Mol. Pharmacol., 34,* 605-613.

Dewey, W.L. (1986). Cannabinoid pharmacology. *Pharmacol. Rev., 38,* 151-178.

Di Chiara, G., & Imperato, A. (1988). Drugs abused by humans preferentially increase synaptic dopamine concentrations in the mesolimbic system of freely moving rats. *Proc. Natl. Acad. Sci. USA., 85,* 5274-5278.

Douglas, R.J. (1967). The hippocampus and behavior. *Psychol. Bull., 67,* 416-442.

Eichenbaum, H., & Cohen, N.J. (1988). Representation in the hippocampus: What do hippocampal neurons encode? *Trends Neurosci., 11,* 244-248.

Gaoni, Y., & Mechoulam, R. (1964). Isolation, structure, and partial synthesis of an active constituent of hashish. *J. Am. Chem. Soc., 86,* 1646.

Gardner, E.L., Paredes, W., Smith, D., Donner, A., Milling, C., Cohen, D., & Morrison, D. (1988). Facilitation of brain stimulation reward by Δ^9-tetrahydrocannabinol. *Psychopharmacology, 96,* 142-144.

Gardner, E.L., Chen, J., Paredes, W., Li, J., & Smith, D. (1989). Strain-specific facilitation of brain stimulation reward by Δ^9-tetrahydrocannabinol in laboratory rats is mirrored by strain-specific facilitation of presynaptic dopamine efflux in nucleus accumbens. *Soc. Neurosci. Abst., 15,* 638.

Greenamyre, J.T., Young, A.B., & Penney, J.B. (1984). Quantitative autoradiographic distribution of L-[^{3}H]glutamate binding sites in rat central nervous system. *J. Neurosci., 4,* 2133-2144.

Harris, R.T., Waters, W., & McLendon, D. (1974). Evaluation of reinforcing capability of Δ^9-tetrahydrocannabinol in rhesus monkeys. *Psychopharmacologia, 37,* 23-29.

Harris, L.S., Dewey, W.L., & Razdan, R.K. (1977). Cannabis. Its chemistry, pharmacology, and toxicology. In W.R. Martin (Ed.), *Handbook of experimental pharmacology* (pp. 371-429). New York: Springer-Verlag.

Herkenham, M. (1991). Characterization and localization of cannabinoid receptors in brain: An in vitro technique using slide-mounted tissue sections. *NIDA Res. Monogr., 112,* 129-145.

Herkenham, M., Lynn, A.B., Little, M.D., Johnson, M.R., Melvin, L.S., de Costa, B.R., & Rice, K.C. (1990). Cannabinoid receptor localization in brain. *Proc. Natl. Acad. Sci. USA., 87,* 1932-1936.

Herkenham, M., Lynn, A.B., de Costa, B., & Richfield, E.K. (1991a). Neuronal localization of cannabinoid receptors in the basal ganglia of the rat. *Brain Res., 547,* 267-274.

Herkenham, M., Lynn, A.B., Johnson, M.R., Melvin, L.S., de Costa, B.R., & Rice, K.C. (1991b). Characterization and localization of cannabinoid receptors in rat brain: A quantitative in vitro autoradiographic study. *J. Neurosci., 11,* 563-583.

Hilliard, C.J., Harris, R.A., & Bloom, A.S. (1985). Effects of the cannabinoids on physical properties of brain membranes and phospholipid vesicles: Fluorescent studies. *J. Pharmacol. Exp. Ther., 232,* 579-588.

Hollister, L.E. (1986). Health aspects of cannabis. *Pharmacol. Rev., 38,* 1-20.

Hollister, L.E., Gillespie, H.K., Mechoulam, R., & Srebnik, M. (1987). Human pharmacology of 1S and 1R enantiomers of delta-3-tetrahydrocannabinol. *Psychopharmacology, 92,* 505-507.

Hooker, W.D., & Jones, R.T. (1987). Increased susceptibility to memory intrusions and the Stroop interference effect during acute marijuana intoxication. *Psychopharmacology, 91,* 20-24.

Howlett, A.C., Johnson, M.R., Melvin, L.S., & Milne, G.M. (1988). Nonclassical cannabinoid analgesics inhibit adenylate cyclase: Development of a cannabinoid receptor model. *Mol. Pharmacol., 33,* 297-302.

Howlett, A.C., Bidaut-Russell, M., Devane, W.A., Melvin, L.S., Johnson, M.R., & Herkenham, M. (1990). The cannabinoid receptor: Biochemical, anatomical and behavioral characterization. *Trends Neurosci., 13,* 420-423.

Johnson, M.R., & Melvin, L.S. (1986). The discovery of nonclassical cannabinoid analgetics. In R. Mechoulam (Ed.), *Cannabinoids as therapeutic agents* (pp. 121-145). Boca Raton, FL: CRC Press.

Köhler, C., & Schwarcz, R. (1983). Comparison of ibotenate and kainate neurotoxicity in rat brain: A histological study. *Neuroscience, 8,* 819-835.

Kornetsky, C. (1985). Brain-stimulation reward: A model for the neuronal bases for drug-induced euphoria. *NIDA Res. Monogr., 62,* 30-50.

Kozel, N.J., & Adams, E.H. (1986). Epidemiology of drug abuse: An overview. *Science, 234,* 970-974.

Leite, J.R., & Carlini, E.A. (1974). Failure to obtain "cannabis-directed behavior" and abstinence syndrome in rats chronically treated with cannabis sativa extracts. *Psychopharmacologia, 36,* 133-145.

Little, P.J., Compton, D.R., Johnson, M.R., & Martin, B.R. (1988). Pharmacology and stereoselectivity of structurally novel cannabinoids in mice. *J. Pharmacol. Exp. Ther., 247,* 1046-1051.

Marsden, C.D. (1981). Treatment of torsion dystonia. In A. Barbeau (Ed.), *Disorders of movement: Current status of modern therapy,* Vol. 8 (pp. 81-104). Philadelphia: JB Lippincott.

Martin, B.R. (1986). Cellular effects of cannabinoids. *Pharmacol. Rev., 38,* 45-74.

Martin, B.R., Balster, R.L., Razdan, R.K., Harris, L.S., & Dewey, W.L. (1981). Behavioral comparisons of the stereoisomers of tetrahydrocannabinols. *Life Sci., 29,* 565-574.

Mechoulam, R. (1973). Cannabinoid chemistry. In R. Mechoulam (Ed.), *Marihuana: Chemistry, pharmacology, metabolism, and clinical effects* (pp. 1-99). New York: Academic Press.

Mechoulam, R. (1986). The pharmacohistory of *Cannabis sativa.* In R. Mechoulam (Ed.), *Cannabinoids as therapeutic agents* (pp. 1-19). Boca Raton, FL: CRC Press.

Mechoulam, R., Shani, A., Edery, H., & Grunfeld, Y. (1970). Chemical basis of hashish activity. *Science, 169,* 611-612.

Meinck, H.-M., Schonle, P.W., & Conrad, B. (1989). Effect of cannabinoids on spasticity and ataxia in multiple sclerosis. *J. Neurol., 236,* 120-122.

Miller, L.L. (1984). Marijuana: Acute effects on human memory. In S. Agurell, W.L. Dewey, & R.E. Willette (Eds.), *The cannabinoids: Chemical, pharmacologic, and therapeutic aspects* (pp. 21-46). New York: Academic Press.

Ng Cheong Ton, J.M., Gerhardt, G.A., Friedemann, M., Etgen, A.M., Rose, G.M., Sharpless, N.S., & Gardner, E.L. (1988). The effects of Δ^9-tetrahydrocannabinol on potassium-evoked release of dopamine in the rat caudate nucleus; an in vivo electrochemical and in vivo microdialysis study. *Brain Res., 451,* 59-68.

Pertwee, R.G. (1988). The central neuropharmacology of psychotropic cannabinoids. *Pharmacol. Ther., 36,* 189-261.

Petro, D.J., & Ellenberger, C.E. (1981). Treatment of human spasticity with delta-9-tetrahydrocannabinol. *J. Clin. Pharmacol., 21,* 413s-416s.

Reichman, M., Nen, W., & Hokin, L.E. (1988). Δ^9-Tetrahydrocannabinol increases arachnadonic acid levels in guinea pig cerebral cortex slices. *Mol. Pharmacol., 34,* 823-828.

Richfield, E.K. (1990). Quantitative autoradiography of the dopamine uptake complex in rat brain using [^{3}H]GBR 12935: Binding characteristics. *Brain Res., 540,* 1-13.

Richfield, E.K., & Herkenham, M. (1989). Quantitative autoradiography of the dopamine uptake complex in the central nervous system. *Soc. Neurosci. Abst., 15,* 1230.

Richfield, E.K., Young, A.B., & Penney, J.B. (1986). Properties of D$_2$ dopamine receptor autoradiography: High percentage of high-affinity agonist sites and increased nucleotide sensitivity in tissue sections. *Brain Res., 383,* 121-128.

Richfield, E.K., Young, A.B., & Penney, J.B. (1987). Comparative distribution of dopamine D-1 and D-2 receptors in the basal ganglia of turtle, pigeon, rat, cat, and monkey. *J. Comp. Neurol., 262,* 446-463.

Schulze, G.E., McMillan, D.E., Bailey, J.R., Scallet, A., Ali, S.F., Slikker, W.J., & Paule, M.G. (1988). Acute effects of Δ-9-tetrahydrocannabinol in rhesus monkeys as measured by performance in a battery of complex operant tests. *J. Pharmacol. Exp. Ther., 245,* 178-186.

Stark, P., & Dews, P.B. (1980). Cannabinoids. I. Behavioral Effects. *J. Pharmacol. Exp. Ther., 214,* 124-130.

Wilson, R.S., & May, E.L. (1975). Analgesic properties of the tetrahydrocannabinols, their metabolites, and analogs. *J. Med. Chem., 18,* 700-703.

Wilson, R.S., May, E.L., Martin, B.R., & Dewey, W.L. (1976). 9-Nor-9-hydroxy-hexahydrocannabinols. Synthesis, some behavioral and analgesic properties, and comparison with the tetrahydrocannabinols. *J. Med. Chem., 19,* 1165-1167.

Wilson, R.S., May, E.L., & Dewey, W.L. (1979). Some 9-hydroxycannabinoid-like compounds. Synthesis and evaluation of analgesic and behavioral properties. *J. Med. Chem., 22,* 886-888.

Zezula, J., Cortés, R., Probst, A., & Palacios, J.M. (1988). Benzodiazepine receptor sites in the human brain: Autoradiographic mapping. *Neuroscience, 25,* 771-795.

14

Effects of Cannabinoids and Nicotine on Central Nervous System Neurons

SAM A. DEADWYLER, ROBERT HAMPSON,
BARBARA BENNETT, SHAO WANG, CHARLES HEYSER,
AND JIAN MU

Nicotine and cannabinoids, two substances associated with compulsive use, are normally smoked and therefore have high potency as well as rapid access to neurons in the brain via the pulmonary vascular system. It is important to understand how occupancy by nicotine and cannabinoids of their specific receptors in central neurons produces changes in membrane conductances. One method of acquiring detailed information on these actions is to assess them in cultures of CNS neurons prepared from different brain regions. Under these conditions, it is possible to isolate the direct actions of the substance to determine accurately the potency and time course of effects on identified cellular processes.

Several aspects of cannabinoid and nicotinic actions on specific neuronal processes are described in this chapter. Where possible, the functional implications of these cellular actions for cognitive and behavioral processes are addressed.

EFFECTS OF PSYCHOACTIVE CANNABINOIDS ON CNS NEURONAL ACTIVITY

The effects of cannabinoids on the human nervous system range from the hallucinations and euphoria that underlie the abuse potential of *Cannabis* extracts, to potentially therapeutic analgesic, antiemetic, and antiglaucoma properties (Dewey, 1986; Martin, 1986; Howlett et al., 1990). Until quite recently, research into the mechanisms by which cannabinoids affect the CNS concen-

This work was supported by grants from the National Institute on Drug Abuse (DA03502, DA04441, DA00119 [S.A.D.], DA05073 [B.A.B.]) and gifts from the R.J. Reynolds Tobacco Co. and Sterling Drug Co. to S.A.D.

trated on neural membrane anesthetic effects (Karler et al., 1984, 1986; Turkanis & Karler, 1983).

Growing evidence of the existence of a cannabinoid receptor (Devane et al., 1988; Nye et al., 1985; Turkanis & Karler, 1983), was confirmed by the recent labeling, isolation, and cloning of the receptor (Herkenham et al., 1990; Howlett et al., 1990; Matsuda et al., 1990). Given this discovery, the focus of research has shifted to reconciling the wide range of pharmacological effects of cannabinoids. Now that specific cannabinoid-receptor interactions can be investigated, it is especially important to determine the cellular mechanisms affected by occupancy of this receptor. Such knowledge may eventually make it possible to isolate therapeutic from psychogenic effects of cannabinoids.

The cellular effects of cannabinoids were originally believed to result from their anesthetic properties, leading to considerable interest in the development of a cannabinoid-based analgesic. However, the finding that cannabinoids inhibit adenylyl cyclase in NG108-15 neuroblastoma x glioma cells (Howlett, 1985) suggested that these compounds may bind to G-protein-coupled receptors. Larry Melvin and Ross Johnson at Pfizer Central Research synthesized a number of compounds from the parent drug levonantradol and, in collaboration with Allyn Howlett, demonstrated their increased potency as analgesic agents and inhibitors of cAMP accumulation (Howlett, 1990; Howlett et al., 1988). The most potent of these compounds, designated CP 55,940 and CP 55,244, were later tested in a number of bioassay systems (Johnson et al., 1988). This group of researchers published a characterization of the cannabinoid receptor based on structure-activity data from Δ^9-THC and the analog compounds, including their binding potency to crude brain membrane fractions and their ability to decrease cAMP levels in brain tissue slices (Devane et al., 1988). The chemical structure of these compounds suggested three main areas of attachment of the ligand to the cannabinoid receptor (Howlett et al., 1988).

This three-position binding model (Howlett et al., 1988, 1990; Johnson et al., 1988) has remained the primary model for the ligand-specific actions of cannabinoids under a number of test conditions. More recently Susan Ward (Sterling Drug Co.), Steve Childers (Bowman Gray School of Medicine), and their co-workers (Pacheco et al., 1992) reported that the aminoalkylindoles, synthesized by Sterling, are potent cannabinoid receptor ligands. The fact that the aminoalkylindoles WIN 55,212-2, are somewhat dissimilar in structure to the Pfizer analogs suggests there may be different configurations of the cannabinoid receptor.

The cannabinoid receptor is a G-protein-coupled receptor, with seven transmembrane segments and numerous conserved residues typifying G-protein-coupled receptors (Matsuda et al., 1990). The binding of cannabinoid analogs, such as [^{3}H]-CP-55,940, and such aminoalkylindoles as [^{3}H]-WIN-55,212-2 is sensitive to sodium and guanine nucleotides (Howlett, 1990; Ward, unpublished data). Moreover, agonist occupation of cannabinoid receptors produces GTP-dependent inhibition of adenylyl cyclase, as determined in NG108 cells (Howlett, 1985), and brain membrane homogenates (Howlett, 1990; Pacheco et al., 1991).

The distribution of the cannabinoid receptor in brain has recently been reported by Miles Herkenham and co-workers (1990, 1991; see Chapter 13). The receptor is enriched in such areas as substantia nigra (pars reticulata), hippo-campus (dentate gyrus), and cerebellum (molecular layer). In these areas, the density of cannabinoid receptor binding sites is high compared to other G-protein-coupled receptors. Moreover, the distribution and density of the receptor vary among mammalian species (Herkenham et al., 1990).

ACTIONS OF CANNABINOIDS AND CANNABINOID ANALOGS ON CNS NEURONS IN CULTURE

In vitro systems provide one of the best approaches for testing the actions of unknown compounds on neural processes. Our initial studies used the in vitro hippocampal slice preparation to examine the effects of Δ^9-THC on cellular and synaptic processes (Deadwyler, 1986; Deadwyler et al., 1985). More recent studies of the actions of cannabinoids have utilized a well-studied tissue culture system to minimize alternative interpretations of electrophysiological effects. Briefly, cells from fetal hippocampus and cerebral cortex were dissociated after removal from 18-day-old fetal rat brains and grown in culture for 5-17 days. Preservation of neuronal activity was determined by assessment of intact volt-age-sensitive currents and the response to exogenously applied neurotransmit-ters with known postsynaptic actions. Only cells in which stable active currents were present were used in tests of cannabinoid action.

We used local pipette as well as bath application of cannabinoid sub-stances. Because cannabinoid substances do not dissolve in aqueous media, they were prepared in suspension. Complications introduced by detergents used in the suspension were minimized by the use of a nondetergent suspension vehicle, cyclodextrin (Howlett, 1985). The delivery pipette was positioned within 20-30 μm of the cell for most recordings. This technique has been found to reflect true dose-response relationships in cultured cells (Dichter, 1986). The use of physiological doses of cannabinoids was validated by increasing the distance between the drug delivery pipette and the cell and observing a corre-sponding proportional decrease in time course and magnitude of cannabinoid effects.

Results were obtained using whole-cell patch-clamp recording. The tech-niques utilized to form gigaseals and to excise membrane from the interior of the electrode were similar to that described by Hamill et al. (1981). Under these recording conditions it was necessary for the patch pipette to contain a differ-ent concentration of electrolytes than normally found in the cell interior; there-fore, the cell was dialyzed with the media in the pipette. In the studies pre-sented below, this dialysis changed the intracellular chloride concentration, causing the equilibrium potential for chloride (E_{Cl}) to be shifted from -90 mV to between 0 and $+10$ mV.

An important question concerning cannabinoid receptor function was whether Δ^9-THC or the high-potency cannabinoid analogs produced a change in membrane conductance or more specifically a ligand-gated current. We de-termined this by applying cannabinoids to cultured hippocampal and cortical neurons under voltage-clamp conditions. The cannabinoid-gated current re-flected a flow of ions as evidenced by the reduction in the inward current and reversal to outward current as the membrane was stepped to more depolarized levels. This is shown for the three cannabinoid receptor ligands (Δ^9-THC, levonantradol, and CP 55,940) in Figure 14-1. The deflections associated with drug application represent inward currents of similar magnitude and duration for each ligand. The duration of cannabinoid-gated current was magnitude-dependent and ranged between 1-3 seconds. The reversal potential for THC, CP 55,940, and levonantradol currents ranged from $+10$ to $+14$ mV, which was near E_{Cl} (0 mV) in this preparation. The cannabinoid current was very large at extreme hyperpolarized membrane levels, reflecting the increased driving force on chloride ions. The whole-cell conductance during the levonantradol-gated

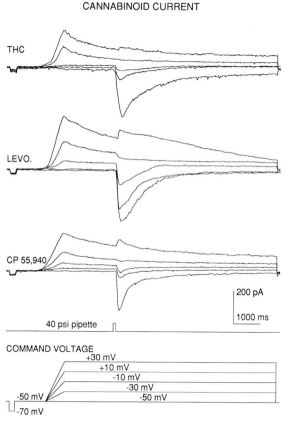

Figure 14-1. Reversal potentials for currents gated by cannabinoid receptor ligands, Δ^9-THC, and the synthetic analogs, levonantradol and CP55,940 (Pfizer). Application of Δ^9-THC resulted in an inward current at resting membrane potential (-50 mV). The current decreased as the membrane was depolarized, and it reversed at membrane potentials between $+10$ and $+30$ mV. The voltage command profile is shown in the bottom panel. Voltage steps were "ramped" to avoid activation of rate-sensitive currents. Rectification was apparent at more depolarized step commands. The pressure pulse to the pipette was the same duration (25 ms) and intensity (40 PSI) for each compound, and the concentration of the substances were the same (1.0 mM) in each delivery pipette.

current was 4.2 ns, whereas CP 55,940 and Δ^9-THC currents ranged between 2.6-2.9 ns respectively.

The ionic basis of the inward current was investigated in two ways—by ion substitution and by changing E_{Cl} in the preparation. First, chloride in the recording pipette was replaced by acetate, which maintained the normal chloride concentration in the cell (<5.0 mM). Under these conditions, the cannabinoid-gated current did not reverse until -90 mV, which was the calculated E_{Cl} for this cell. Subsequently reducing the extracellular chloride concentration to 5.0 mM in the bathing medium completely eliminated the outward current. These two manipulations strongly suggest that the cannabinoid-gated current in these neurons is mediated, at least in part, by chloride ions (Huguenard & Alger, 1986; Ozawa & Yuzaki, 1984; Zhang et al., 1990).

The cannabinoid gated-current was insensitive to blockade of voltage-sensitive sodium channels by tetrodotoxin (TTX, 1-10 μM). The lower traces in Figure 14-2 indicate that the voltage-sensitive inward sodium current in the same cell was blocked by TTX. Thus, the cannabinoid current was TTX-insensitive, indicating that invasion of presynaptic terminals by action potentials is not a necessary condition for production of the chloride conductance change.

The cannabinoid current was compared to GABA and glutamate-gated currents in the same hippocampal and cortical cell cultures. Glutamate current (2.7 nS) was inward (depolarizing) at resting potential (-50 mV) and reversed when applied at membrane potentials of $\geq +26$ mV. This depolarizing glutamate current has been documented by several investigations as being mediated by both sodium and calcium ions (Brown et al., 1990; Jahr & Stevens, 1987; Tsuzuki et al., 1989). Elimination of chloride did not affect the magnitude or duration of the glutamate-gated current. Therefore, the cannabinoid current could not have resulted from the nonspecific activation of glutamate receptor channels.

Figure 14-3 shows the production of a large GABA current recorded in a cultured hippocampal neuron. This current was also inward, but as with cannabinoid currents, it was produced by the outward movement of chloride ions. The similarity of GABA-evoked current to the cannabinoid current was apparent in that the reversal potentials for both currents were nearly the same ($+10$ mV), and the whole-cell conductance for GABA (4.7 nS) was similar to levonantradol (4.2 nS). The similarity between the GABA and cannabinoid-gated currents implicates a chloride current in cannabinoid receptor-mediated effects on CNS neurons. This result also suggests that the cannabinoid current is possibly mediated by activation of a $GABA_A$ receptor-mediated conductance. Further investigation of this relationship with other cannabinoid analogs is required before such a possibility can be confirmed.

The recently cloned cannabinoid receptor has been identified as a G-protein-coupled receptor (Matsuda et al., 1990). To compare the cannabinoid currents described above with those of known G-protein-coupled receptors, neurons in hippocampal culture were exposed to the $GABA_B$ agonist baclofen. The $GABA_B$ receptor in hipocampal cells controls a potassium current, and baclofen gates this current (Thalmann, 1988). The current produced by this ligand was quite different from either the cannabinoid or GABA current. The reversal

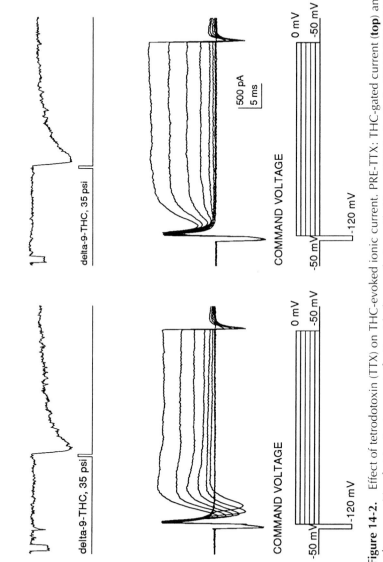

Figure 14-2. Effect of tetrodotoxin (TTX) on THC-evoked ionic current. PRE-TTX: THC-gated current (**top**) and voltage-sensitive fast (active) currents (**bottom**) before perfusion with 10 μm TTX in the bath. POST-TTX: THC-gated current (**top**) and voltage-sensitive fast (active) currents (**bottom**) after perfusion with 10 μm TTX in the bath. THC-gated current was unchanged, although the fast inward (action potential) current was blocked by TTX.

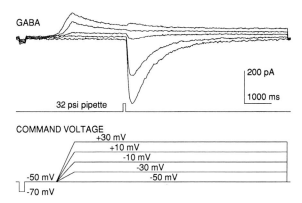

Figure 14-3. GABA-gated chloride current. Pressure pipette application of GABA (1.0 mM) resulted in an inward current at resting membrane potential. The magnitude and duration of the current were similar to that of the cannabinoid-gated current. The GABA-gated current reversal potential (+10 mV) was also similar to that produced by Δ^9-THC.

potential for the baclofen-gated current (between −70 and −90 mV) was indicative of outward potassium ion flux shown to be G-protein-coupled in other preparations (Lacey et al., 1988; Tatsumi et al., 1990). Thus, the presence of baclofen-gated currents in these cells indicates the presence of a G-protein-mediated conductance (Deadwyler et al., 1993).

The above findings suggest that cannabinoid and cannabinoid-like substances change chloride conductances in CNS neurons. However, several questions remain to be answered before the mode of cannabinoid action at the cellular level can be completely understood. First, it is necessary to determine the dose- and potency-related effects of cannabinoids and cannabinoid analogs on these electrophysiological indicators of neuronal activity and whether potencies match the binding and biochemical potencies in terms of effects on inhibition of adenylyl cyclase and other measures. It is important to assess the exact manner in which cannabinoids influence the affected channels and other cellular processes controlling chloride conductances. Second, it is necessary to ascertain whether cannabinoids produce a change in chloride conductance as a direct result of receptor occupancy and whether G-protein-coupling is required (Deadwyler et al., 1993). The similarity in electrophysiological action and potency of the cannabinoid substances to GABA$_A$ effects suggests that both exert potentially powerful influences over cellular excitability in both hippocampal and cortical neurons.

EFFECTS OF CANNABINOIDS ON MEMORY AND HIPPOCAMPAL CELL ACTIVITY

Many of the effects of cannabinoids in human and experimental animals are biphasic in character. These effects tend to be a mix of inhibition and excitation at low doses, and primarily inhibition at higher doses. Euphoria, hallucinations, and time dilation are typical subjective impressions reported by marijuana smokers, although sedation, delayed reaction time, memory impairment, and decreased psychomotor performance are also associated with its use (Hollister, 1986; Martin, 1986). Although the subjective effects of cannabinoids cannot be tested directly in experimental models, behavioral measures of these phenomena have been assessed experimentally. Decreased performance in behavioral tasks (Martin, 1986), increased "interference" with selective attention (Hooker & Jones, 1987), and increased reaction time (Hollister, 1986) have been demonstrated in human and animal models. The reported dysphoria in humans is paralleled experimentally by decreased performance in signal detection and discrimination tasks in animals with no impairments in primary auditory pathway responsiveness to the stimulus (Deadwyler et al., 1990; Hampson et al., 1989). Short-term memory loss is the most consistently reported effect of Δ^9-THC in humans (Miller & Branconnier, 1983). It is rare that reports of the other types of behavioral disruptions in humans cited above are not accompanied by indications of short-term memory loss.

Several of the above behavioral and cognitive effects of Δ^9-THC are accompanied by biphasic dose-dependent changes in neural activity. Cannabinoids have been demonstrated to stimulate synchronous activity in the EEG at low doses, yet they act as anticonvulsants and depress EEG indicators at higher doses (Karler & Turkanis, 1981). Similarly, postsynaptic potentials and neural spikes recorded from in vitro neuronal preparations are excited by low doses (Karler et al., 1986) and inhibited by high doses of cannabinoids (Kujtan et al., 1983; Nowicky et al., 1987; Turkanis & Karler, 1983). Cannabinoids have also been shown to decrease behaviorally correlated firing of individual hippocampal neurons (Campbell et al., 1986; Heyser et al., 1989, 1993) and to reduce the amplitude of synaptic potentials evoked by sensory stimuli during performance of behavioral tasks (Campbell et al., 1986a & b). Results of evoked potential studies in rats suggest that cannabinoids interfere with the normal processing of sensory information by interrupting the transmission of sensory activity between specific brain regions (Deadwyler et al., 1990; Hampson et al., 1989).

Previous studies from this laboratory determined that Δ^9-THC disrupted auditory evoked neural activity in the dentate gyrus of the hippocampus; this was associated with disruption of tone discrimination performance in the same animals (Campbell et al., 1986a & b; Deadwyler et al., 1990; Hampson et al., 1989). We did not determine whether these effects were the result of changes in the ability to (1) *detect* the tone stimulus or (2) to *store* or (3) *retrieve* critical information relative to the tone stimulus once detected. In more recent studies, a delayed match to sample (DMTS) task was implemented that would allow separation of the effects of Δ^9-THC into one or more of the above categories.

The DMTS task as originally designed for rats by Dunnett (1985) provides a basis for precise correlations between behavioral and memory-related changes in performance and hippocampal electrical events. The task is designed to test two different aspects of sensory processing: *storage* and *retrieval*. In this task, responding on one of two spatially distinct levers requires a "matching" response on that same lever after an interpolated 1-30 second delay when both levers are represented. Animals with hippocampal lesions show deficits in this task at longer (≥ 5 seconds) but not shorter (≤ 5 seconds) delay intervals (Dunnett, 1985; Eichenbaum & Cohen 1988; Olton et al., 1978). Figure 14-4 shows a dose-dependent decrease in performance on the DMTS task over the same dose ranges (0.5-2.0 mg/kg) found to be effective in the previously described tone discrimination studies (Campbell et al., 1986a & b). There was also a statistically significant dose-by-delay interaction ($F_{(5,342)} = 6.1$, $P < 0.001$), reflecting the fact that increasing doses of Δ^9-THC produced a greater retention deficit as the delay interval became longer (Fig. 14-4). This finding indicates that Δ^9-THC had less effect on performance when retrieval of sample information was immediate (≤ 5 seconds) than when retrieval was delayed up to 30 seconds.

Striking effects of Δ^9-THC on differentiated hippocampal cell activity recorded during performance of the DMTS task were found in these same animals. Recordings made from specific classes of hippocampal CA1 complex spike cells (Heyser et al., 1993) revealed marked changes in the behavioral correlates of the DMTS task. Complex spike cells recorded from the CA1 and

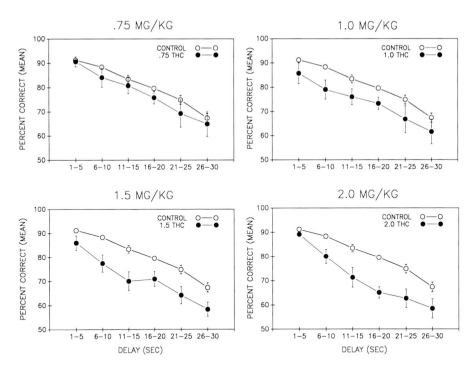

Figure 14-4. Effects of Δ^9-THC on rat DMTS performance. DMTS performance curves after administration of Δ^9-THC are compared to control behavior for each of four doses (0.75, 1.0, 1.5, 2.0 mg/kg i.p.). Data was combined from eight animals that received vehicle (control) and drug injections on alternate days. Each of the curves shows a delay-dependent decrease with minimal disruption of behavioral performance at the 1 to 5 second delays and maximal disruption at 26- to 31-second delays. The performance deficit increases with increasing dosage of Δ^9-THC. All values are mean $\pm$ SE. (From Heyser et al., 1993.)

CA3 region of the hippocampus fired only during specific phases of the task. At least two types of cells could be differentiated on the basis of phases of the task in which firing occurred. One cell type fired during the SAMPLE *and* MATCH phase of the task, whereas another fired only during the MATCH phase of the task. The presence of these cell types illustrates the tendency for principal cells in the hippocampus to fire only during the critical "decision-making" stages of the DMTS task. Figure 14-5 shows a comparison between cells recorded in the

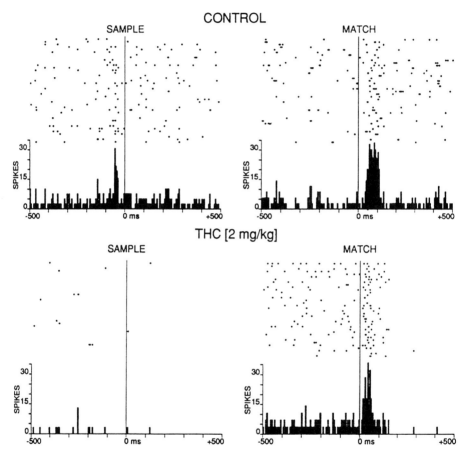

Figure 14-5. Δ-9-THC alters hippocampal neural correlates of the DMTS task. Individually isolated hippocampal cells were identified as pyramidal cells and recorded for the duration of the 100-trial session (Heyser et al., 1993). Examples of SAMPLE and MATCH phase cell firing (rasters and histograms) during control (vehicle) and drug (THC) sessions. **Top,** Note the concentration of firing before the SAMPLE (left) and after the MATCH (right) responses (see histograms) typical of many cells of this type. Identified complex spike cells did not fire on MISMATCH (error) trials. **Bottom,** Hippocampal cell firing recorded from a different cell in the same animal in which Δ⁹-THC (2.0 mg/kg) was injected at the beginning of the DMTS session. There was virtually no correlated increased firing in this cell during the SAMPLE (response) phase of the task (*left*). The absence of SAMPLE-related firing was typical of drug sessions. However, MATCH (*right*) response-correlated firing was preserved in the same cell on correct (MATCH) trials (compare with top).

vehicle control sessions and those recorded after Δ^9-THC injection in an animal whose behavioral performance under both conditions was similar to that shown in Figure 14-4 (2 mg/kg). In the Δ^9-THC recording sessions when performance was impaired at delay intervals longer than 10 seconds, identified hippocampal complex spike cells did not fire in the SAMPLE phase of the task (Fig. 14-5, post vs. pre-THC), but cells were encountered that did fire during the MATCH phase of the DMTS task. SAMPLE phase firing was quite prominent in cells sampled from the same animal during vehicle control sessions (Fig. 14-5, pre-THC).

It is likely that the deficit in performance in the DMTS task produced by Δ^9-THC resulted from the lack of hippocampal cell firing in the SAMPLE phase of the task (Heyser et al., 1992). Loss of cell firing associated with *registration* of lever position and impaired recall of that critical information at the end of the interpolated delay would account for the deficit in DMTS performance (Hampson et al., 1993). The appearance of hippocampal cell discharges during the MATCH phase of the task verified that hippocampal cell firing was selectively and not universally depressed by Δ^9-THC. One mechanism whereby SAMPLE phase firing in CA1 and CA3 hippocampal neurons could be eliminated is the previously demonstrated THC-induced suppression of sensory activation of dentate granule cells (Campbell et al., 1986b). The granule cells provide a critical link in the transmission of sensory information between entorhinal cortex and hippocampus (Deadwyler et al., 1987, 1988; Hampson & Deadwyler, 1992) and would therefore be necessary for the *registration* of (SAMPLE) lever position information. Decreased activation of granule cells by cannabinoids would not be critical to firing in the *recall* (MATCH) phase of the task since presumably lever position information would already be "stored" in the hippocampus or related structures at the time of retrieval.

Whatever the mechanism of cannabinoid disruption of memory-related cellular activity in the hippocampus, it is clear that the effects are specific, dose-dependent, and highly replicable. It is also significant to note that the dentate gyrus, the region where sensory transmission via a well-characterized synaptic process is disrupted by cannabinoids (Campbell et al., 1986a), is also one of three brain areas described by Herkenham et al. (1990, 1991) as containing the highest density of cannabinoid receptors in all mammalian species, including humans (see Chapter 13). Taken together with the information presented on the potential cellular effects of cannabinoids, the selective suppression of hippocampal cellular activity by cannabinoid receptor-mediated membrane actions could provide a neural basis for the well-documented memory impairments that accompany exposure to this substance in humans.

EFFECTS OF NICOTINE ON IN VITRO CNS CELLULAR ACTIVITY

Cell patch-clamp technology has recently been applied to the study of the actions of nicotine in mammalian CNS neurons. Although the nicotinic acetylcholine receptor is one of the best understood membrane conductance mechanisms (Changeux et al., 1984), the role of this receptor in the brain remains relatively obscure. Recent molecular biological analyses have demonstrated several nicotinic receptor subtypes in brain with potentially different functional roles based on regional, cellular, and pharmacological differences (Luetje & Patrick, 1991; Luetje et al., 1990; see Chapter 6).

This section describes the actions of nicotine on two major CNS cell types tested in vitro as a means of determining the manner in which nicotine receptors influence the activity of these cells in vivo. Such experiments complement data derived from artificial expression systems, such as the frog oocyte (Luetje & Patrick, 1991), as well as information from in vivo recordings in anesthetized and awake animals (Garza et al., 1987). Whole-cell voltage-clamp recordings of hippocampal and cortical neurons grown in culture were performed. Nicotine was delivered to the cells by pipette and bath application. In this case nicotine could be applied feasibly by either method, as the only critical factor was the potential receptor desensitization resulting from long-term exposure as described previously (Gribkoff et al., 1988).

The cortical cells grown in culture for use in these studies express nicotinic receptors (Fluhler et al., 1989; Lippiello et al., 1989). These receptors appear within 5 days and show functional significance within 7 days, permitting analysis of the effects of nicotine on both voltage-sensitive and receptor-mediated currents, and possible interactions with other transmitters and cellular mechanisms affected by nicotine.

Nicotine-Gated Currents in Cortical Neurons

In whole-cell voltage-clamp cortical neurons, nicotine causes a depolarizing inward current that is antagonized by d-tubocurarine (dTC), dihydro-beta-erythroidine (DBE), and hexamethonium. Nicotine caused firing in cells that are silent when studied in current clamp mode. The application of nicotine in brief pulses produced currents lasting 0.5-2.0 seconds reaching peak magnitudes ranging between 0.2-1.0 nA (Fig. 14-6). Conductances ranged between 7.8 and 8.3 ns. The nicotine current reversed near the sodium equilibrium potential ($E_{Na} = +20$ mV) for these cells. The effective dose for this current ranged between 20 and 100 μm, which may not reflect the effective concentration at the receptor during pipette (0.5-1.0 mm) delivery of nicotine. The nicotine-provoked current was mediated by nicotinic receptors since total blockade was achieved with lower concentrations (30-60 μM) of dTC in the bathing medium.

A quite unexpected finding was that nicotine-gated currents of this type were completely absent in hippocampal neurons tested from cultures of the same age (6 days). Figure 14-7 shows this comparison for two neurons: one from a cortical culture and one from a hippocampal culture. These cells were obtained from the same hippocampal cultures that exhibited the cannabinoid, GABA and glutamate currents described above. At the same dose, nicotine did not produce a detectable change in membrane conductance in the hippocampal neuron. Thus, hippocampal neurons at this stage (6 days) in culture apparently do not have the nicotinic receptor-mediated conductance mechanisms observed in cortical neurons of the same age (Alkondon & Albuquerque, 1991).

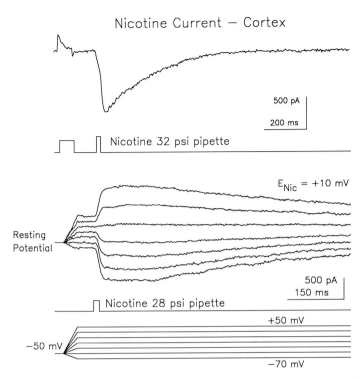

Nicotine Current − Cortex

500 pA

200 ms

Nicotine 32 psi pipette

E_{Nic} = +10 mV

Resting
Potential

500 pA
150 ms

Nicotine 28 psi pipette

+50 mV

−50 mV

−70 mV

Figure 14-6. Nicotine-gated currents in cultured cortical neurons (age 7 days). **Top,** Pressure pipette application of nicotine (1.0 mm) resulted in an inward current at resting membrane potential. **Bottom,** Reversal potential for the nicotine-gated current was +10 mV. Membrane potential (−55 mV) was changed in ramped 20-mV increments on successive applications to a maximum depolarization of +50 mV (voltage steps: bottom trace). The nicotine current decreased in magnitude with depolarization, and reversed above +10 mV.

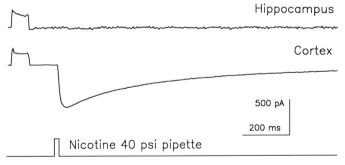

Hippocampus

Cortex

500 pA

200 ms

Nicotine 40 psi pipette

Figure 14-7. Comparison of nicotine-gated current in neurons from hippocampal versus cortical cultures. Application of nicotine (1.0 mm) failed to evoke a current in cultured hippocampal neurons, whereas the same nicotine-filled pipette provoked a nicotine-gated current in a neuron from a cortical cell culture of the same age (6 days). Both neurons exhibited stable voltage-sensitive currents, as well as ligand-gated currents evoked by other neurotransmitters. Hippocampal neurons failed to exhibit receptor-mediated nicotinic responses under these conditions.

Effects of Nicotine on Calcium-Mediated Potassium Conductance

The specific channel kinetics of the actions of nicotine on CNS neurons has not been determined. However, recent findings from oocyte expression studies of nicotinic receptor subunits suggest that receptor-coupled conductances vary among nicotine receptor subtypes with different combinations of subunits (Luetje & Patrick, 1991; see Chapter 6). Several recent investigations employing iontophoretic applications of nicotine onto cells both in vivo and in vitro suggest that nicotine delivered in moderate concentrations can produce depolarization and cell firing (Egan & North, 1986; Garza et al., 1987) or hyperpolarization (Wong & Gallagher, 1989). However, it is also well established that the nicotine concentration in brain achieved through smoking is in the low micromolar range (Warburton, 1985). If the concentration of nicotine required for such currents is not sufficient to produce threshold depolarization for the action potential, the role of this substance in brain could be primarily modulatory. Such modulation could act on other conductance mechanisms within the cell to alter excitability in a manner analogous to that proposed for the muscarinic acetylcholine receptor M_2 subtype (Christie & North, 1988).

Therefore, studies were designed to test the possibility that nicotine could alter the level of calcium (Ca^{2+}) in the cell by determining whether calcium-mediated conductance processes could be activated by nicotine. Initial investigation of this possibility revealed the presence of voltage-sensitive potassium currents in cultured cortical neurons that were enhanced by nicotine (20–100 μm) in the bathing medium (Fig. 14-8). A fast, voltage-sensitive outward potassium current was markedly enhanced by the receptor-specific action of nicotine. The time course and magnitude of this outward current corresponded closely to I_{Kc}, the calcium-mediated fast potassium conductance that is partially responsible for action potential repolarization in most CNS neurons (Storm, 1990). The I_{Kc} is blocked by low concentrations (≤ 10 mM) of tetraethylammonium (TEA) and is voltage-dependent in the range of -90 to -20 mV. Depolarization activates I_{Kc}, then calcium inactivates it in cortical neurons (McCormick, 1989, 1991; McCormick & Williamson, 1989).

One potential explanation for the increase in I_{Kc} is that intracellular Ca^{2+} levels are increased by a nicotine-gated sodium-calcium channel. The increased level of Ca^{2+} in the cell required to activate I_{Kc} presumably results from Ca^{2+} influx through a nicotine receptor-controlled channel. As stated above, the I_{Kc} is the most likely candidate for such Ca^{2+}-dependent effects since the potassium currents that are not mediated by Ca^{2+} are relatively insensitive to TEA and to calcium blockers (Brown et al., 1990; Storm, 1990). To test this assumption further, two manipulations of Ca^{2+} entry into the cell were implemented: (1) enhancement of the Ca^{2+} effect on potassium conductance by substitution of barium in the bathing medium and (2) reduction of the nicotine effects on I_{Kc} by blockade of Ca^{2+} entry into the cell with cadmium, a well-known Ca^{2+} channel blocking agent (Llinas, 1988).

Exchange of the standard bath solution for one containing barium (2.0 mm $BaCl_2$ and 0.5 mm $CaCl_2$) produces effects similar to those of nicotine in that the $BaCl_2$ medium enhanced I_{Kc} in cultured neocortical neurons (Deadwyler et

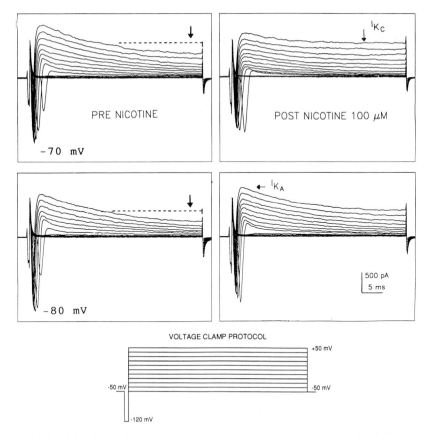

Figure 14-8. Nicotine enhances voltage-sensitive potassium current. **Left,** Voltage-sensitive currents evoked in normal bathing medium by progressive increased depolarizing steps. **Right,** Voltage-sensitive currents after addition of 100 μM nicotine to the bathing medium. Nicotine enhanced the inactivating outward current in response to depolarizing voltage steps. Dotted line in left panel shows the degree of enhancement and voltage sensitivity of nicotine-induced increase in late outward potassium current. I_{Ka} shows time domain of early TEA-insensitive potassium current not affected by nicotine. I_{Kc} shows time domain of late potassium current mediated by intracellular calcium levels. The I_{Kc} was voltage dependent in the -90 to -20 mV range and was blocked by 10 mm TEA. Voltage step command protocol is the same as shown in Figure 14-4.

al., 1992). These data agree with other reports in which barium has been shown to enhance I_{Kc} in hippocampal and sympathetic ganglion cells (Adams & Halliwell, 1982; Brown et al., 1990; Hotson & Prince, 1980). The converse manipulation, addition of cadmium to the bathing medium to block Ca^{2+} entry into the cell, prevents the increase in I_{Kc} provoked by nicotine (Deadwyler et al., 1992). These findings indicate that calcium entry into the cell is responsible for the nicotine-produced activation of I_{Kc} in cortical neurons in culture (Fig. 14-8).

The availability of other types of cultured CNS neurons to test these effects of nicotine provides an important control for possible nonspecific actions within the culture system. Hippocampal neurons exposed to the exact same concentrations of nicotine did not show an increase in I_{Kc}. However, when they were exposed to the $BaCl_2$-containing medium there was an increased I_{Kc} in the same manner as in neocortical neurons, similar to the effect provoked by nicotine.

Three possible explanations could account for this difference in I_{Kc} responsiveness between cortical and hippocampal neurons in culture: (1) neurons from hippocampal cultures may not express nicotinic receptors at this age in culture, (2) hippocampal neurons may not possess the same type of Ca^{2+} channels as cortical neurons, or (3) I_{Kc} in hippocampal-cultured neurons may be coupled through second-messenger systems that are not activated by nicotinic receptors. The most parsimonious explanation for these differences would be the first; that is, there are no nicotinic cholinergic receptors on hippocampal neurons in culture at 6-7 days (Alkondon & Albuquerque, 1991).

EFFECTS OF NICOTINE ON GLUTAMATE AND GABA-GATED CURRENTS

Interaction with Other Transmitter-Gated Currents

There are further implications of the nicotine-mediated changes in membrane conductance in CNS neurons. It can be expected that cells that possess nicotinic receptor-gated conductances would also have conductances coupled to other types of neurotransmitter receptors. Nicotine receptor occupancy during temporally overlapping currents produced by synaptic release of other transmitters could significantly modulate membrane reactivity to those transmitter substances. In addition, the Ca^{2+} conductance produced by nicotinic receptor occupancy has significant implications for those transmitters that may also modulate Ca^{2+} conductances. Ca^{2+} entry into the cell provoked by nicotine would decrease the Ca^{2+} conductance required to initiate Ca^{2+}-triggered events, such as I_{Kc}, by other contiguously active transmitters (Llinas, 1988).

This potential interaction was tested by examining the responsiveness of cortical neurons in culture to brief pipette applications of glutamate and GABA in the presence of nicotine in the bathing medium. The tests were performed after only brief exposure (1-2 minutes) to nicotine since receptor desensitization was a possible problem in these studies (Gribkoff et al., 1988). In all cases, nicotine in the bath enhanced currents produced by pipette application of glutamate or GABA as shown in Figure 14-9. In the case of glutamate the current was carried mostly by an inward flow of Na^+ and/or possibly Ca^{2+} ions. Nicotine increased the magnitude of the glutamate current, but did not alter its time course. Because of the change in chloride gradient produced by dialysis of the cell by the pipette solution, the GABA current was inward, reflecting an outward movement of chloride ions (see Cannabinoids above). In the presence of nicotine, $GABA_A$-produced chloride current was enhanced (Fig. 14-9). The effects of nicotine on glutamate and GABA currents were shown to be nicotine receptor-specific since they were blocked when dTC or DBE (60 μm) were included in the bath.

Glutamate Current

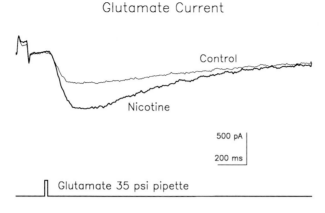

GABA Current

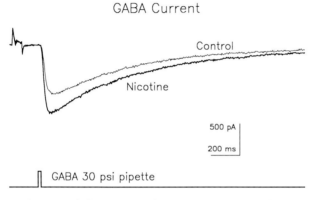

Figure 14-9. Modulation of glutamate- and GABA-gated currents by nicotine. **Top,** Pressure pipette application of glutamate (1.0 mm) produced an inward current at resting membrane potential. The reversal potential (not shown) for this current was +30 mV. Addition of 50 μM nicotine to the bathing medium resulted in an increase in the glutamate-evoked current. **Bottom,** Current evoked by pressure pipette application of GABA (1.0 mm) was also inward at resting potential (E_{Cl} = 0 mV). Nicotine added to the bathing medium (50 μm) produced an enhancement of the GABA current similar to that observed for the glutamate current.

These findings suggest that nicotine could play both a modulatory and a direct role in altering the excitability of neurons in the CNS. It is not possible without additional study to predict the exact manner by which the presence of nicotine might alter neuronal responsiveness to other transmitter agents. Recently, McCormick (1989, 1991) has suggested that several different receptors on the same neocortical neuron might couple to the same channel, as originally demonstrated for opiate and catecholamine receptors in other types of cells (North, 1989). The mechanism responsible for enhanced glutamate and GABA currents would have to be somewhat different since there are no reports of coupling between the cholinergic nicotinic receptor on these cells and other receptors, such as excitatory amino acid or GABA receptor subtypes. However, Ca^{2+} entry into the cell produced by nicotine would definitely implicate several well-known mechanisms that could alter the responsiveness of CNS neurons to other simultaneously active transmitters.

REFERENCES

Adams, P.R., & Halliwell, J.V. (1982). A hyperpolarization-induced inward current in hippocampal pyramidal cells. *J. Physiol., 324,* 62-63P.

Alkondon, M., & Albuquerque, E.X. (1991). Initial characterization of the nicotinic acetylcholine receptor in rat hippocampal neurons. *J. Receptor Res., 11,* 1001-1021.

Brown, D.A., Gahwiler, B.H., Griffith, W.H., & Halliwell, J.V. (1990). Membrane currents in hippocampal neurons. *Prog. Brain Res., 83,* 141-160.

Campbell, K.A., Foster, T.C., Hampson, R.E., & Deadwyler, S.A. (1986a). Effects of delta-9-tetrahydrocannabinol on sensory-evoked discharges of granule cells in the dentate gyrus of behaving rats. *J. Pharmacol. Exp. Ther., 239,* 941-945.

Campbell, K.A., Foster, T.C., Hampson, R.E., & Deadwyler, S.A. (1986b). Delta-9-tetrahydrocannabinol differentially affects sensory-evoked potentials in the rat dentate gyrus. *J. Pharmacol. Exp. Ther., 239,* 936-940.

Changeux, J.P., Devillers-Thiery, A., & Chemouilli, P. (1984). Acetylcholine receptor: An allosteric protein. *Science, 225,* 1335-1345.

Christie, M.J., & North, R.A. (1988). Control of ion conductances by muscarinic receptors. *Trends Pharmacol. Sci.,* Suppl:30-34.

Deadwyler, S.A., Hampson, R.E., Bennett, B.A., Edwards, T.A., Mo, J., Pacheco, M.A., Ward, S.J., & Childers, S.R. (1993). Cannabinoids modulate potassium current in cultured hippocampal neurons. *Receptors and Channels* (in press).

Devane, W.A., Dysarz, F.A.I., Johnson, M.R., Melvin, L.S., & Howlett, A.C. (1988). Determination and characterization of a cannabinoid receptor in rat brain. *Mol. Pharmacol., 34,* 605-613.

Dewey, W.L. (1986). Cannabinoid pharmacology. *Pharmacol. Rev., 38,* 151-178.

Dichter, M.A. (1986). The pharmacology of cortical neurons in tissue culture. In H.M. Geller (Ed.), *Electrophysiological techniques in pharmacology* (pp. 121-147). New York: Alan R. Liss.

Dunnett, S.B. (1985). Comparative effects of cholinergic drugs and lesions of nucleus basalis or fimria-fornix on delayed matching in rats. *Psychopharmacology, 87,* 357-363.

Eichenbaum, H., & Cohen, N.J. (1988). Representation in the hippocampus: What do hippocampal neurons code? *TINS, 11,* 244-248.

Egan, T.M., & North, R.A. (1986). Acetylcholine hyperpolarizes central neurones by acting on an M_2 muscarinic receptor. *Nature, 319,* 405-407.

Fluhler, E.N., Lippiello, P.M., & Fernandes, K.G.(1989). Nicotine-evoked calcium changes in single fetal rat cortical neurones measured with the fluorescent probe Fura-2. *Soc. Neurosci. Abst., 15,* 679.

Garza, R. de la, Bickford-Winer, P.C., Hoffer, B.J., & Freedman, R. (1987). Heterogeneity of nicotine actions in the rat cerebellum: An in vivo electrophysiological study. *J. Pharmacol. Exp. Ther., 240,* 689-695.

Gribkoff, V.K., Christian, E.P., Robinson, J.H., Deadwyler, S.A, & Dudek, F.E. (1988). Cholinergic excitation of supraoptic neurons in hypothalamic slices of rat. *Neuropharmacology, 27,* 721-727.

Hamill, O.P., Neher, A., Sakmann, B., & Sigworth, F.J. (1981). Improved patch-clamp techniques for high-resolution current recording from cells and cell-free membrane patches. *Pflugers Arch., 391*, 85-100.

Hampson, R.E., & Deadwyler, S.A. (1992). Information processing in the dentate gyrus. In C. Gall & I. Mody (Eds.), *The dentate gyrus and its role in seizures* (pp. 291-299). Amsterdam: Elsevier.

Hampson, R.E., Willis, H.H., Breese, C.R., & Deadwyler, S.A. (1989). Tone-evoked potentials indicate differential processing of sensory information in the hippocampus and neocortex of the rat. *Soc. Neurosci. Abst., 15*, 81.

Herkenham, M., Lynn, A.B., Little, M.D., Johnson, M.R., Melvin, L.S., de Costa, B.R., & Rice, K.C. (1990). Cannabinoid receptor localization in brain. *Proc. Natl. Acad. Sci. USA, 87*, 1932-1936.

Herkenham, M., Lynn, A.B., Johnson, M.R., Melvin, L.S., de Costa, B.R., & Rice, K.C. (1991). Characterization and localization of cannabinoid receptors in rat brain: A quantitative in vitro autoradiographic study. *J. Neurosci., 11*, 563-583.

Heyser, C.J., Hampson, R.E., & Deadwyler, S.A. (1989). Characteristics of hippocampal complex spike neurons during performance of a delayed match to sample task. Selective influences of delta-9-THC. *Soc. Neurosci. Abst., 15*, 1170.

Heyser, C.J., Hampson, R.E., & Deadwyler, S.A. (1993). The effects of delta-9-THC on delayed match to sample performance in rats: Alterations in short-term memory produced by changes in task specific firing of hippocampal cells. *J. Pharm. Exp. Ther. 264*, 294-307.

Hollister, L.E. (1986). Health aspects of Cannabis. *Pharmacol. Rev., 38*, 1-20.

Hooker, W.D., & Jones, R.T. (1987). Increased susceptibility to memory intrusions and the Stroop interference effect during acute marijuana intoxication. *Psychopharmacology, 91*, 20-24.

Hotson, J.R., & Prince, D.A. (1980). A calcium-activated hyperpolarization follows repetitive firing in hippocampal neurons. *J. Neurophysiol., 43*, 409-419.

Howlett, A.C. (1985). Cannabinoid inhibition of adenylate cyclase. Biochemistry of the response in neuroblastoma cell membranes. *Mol. Pharmacol., 27*, 429-436.

Howlett, A.C. (1990). Reverse pharmacology applied to the cannabinoid receptor. *Trends. Pharmacol. Sci., 11*, 395-397.

Howlett, A.C., Johnson, M.R., Melvin, L.S., & Milne, G.M. (1988). Nonclassical cannabinoid analgetics inhibit adenylate cyclase: Development of a cannabinoid receptor model. *Mol. Pharmacol., 33*, 297-302.

Howlett, A.C., Bidaut-Russell, M., Devane, W.A., Melvin, L.S., Johnson, M.R., & Herkenham, M. (1990). The cannabinoid receptor: Biochemical, anatomical and behavioral characterization. *Trends. Neurosci., 13*, 420-423.

Huguenard, J.R., & Alger, B.E. (1986). Whole-cell voltage-clamp study of fading of GABA-activated currents in acutely dissociated hippocampal neurons. *J. Neurophysiol., 56*, 1-18.

Jahr, C.F., & Stevens, C.F. (1987). Glutamate activates multiple single channel conductances in hippocampal neurons. *Nature, 325*, 522-525.

Johnson, M., Devane, W., Howlett, A., Melvin, L., & Milne, G. (1988). Structural studies leading to the discovery of a cannabinoid binding site. *NIDA Res. Monogr., 90*, 129-135.

Karler, R., & Turkanis, S.A. (1981). The cannabinoids as potential antiepileptics. *J. Clin. Pharmacol., 21*, 437S-448S.

Karler, R., Calder, L.D., & Turkanis, S.A. (1984). Changes in CNS sensitivity to cannabinoids with repeated treatment: Tolerance and auxoesthesia. *NIDA. Res. Monogr., 54*, 312-322.

Karler, R., Calder, L.D., & Turkanis, S.A. (1986). Prolonged CNS hyperexcitability in mice after a single exposure to delta-9-tetrahydrocannabinol. *Neuropharmacology, 25,* 441-446.

Kujtan, P.W., Carlen, P.L., & Kapur, B.M. (1983). delta 9-Tetrahydrocannabinol and cannabidiol: Dose-dependent effects on evoked potentials in the hippocampal slice. *Can. J. Physiol. Pharmacol., 61,* 420-426.

Lacey, M.G., Mercuri, N.B., & North, R.A. (1988). On the potassium conductance increase activated by GABA and dopamine D2 receptors in rat substantia nigra neurones. *J. Physiol. (Lond.), 401,* 437-453.

Lippiello, P.M., Fernandes, K.G., Langone, J.J., & Bjercke, R.J. (1989). Identification of nicotinic receptors on cultured cortical neurons using anti-idiotypic antibodies. *Soc. Neurosci. Abstr., 15,* 677.

Llinas, R.R. (1988). The intrinsic electrophysiological properties of mammalian neurons: Insights into central nervous system function. *Science, 242,* 1654-1664.

Luetje, C.W., & Patrick, J. (1991). Both alpha and beta-subunits contribute to the agonist sensitivity of neuronal nicotinic acetylcholine receptors. *J. Neurosci., 11,* 837-845.

Luetje, C.W., Wada, K., Rogers, S., Abramson, S.N., Tsuji, K., Heinemann, S., & Patrick, J. (1990). Neurotoxins distinguish between different neuronal nicotinic acetylcholine receptor subunit combinations. *J. Neurochem., 55,* 632-640.

Martin, B.R. (1986). Cellular effects of cannabinoids. *Psychol. Rev., 38,* 45-74.

Matsuda, L.A., Lolait, S.J., Brownstein, M.J., Young, A.C., & Bonner, T.I. (1990). Structure of a cannabinoid receptor and functional expression of the cloned cDNA [see comments]. *Nature, 346,* 561-564.

McCormick, D.A. (1989). Cholinergic and noradrenergic modulation of thalamocortical processing. *Trends. Neurosci., 12,* 215-221.

McCormick, D.A. (1991). Refinements in the in vitro slice technique and human neuropharmacology. *Trends. Pharmacol. Sci., 11,* 53-56.

McCormick, D.A., & Williamson, A. (1989). Convergence and divergence of neurotransmitter action in human cerebral cortex. *Proc. Natl. Acad. Sci. USA., 86,* 8098-8102.

Miller, L.L., & Branconnier, R.J. (1983). Cannabis: Effects on memory and the cholinergic limbic system. *Psychol. Bull, 93,* 441-456.

North, R.A. (1989). Twelfth Gaddum memorial lecture. Drug receptors and the inhibition of nerve cells. *Br. J. Pharmacol., 98,* 13-28.

Nowicky, A.V., Teyler, T.J., & Vardaris, R.M. (1987). The modulation of long-term potentiation by delta-9-tetrahydrocannabinol in the rat hippocampus, in vitro. *Brain Res. Bull., 19,* 663-672.

Nye, J.S., Seltzman, H.H., Pitt, C.G., & Snyder, S.H. (1985). High-affinity cannabinoid binding sites in brain membranes labeled with [3H]-5'-trimethylammonium delta 8-tetrahydrocannabinol. *J. Pharmacol. Exp. Ther., 234,* 784-791.

Olton, D.S., Walker, J.A., & Gage, F.H. (1978). Hippocampal connections and spatial discrimination. *Brain Res., 139,* 295-308.

Ozawa, S., & Yuzaki, M. (1984). Patch-clamp studies of choloride channels activated by gamma-aminobutyric acid in cultured hippocampal neurones of the rat. *Neurosci. Res., 1,* 275-293.

Pacheco, M., Childers, S.R., Arnold, R., Casiano, F., & Ward, S.J. (1991). Aminoalkylindoles: Actions on specific G-protein-linked receptors. *J. Pharmacol. Exp. Ther., 257,* 170-183.

Storm, J.F. (1990). Potassium currents in hippocampal pyramidal cells. *Prog. Brain Res., 83,* 161-187.

Tatsumi, H., Costa, M., Schimerlik, M., & North, R.A. (1990). Potassium conductance increased by noradrenaline, opioids, somatostatin, and G-proteins: Whole-cell recording from guinea pig submucous neurons. *J. Neurosci., 10,* 1675-1682.

Thalmann, R.H. (1988). Evidence that guanosine triphosphate (GTP)-binding proteins control a synaptic response in brain: Effect of pertussis toxin and GTP-gamma-S on the late inhibitory postsynaptic potential of hippocampal CA3 neurons. *J. Neurosci., 8,* 4589-4602.

Tsuzuki, K., Iino, M., & Ozawa, S. (1989). Ion channels activated by quinolinic acid in cultured rat hippocampal neurons. *Brain Res., 481,* 258-264.

Turkanis, S.A., & Karler, R. (1983). Effects of delta 9-tetrahydrocannabinol on cat spinal motoneurons. *Brain Res., 288,* 283-287.

Warburton, D.M. (1985). Nicotine and the smoker. *Rev. Environ. Health., 5,* 343-390.

Wong, L.A., & Gallagher, J.P. (1989). A direct nicotine receptor mediated inhibition recorded intracellularly in vitro. *Nature, 341,* 439-442.

Zhang, L., Spigelman, I., & Carlen, P.L. (1990). Whole-cell patch study of gabaergic inhibition in CA1 neurons of immature rat hippocampal slices. *Dev. Brain Res., 56,* 127-130.

15

Long-Term Potentiation of Synaptic Transmission

ROBERT C. MALENKA

Learning, the acquisition of new information, and memory, the retention and retrieval of information, are of fundamental importance to the development and organization of both adaptive and maladaptive behavior. Substance abuse and addiction provide perhaps the most poignant example of the critical role of learning and memory in the development of a maladaptive behavior that has profound individual and societal consequences. Behavioral experimentation has demonstrated that some of the most basic forms of learning, including both classical and operant conditioning, are involved in aspects of substance abuse, such as the development of tolerance and sensitization (Goudie & Emmett-Oglesby, 1989). Although learning and memory are critical for the addictive process, virtually all of the self-administered drugs that lead to psychological or physical dependence may interfere with normal, adaptive learning and memory. Clearly, a more comprehensive understanding of the neural mechanisms responsible for learning and memory will greatly facilitate research on the biological basis of substance abuse and addiction.

Delineating the biophysical and biochemical mechanisms underlying learning and memory in the mammalian brain has been a major goal of neurobiology for several decades. Several different experimental strategies have been employed to study the cellular basis of learning and memory. One approach involves determining the neural circuit responsible for a well-defined behavioral response and then searching for biophysical and biochemical changes occurring in this circuit and that are causally related to the learning process. This strategy has been applied successfully to simple invertebrate preparations (Alkon, 1984; Kandel et al., 1987), but it has been more difficult to apply to the mammalian CNS because of the inherent complexity of the neural circuits in the mammalian brain.

This work is supported by grants from the National Institute of Mental Health, the Klingenstein Foundation, the Sloan Foundation, The National Alliance for Research on Schizophrenia and Depression, and a Scholars Award from the McKnight Foundation.

Another strategy is based on the hypothesis (Cajal, 1911; Eccles, 1953; Hebb, 1949) that learning and memory depend on changes due to usage in the strength of synaptic transmission at certain critical synapses in the brain. This strategy involves searching for neural circuits that exhibit long-lasting changes in synaptic efficacy in response to brief experimental manipulations. A disadvantage of this approach is that it often ignores the question of whether the organism ever actually uses the phenomenon under study. However, a major advantage is that it allows the use of reduced experimental preparations (e.g., brain slices) that are amenable to more rigorous cellular analysis.

The most striking example of this second approach is the study of long-term potentiation of synaptic transmission (LTP) in the hippocampus. LTP, first observed in vivo in the dentate gyrus by Lomo (1966) and characterized in greater detail by Bliss and Lomo (1973), is a long-lasting enhancement of synaptic transmission elicited by brief, repetitive activation of excitatory afferents. Since its discovery, LTP has become the most compelling model of a synaptic mechanism related to learning and memory and thus has been the subject of much research aimed at determining its underlying cellular mechanisms. This effort was greatly facilitated by the demonstration that the in vitro hippocampal slice preparation was capable of generating LTP.

The in vitro hippocampal slice retains three excitatory synaptic relays, all of which can exhibit phenomenologically similar LTP. However, some of the most fundamental mechanistic properties of these different forms of LTP are quite distinct (Zalutsky & Nicoll, 1990). The chapter focuses on the cellular mechanisms underlying the most extensively studied form of LTP, which occurs at the synapse between the Schaffer collateral/commissural fibers of CA3 pyramidal cells and CA1 pyramidal cells. Several recent reviews cover much of the following material in greater detail (Brown et al., 1990; Gustafsson & Wigstrom, 1988; Madison et al., 1991; Malenka & Nicoll, 1990; Malenka et al., 1989a).

PROPERTIES OF LTP INDUCTION

Two requirements must be fulfilled to elicit LTP: The activation of the excitatory afferents must be both above a certain critical threshold level and above a certain frequency (Dunwiddie & Lynch, 1978; McNaughton et al., 1978). Under normal recording conditions, low-frequency stimuli, no matter how strong, will not induce LTP. Figure 15-1 shows an example of LTP in the CA1 region of a hippocampal slice preparation. A single 1-second stimulation at 100 Hz caused an increase in synaptic strength as measured by changes in the shape and size of the excitatory postsynaptic potential (EPSP) that lasted for over an hour.

Two other features of LTP gave important clues to the cellular mechanisms underlying its induction. An individual postsynaptic cell receives many independent afferent synapses spread over the extent of its dendritic tree. Taking advantage of the ability to stimulate completely independent populations of afferent fibers synapsing on the same postsynaptic cell, it was found

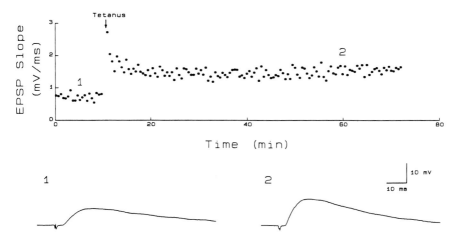

Figure 15-1. Graph showing LTP in the CA1 region of the hippocampus. The slope of the intracellularly recorded EPSP is plotted against time. Test stimuli were given every 10 seconds (each point is the average of three successive measurements). To elicit LTP, a 100 hz-1 second tetanus was given. Below the graph are raw data traces taken at the times indicated by the numbers on the graph.

that LTP occurred only at synapses that were activated during the tetanus and not at adjacent synapses. This "synapse specificity" of LTP indicates that some general, nonspecific change in the postsynaptic cell's properties cannot account for LTP.

Despite the restrictions imposed by the occurrence of synapse specificity, different afferents that synapse on the same postsynaptic cell can interact in quite remarkable ways. It was demonstrated that when tetanic stimulation of a "weak" input, which was incapable of inducing LTP by itself, was given at approximately the same time as a "strong" tetanus which was applied to an independent pathway capable of generating LTP, the response to the weak input was also potentiated. This action can occur even when the two inputs terminate on dendritic trees located on opposite sides of the cell body. This pairing of two inputs or the so-called associative induction of LTP is reminiscent of certain features of behavioral classical conditioning and puts constraints on the potential underlying mechanisms of LTP.

Role of Postsynaptic Depolarization

How does the associative induction of LTP occur? Attention immediately focused on the postsynaptic cell since it was the most obvious anatomical structure connecting the two sets of afferents. It seemed unlikely that some diffusible factor played a critical role since the two inputs had to be activated within a narrow temporal window of approximately 100 ms to induce LTP. Instead, this temporal constraint made postsynaptic depolarization a likely candidate since strong depolarization in one part of the cell could rapidly affect (i.e., depolarize) other parts of the cell.

Depolarization of the postsynaptic cell is indeed an essential requirement for LTP generation. LTP can be blocked by preventing the depolarization that normally occurs during a tetanus (Kelso et al., 1986; Malinow & Miller, 1986). Conversely, LTP can be generated simply by "pairing" low-frequency stimulation with postsynaptic depolarization (Gustafsson et al., 1987). Thus, experimentally depolarizing the postsynaptic cell abolishes the need for high-frequency stimulation to induce LTP. A "weak" tetanus by itself simply cannot depolarize the cell sufficiently to support LTP induction.

Role of NMDA Receptors

Although the requirement for postsynaptic depolarization can explain the associative induction of LTP and the requirements for a high-frequency, "strong" stimulation, it does not explain synapse specificity. Glutamate, the presumptive excitatory neurotransmitter at these synapses, can activate several different subtypes of receptors (Collingridge & Lester, 1989). Some of these originally were named and defined by the relatively selective agonists N-methyl-D-aspartate (NMDA), kainate, and quisqualate. Kainate and quisqualate receptors are often together referred to as "non-NMDA" receptors and can be potently antagonized by the quinoxalinedione, CNQX. NMDA receptors are selectively blocked by the competitive antagonist, D-2-amino-5-phosphonovalerate (D-APV).

At negative membrane potentials close to the normal resting membrane potential, CNQX greatly reduces the EPSP evoked by single stimuli, whereas APV has very little, if any, effect. This finding indicates that, during normal low-frequency stimulation, synaptically released glutamate preferentially opens non-NMDA receptor channels. However, it has been clearly established that APV blocks the induction of LTP, indicating that NMDA receptors also can be activated by synaptically released glutamate and that this activation is required for LTP (Collingridge et al., 1983).

Why can NMDA receptors be activated by high-frequency stimulation, but not by low-frequency stimulation? The answer came from studies of the biophysical properties of the responses to glutamate and NMDA (Mayer et al., 1984; Nowak et al., 1984). It was demonstrated that physiological levels of extracellular magnesium (Mg^{2+}) exert a voltage-dependent block of the NMDA receptor ionophore. At negative membrane potentials, Mg^{2+} sits in the ion channel and greatly inhibits current flow, even though the NMDA receptor is activated. As the membrane potential is depolarized, Mg^{2+} is expelled from the channel, thereby allowing current to flow. Synaptically released glutamate normally binds to both non-NMDA and NMDA receptors, but only the non-NMDA receptors contribute significantly to the generation of the EPSP. As the cell is depolarized either by a strong tetanus or by direct current injection, the NMDA receptor ionophore is able to generate a synaptic response. Thus, the NMDA receptor serves as a "voltage sensor." Since it must be activated by synaptically released glutamate for the induction of LTP, only those synapses sufficiently depolarized *during* synaptic transmission will exhibit LTP (synapse specificity).

Role of Postsynaptic Calcium

The requirement for NMDA receptor activation and its inherent biophysical properties can explain all the features of LTP discussed to this point, including synapse specificity and associativity. Which features of current flow through the NMDA receptor channel are critical for LTP induction? Unlike non-NMDA receptor channels, which are fairly nonselective monovalent cation-carrying pores permeable primarily to sodium and potassium (Collingridge & Lester, 1989), the NMDA receptor channel is also able to pass calcium into the cell. The first direct evidence supporting a role for postsynaptic calcium in LTP induction was the demonstration that injection into the postsynaptic cell of EGTA, a calcium chelator, prevented the generation of LTP (Lynch et al., 1983). Figure 15-2 shows an experiment (Malenka et al., 1988) in which a more potent and rapid chelator of calcium than EGTA, known as Nitr-5, was injected into a CA1 pyramidal cell. After a strong tetanus, the cell filled with Nitr-5 exhibited only post-tetanic potentiation (lasting at most 1-2 minutes), whereas all the surrounding cells exhibited robust LTP (measured with an extracellular recording microelectrode).

Although the ability of calcium chelators to block LTP provides reasonable evidence that a postsynaptic increase in calcium is required for LTP induction, this result does not differentiate between calcium increases due to the influx of calcium across the membrane (as would be expected for calcium entering via the NMDA receptor ionophore) and release of calcium from intracellular stores. In cultured CNS neurons, the NMDA receptor-mediated influx of calcium can be suppressed by holding the membrane potential at depolarized levels (Mayer et al., 1987). Consistent with this result, it was found that strongly depolarizing the cell beyond the EPSP reversal potential could prevent LTP, even though subsequently it was possible, in the same cell, to induce LTP by pairing more modest depolarization with synaptic stimulation (Malenka et al., 1988). Thus, calcium influx is necessary for LTP induction, although a role for the release of calcium from intracellular stores still must be considered.

Another experiment that further tested the role of postsynaptic calcium in LTP induction again utilized the photolabile calcium chelator, Nitr-5. This compound normally binds calcium with high affinity, but undergoes photolysis when exposed to UV light, resulting in the release of calcium. EPSPs recorded from cells filled with calcium-loaded Nitr-5 became larger when exposed to UV light (Malenka et al., 1988). Control experiments indicated that this effect was indeed due to the release of calcium and not to the photolysis of Nitr-5. Thus, consistent with the hypothesis that a rise in calcium is a necessary and perhaps sufficient trigger to induce LTP, directly increasing postsynaptic calcium potentiated synaptic transmission.

Role of Dendritic Spines

Excitatory synapses in the CA1 region of the hippocampus occur on dendritic spines, small protuberances connected to the main dendritic shaft via thin necks. Several theoretical studies suggest that these spines may serve both to amplify NMDA receptor-mediated calcium increases and to isolate them from

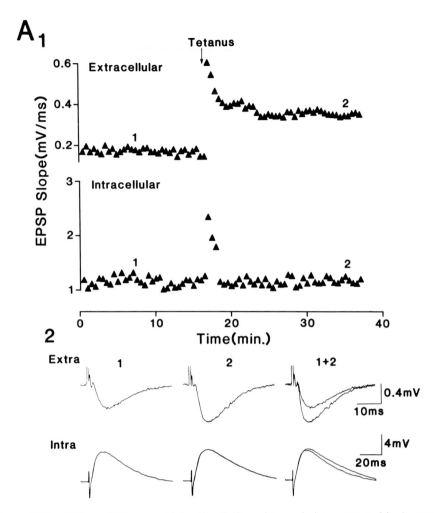

Figure 15-2. Filling a CA1 pyramidal cell with the calcium-chelator, Nitr-5, blocks LTP. A1. These are graphs of the initial slopes of a field EPSP recorded extracellularly in stratum radiatum of the rat hippocampal slice preparation and the simultaneously recorded intracellular EPSP. The cell was penetrated with an electrode containing Nitr-5 (100 mM) 15 minutes before time 0 on the graph. Each point on the graphs is the average of three successive measurements. Stimulation was applied at 0.1 hz. At the time indicated by the arrow two tetani (100 hz, 1 second) separated by 30 seconds were given. Only post-tetanic potentiation was elicited in the Nitr-5 filled cell while LTP was generated in all the surrounding cells as evidenced by the stable increase in the field EPSP. A2 shows sample records taken at the times indicated by the numbers on the graphs in A1. Each trace is the average of 6 sweeps. In the right column, the traces are superimposed. (From Malenka et al., 1988, with permission.)

increases occurring in adjacent synapses or in the main dendritic shaft (Holmes & Levy, 1990; Zador et al., 1990). Experimental evidence suggests that NMDA receptors are co-localized with non-NMDA receptors on dendritic spines (Bekkers & Stevens, 1989). Thus, each synapse may be able to generate its own private source of calcium.

BIOCHEMICAL MECHANISMS INVOLVED IN LTP

Role of Protein Kinases

Given that a rise in calcium in the dendritic spine is required for the generation of LTP, a critical question is what biochemical mechanisms are activated by calcium and are involved in LTP. Much of the most recent work has focused on the potential role of protein kinases, enzymes that modify protein function by phosphorylation and that play a critical role in a myriad of cell functions. Application of any one of a battery of nonselective kinase inhibitors, including polymyxin B, K-252b, sphingosine, and H-7, suppresses LTP (see Malenka & Nicoll, 1990 or Madison et al., 1991 for specific references). A protein kinase localized specifically to the postsynaptic cell has been implicated in LTP induction by the finding that injection of H-7 directly into the postsynaptic cell suppresses LTP (Malenka et al., 1989b; Malinow et al., 1989).

Two specific protein kinases have been the focus of most experimental work. Calcium/calmodulin-dependent protein kinase II (CaMKII) makes up approximately 20-40% of the protein in the postsynaptic density (an anatomical structure found in the subsynaptic region of dendritic spines) (Kelly et al., 1984; Kennedy et al., 1983); and therefore should be readily accessible to the NMDA receptor-mediated calcium rise required for LTP induction. Calmodulin antagonists have been reported to suppress LTP (for references, see Madison et al., 1991; Malenka & Nicoll, 1990), but all of these compounds may have had actions in addition to calmodulin inhibition. A more convincing demonstration of the potential importance of CaMKII in LTP came from experiments that used synthetic peptides specifically designed to inhibit calmodulin or CaMKII (Malenka et al., 1989b; Malinow et al., 1989). Figure 15-3 shows that the direct injection into postsynaptic cells of a calmodulin-binding peptide suppressed LTP, whereas injection of a control peptide had no effect.

The calcium- and phospholipid-dependent protein kinase known as protein kinase C (PKC) may also play an important role in LTP. Phorbol esters, exogenous activators of PKC, potentiate synaptic transmission (Malenka et al., 1986) although there are differences between LTP and the effects of phorbol ester application (for references, see Malenka & Nicoll, 1990). In the dentate gyrus, translocation of PKC from the cytosol to the membrane has been associated with LTP, as has increased phosphorylation of a presynaptic PKC substrate known as F-1, B-50, GAP-43, or P-57 (see Linden & Routtenberg, 1989 for a review of this work). Perhaps the most direct evidence in support of a role for PKC in LTP comes from the demonstration that LTP can be suppressed by injection into the postsynaptic cell of a peptide that inhibits substrate phosphorylation by PKC (Malinow et al., 1989).

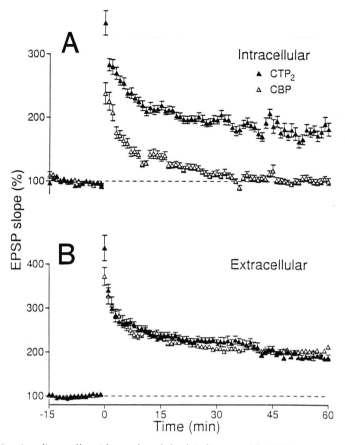

Figure 15-3. Loading cells with a calmodulin-binding peptide (CBP) suppresses LTP. **A.** Summary graphs comparing the effect of a LTP-inducing tetanus on the EPSP slope recorded from cells filled with either CBP (open triangles; 190 uM: n = 11) or the control peptide CTP₂ (closed triangles; 190 uM: n = 8). At time 0, two 100 hz-1 second tetani separated by 30 seconds were given. **B.** Summary graphs of the initial slopes of the field EPSPs recorded at the same time as the intracellularly recorded EPSPs shown in **A.** This graph shows that the magnitude of LTP generated in the two populations of slices was indistinguishable. (From Malenka et al., 1989b, with permission.)

How could activation of protein kinases mediate the long-lasting increase in synaptic efficacy that occurs during LTP? One possibility, proposed several years ago, is that a kinase activated by phosphorylation and capable of autophosphorylation may be able to serve as a "molecular switch" that could store information for long periods (Lisman, 1985). Subsequently, it was demonstrated that both PKC and CaMKII have biochemical properties that permit them to become constitutively active (for references, see Malenka & Nicoll, 1990; Madison et al., 1991). If persistent kinase activity is required for LTP, then application of kinase inhibitors that inhibit substrate phosphorylation should specifically reverse established LTP. The results of this sort of experiment have been inconsistent (see Malenka & Nicoll, 1991). The role of a constitutively active protein kinase in LTP remains an intriguing hypothesis.

OTHER BIOCHEMICAL MECHANISMS IN LTP

One of the first comprehensive hypotheses attempting to outline the biochemical steps involved in LTP proposed that a rise in calcium activated the calcium-dependent protease, calpain (Lynch and Baudry, 1984). This in turn degraded fodrin, a cytoskeletal protein, and might result in changes in dendritic spine structure, such as uncovering a covert population of glutamate receptors. Experimental evidence in support of this hypothesis includes the recent finding that incubating hippocampal slices in specific calpain inhibitors can suppress LTP (del Cerro et al., 1990).

The roles of new protein synthesis and gene expression in LTP have also begun to receive experimental attention. Protein synthesis inhibitors seem to disrupt LTP, although the exact mechanism and timing of this effect are not clear (Malenka & Nicoll, 1990). Similarly, several immediate-early genes, such as c-fos, jun-B, and zif/268, can be "turned on" by LTP-inducing stimuli, although this transcriptional activation does not seem to be specific for LTP (Malenka & Nicoll, 1990).

ARE THERE MULTIPLE FORMS OF LTP?

Although LTP is considered a stable, long-lasting enhancement of synaptic transmission, it is clear that shorter, decremental forms of synaptic potentiation occur. Figure 15-4 shows that, in the presence of the NMDA receptor

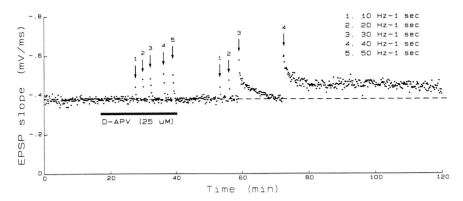

Figure 15-4. Distinct forms of synaptic potentiation can be elicited by NMDA receptor activation. Graph is from an experiment in which the effects of single tetani (1-5) on the strength of synaptic transmission were examined in the presence and absence of the NMDA receptor antagonist, D-APV. When NMDA receptors are blocked, a tetanus elicits only posttetanic potentiation lasting less than one minute. Under normal conditions, the same tetani can cause either PTP (1,2), a decremental synaptic enhancement (3) or stable LTP (4).

antagonist D-APV, a tetanus elicits a very short-lasting enhancement of synaptic transmission known as post-tetanic potentiation. The same sort of tetanus applied in the absence of NMDA receptor antagonists can induce post-tetanic potentiation, a longer-lasting decremental synaptic enhancement often referred to as short-term potentiation (STP) or stable LTP. Recent work suggests that the duration of NMDA receptor-dependent synaptic enhancement may depend on the magnitude of the calcium increase in the dendritic spine and that the induction of nondecremental, stable LTP requires some critical, "threshold" level of postsynaptic calcium (Malenka, 1991). This threshold level of calcium may activate biochemical processes not activated by lower levels of calcium. Thus, the intracellular processes responsible for STP may be a necessary, but not sufficient step for the generation of stable LTP. No matter what the under-

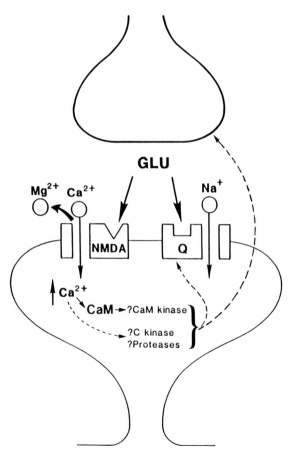

Figure 15-5. Possible postsynaptic events leading to the generation of LTP in a dendritic spine on a hippocampal CA1 pyramidal cell. During depolarization, Mg^{2+} is expelled from the NMDA receptor channel allowing calcium to enter the spine. This rise in calcium activates calmodulin and perhaps other biochemical events. This leads to the modification of non-NMDA receptors (Q) and the release of some substance which acts on the presynaptic terminal. (Modified from Malenka et al., 1989a, with permission.)

lying mechanisms, the ability to generate forms of synaptic enhancement with distinct time courses is likely to be important for many aspects of nervous system function, including learning and memory.

WHERE IS THE SITE OF CHANGE RESPONSIBLE FOR LTP?

An increase in the strength of synaptic transmission can occur either because of an increase in transmitter release from the presynaptic terminal or because the postsynaptic cell generates a larger response to a constant presynaptic input. There is evidence that both of these mechanisms may be important for LTP (Madison et al., 1991; Malenka & Nicoll, 1990). Figure 15-5 shows a schematic summary of some of the steps that may be involved in LTP. Activation of a number of calcium-dependent biochemical processes may somehow modify the postsynaptic glutamate receptors (Q; quisqualate) responsible for EPSP generation, perhaps via phosphorylation. In addition, if transmitter release is enhanced during LTP, some "retrograde" messenger must be released from the postsynaptic cell and act on the presynaptic terminal since all of the steps necessary for LTP "induction" reside in the postsynaptic cell. Clearly, we are just beginning to unravel the intracellular machinery responsible for LTP.

CONCLUSIONS

This chapter focuses on the mechanisms underlying the generation of the NMDA receptor-dependent form of LTP found in the CA1 region of the hippocampus. Why has this simple form of synaptic plasticity generated so much interest and research? It has become apparent that NMDA receptors are involved in a myriad of different forms of normal and pathological (e.g., seizures) synaptic plasticity in a variety of brain regions and during development (Watkins & Collingridge, 1989). Therefore, a detailed understanding of the mechanisms underlying LTP should yield important clues to the mechanisms responsible for all forms of NMDA receptor-dependent synaptic plasticity. With the advent of more sophisticated molecular and electrophysiological techniques, it may soon be possible to determine in much greater detail the biochemical and molecular events responsible for LTP. This eventually may lead to the development of agents that enhance the ability to learn and remember or retard the inevitable deterioration of this ability.

Do NMDA receptors and LTP have any direct relevance to investigations of the biological basis of substance abuse and addiction? NMDA receptors have already been directly implicated in the mechanism of action of the psychotomimetic phencyclidine (PCP) (Collingridge & Lester, 1989). Whether other commonly abused substances affect NMDA receptor function or LTP has not been investigated but may be important, especially for those compounds that are known to interferre with the learning process or cause seizures. Perhaps the most fruitful line of inquiry will be to investigate the forms and mechanisms of synaptic plasticity occurring in the neural circuits directly involved in drug-seeking behavior.

REFERENCES

Alkon, D.L. (1984). Calcium-mediated reduction of ionic currents: A biophysical memory trace. *Science, 226,* 1037-1045.

Bekkers, J.M., & Stevens, C.F. (1989). NMDA and non-NMDA receptors are co-localized at individual excitatory synapses in cultured rat hippocampus. *Nature, 341,* 230-233.

Bliss, T.V.P., & Lømo, T. (1973). Long-lasting potentiation of synaptic transmission in the dentate area of the anaesthetized rabbit following stimulation of the perforant path. *J. Physiol., 232,* 331-356.

Brown, T.H., Kairiss, E.W., & Keenan, C.L. (1990). Hebbian synapses: Biophysical mechanisms and algorithms. *Annu. Rev. Neurosci., 13,* 475-511.

Cajal, S.R. (1911). *Histologie du systeme nerveux de l'homme et des vertebres,* Vol. II (p. 993). Paris: Maloine.

Collingridge, G.L., & Lester, R.A.J. (1989). Excitatory amino acid receptors in the vertebrate central nervous system. *Pharmacol. Rev., 40,* 143-210.

Collingridge, G.L., Kehl, S.J., & McLennan, H. (1983). Excitatory amino acids in synaptic transmission in the Schaffer collateral-commissural pathway of the rat hippocampus. *J. Physiol., 334,* 33-46.

del Cerro, S., Larson, J., Oliver, M.W., & Lynch, G. (1990). Development of hippocampal long-term potentiation is reduced by recently introduced calpain inhibitors. *Brain Res., 530,* 91-95.

Dunwiddie, T.V., & Lynch, G. (1978). Long-term potentiation and depression of synaptic responses in the rat hippocampus: Localization and frequency dependency. *J. Physiol., 276,* 353-367.

Eccles, J.C. (1953). *The neurophysiological basis of mind. The principles of neurophysiology* (p. 314). Oxford: Clarendon Press.

Goudie, A.J., & Emmett-Oglesby, M.W. (Eds.). (1989). *Psychoactive drugs: Tolerance and sensitization.* Clifton, NJ: Humana Press.

Gustafsson, B., & Wigström, H. (1988). Physiological mechanisms underlying long-term potentiation. *Trends Neurosci., 11,* 156-162.

Gustafsson, B., Wigström, H., Abraham, W.C., & Huang, Y.-Y. (1987). Long-term potentiation in the hippocampus using depolarizing current pulses as the conditioning stimulus to single volley synaptic potentials. *J. Neurosci., 7,* 774-780.

Hebb, D.O. (1949). *The organization of behavior.* New York: John Wiley & Sons, Inc.

Holmes, W.R., & Levy, W.B. (1990). Insights into associative long-term potentiation from computational models of NMDA receptor-mediated calcium influx and intracellular calcium concentration changes. *J. Neurophysiol., 63,* 1148-1168.

Kandel, E.R., Castellucci, V.F., Goelet, P., & Schacher, S. (1987). Cell-biological interrelationships between short-term and long-term memory. In E.R. Kandel (Ed.), *Molecular neurobiology in neurology and psychiatry* (pp 111-132). New York: Raven Press.

Kelly, P.T., McGuinness, T.L., & Greengard, P. (1984). Evidence that the major postsynaptic density protein is a component of Ca^{2+}/calmodulin-dependent protein kinase. *Proc. Natl. Acad. Sci. USA., 81,* 945-949.

Kelso, S.R., Ganong, A.H., & Brown, T.H. (1986). Hebbian synapses in hippocampus. *Proc. Natl. Acad. Sci. USA., 83,* 5326-5330.

Kennedy, M.B., Bennett, M.K., & Erondu, N.E. (1983). Biochemical and immunochemical evidence that the "major postsynaptic density protein" is a subunit of a calmodulin-dependent protein kinase. *Proc. Natl. Acad. Sci. USA., 80,* 7357-7361.

Linden, D.J., & Routtenberg, A. (1989). The role of protein kinase C in long-term potentiation: A testable model. *Brain Res. Rev., 14*, 279-296.

Lisman, J.E. (1985). A mechanism for memory storage insensitive to molecular turnover: A bistable autophosphorylating kinase. *Proc. Natl. Acad. Sci. USA., 82*, 3055-3057.

Lømo, T. (1966). Frequency potentiation of excitatory synaptic activity in the dentate area of the hippocampal formation. *Acta Physiol. Scand., 68* (Suppl. 277), 128.

Lynch, G., & Baudry, M. (1984). The biochemistry of memory: A new and specific hypothesis. *Science, 224*, 151-153.

Lynch, G., Larson, J., Kelso, S., Barrionuevo, G., & Schottler, F. (1983). Intracellular injections of EGTA block induction of hippocampal long-term potentiation. *Nature, 305*, 719-21.

Madison, D.V., Malenka, R.C., & Nicoll, R.A. (1991). Mechanisms underlying long-term potentiation of synaptic transmission. *Annu. Rev. Neurosci., 14*, 379-397.

Malenka, R.C. (1991). Postsynaptic factors control the duration of synaptic enhancement in area CA1 of the hippocampus. *Neuron, 6*, 53-60.

Malenka, R.C., & Nicoll, R.A. (1990). Intracellular signals and LTP. *Sem. Neurosci., 2*, 335-343.

Malenka, R.C., Madison, D.V., & Nicoll, R.A. (1986). Potentiation of synaptic tansmission in the hippocampus by phorbol esters. *Nature, 321*, 175-177.

Malenka, R.C., Kauer, J.A., Zucker, R.J., & Nicoll, R.A. (1988). Postsynaptic calcium is sufficient for potentiation of hippocampal synaptic transmission. *Science, 242*, 81-84.

Malenka, R.C., Kauer, J.A., Perkel, D.J., & Nicoll, R.A. (1989a). The impact of postsynaptic calcium on synaptic transmission—its role in long-term potentiation. *Trends Neurosci., 12*, 444-450.

Malenka, R.C., Kauer, J.A., Perkel, D.J., Mauk, M.D., Kelly, P.T., Nicoll, R.A., & Waxham, M.N. (1989b). An essential role for postsynaptic calmodulin and protein kinases activity in long-term potentiation. *Nature, 340*, 554-557.

Malinow, R., & Miller, J.P. (1986). Postsynaptic hyperpolarization during conditioning reversibly blocks induction of long-term potentiation. *Nature, 321*, 529-530.

Malinow, R., Schulman, H., & Tsien, R.W. (1989). Inhibition of postsynaptic PKC or CaMKII blocks induction but not expression of LTP. *Science, 245*, 862-866.

Mayer, M.L., Westbrook, G.L., & Guthrie, P.B. (1984). Voltage-dependent block by Mg^{2+} of NMDA responses in spinal cord neurones. *Nature, 309*, 262-263.

Mayer, M.L., MacDermott, A.B., Westbrook, G.L., Smith, S.J., & Barker, J.L. (1987). Agonist- and voltage-gated calcium entry in cultured mouse spinal cord neurons under voltage clamp measured using arsenazo III. *J. Neurosci., 7*, 3230-3244.

McNaughton, B.L., Douglas, R.M., & Goddard, G.V. (1978). Synaptic enhancement in fascia dentata: Cooperativity among coactive afferents. *Brain Res., 157*, 277-293.

Nicoll, R.A., Kauer, J.A., & Malenka, R.C. (1988). The current excitement in long-term potentiation. *Neuron, 1*, 97-103.

Nowak, L., Bregestovski, P., Ascher, P., Herbet, A., & Prochiantz, A. (1984). Magnesium gates glutamate-activated channels in mouse central neurones. *Nature, 307*, 462-465.

Watkins, J.C., & Collingridge, G.L. (Eds.). (1989). *The NMDA receptor.* Oxford: Oxford University Press.

Zador, A., Koch, C., & Brown, T.H. (1990). Biophysical model of a Hebbian synapse. *Proc. Natl. Acad. Sci. USA., 87*, 6718-6722.

Zalutsky, R.A., & Nicoll, R.A. (1990). Comparison of two forms of long-term potentiation in single hippocampal neurons. *Science, 248*, 1619-1624.

III

NEUROPHARMACOLOGY

While much of this volume can be described as neuropharmacology, we have chosen to include several contributions that relate specifically to that discipline in this section.

One of the key aspects of the study of drugs is to determine their effects on neurotransmitter release. Such studies have been extremely difficult with the peptide neuroregulators due to their limited concentrations. Maidment and Bertolucci describe the problem, the potential value of such measurements for the study of co-release of various substances, and improvements in the assay methods that make such studies possible. Assay methods are also key to the chapter by Faull, who describes the use of mass spectrographic techniques to determine whether morphine alkaloids are normally present in the brain.

Three chapters examine neuropharmacological aspects of a significant drug of abuse. Pechnick discusses the neural substrates for phencyclidine (PCP), a particularly devastating drug that has importance as a model of psychosis. The chemistry and actions of d-methamphetamine (Ice), which is undergoing a resurgence of abuse, is reviewed by Cho. Broad questions about the neuropharmacology of the most important and least well understood major drug, alcohol, are considered by Henriksen.

16

Neurochemical Circuitry of Drug Abuse: The Potential of In Vivo Microdialysis

NIGEL T. MAIDMENT AND MAGALI BERTOLUCCI

In the literature on drug abuse, one repeatedly comes across the terms *tolerance* and *dependence,* which are used to define two aspects of the addiction process that have historically been differentiated. Tolerance can be defined simply as a drug-induced state in which the dose of the drug has to be increased from the pretolerant level to produce an equivalent effect. It might be considered in terms of a homeostatic mechanism in the brain returning the organism to a state equivalent to the drug-free condition. Dependence is often subdivided into "physical" and "psychic" forms. Physical dependence is a state that develops in both animals and humans after they are exposed for a sufficiently long period of time to high doses of certain kinds of addictive drugs, such as heroin. When these substances are withdrawn suddenly, severe physical disturbances are experienced, the symptoms of which vary depending on the drug. Often, they result from actions of the drug in the peripheral nervous system and so may include gastrointestinal disorder, nausea, chills, etc. Since these symptoms are abolished by administration of the drug, they provide an impetus for continued drug use. However, the observation that alleviation of these adverse side effects by appropriate drugs does not prevent continued taking of the abused drug, coupled with the fact that not all drugs of abuse produce such severe physical disturbances on withdrawal (e.g., cocaine), suggests another component to the addictive process. Thus, adverse psychological mood perturbations precipitated by drug withdrawal combined with a craving for the pleasurable effects of the drug are seen as another, perhaps more important, driving force for continued administration. It is this phenomenon that has been termed psychic dependence, and an understanding of its neurochemical and neuroanatomical basis is the major challenge for neuroscientists studying drug abuse.

This work was supported by grants from the NIDA (DA-05010), NSF (BNS-8618972), The Lucille P. Markey Charitable Trust, and The National Alliance for Research on Schizophrenia and Depression, and the W.M. Keck Foundation.

We are currently some way from being able to piece together this functional neurochemical circuitry, which is both common and specific to the addictive processes associated with various classes of abused drugs. A number of experimental approaches are being taken to address this issue. This chapter briefly reviews the literature on the neurochemical anatomy of drug abuse and emphasizes the potential of the recently popularized technique of microdialysis for providing insight into the complex neurochemical interactions taking place in discrete brain nuclei after repeated administration of abused drugs. In particular, we highlight the potential application of this method to in vivo monitoring of neuropeptide release under such conditions.

IS THERE A "CENTER FOR DRUG ABUSE" IN THE BRAIN?

Drugs of abuse have been categorized into several pharmacological classes, including central stimulants (e.g., amphetamine and cocaine), opiates (e.g., morphine), central depressants (e.g., ethanol, barbiturates), and cholinergic agonists, e.g., nicotine. Although biochemical studies have established that these drugs act, at least initially, through different receptor mechanisms in the brain and so may involve several different neurotransmission systems in the mediation of their effects, there is a growing consensus that there exists, possibly in the form of the limbic dopamine system, a common neurochemical/ neuroanatomical substrate for the reinforcing properties of many abused drugs. That is, it can be postulated that the tendency for any particular drug to be abused results from that drug's ability to interact at one level or another with the brain's endogenous reward or reinforcement center. That such an endogenous positive reinforcement substrate exists in the brain is supported by the behaviorally reinforcing properties of certain natural stimuli. A common example given is the observation that fasted animals will administer sweet solutions containing only saccharin in preference to neutrally tasting nutritive solutions even as the level of food deprivation becomes extreme (Jacobs & Sharma, 1969). This observation is interpreted as evidence for the existence of a substrate in the brain mediating certain kinds of pleasurable sensations, and it is postulated that abused drugs may directly affect this system.

Self-Stimulation Paradigm

An indication that mesencephalic dopaminergic neurons might have a pivotal role in natural reward processes came originally from intracranial self-stimulation experiments and associated pharmacological manipulations. Several sites in the brain are able to sustain self-stimulation behavior when implanted with stimulating electrodes (Crow, 1972; Routtenberg & Malsbury, 1969). Routtenberg (1964) initially demonstrated how powerful these stimulations could be by showing that animals will neglect food, even when they are starving, if they are allowed to self-stimulate certain regions of their brain by pressing a bar in their cage. Subsequently, the distribution of positive sites for intracranial self-stimulation was found to be closely associated with the region of the dopaminergic cell bodies in the mesencephalon (substantia nigra and ventral tegmentum) from which high rates of self-stimulation could be obtained (Corbett & Wise, 1980; Wise, 1981). More convincing evidence for the involvement of dopamine neurons in this behavior comes from several studies utilizing pharmacological interventions. Thus, 6-hydroxydopamine (6-OHDA) lesions of the ascending fibers of the mesencephalic dopaminergic projections induce marked decreases in rates of self-stimulation obtained from electrodes in the ventral tegmental area (VTA) (Fibiger et al., 1987; Phillips & Fibiger, 1978). Similarly, systemic administration of dopaminergic receptor antagonists decreases the self-stimulation rates in a dose-related manner (Fibiger, 1978; Fibiger & Phillips, 1986; Wise, 1978). It has been argued, however, that since dopamine systems are known to be important in locomotor and motivational behavior, such effects could be due to a reduction in the ability of the animal to respond, rather than any impact on the efficacy of the rewarding stimulus itself. Several experimental models, including threshold, extinction, and curve-shift paradigms, have been used to support the idea that neuroleptic-induced motor impairments alone cannot account for the observed decrease in self-stimulation rates, rather, dopaminergic receptor blockade specifically reduces the rewarding properties of brain stimulation (see Wise, 1987 for a summary of this data). This continues to be a subject of debate, however (Ettenberg, 1989), and it is worthwhile to note that there are apparently no reports demonstrating an initial increase in electrical self-stimulation rates in the presence of low doses of neuroleptics. Such an effect could be predicted if the animal's motor capability was not impaired since one would expect the animal to attempt to overcome the partial dopamine receptor blockade by increasing the rate of stimulation. Such a phenomenon is in fact the predominant effect of neuroleptic administration reported in psychostimulant drug self-administration studies (see below). It is interesting that two apparently opposite effects of these drugs in two reinforcement paradigms—electrical self-stimulation and drug self-administration—have both been used to support the involvement of dopamine systems in reinforcing behavior.

Dopaminergic cells in the ventral tegmentum and substantia nigra innervate several major forebrain structures, including the nucleus accumbens, prefrontal cortex, and caudate. The next logical question to be asked therefore was whether one of these terminal fields could be singled out as being the reward area. Using local drug injections, the nucleus accumbens has emerged as the prime candidate. Thus, a significant reduction in self-stimulation of the VTA is observed when neuroleptics are injected into the ipsilateral nucleus accumbens, but not the prefrontal cortex or caudate (Mogenson et al., 1979; Mora et al., 1977; Stellar & Corbett, 1989).

However, the direct activation of dopamine neurons as a mediator of self-stimulation reward behavior is questionable in view of studies examining the excitability properties of these cells. It has been demonstrated that the unmyelinated dopamine axons have very high thresholds for excitation so that they are activated only when high currents, long duration pulses and/or small electrode tips are used (Yeomans, 1989; Yeomans et al., 1988). Since the majority of self-stimulation experiments have used parameters that are subthreshold for dopamine neuronal excitation, a direct role for the ascending dopaminergic pathways in brain stimulation reward is unlikely (Yeomans, 1989). Indeed, it has been suggested that the specific fibers of the reward system might extend down the medial forebrain bundle to connect with the dopaminergic cells of that region, in the opposite direction of the projection of the catecholamine fibers (Bielajew & Shizgal, 1986). Regardless of the above caveat, the neuroleptic blockade experiments described above suggest that activation of dopamine receptors in the terminal fields of dopamine neurons, predominantly if not exclusively in the nucleus accumbens, is necessary for the maintenance of medial forebrain bundle (MFB) self-stimulation behavior.

However, on the basis of the above data alone, it could still be argued that dopamine systems may play a purely permissive role in the reinforcing behavior, rather than being a primary driving force. The first indication that dopamine release is indeed activated by self-stimulation behavior was provided by ex vivo measurements of dopamine and its metabolites in brain tissue (Simon et al., 1979). The use of postmortem total tissue content measurements as estimations of release events is, however, fraught with interpretational problems. For instance, an increase in the tissue content of dopamine may reflect a decreased release, which would result in increased neuronal stores, or it might be due to an increase in synthesis with little change in release. Measurement of dopamine metabolites in addition to dopamine, and the expression of a dopamine : DOPAC ratio is often used as an index of release. However, this does not consider the possibility that dopamine turnover within the terminal may change in the absence of changes in release. What is required therefore is a direct and continual measurement of the extracellular content of the transmitter during the behavior, which is provided most effectively by microdialysis and voltammetry procedures (for reviews, see Adams & Justice, 1987; Joseph et al., 1986; Marsden, 1984; Robinson & Justice, 1991).

Briefly, microdialysis involves implanting a hollow tubular dialysis membrane into the brain region of interest, which is continually perfused with an artificial CSF. Compounds in the extracellular fluid simply diffuse across the membrane along their concentration gradient and are analyzed in the collected perfusate. This technique has the advantage of being able to estimate the extracellular content of any compound small enough to cross the membrane and for which there is a sufficiently sensitive assay procedure. Voltammetry is more restricted in its scope because it depends on the electroactivity of the compound detected, which effectively limits its application to catechol and indole transmitters and their metabolites. Its major advantages over microdialysis are an increased potential sampling frequency and greatly improved spatial resolution with an associated reduction in tissue trauma. There are several reports demonstrating the capability of both of these methodologies to detect increases in dopamine release in the nucleus accumbens and caudate during forced stimulation of the MFB at current intensities and pulse durations sufficient to directly activate dopamine cells (Gonon & Buda, 1985; Imperato & Di Chiara, 1984; Stamford et al., 1986). However, studies applying these powerful techniques directly to the self-stimulation paradigm, in which, as noted above, more subtle stimulation parameters are employed, are few in number. Gratton et al. (1988)

used an indirect approach—first training rats to self-stimulate the VTA or MFB and then conducting voltammetric experiments in the same animals under anesthesia using identical, but forced, stimulation parameters. In this way they were able to demonstrate small transient increases in dopamine release in the nucleus accumbens, caudate, and prefrontal cortex. Similar but more direct experiments in unanesthetized behaving animals were conducted by Phillips et al. (1989). These authors also reported increased chronoamperommetric current that was attributed to dopamine during self-stimulation behavior. It should be noted, however, that the specificity for dopamine of the stearate-modified electrodes employed in this study has been questioned (Marsden et al., 1988). Finally, Nakahara et al. (1989), using microdialysis, reported increases in recovered dopamine during self-stimulation of the MFB over 1-hour periods if nomifensine was administered to inhibit dopamine uptake. The responses were, however, somewhat variable, and the number of experiments was too limited to enable firm conclusions to be drawn from the data.

In summary, evidence that dopamine release is significantly elevated during self-stimulation behavior is less than convincing and requires further investigation. This could reflect limitations of the current in vivo methodology in measuring subtle, but nonetheless behaviorally relevant, changes in synaptic release—changes that may not produce significant elevations in the general extracellular content of dopamine due to the effective uptake mechanism in the synapse. In the absence of such data, whether dopamine plays an active role in the self-stimulation process or instead serves some kind of permissive function remains an issue for debate. If an activation of dopamine release is important, it is becoming increasingly clear that these neurons are activated indirectly via transynaptic mechanisms.

Interaction of Abused Drugs with Self-Stimulation Behavior

Having postulated the existence of an endogenous reward center with its locus in the mesolimbic dopamine system, the next logical step in the search for a common neurochemical/neuroanatomical substrate for drug abuse was to determine if such drugs could be shown to interact in some way with this system. Most of the different pharmacological classes of abused drugs have indeed been shown to interact with brain self-stimulation in one way or another. When psychomotor stimulants, such as amphetamine (Stein & Ray, 1960; Wise & Stein, 1970) and cocaine (Crow, 1970; Wauquier & Niemegeers, 1974), opiates (Adams et al., 1972), ethanol (De Witte & Bada, 1983; Lorens & Sainati, 1978), barbiturates (Mogenson, 1964), benzodiazepines (Olds, 1966), and nicotine (Clarke & Kumar, 1984) are administered peripherally at selected low doses, they facilitate responding for brain stimulation. The interaction sites of these drugs with the reward system have only been studied in the case of the opiates and the psychostimulants. The sites where the opiates facilitate the medial forebrain bundle self-stimulation seem to be in the VTA, since local injections of morphine in this area, as opposed to the nucleus accumbens and the caudate nucleus, enhance the animals' response rates (Broekkamp & Van Rossum, 1975; Broekkamp et al., 1976, 1979). With regard to psychostimulants, amphetamine has been shown to increase brain stimulation rates when locally injected in the nucleus accumbens, but not in the neostriatum (Broekkamp et al., 1975).

Drug Self-Administration

Of course, demonstrating that abused drugs potentiate the electrical activation of the apparent endogenous reward center does not, in and of itself, provide sufficient evidence that this is the active site of action for the rewarding properties of the drugs in the brain. It was therefore necessary to develop ways of assessing the locus of drug action when administered to animals alone, in the absence of electrical self-stimulation, and in a repeated regimen approximating, as close as possible, that occurring in the human drug abuser. The self-administration paradigm was developed for this purpose and has been used extensively to study the reinforcing properties of abused drugs. In this behavioral model, the animals receive an injection of a drug when demonstrating a correct operant response—most commonly, bar pressing. The question of anatomical specificity can be approached in two ways. Either the drugs can be tested for their reinforcing properties when injected directly into specific brain regions or they can be administered peripherally, and attempts to block their effects can be made by central injection of known antagonists or by selective neurotoxic lesions. Such studies have only been carried out extensively for the psychostimulants and opiates and are reviewed below.

Psychostimulants

Biochemical in vitro studies made in the 1960s (Carr & Moore, 1969; Stein, 1964; Van Rossum et al., 1962) indicated that amphetamine is capable of releasing biogenic amines, including norepinephrine, serotonin, and dopamine, from nerve terminals. Amphetamine is believed to release the amines from a newly synthesized pool through an as yet undetermined mechanism, although recent experiments conducted both in vivo with microdialysis and in cultured mesencephalic dopamine cells suggest that it may act via a weak base mechanism to disrupt the vesicular-cytoplasmic proton gradient necessary for the sequestration and retention of dopamine within synaptic vesicles (Sulzer et al., 1991, 1992; Sulzer, Maidment, & Rayport, 1993). Similar in vitro experiments using brain slices (Heikkila et al., 1975) showed that cocaine is not a releasing agent like amphetamine, but rather increases synaptic levels of catecholamines by blocking the reuptake mechanism, which is the main route of catecholaminergic inactivation in the synapse. The recent cloning of the gene for this transporter (Kilty et al., 1991; Shimada et al., 1991) will make possible molecular studies of the specific interaction of cocaine with the transporter protein and provide information on the regulation of transporter synthesis during chronic cocaine administration.

In studies using the peripheral self-administration paradigm, the observation that alpha-methyl-para-tyrosine, an inhibitor of catecholamine synthesis, attenuates the rewarding properties of the psychostimulants confirmed the catecholaminergic mediation of their effects (Davis & Smith, 1973; Jonsson et al., 1971; Pickens et al., 1968). Evidence for the primary involvement of dopamine systems, as opposed to norepinephrine or serotonin, in the rewarding properties of psychostimulants has come from several sources. First and foremost, antagonists of dopamine, but not of noradrenaline or serotonin, increase in a dose-dependent manner the rate of self-administration responses for amphetamine and cocaine (Davis & Smith, 1975; Dewit & Wise, 1977; Risner & Jones, 1976, 1980; Yokel & Wise, 1975, 1976). As discussed above, this result has been taken to reflect a reduction of the reinforcing potential of the drugs as a result of dopamine receptor blockade whereby the animal increases its response rate in an attempt to overcome the effect of the antagonist. Higher doses of neuroleptics do in fact produce an extinction of the reinforcing behavior, presumably because the animal "learns" that increases in lever pressing no longer result in the desired pleasurable response. Similarly, lesion studies confirmed the importance of the dopaminergic as opposed to norepinephrine pathways in amphetamine and cocaine reinforcement and provided insight into the particular structures involved. Thus, Roberts et al. (1977) were the first to show that 6-OHDA lesions of the ascending norepinephrine projections failed to affect intravenous cocaine self-administration, whereas similar lesions of the nucleus accumbens produced a significant reduction in the self-administration of cocaine. Subsequent 6-hydroxydopamine lesion studies have strengthened the case for the importance of the VTA-nucleus accumbens dopamine pathway to the reinforcement-inducing effects of amphetamine and cocaine (Bozarth & Wise, 1985; Lyness et al., 1979; Pettit et al., 1984; Roberts & Koob, 1982). However, Roberts and Koob (1982) add a cautionary note in the discussion of their results, which showed that cocaine reinforcement was attenuated by VTA 6-hydroxydopamine lesions. They observed a lack of correlation between nucleus accumbens dopamine depletion and the degree of change in cocaine intake and noted that several animals sustained a severe depletion of dopamine but continued to administer cocaine at high rates. One explanation offered for this finding was that dopamine depletion in other terminal regions, such as the prefrontal cortex or amygdala, may be more critical. The caudate is apparently not involved since several review articles state the ineffectiveness of 6-hydroxydopamine lesions in this structure in attenuating cocaine reward (Pulvirenti & Koob, 1990; Roberts & Koob, 1982), although original articles supporting this statement are elusive! In a similar vein, although local injection of a selective dopamine antagonist into the nucleus accumbens was able to block cocaine peripheral self-administration (Phillips et al., 1983), direct injection of cocaine into this region failed to promote self-administration behavior (Goeders & Smith, 1983). Similar injections of cocaine into the prefrontal cortex (Goeders & Smith, 1983, 1986) were, however, effective in inducing self-administration. Contrarily, amphetamine is self-administered into the nucleus accumbens, but not the striatum or prefrontal cortex (Hoebel et al., 1983). Such anomalous findings are difficult to reconcile in view of the proposed similar end-effect of these drugs—an elevation in extracellular dopamine. In view of these data it seems that the long-standing promotion of the VTA-nucleus accumbens dopamine pathway as the sole locus for the reinforcing properties of psychostimulants may be somewhat simplistic.

Microdialysis has begun to be used to address the issue of psychostimulant action on dopamine release both in acute situations and, more recently and most importantly, in the self-administration paradigm. First, Di Chiara and co-workers (Carboni et al., 1989; Di Chiara & Imperato, 1988) carried out a systematic survey of the effects of various categories of drugs of abuse on the extracellular concentration of dopamine and its metabolites in both the nucleus accumbens and the caudate nucleus of freely moving rats. Their data showed that drugs abused by humans, such as opiates, ethanol, nicotine, amphetamine, and cocaine, increased extracellular dopamine levels significantly in both areas. Percentage increases above basal concentrations were, however, up to two times greater in the accumens than in the caudate, which, the authors argue, supports a role for the accumbens rather than the caudate in the reinforcing properties of these drugs. Such a conclusion is questionable, particularly when one considers the fact that the basal dopamine concentration before drug administration was twice as high in the caudate as in the accumbens. Similar studies have confirmed the dopamine-elevating properties of both cocaine and amphetamine in acute preparations in the nucleus accumbens, caudate, and prefrontal cortex (Maisonneuve et al., 1990; Pettit & Justice, 1989; Sharp et al., 1987).

Whereas the above microdialysis data largely confirmed what was already known about psychostimulant effects on dopamine release, more recently, new and interesting information has been forthcoming from microdialysis studies in chronically administered and self-administering animals. For example, it has long been recognized that animals self-administering psychostimulants will adjust their rate of administration according to the dose so that higher doses result in lower frequencies of responding (Pickens & Thompson, 1968). It could be postulated that such titration of responding results in the maintenance of a fixed, optimally elevated level of extracellular dopamine in the nucleus accumbens. This hypothesis was tested by Pettit and Justice (1989; Pettit et al., 1990) using a range of cocaine doses in a self-administration paradigm. Their data showed that the animals did indeed self-administer at a rate sufficient to maintain a constant elevated level of dopamine in the nucleus accumbens for any given dose. Furthermore, their lever pressing response was reduced as the dose of self-administered cocaine was increased. However, this reduction was not sufficient to prevent both an increase in cocaine intake and an associated increase in the magnitude of the elevation in extracellular dopamine in the nucleus accumbens. This raises the question of why animals on the lower dose do not increase their response rate in order to achieve levels comparable to those attained with higher doses. One plausible explanation offered by the authors is that it is in some way the kinetics of the dopamine increase that is important so that higher doses produce more rapid elevations in dopamine. This is an interesting concept that may be worthy of further investigation.

It has been known for some time that repeated administration of cocaine results in a potentiation of the behavioral effects of the drug (Downs & Eddy, 1932; Kalivas et al., 1988; Tatum & Seevers, 1929). This sensitization or "reverse tolerance" at the behavioral level appears when the animal is challenged with cocaine after just one previous exposure to the drug (Lin-Chu et al., 1985). Particularly interesting is the observation that this sensitization phenomenon persists for several months after withdrawal of the drug (Kilby & Ellinwood,

1977; Post et al., 1985), suggesting the inducement of some kind of long-term change in neurochemical function. Petit et al. (1990) therefore sought to find out if the effect of a challenge dose of cocaine on extracellular dopamine in the accumbens was altered by previous exposure to the drug and also if the concentration of cocaine attained in the extracellular fluid in this brain region and in the plasma was itself affected. They found that after 10 or 30 daily injections the increase in dialysate dopamine levels produced by a challenge dose was significantly potentiated compared to chronic saline controls. However, there was a corresponding increase in the concentration of cocaine attained in the dialysates and in the plasma. When dopamine: cocaine ratios were calculated, there was no difference between the two groups, indicating that the potentiation of the dopamine response could be entirely accounted for by an increase in the availability of cocaine. Since plasma levels of the drug were also elevated, it would seem that the cocaine sensitization phenomenon can be explained, in part if not completely, in terms of a change in the peripheral management of the drug. The sensitization phenomenon with regard to dopamine release was subsequently confirmed by Kalivas and Duffy (1990), using a forced injection paradigm, and similar findings have been reported for amphetamine (see Chapter 24). However, the data of Hurd et al., (1989, 1990) are directly contradictary. These authors reported that chronic exposure to cocaine (10-day period of self-administration) resulted in complete tolerance to the dopamine-elevating effects of a challenge dose both in the nucleus accumbens and striatum. As always, such diammetrically opposing findings are perplexing and demonstrate the complexity of the systems under investigation. An explanation tentatively offered by Pettit and co-workers concerns differences in probe placement within the accumbens. Whereas these authors placed their probes in the anterior of this structure, Hurd et al. (1990) studied the posterior region, the dopamine terminals of which have been shown to co-localize CCK and/or neurotensin. It is tempting to postulate that these neurons may possess additional regulatory mechanisms resulting from their peptide content (see discussion below).

Opiates

Whereas the psychostimulants clearly interact with dopamine systems directly at the level of the presynaptic dopamine terminal, the opiates are proposed to have more indirect influences on dopamine transmission in this hypothetical reward pathway. The VTA was the first region to be studied as a potential anatomical substrate for opiate reward since, as described above, it had been identified as the locus of interactions between opiates and electrical self-stimulation. As predicted, local injections of opiates into the VTA were able to sustain self-administration (Bozarth & Wise, 1981; Phillips & Lepiane, 1980, 1982). Using the same paradigm, Britt and Wise (1983) showed that local injections of opiate antagonists into the VTA induced a higher rate of intravenous heroin self-administration, which was thought to reflect a decrease in the rewarding effects of heroin and an attempt on the part of the animal to overcome the effect of the antagonist. However, the VTA is not the only site at which opiates are self-administered. Rats will also self-administer morphine (Olds,

1982) and met-enkephalin (Goeders et al., 1984) directly into the nucleus accumbens, and the rewarding properties of intravenously self-administrated heroin are decreased after injection of opiate antagonists into this region of the brain (Vaccarino et al., 1985). However, the direct involvement of dopamine neurons in mediating these actions is an area of some controversy. Clearly, intra-VTA administration of opiates activates the ascending dopamine fibers as demonstrated by electrophysiological (Hu & Wang, 1984; Matthews & German, 1984) and behavioral studies (Holmes et al., 1983; Joyce & Iversen, 1979). Similarly, locomotor activity is enhanced by local injections of opiates into the nucleus accumbens (Kalivas et al., 1983; Pert & Sivit, 1977; Swerdlow et al., 1987), which might indicate a potentiation of dopamine release.

All of the above is circumstantial evidence, however. The real test is whether dopamine antagonists and/or lesions of dopamine pathways are able to influence opiate reinforcement. It is in this matter that there seems to be some disagreement in the literature. Early studies by Schwartz and Marchok (1974) and Sherman et al. (1980) suggested an attenuating effect of neuroleptics on intravenous opiate self-administration and place preference. However, subsequently Ettenberg et al. (1982) were unable to demonstrate any effect of a dopamine antagonist on heroin self-administration. Moreover, Pettit et al. (1984) and Dworkin et al. (1988a) have reported the persistence of heroin self-administration after 6-OHDA lesions of the nucleus accumbens, suggesting that the rewarding properties of heroin are independent of dopamine activation, at least of this particular dopamine pathway. A logical conclusion is that opiates are able to act at a site distal to the dopamine terminals. In support of this concept, Dworkin et al. (1988b) and Zito et al. (1985) used a different neurotoxin in the nucleus accumbens—kainic acid—which selectively destroys the cell perikarya while sparing the terminals or fibers of passage. Such lesions attenuated the reinforcing property of morphine, heroin, and cocaine in self-administration paradigms, suggesting the involvement of a common nucleus accumbens efferent pathway mediating psychostimulant and opiate reward, a topic discussed further in the following section.

AFTER DOPAMINE, WHAT NEXT?

Regardless of its implicated central importance as a site of action for the reinforcing properties of abused drugs, continued consideration of limbic dopamine neurotransmission in isolation is unlikely to further our understanding of the mechanisms of reinforcement to a significant degree. Achieving this goal and ultimately that of elucidating the neurochemical processes leading to addiction will surely require insight into the neurochemical changes induced in associated pathways by repeated drug administration. Such research is in its infancy and perhaps represents an area where microdialysis has the potential to have the most significant impact on the drug abuse field. However, from what is already known of the basic neurochemical circuitry of the basal ganglia and limbic systems, it is clear that such investigations will have to be capable of encompassing neuropeptides. Indeed, subpopulations of mesocorticolimbic dopamine neurons themselves are known to co-localize one or both of two neuropeptides—cholecystokinin (CCK_8) and neurotensin (Hökfelt et al., 1980, 1984; Seroogy et al., 1988). The functional significance of this coexistence has yet to be fully understood, but both of these peptides have been linked to the reinforcement process. Thus, a decrease in self-stimulation rates of the MFB has been described after systemic (De Witte et al., 1985) or intra-accumbens (Vaccarino & Koob, 1984) administration of CCK_8. Similar effects were observed with the CCK analog: BOC-CCK-27-33 (Heidbreder et al., 1989). Conversely, Vaccarino and Vaccarino (1989) demonstrated a facilitation of self-stimulation by the CCK antagonist proglumide when injected into the rostral part of the nucleus accumbens. Preliminary data (Vaccarino et al., 1989) also indicate that intra-accumbens infusion of CCK_8 may attenuate the rewarding properties of cocaine. These data open up the intriguing possibility that increases in the release of the CCK_8 component of the available neurotransmitter repertoire of dopamine neurons may represent part of the neurochemical homeostatic mechanism initiated by repeated psychostimulant administration. The action of this peptide within the accumbens seems to be more complex, however, since facilitatory responses have been reported in caudal parts of this structure (Vaccarino & Vaccarino, 1989). In contrast, neurotensin has been shown to possess reinforcing properties when injected into the VTA (Glimcher et al., 1987), probably reflecting an activation of dopamine neurons (Kalivas et al., 1983).

Surprisingly little is known about changes induced in the endogenous opioid peptide systems themselves after self-administration of abused drugs. Such information may be particularly important considering the implication, alluded to above, that not only opiate alkaloid self-administration but also that of psychostimulants may involve endogenous opioid systems. Evidence for this is provided by the observation that opiate antagonists attenuate the ability of cocaine to decrease the threshold for self-stimulation (Bain & Kornetsky, 1987) and may reduce the rewarding property of cocaine self-administration (Carroll et al., 1986), although this effect is disputed (Ettenberg et al., 1982). More recently, the possible involvement of opioid systems in cocaine reward was suggested by the interesting findings of Hammer (1989) that opiate receptors (measured by ^{3}H-naloxone autoradiography) are upregulated in the nucleus accumbens and ventral pallidum after chronic cocaine administration. Such changes are particularly intriguing in light of the fact that ibotenic acid lesions of the ventral pallidum produce significant decreases in both cocaine and heroin self-administration (Hubner & Koob, 1990). This data, taken together with that showing similar effects after kainic acid lesions of the nucleus accumbens (Dworkin et al., 1988b; Zito et al., 1985), suggest that the nucleus accumbens-ventral pallidal pathway may represent a point of convergence of the neural substrates mediating opiate and psychostimulant reinforcement. Indeed, dopamine terminals in the nucleus accumbens have been shown to make synaptic contact with opioid peptide-containing cells (Sesack & Pickel, 1990), which themselves are believed to project to the ventral pallidum (Zahm et al., 1985). It would clearly be of interest to know whether opioid peptide release is modified during psychostimulant self-administration. Indications that opioid peptidergic systems in the forebrain (more specifically the striatum) are under the control of dopamine arise from studies showing increased pro-enkephalin message production in these regions after the administration of dopamine agonists (Bannon et al., 1989). Similarly, there is little information concerning adaptations of endogenous opioid peptide release during chronic opioid alkaloid administration, which might be important in understanding the mechanisms of opiate tolerance. Sweep et al. (1988, 1989) demonstrated decreases in the total tissue content of beta-endorphin in limbic structures after heroin or cocaine self-administration but, again, such measurements are not readily interpretable in terms of release for the reasons discussed above. To answer these and other questions related to the role of neuropeptide release in the drug abuse process it is necessary to develop the application of in vivo extracellular sampling techniques, such as microdialysis, to neuropeptides.

MONITORING NEUROPEPTIDE RELEASE WITH MICRODIALYSIS

Although microdialysis has become a method of choice for monitoring the extracellular content of dopamine and several other "classical" neurotransmitters in the brain, neuroactive peptides have received much less scrutiny by this promising technique. This is largely due to the insufficient sensitivity offered by the currently available physical techniques for their quantitative analysis, e.g., UV absorbance, fluorescence spectroscopy, mass spectrometry. Immunoassay is therefore the only alternative at this time, but this procedure is generally tedious to carry out and, unless the correct precautions are observed, the specificity of the measurement is subject to a degree of uncertainty. Additional problems are posed by the propensity of many neuropeptides to bind nonspecifically to the polymers used in the fabrication of dialysis membranes, so that recovery of the peptide becomes a major issue. In recent years we have attempted to address these problems while focusing our attention, for the reasons discussed above, on the measurement of endogenous opioids, CCK, and neurotensin in the basal ganglia and limbic system of the rat brain.

The first question we addressed was that of efficiency of recovery of the peptides across the various types of dialysis membrane available. Concentric cannula style microdialysis probes were constructed, and the following types of membrane tested: cellulose (Gambro), cellulose acetate (Cordis Dow), cuprophan (Enka Glanzstoff), polyacrylonitrile (Hospal), and polysulphone (Amicon). These probes were compared with the similarly constructed commercially available polycarbonate variety (CMA/10 Carnegie Medicin) in vitro in the normal way using an unstirred artificial CSF as the medium. Initial experiments used ^{125}I-labeled peptides in the presence of suitable amounts of unlabeled material. Doing so allowed relative recovery to be estimated rapidly using a gamma counter. Subsequently, unlabeled peptide was used alone, which required the use of the radioimmunoassay described below. The results are summarized in Table 16-1. The three most efficient membranes were the cuprophan thin wall, the polyacrylonitrile (PAN), and the polycarbonate used in the Carnegie Medicin probes. The polysulphone membrane was found to be unsuitable for the probe design used since ultrafiltration occurred at flow rates

Table 16-1.   Relative recovery (%) of labeled and unlabeled peptides

Membrane	Mol. wt. cut-off	O.D. (um)	^{125}I-Leu-enk	Leu-enk	^{125}I-CCK$_8$	CCK$_8$	^{125}I-NT	NT
Cellulose	5000	250	3.2	2.4				
Cuprophan	12000	215	5.6	5.1				
Polyacrylonitrile	40000	300	8.0	8.8	4.7	9.2	9.1	12.3
Polycarbonate	20000	500	6.4	5.0	12.0	21.3	10.4	5.7

A comparison of the relative recovery of labeled and unlabeled peptides across several types of membrane. Continuously perfused (2 μl/min) dialysis probes (4 mm active length) were immersed in 5 ml unstirred solutions at room temperature, and samples were collected every 10 or 20 minutes. The amount of material in the dialysate was compared with that measured in an equal volume of the external solution with the result expressed as a percentage. The concentration of peptide in each case was 1 nM. In the radiolabeled experiments approx. 5,000 cpm in 20 μl of tracer peptide was added to the 1 nM solutions.

as low as 1 μl/min. The polycarbonate membrane, although in general giving the highest relative recovery values, also has the largest diameter and thus exhibits a greater surface area for diffusion for a given length of membrane. Carnegie Medicin recently introduced a smaller diameter (200 μm) probe with a polycarbonate membrane that we had not tested at the time of writing. It is worth pointing out that the two methods used—radiolabeled versus unlabeled—were not always in close agreement. For instance, although the polycarbonate membrane was approximately twice as efficient as the PAN membrane at recovering CCK$_8$ regardless of the method used, the absolute percentage recovery values for both membranes were significantly higher for the unlabeled peptide than for the ^{125}I-Boltan-Hunter-labeled peptide. Similarly, unlabeled NT seemed to be recovered less efficiently across polycarbonate membranes when compared to its iodinated counterpart. Clearly, changes in the charge and/or hydrophobicity of a peptide produced by iodination are capable of producing marked changes in its recovery across different membranes. These concerns are, of course, heightened in the case of Boltan-Hunter labeled peptides. Hence, despite the convenience of using the iodinated RIA tracer peptide to assess a peptide's recovery, it would seem pertinent to validify this method for each peptide and for each membrane using unlabeled material (see Maidment et al., 1991a for more details).

Commonly used radioimmunoassay procedures are generally tedious to carry out and usually provide detection limits of the order of 1–10 fmol of peptide. Therefore, in view of the low concentration of neuropeptides in the extracellular environment and their relatively low recovery across the dialysis membrane, it was necessary to make several improvements to the procedure. To this end, in collaboration with Dr. Chris Evans, solid-phase radioimmunoassays were developed whereby the antibody is immobilized on the surface of 96-well Immulon II-coated plates via attachment of the constant region of the immunoglobulin (Ig) molecule to protein A or G. Doing so negates the need for time-consuming procedures for separation of antibody-bound from free tracer peptide (e.g., second antibody precipitation or charcoal absorption) since separation can now be achieved simply by washing the plate. The individual wells containing Ab-bound tracer peptide are then physically separated and counted in a gamma counter. To maximize the sensitivity of the assay, iodinated tracer peptide must be prepared on a regular basis (preferably each month) and must be purified by HPLC. In this way we have achieved IC_{50} values for our peptide assays as low as 1 fmole with limits of detection down to 0.1 fmole. An example of a calibration curve for Met-enkephalin and a diagram of the components of the solid-phase assay are shown in Figure 16-1. The antiserum used in this assay was raised in rabbits using alpha-N-acetyl-alpha-endorphin as the antigen and cross-reacts 100% with the alpha-N-acetylated Tyr.Gly.Gly.Phe.X sequence, thereby recognizing all known active endogenous opioid peptides after chemical acetylation of the sample. For this reason we refer to this assay as a "universal opioid peptide" radioimmunoassay.

In addition to its speed and simplicity, the solid-phase method offers one other important advantage, and that is in the matter of nonspecific binding.

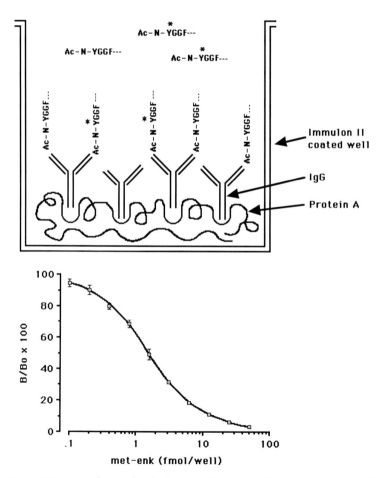

Figure 16-1. Diagram of an individual well of the solid-phase universal opioid peptide assay together with a typical displacement curve for Met-enkephalin after acetylation. Standards were conducted in quadruplet, and each point represents the mean and SEM. (From Robinson, T.E., & Justice, J.B. (eds.). (1991). *Microdialysis in the neurosciences*. New York: Elsevier, with permission.)

Since there is no precipitation/adsorption step during which tracer peptide can become nonspecifically entrapped, nonspecific binding becomes negligible. This characteristic enables the transfer of individual well contents before the final wash (i.e., sample plus iodinated peptide) into wells containing immobilized antibody to a second peptide. In this way it is possible to sequentially assay several peptides in a single biological sample. This is particularly advantageous where the amount of peptide material available is close to the detection limits of the assay so that division of the sample is undesirable. Of course, microdialysis is a prime example of this situation, and we have used this sequential multiple antigen radioimmunoassay technique (SMART) to measure CCK and neurotensin fragments in single dialysis samples collected from rat brain. Full details of the assay procedure are reported elsewhere (Maidment et al., 1991a).

Figure 16-2 demonstrates several features of the releasable immunoreactive material detected with the universal opioid assay in dialysates of the globus

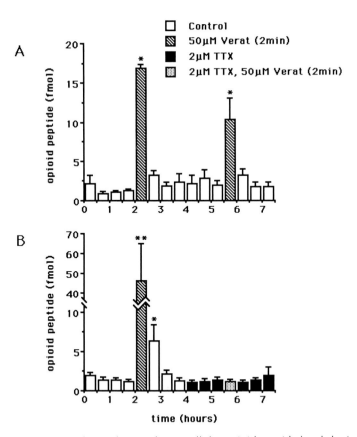

Figure 16-2.   **A,** Repeated stimulation of extracellular opioid peptide levels by incorporation of veratridine (50 μM) in the perfusion medium for 2 minutes of a 30-minute sampling period. Values expressed as in Figure 16-3, n = 4. **B,** Blockade of the second veratridine stimulation by continuous perfusion with tetrodotoxin (2 μM). No significant effect on basal levels was observed (n = 5). (From Maidment et al., 1989, with permission.)

pallidus/ventral pallidum of Halothane-anesthetized rats. First, basal unstimulated extracellular quantities were well within the detection limits of the RIA with 30-minute sampling periods, in the absence of peptidase inhibitors. Second, extracellular levels were greatly increased by incorporation of the voltage-dependent sodium channel activator—veratridine—in the perfusion medium, an effect that was blocked by tetrodotoxin. Similar experiments (Maidment et al., 1989) revealed similar effects with 100 mM K^+, which could be blocked with the calcium ion chelator EGTA. However, it should be noted that neither EGTA nor tetrodotoxin reduced the amount of opioid peptides recovered under basal conditions. The lack of calcium dependence probably reflects the presence of adequate intraneuronal stores for maintaining a low level of vesicular release, with EGTA not being capable of entering the cell. The insensitivity of basal levels to tetrodotoxin suggests that a certain amount of leakage of opioid peptide from neurons (or from extraneuronal compartments) occurs independent of impulse flow. Alternatively, the basal release may be a function of tissue damage inherent in the acute preparation. This question will be resolved by the use of chronic implants. The all-important verification of the identity of the immunoreactivity was achieved by linking the RIA to reverse-phase HPLC, which revealed the expected major contribution of Met- and Leu-enkephalin to the recovered immunoreactivity as shown in Figure 16-3. Full details of this procedure are reported elsewhere (Maidment et al., 1989, 1991a).

Similar preliminary experiments have been carried out to validate the method for measurement of CCK and neurotensin release; these have linked microdialysis in basal forebrain regions to the sequential multiple antigen radioimmunoassay technique detailed above. Recovered amounts of immunoreactivity for both CCK and neurotensin under basal, prestimulus conditions in the medial nucleus accumbens-septum of anesthetized rats were very low (on average approximately 0.3 fmol per 30-minute sample) and were sometimes below detection limits (Fig. 16-4). Similar amounts of CCK immunoreactivity were also recovered from the medial caudate nucleus and medial prefrontal cortex, but no immunoreactive neurotensin was detected in these regions (Maidment et al., 1991a). Significant amounts of material were detected after stimulation with high potassium, and this release was calcium dependent (Fig. 16-4). To have confidence in the RIA measurement, it was necessary to verify the identity of the immunoreactive material by demonstrating co-elution with known standards on rpHPLC. This was not a trivial task due to the low amounts of material recovered (the procedure is described fully in Maidment et al., 1991a). However, it revealed the nature of the CCK immunoreactivity as sulphated CCK_8. The neurotensin immunoreactive material consisted of a mixture of N-terminal fragments (1-8, 1-10 and 1-11) in addition to neurotensin itself (1-13).

Figure 16-4 also demonstrates the large increase in both CCK and NT release occurring immediately postmortem. Similar dramatic increases in the extracellular content of amino acid (Globus et al., 1988), biogenic amine neurotransmitters (Gonzalez-Mora et al., 1989), and opioid peptides (Maidment et al., 1991b) have been reported after terminal or transient ischemia. These findings highlight the problems of using postmortem tissue for studying release

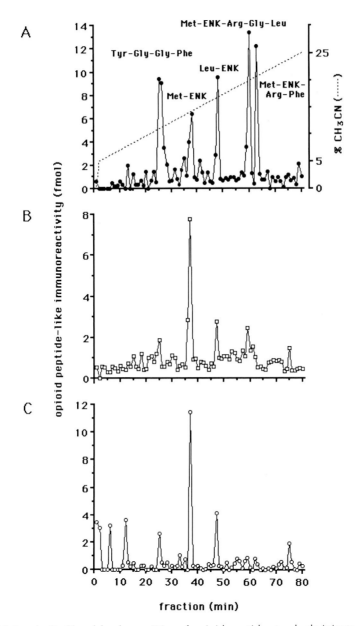

Figure 16-3. **A,** Profile of fmol quantities of opioid peptide standards injected onto reverse-phase HPLC as described in the text and eluted with the acetonitrile gradient shown. Each 10 minute fraction was assayed by RIA. Recovery of injected material was estimated as 80-100%. **B,** Example of an elution profile of baseline release collected from the globus pallidus/ventral pallidum of a single rat over a 10-hour period demonstrating clear peaks coeluting with Met- and Leu-enkephalin together with smaller peaks coinciding with Tyr.Gly.Gly.Phe. and Met-enkephalinArg.Gly.Leu. **C,** Elution profile of opioid peptide immunoreactivity recovered over a 1-hour period of continual stimulation with 100 mM K+-containing artificial CSF showing a similar profile to that under baseline conditions. Small peaks of immunoreactivity were occasionally observed in the first 10-15 fractions, but their precise elution times were not consistent. (From Maidment et al., 1989, with permission.)

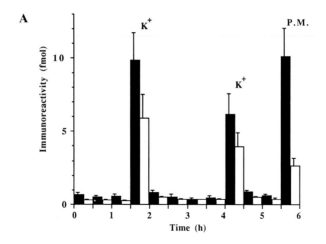

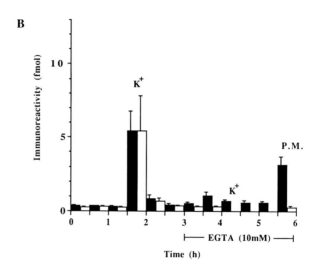

Figure 16-4. **A,** Repeated stimulation of extracellular CCK (*solid bars*) and neurotensin (*open bars*) immunoreactive material recovered from the medial nucleus accumbens/ septum by incorporation of 200 mM potassium in the perfusion fluid for 10 minutes of a 30-minute sampling period and the elevated amounts of such material recovered in the first post mortem sample (P.M.). **B,** A separate series of experiments demonstrating that incorporating EGTA in the perfusion medium prevents the second stimulation of both CCK and neurotensin immunoreactive material and attenuates the post mortem (P.M.) increases. (From Maidment et al., 1991a, with permission.)

processes since not only will the releasable pool be depleted severely but also it is likely that the exposure of receptors to unusually high concentrations of neurotransmitters at the time of sacrifice will have consequences for their subsequent function in vitro.

SUMMARY

Although drugs that are abused by humans fall into several pharmacological categories and therefore must act initially at different receptor sites in the brain, it is nevertheless possible to envisage a core circuitry mediating the reinforcement properties of all such drugs, with different drugs feeding into the system at separate loci. The mesolimbic dopamine system has been proposed as a prime candidate for being part of such a system on the basis of the evidence reviewed above. It is now necessary to direct research efforts into elucidating the remaining parts of this neurochemical circuitry if we are to further our understanding of the reinforcement process and ultimately the mechanisms of drug addiction. We are beginning to gain insight into the changes in receptor and second-messenger regulatory processes induced by repeated drug administration (see Chapters 2 and 3), and it is logical to propose that such adaptive changes, in addition to being responsible for the development of tolerance, are also involved in the phenomenon of dependence. That is, on withdrawal of the drug the system is in an overcompensated state, which results in adverse physical or mood symptoms. However, it is perhaps somewhat naive to consider these adaptive processes in the primary affected cells as solely responsible for the production of a rebound over compensation response on drug withdrawal leading to the inducement for continued drug administration. Thus, a second, "between-systems" explanation has been proposed whereby the adaptation to the drug takes the form of compensatory changes in other neuronal circuits. Although the activation of mesolimbic dopamine may be central to the development of initial repeated drug-seeking behavior and is the primary site for generation of pleasurable effects, it is quite likely that once repeated administration is established, neuronal mechanisms distal to the dopamine system that undergo plastic changes as a result of dopamine bombardment, become the important substrates for mediation of anhedonia associated with withdrawal and contribute strongly to relapse into continued drug use. An understanding of these phenomena and the neurochemical circuitry involved could prove valuable in developing medications useful in the treatment of addiction.

Microdialysis is a powerful technique that is becoming widely used for monitoring a growing number of neuroactive substances in the brain extracellular environment. As such, it is already making significant contributions to this area. However, the realization of its full potential in the area of drug abuse will require the development of its application to neuropeptides. Our preliminary results demonstrate the general feasibility of such an approach while emphasizing the requirement for still further increments in the sensitivities of peptide assay technologies, as the levels measured in the dialysates are some 100 to 1000 times less than those of, for instance, dopamine. Thus, although we have been able to reliably measure basal extracellular levels of met- and leu-enkephalin in the basal ganglia, the measurement of CCK_8 and neurotensin is less satisfactory. Basal amounts of these peptides seem to be close to the limit of detection, so that depolarizing stimuli are required to obtain reliable signals at present. It will also be necessary to establish the feasibility of measuring these low amounts of material over extended periods of time in the freely moving animal. Doing so will likely require the employment of chronic guide cannula and replacable dialysis probes as has been done for dopamine (see Chapter 24).

ACKNOWLEDGMENTS

We would like to thank Brenda Siddall, Elizabeth Erdelyi, and Daniel Brumbaugh for their excellent technical advice and assistance in the execution of the neuropeptide dialysis studies. We also thank Dr. Jack D. Barchas for his constant support and encouragement. The gift of neurotensin antibody from Dr. Geoff Bennett is gratefully acknowledged.

REFERENCES

Adams, R.N., & Justice, J.B. (Eds.). (1987). *Voltammetry in the neurosciences: Principles, methods and applications*. Clifton, NJ: Humana Press.

Adams, W.J., Lorens, S.A., & Mitchell, C.L. (1972). Morphine enhances lateral hypothalamic self-stimulation in the rat. *Proc. Soc. Exp. Biol.*,

Bain, G.T., & Kornetsky, C. (1987). Naloxone attenuation of the effect of cocaine on rewarding brain stimulation. *Life Sci., 40*, 1119-1125.

Bannon, M.J., Kelland, M., & Chiodo, L.A. (1989). Medial forebrain bundle stimulation or D_2 dopamine receptor activation increase preproenkephalin mRNA in rat striatum. *J. Neurochem., 52*, 859-862.

Bielajew, C., & Shizgal, P. (1986). Evidence implicating descending fibers in self-stimulation of the medial forebrain bundle. *J. Neurosci., 6*, 919-929.

Bozarth, M.A., & Wise, R.A. (1981). Intracranial self-administration of morphine into the ventral tegmental area in rats. *Life Sci., 28*, 551-555.

Bozarth, M.A., & Wise, R.A. (1985). Involvement of the ventral tegmental dopamine system in opioid and psychomotor stimulant reinforcement. *NIDA Res. Monogr., 67*, 190-196.

Britt, M.D., & Wise, R.A. (1983). Ventral tegmental site of opiate reward: Antagonism by a hydrophillic opiate receptor blocker. *Brain Res., 258*, 105-108.

Broekkamp, C.L.E., & Van Rossum, J.M. (1975). The effect of microinjections of morphine and haloperidol into the neostriatum and the nucleus accumbens on self-stimulation behaviour. *Arch. Int. Pharmacodyn., 217*, 110-117.

Broekkamp, C.L.E., Pijneburg, A.J.J., Cools, A.R., & Van Rossum, J.M. (1975). The effect of microinjections of amphetamine into the neostriatum and the nucleus accumbens on self-stimulation behavior. *Psychopharmacologia, 42*, 179-183.

Broekkamp, C.L.E., Van Den Boggard, J.H., Heijnen, H.J., Rops, R.H., Cools, A.R., & Van Rossum, J.M. (1976). Separation of inhibiting and stimulating effects of morphine on self-stimulation behavior by intracerebral microinjections. *Eur. J. Pharmacol., 36*, 443-446.

Broekkamp, C.L., Phillips, A.G., & Cools, A.R. (1979). Facilitation of self-stimulation behavior following intracerebral microinjections of opioids into the ventral tegmental area. *Pharmacol. Biochem. Behav., 11*, 289-295.

Carboni, E., Imperato, A., Perezzani, L., & Di Chiara, G. (1989). Amphetamine, cocaine, phencyclidine and nomifensine increase extracellular dopamine concentrations preferentially in the nucleus accumbens of freely moving rats. *Neuroscience, 28,* 653-661.

Carr, L.A., & Moore, K.E. (1969). Norepinephrine: Release from brain by d-amphetamine in vivo. *Science, 164,* 322-323.

Carroll, M.E., Lac, S.T., Walker, M.J., Kragh, R., & Newman, T. (1986). Effects of naltrexone on intravenous cocaine self-administration in rats during food satiation and deprivation. *J. Pharmacol. Exp. Ther., 238,* 1-7.

Clarke, P.B.S., & Kumar, R. (1984). Effects of nicotine and d-amphetamine on intracranial self-stimulation in a shuttle box test in rats. *Psychopharmacology, 84,* 109-114.

Corbett, D., & Wise, R.A. (1980). Intracranial self-stimulation in relation to the ascending dopaminergic systems of the midbrain: A moveable electrode mapping study. *Brain Res., 185,* 1-15.

Crow, T.J. (1970). Enhancement by cocaine of intra-cranial self-stimulation in the rat. *Life Sci., 9,* 375-381.

Crow, T.J. (1972). Catecholamine-containing neurones and electrical self-stimulation. 1. A review of some data. *Psychol. Med., 2,* 414-421.

Davis, W.H., & Smith, S.G. (1973). Blocking effect of alpha-methyltyrosine on amphetamine based reinforcement. *J. Pharmacol. Pharmac., 25,* 174-177.

Davis, W.H., & Smith, S.G. (1975). Effect of haloperidol on (+)-amphetamine self-administration. *J. Pharmacol. Pharmac., 27,* 540-542.

De Wit, H., & Wise, R.S. (1977). Blockade of cocaine reinforcement in rats with the dopamine receptor blocker pimozide, but not with the noradrenergic blockers phentolamine and phenoxybenzamine. *Can. J. Psychol., 31,* 195-203.

De Witte, P., & Bada, M.F. (1983). Self-stimulation and alcohol administered orally or intraperitoneally. *Exp. Neurol., 82,* 675-682.

De Witte, P.H., Swanet, E., Gewiss, M., Goldman, S., Roques, B.P., & Vanderhaegen, J.J. (1985). Psychopharmacological profile of cholecystokinin using the self-stimulation and the drug discrimination paradigms. *Ann. N.Y. Acad. Sci., 448,* 470-487.

Di Chiara, G., & Imperato, A. (1988). Drugs of abuse preferentially stimulate dopamine release in the mesolimbic system of freely moving rats. *Proc. Natl. Acad. Sci. USA., 85,* 5274-5278.

Downs, A.W., & Eddy, N.B. (1932). The effect of repeated doses of cocaine on the rat. *J. Pharmacol. Exp. Ther., 46,* 199-202.

Dworkin, S.I., Guerin, G.F., Co, C., Goeders, N.E., & Smith, J.E. (1988a). Lack of an effect of 6-hydroxydopamine lesions of the nucleus accumbens on intravenous morphine self-administration. *Pharmacol. Biochem. Behav., 30,* 1051-1057.

Dworkin, S.I., Guerin, G.F., Goeders, N.E., & Smith, J.E. (1988b). Kainic acid lesions of the nucleus accumbens selectively attenuate morphine self-administration. *Pharmacol. Biochem. Behav., 29,* 175-181.

Ettenberg, A. (1989). Dopamine, neuroleptics and reinforced behavior. *Neurosci. Biobehav. Rev., 13,* 105-111.

Ettenberg, A., Pettit, H.O., Bloom, F.E., & Koob, G.F. (1982). Heroin and cocaine intravenous self-administration in rats: Mediation by separate neural systems. *Psychopharmacology, 78,* 204-209.

Fibiger, H.C. (1978). Drugs and reinforcement: A critical review of the catecholamine theory. *Annu. Rev. Pharmacol. Toxicol., 18,* 37-56.

Fibiger, H.C., & Phillips, A.G. (1986). Reward, motivation, cognition: Psychobiology of mesotelencephalic dopamine systems. In F.E. Bloom & S.R. Geiger (Eds.),

Handbook of physiology: The nervous system IV, (pp. 647-675). Bethesda, MD: American Physiological Society.

Fibiger, H.C., Lepiane, F.G., Jakubovic, A., & Phillips, A.G. (1987). The role of dopamine in intracranial self-stimulation of the ventral tegmental area. *J. Neurosci., 7*, 3888-3896.

Glimcher, P.W., Giovino, A.A., & Hoebel, B.G. (1987). Neurotensin self-injection in the ventral tegmental area. *Brain Res., 403*, 147-150.

Globus, M.Y.T., Busto, R., Dietrich, W.D., Martinez, E., Valdes, I., & Ginsberg, M.D. (1988). Effect of ischemia on the in vivo release of striatal dopamine, glutamate and gamma-aminobutyric acid studied by microdialysis. *J. Neurochem., 51*, 1455-1464.

Goeders, N.E., & Smith, J.E. (1983). Cortical dopaminergic involvement in cocaine reinforcement. *Science, 221*, 773-775.

Goeders, N.E., & Smith, J.E. (1986). Reinforcing properties of cocaine in the medial prefrontal cortex: Primary action on presynaptic dopaminergic terminals. *Pharmacol. Biochem. Behav., 25*, 191-199.

Goeders, N.E., Lane, J.D., & Smith, J.E. (1984). Self-administration of methionine enkephalin into the nucleus accumbens. *Pharmacol. Biochem. Behav., 20*, 451-455.

Gonon, F.G., & Buda, M.J. (1985). Regulation of dopamine release by impulse flow and by autoreceptors as studied by in vivo voltammetry in the rat striatum. *Neuroscience, 14*, 765-774.

Gonzales-Mora, J.L., Maidment, N.T., Guadalupe, T., & Mas, M. (1989). Post-mortem dopamine dynamics assessed by voltammetry and microdialysis. *Brain Res. Bull., 23*, 323-327.

Gratton, A., Hoffer, B.J., & Gerhardt, G.A. (1988). Effects of electrical stimulation of brain reward sites on release of dopamine in rat: An in vivo electrochemical study. *Brain Res. Bull., 21*, 319-324.

Hammer, R.P. (1989). Cocaine alters opiate receptor binding in critical brain reward regions. *Synapse, 3*, 55-60.

Heidbreder, C., Roques, B.P., & De Witte, P. (1989). Similar potencies of CCK_8 and its analogue BOC(Nle28;Nle31) CCK27-33 on the self-stimulation behavior: Both are antagonized by a newly synthesized cyclic CCK analogue. *Neuropeptides, 13*, 89-94.

Heikkila, R.E., Orlansky, H., & Cohen, G. (1975). Studies on the distinction between uptake inhibition and release of 3H-dopamine in rat brain tissue slices. *Biochem. Pharmacol., 24*, 847-852.

Hoebel, B.G., Monaco, A., Hernandes, L., Aulisi, E., Stanley, B.G., & Lenard, L. (1983). Self-injection of amphetamine directly into the brain. *Psychopharmacology, 81*, 158-163.

Hökfelt, T., Skirboll, L., Rehfeld, J.F., Goldstein, M., Markey, K., & Dann, O. (1980). A subpopulation of mesencephalic dopamine neurons projecting to limbic areas contain a cholecystokinin-like peptide: Evidence from immunohistochemistry combined with retrograde tracing. *Neuroscience, 5*, 2093-2124.

Hökfelt, T., Everitt, B.J., Theodorsson-Norheim, E., & Goldstein, M. (1984). Occurrence of neurotensinlike immunoreactivity in subpopulations of hypothalamic, mesencephalic and medullary catecholamine neurons. *J. Comp. Neurol., 22*, 543-559.

Holmes, L.J., Bozarth, M.A., & Wise, R.A. (1983). Circling from intracranial morphine applied to the ventral tegmental area in rats. *Brain Res. Bull., 11*, 295-298.

Hu, X.T., & Wang, R.Y. (1984). Comparison of morphine-induced effects on dopamine and non-dopamine neurons in the rat ventral tegmental area. *Soc. Neurosci. Abst., 10,* 66.

Hubner, C.B., & Koob, G.F. (1990). The ventral pallidum plays a role in mediating cocaine and heroin self-administration in the rat. *Brain Res., 508,* 20-29.

Hurd, Y., Weiss, F., Koob, G., Erik, N., & Ungerstedt, U. (1989). Cocaine reinforcement and extracellular dopamine overflow in rat nucleus accumbens: An in vivo microdialysis study. *Brain Res., 498,* 199-203.

Hurd, Y., Weiss, F., Koob, G., & Ungerstedt, U. (1990). The influence of cocaine self-administration on in vivo dopamine and acetylcholine neurotransmission in rat caudate-putamen. *Neurosci. Lett., 109,* 227-233.

Imperato, A., & Di Chiara, G. (1984). Trans-striatal dialysis coupled to reverse phase high performance liquid chromatography with electrochemical detection: A new method for the study of the in vivo release of endogenous dopamine and metabolites. *J. Neurosci., 4,* 966-967.

Jacobs, H.L., & Sharma, K.N. (1969). Taste versus calories: Sensory and metabolic signals in the control of food intake. *Ann. N. Y. Acad. Sci., 157,* 1084-1125.

Jonsson, L.E., Anggard, E., & Gunne, L.M. (1971). Blockade of intravenous amphetamine euphoria in man. *Clin. Pharmacol. Ther., 12,* 889-896.

Joseph, M.H., Fillenz, M., MacDonald, I.A., & Marsden, C.A. (Eds.). (1986). Monitoring neurotransmitter release during behavior. Chichester (England): *Ellis Horwood Health Science Series. Ltd.*

Joyce, E.M., & Iversen, S.D. (1979). The effect of morphine applied locally to mesencephalic dopamine cell bodies on spontaneous motor activity in the rat. *Neurosci. Lett., 14,* 207-212.

Kalivas, P., & Duffy, P. (1990). Effect of acute and daily cocaine treatment on extracellular dopamine in the nucleus accumbens. *Synapse, 5,* 48-58.

Kalivas, P.W., Widerlov, E., Stanley, D., Breese, G., & Prange, A.J. (1983). Enkephalin action on the mesolimbic system: A dopamine-dependent and a dopamine-dependent increase in locomotor activity. *J. Pharmacol. Exp. Ther., 227,* 229-237.

Kalivas, P.W., Duffy, P., Dumars, L.A., & Skinner, C. (1988). Behavioral and neurochemical effects of acute and daily cocaine administration in rats. *J. Pharmacol. Exp. Ther., 245,* 485-492.

Kilby, M.M., & Ellinwood, E.H. (1977). Reverse tolerance to stimulant-induced abnormal behavior. *Life Sci., 20,* 1063-1076.

Kilty, J.E., Lorang, D., & Amara, S.G. (1991). Cloning and expression of a cocaine-sensitive rat dopamine transporter. *Science, 254,* 578-579.

Lin-Chu, G., Robinson, T.E., & Becker, J.B. (1985). Sensitization of rotational behavior produced by a single exposure to cocaine. *Pharmacol. Biochem. Behav., 22,* 901-903.

Lorens, S.A., & Sainati, S.M. (1978). Naloxone blocks the excitatory effect of ethanol and chlordiazepoxide on lateral hypothalamic self-stimulation in the rat. *Life Sci., 23,* 1359-1363.

Lyness, W.H., Friedle, N.M., & Moore, K.E. (1979). Destruction of dopaminergic nerve terminals in nucleus accumbens: Effect on amphetamine self-administration. *Pharmacol. Biochem. Behav., 11,* 553-556.

Maidment, N.T., Brumbaugh, D.R., Rudolph, V.D., Erdelyi, E., & Evans, C. (1989). Microdialysis of extracellular endogenous opioid peptides from rat brain in vivo. *Neuroscience, 33,* 549-557.

Maidment, N.T., Siddall, B.J., Rudolph, V.R., Erdelyi, E., & Evans, C. (1991a). Dual determination of extracellular cholecystokinin and neurotensin fragments in rat forebrain: Microdialysis combined with a sequential multiple antigen radioimmunoassay. *Neuroscience, 45,* 81-93.

Maidment, N.T., Siddall, B., Rudolph, V.D., & Evans, C.J. (1991b). Post-mortem changes in rat brain extracellular opioid peptides revealed by microdialysis. *J. Neurochem., 56,* 1980-1984.

Maisonneuve, I., Keller, R., & Glick, S. (1990). Similar effects of d-amphetamine and cocaine on extracellular dopamine levels in medial prefrontal cortex of rats. *Brain Res., 535,* 221-226.

Marsden, C.A. (Ed.). (1984). *Measurement of neurotransmitter release in vivo.* New York: John Wiley & Sons Ltd.

Marsden, C.A., Joseph, M.H., Kruk, Z.L., Maidment, N.T., O'Neill, R.D., Schenk, J.O., & Stamford, J.A. (1988). In vivo voltammetry-Present electrodes and methods. *Neuroscience, 25,* 389-400.

Matthews, R.T., & German, D.C. (1984). Electrophysiological evidence for excitation of rat ventral tegmental area dopaminergic neurons by morphine. *Neuroscience, 11,* 617-626.

Mogenson, G.J. (1964). Effects of sodium pentobarbital on brain self-stimulation. *J. Comp. Physiol. Psychol., 58,* 461-462.

Mogenson, G.J., Takigawa, M., Robertson, A., & Wu, M. (1979). Self-stimulation of the nucleus accumbens and ventral tegmental area of Tsai attenuated by microinjections of spiroperidol into the nucleus accumbens. *Brain Res., 171,* 247-259.

Mora, F., Myers, R.D., & Sanguinetti, A.M. (1977). Self-stimulation of the MFB or VTA after microinjection of haloperidol into the prefrontal cortex of the rat. *Pharmacol. Biochem. Behav., 6,* 239-241.

Nakahara, D., Ozaki, N., Kapoor, V., & Nagatsu, T. (1989). The effect of uptake inhibition on dopamine release from the nucleus accumbens of rats during self- or forced stimulation of the medial forebrain bundle: A microdialysis study. *Neurosci. Lett., 104,* 136-140.

Olds, J. (1966). Facilitatory action of diazepam and chlordiazepoxide on hypothalamic reward behavior. *J. Comp. Physiol. Psychol., 62,* 136-140.

Olds, M.E. (1982). Reinforcing effects of morphine in the nucleus accumbens. *Brain Res., 237,* 429-440.

Pert, A., & Sivit, C. (1977). Neuroanatomical focus for morphine and enkephalin-induced hypermotility. *Nature, 265,* 645-647.

Pettit, H.O., & Justice, J.B. (1989). Dopamine in the nucleus accumbens during cocaine self-administration as studied by in vivo microdialysis. *Pharmacol. Biochem. Behav., 34,* 899-904.

Pettit, H.O., Ettenberg, A., Bloom, F.E., & Koob, G.F. (1984). Destruction of dopamine in the nucleus accumbens selectively attenuates cocaine but not heroin self-administration in rats. *Psychopharmacology, 84,* 167-173.

Pettit, H.O., Pan, H.T., Parsons, L.H., & Justice, J.B. (1990). Extracellular concentrations of cocaine and dopamine are enhanced during chronic cocaine administration. *J. Neurochem., 55,* 798-804.

Phillips, A.G., & Fibiger, H.C. (1978). The role of dopamine in maintaining intracranial self-stimulation in the ventral tegmentum, nucleus accumbens, and medial prefrontal cortex. *Can. J. Physiol., 32,* 58-66.

Phillips, A.G., & Lepiane, F.G. (1980). Reinforcing effects of morphine microinjection into the ventral tegmental area. *Pharmacol. Biochem. Behav., 12,* 965-968.

Phillips, A.G., & Lepiane, F.G. (1982). Reward produced by microinjection of (d-ala)-met enkephalinamide into the ventral tegmental area. *Behav. Brain Res., 5,* 225-229.

Phillips, A.G., Mora, F., & Rolls, E.T. (1981). Intracerebral self-administration of amphetamine by rhesus monkeys. *Neurosci. Lett.*, *24*, 81-86.

Phillips, A.G., Broekkamp, C.L.E., & Fibiger, H.C. (1983). Strategies for studying the neurochemical substrates of drug reinforcement in rodents. *Prog. Neuro-Psychopharmacol. Biol. Psychiat.*, *7*, 585-590.

Phillips, A.G., Blaha, C.D., & Fibiger, H.C. (1989). Neurochemical correlates of brain-stimulation reward measured by ex vivo and in vivo analyses. *Neurosci. Biobehav. Rev.*, *13*, 99-104.

Pickens, R., & Thompson, T. (1968). Cocaine-reinforced behavior in rats: Effects of reinforcement magnitude and fixed-ratio size. *J. Pharmacol. Exp. Ther.*, *161*, 122-129.

Pickens, R., Meisch, R.A., & Dougherty, J.A. (1968). Chemical interactions in metamphetamine reinforcement. *Psychol. Rep.*, *23*, 1267-1270.

Post, R.M., Weiss, S.R.B., Pert, A., & Uhde, T.W. (1987). Chronic cocaine administration: Sensitization and kindling effects. In S. Fisher, A. Raskin, & E.H. Uhlenhuth (Eds.), *Cocaine: Clinical and biobehavioral aspects* (pp. 109-173). New York: Oxford University Press.

Pulvirenti, L., & Koob, G. (1990). The neural substrates of drug addiction and dependence. *Funct. Neurol.*, *5*, 109-116.

Risner, M.E., & Jones, B.E. (1976). Role of noradrenergic and dopaminergic processes in amphetamine self-administration. *Pharmacol: Biochem. Behav.*, *5*, 477-482.

Risner, M.E., & Jones, B.E. (1980). Intravenous self-administration of cocaine and norcocaine by dogs. *Psychopharmacology*, *71*, 83-89.

Roberts, D.C.S., & Koob, G.F. (1982). Disruption of cocaine self-administration following 6-hydroxydopamine lesions of the ventral tegmental area in rats. *Pharmacol. Biochem. Behav.*, *17*, 901-904.

Roberts, D.C.S., Corcoran, M.E., & Fibiger, H.C. (1977). On the role of ascending catecholaminergic systems in intravenous self-administration of cocaine. *Pharmacol. Biochem. Behav.*, *6*, 615-620.

Robinson, T.E., & Justice, J.B. (Eds.). (1991). *Microdialysis in the neurosciences. Techniques in the behavioral and neural sciences*, New York: Elsevier Science Publishers.

Rothman, R.B., McLean, S., Bykov, V., Lessor, R.A., Jacobson, A.E., Rice, K.C., & Holaday, J.W. (1987). Chronic morphine upregulates a mu-opiate binding site labeled by 3(H)cycloFOXY: A novel opiate antagonist suitable for positron emission tomography. *Eur. J. Pharmacol.*, *142*, 73-81.

Routtenberg, A. (1964). Self-starvation caused by "feeding-center" stimulation. *Am. Psychol.*, *19*, 502-507.

Routtenberg, A., & Malsbury, C. (1969). Brainstem pathways of reward. *J. Comp. Physiol. Psychol.*, *68*, 22-30.

Schwartz, A.S., & Marchok, P.L. (1974). Depression of morphine-seeking behavior by dopamine inhibition. *Nature* (Lond), *248*, 257-258.

Seroogy, K.B., Ceccatelli, S., Schalling, M., & Hökfelt, T. (1988). A subpopulation of dopaminergic neurons in the rat ventral mesencephalon contains both neurotensin and cholecystokinin. *Brain Res.*, *455*, 88-98.

Sesack, S.R., & Pickel, V.M. (1990). Ultrastructural evidence for interactions between opioid and dopaminergic neurons in the rat mesolimbic system. In J.M. Van Ree, et al. (Eds.), *New leads in opioid research* (pp. 241-243). Amsterdam: Exerpta Medica.

Sharp, T., Zetterstrom, T., Ljungberg, T., & Ungerstedt, U. (1987). A direct comparison of amphetamine-induced behaviors and regional brain dopamine release in the rat using intracerebral dialysis. *Brain Res., 401,* 322-330.

Sherman, J.E., Pickman, C., Rice, A., Libeskind, J.C., & Holman, E.W. (1980). Rewarding and aversive effects of morphine: Temporal and pharmacological properties. *Pharmacol. Biochem. Behav., 13,* 501-505.

Shimada, S., Kitoyama, S., Lin, C.L., Patel, A., Nanthakumar, E., Gregor, P., Kuhar, M., & Uhl, G. (1991). Cloning and expression of a cocaine-sensitive dopamine transporter complementary DNA. *Science, 254,* 576-578.

Simon, H., Stinus, L., Tassin, J.P., Lavielle, S., Blanc, G., Thierry, A.M., Glowinski, J., & Le Moal, M. (1979). Is the dopaminergic mesocorticolimbic system necessary for intracranial self-stimulation? Biochemical and behavioral studies from A10 cell bodies and terminals. *Behav. Neural. Biol., 27,* 125-145.

Stamford, J.A., Kruk, Z.L., & Millar, J. (1986). In vivo voltammetric characterization of low affinity striatal dopamine uptake: Drug inhibition profile and relation to dopaminergic innervation density. *Brain Res., 373,* 85-91.

Stein, L. (1964). Self-stimulation of the brain and the central stimulant action of amphetamine. *Fed. Proc., 23,* 836-850.

Stein, L., & Ray, O.S. (1960). Brain stimulation reward "thresholds" self-determined in rat. *Psychopharmacology, 1,* 251-256.

Stellar, J.R., & Corbett, D. (1989). Regional neuroleptic microinjections indicate a role for nucleus accumbens in lateral hypothalamic self-stimulation reward. *Brain Res., 477,* 126-143.

Sulzer, D., Maidment, N.T., & Rayport, S. (1991). Reverse action of the plasma membrane transporter mediates weak base-induced dopamine release: Implications for amphetamine action. *Soc. Neurosci. Abstr., 17,* 1552.

Sulzer, D., Maidment, N.T., & Rayport, S. (1993). Amphetamine and other weak bases act to promote reverse transport of dopamine in ventral midbrain neurons. *J. Neurochem.* (in press).

Sulzer, D., Pathos, E., Sung, H.M., Maidment, N.T., Hoebel, B.G., & Rayport, S. (1992). Weak base model of amphetamine action. *Annal. N.Y. Acad. Sci., 654,* 525-528.

Sweep, C.G.J., Van Ree, J.M., & Wiegant, V.M. (1988). Characterization of b-endorphin-immunoreactivity in limbic brain structures of rats self-administering heroin or cocaine. *Neuropeptides, 12,* 229-236.

Sweep, C.G.J., Wiegant, V.M., & De Vry, J. (1989). B-endorphin in brain limbic structures as neurochemical correlate of psychic dependence on drugs. *Life Sci., 44,* 1133-1140.

Swerdlow, N.R., Amalric, M., & Koob, G.F. (1987). Nucleus accumbens opiate dopamine interactions and locomotor activation in the rat: Evidence for a presynaptic locus. *Pharmacol. Biochem. Rehav., 26,* 765-769.

Tatum, A.L., & Seevers, M.H. (1929). Experimental cocaine addiction. *J. Pharmacol. Exp. Ther., 36,* 401-410.

Vaccarino, F.J., & Koob, G.F. (1984). Microinjections of nanogram amounts of sulfated cholecystokinin octapeptide into the rat nucleus accumbens attenuates brain stimulation reward. *Neurosci. Lett., 52,* 61-66.

Vaccarino, F.J., & Vaccarino, A.L. (1989). Antagonism of cholecystokinin function in the rostral and caudal nucleus accumbens: Differential effects on brain stimulation reward. *Neurosci. Lett., 97,* 151-156.

Vaccarino, F.J., Bloom, F.E., & Koob, G.F. (1985). Blockade of nucleus accumbens opiate receptors attenuates intravenous heroin reward in the rat. *Psychopharmacology, 86,* 37-42.

Vaccarino, F.J., Weiss, F., & Koob, G.F. (1989). Neuroleptic-like effect of intra-accumbens cholecystokinin on I.V. cocaine self-administration. *Soc. Neurosci. Abst., 15*, 1097.

Van Rossum, J.M., Van Der Schoot, J.B., & Hurkmans, J.A.T.M. (1962). Mechanisms of action of cocaine and amphetamine in the brain. *Experentia, 18*, 229-231.

Wauquier, A., & Niemegeers, C.J.E. (1974). Intracranial self-stimulation in rats as a function of various stimulation parameters. V. Influence of cocaine on medial forebrain bundle stimulation with monopolar electrodes. *Psychopharmacologia, 38*, 201-210.

Weber, E., Truscott, R.J., Evans, C., Sullivan, S., Angwin, P., & Barchas, J.D. (1981). N-acetyl beta-endorphins in the pituitary: Immunohistochemical localisation using antibodies raised against dynorphin(1-13). *J. Neurochem., 36*, 1977-1985.

Wise, C.D., & Stein, L. (1970). Amphetamine: Facilitation of behavior by augmented release of norepinephrine from the medial forebrain bundle. In E. Costa & S. Gariattini (Eds.), (pp. 463-485). *Amphetamine and related compounds*. New York: Raven Press.

Wise, R.A. (1978). Neuroleptic attenuation of intracranial self-stimulation: Reward or performance deficits? *Life Sci., 22*, 535-542.

Wise, R.A. (1981). Intracranial self-stimulation: Mapping against the lateral boundaries of the dopaminergic cells of the substantia nigra. *Brain Res., 213*, 190-194.

Wise, R.A. (1987). The role of reward pathways in the development of drug dependence. *Pharmacol. Ther., 35*, 227-263.

Yeomans, J.S. (1989). Two substrates for medial forebrain bundle self-stimulation: Myelinated axons and dopamine axons. *Neurosci. Biobehav. Rev., 13*, 91-98.

Yeomans, J.S., Maidment, N.T., & Bunney, B.S. (1988). Excitability properties of medial forebrain bundle axons of A9 and A10 dopamine cells. *Brain Res., 450*, 86-93.

Yokel, R.A., & Wise, R.A. (1975). Increased lever pressing for amphetamine after pimozide in rats: Implications for a dopamine theory of reward. *Science, 187*, 547-549.

Yokel, R.A., & Wise, R.A. (1976). Attenuation of intravenous amphetamine reinforcement by central dopamine blockade in rats. *Psychopharmacology, 48*, 311-318.

Zahm, D.S., Zaborsky, L., Alones, V.E., & Heimer, L. (1985). Evidence for the coexistence of glutamate decarboxylase and met-enkephalin immunoreactivities in axon terminals of the ventral pallidum. *Brain Res., 325*, 317-321.

Zito, K.A., Vickers, G., & Roberts, D.C.S. (1985). Disruption of cocaine and heroin self-administration following kainic acid lesions of the nucleus accumbens. *Pharmacol. Biochem. Behav., 23*, 1029-1036.

17

Mammalian Morphine Alkaloids: Identification and Possible In Vivo Biosynthesis

KYM F. FAULL

Opium, the dried powdered exudate from incised unripe fruiting bodies of the Asian poppy, is legendary for its antidiarrhetic, euphoric, addictive, and analgesic qualities. Although the commonly held image of the opium den has an oriental connotation, the earliest known descriptions of opium collection appear in 7th-century B.C. Assyrian tablets, and the first recorded medicinal use is thought to be Sumerian (300-400 B.C.), probably for the treatment of diarrhea (Terry & Pellens, 1928). Morphine is the chief active ingredient of opium and comprises 10 to 16% of the natural product by weight. Although there is illicit use of morphine, heroin poses a more serious substance abuse problem (Chein et al., 1964; Goldstein & Kalant, 1990). Heroin is the manmade di-acetyl derivative of morphine that was first synthesized in 1874 (Wright, 1874) and introduced into clinical medicine in 1898 (cited from Eddy & May, 1983). The superior potency and greater addictive liability of heroin stem from its improved lipid solubility and the relative ease with which it passes through the blood-brain barrier. Once inside the CNS, heroin is converted to monoacetylmorphine and morphine, which are responsible for its CNS effects.

Opium also contains a variety of other alkaloids, including codeine and thebaine, which are morphine biosynthetic precursors in the poppy and variably comprise up to 3% by weight of opium. Historically morphine and its relatives were thought to occur naturally in only a few species of the genus *Papaver* (Asian poppy), most notably *P. somniferum* and *P. album*. However, a convincing body of recent evidence showing that these alkaloids (collectively referred to here as morphinans) occur naturally in mammals has culminated in the identification of morphine, 6-acetylmorphine, codeine, and thebaine in extracts of mammalian brain. It has also been shown that mammals are capable of carrying out some of the same steps in morphine biosynthesis as the opium

This work was supported by a NIDA grant (DA 0510).

poppy, including the complex conversion of reticuline to salutaridine, which generates the characteristic ring structure and stereochemistry of the morphinan alkaloids. These results challenge the dogma that these alkaloids occur naturally only in the plant kingdom and invite speculation that mammals biosynthesize these compounds. This in turn has led to the suggestion that endogenous morphine alkaloids have a physiological function in mammals. However, additional information is needed before this hypothesis can be accepted. This chapter reviews the recent findings that have renewed interest in this field.

ENDOGENOUS OPIOID SYSTEMS

The demonstration of stereoselective binding sites for narcotic drugs in membrane preparations from brain tissue homogenates (Goldstein et al., 1971; Pert & Snyder, 1973; Simon et al., 1973; Terenius, 1973) revealed the inherent specificity of the recognition sites and led directly to a search for the endogenous mammalian ligand(s). The result was the discovery of the first opioid peptides, the enkephalin pentapeptides, in mammalian brain by Hughes et al. (1975). Some 20 peptides with opioid activity have now been purified from mammalian tissues and sequenced. These are all carboxy-terminal extensions of methionine- and leucine-enkephalin (Akil et al., 1984; Douglass et al., 1984; Evans et al., 1988; Weber et al., 1983), the sequences of which are contained within three precursor molecules—proopiomelanocortin, proenkephalin, and prodynorphin. These precursor molecules undergo differential and tissue-specific post-translational processing to yield a variety of biologically active products with distinct but often overlapping neuroanatomical distributions (see Chapter 9).

Added complexity in the endogenous opioid systems comes from the presence of multiple types of opioid receptors, for which there is convincing pharmacological evidence (Chang & Cuatrecasas, 1979; Lord et al., 1977; Martin et al., 1976; Pasternak, 1988), although their verification as different physical entities awaits elucidation of their primary structures (see Chapter 3). The opioid peptides have a range of selectivity and affinities for the various opioid receptor types with dissociation constants (K_d) in the low nanomolar range as measured by in vitro binding assays (Akil et al., 1984; Evans et al., 1985; Goldstein & James, 1984a & b; Hollt, 1986; Itzhak, 1988; James et al., 1984; Seizinger et al., 1984; Xie & Goldstein, 1987).

The opioid peptides and their receptors are neuroanatomically localized in areas that are presumably significant for many fundamental processes. Opioid peptides, the mRNA encoding their sequences, and opioid receptors are also distributed elsewhere in the body. Recent reports highlight the growing awareness of the role of these systems as mediators of cellular communication in a variety of important physiological phenomena (De Weid, 1990; McCubbin et al., 1991). However, in the context of drug abuse, the major reason for the notoriety of opiates is their addictive liability (Goldstein & Kalant, 1990; Jarvic 1990).

MAMMALIAN MORPHINANS

With the demonstration of stereoselective binding for narcotic drugs in brain membranes, it was not unreasonable to think that the endogenous ligand(s) might be structurally related to the morphine series. However, the pace of discovery of new opioid peptides following identification of the enkephalins subsumed attempts to identify nonpeptide opioids as natural constituents of mammalian tissues. In the decade that followed the enkephalin discovery, research in this area was pursued by only a few laboratories, most notably those of Spector at the Roche Institute in Nutley, New Jersey and Goldstein at the Addiction Research Foundation in Palo Alto, California. Opioid receptor binding assays (Pert et al., 1976; Schulz et al., 1977), tissue bioassays (Schulz et al., 1977), and radioimmunoassays using antisera raised against morphine and related compounds (Gintzler et al., 1976; Goldstein, 1975; Goldstein et al., 1985) have been used to detect nonpeptide opioids in extracts of mammalian tissues. Gintzler et al. (1976), Killian et al. (1981), Hazum et al. (1981), and Goldstein et al. (1985) have all independently reported the presence of substances immunologically related to morphine in mammalian extracts. Each report involved a different antiserum generated against a morphine-related compound, none of which detectably cross-reacted with known opioid peptides.

Identification of Morphine and Codeine in Extracts of Mammalian Brain

Although several of the endogenous opioid peptides have high *affinity* for the mu opioid receptor type, none of the endogenous peptides has high *selectivity* for this receptor type (see Chapter 3), for which morphine itself is historically the prototypical ligand (Goldstein & James, 1984b; James et al., 1984; Kosterlitz, 1985; Martin et al., 1976). This was an important characteristic that revived interest in the existence of nonpeptide opioids in mammalian tissues and led to a resumption of the search interrupted a decade earlier (Goldstein et al., 1985). By 1985 Goldstein's group was able to detect routinely three peaks (named 1, 4, and 5 for historical reasons) with antisera raised against morphine when partially purified extracts of brain and adrenal were chromatographed by reverse phase liquid chromatography (RPLC). To identify these compounds unequivocably, a large-scale purification was carried out (Weitz, 1988; Weitz et al., 1986) from approximately 1200 bovine hypothalami (wet weight about 21 kg). In this work a so-called sequential blank procedure was implemented to control for contamination of extracts with morphinans from laboratory glassware and equipment where they may be present in trace quantities. Using a combination of phase partition, ion exchange, and reverse phase chromatography, about 75 nm of immunoreactive morphine equivalents of peak 1 and 7 nm of immunoreactive morphine equivalents of peak 4 were purified to apparent homogeneity on the basis of the 280 nm UV absorption and immunoreactive RPLC profiles.

Unequivocal identification of peaks 1 and 4 was achieved by combined gas chromatography/mass spectrometry (GC/MS). Aliquots of the final samples (about 1.3% of peak 1 and 14.3% of peak 4) and equivalent proportions of the blank samples were chemically derivatized with N-methylbis(trifluoroacet-amide) and thereby converted to the trifluoroacetyl (TFA) derivatives. As a further precuation against false-positive results, the gas chromatography was carried out with a column naive to morphinans, and retention times and mass spectra of authentic compounds were recorded only after the biological samples had been analyzed. The reconstructed total ion chromatograms from the injection of solvent blanks and sequential blanks were free of peaks, corresponding in retention times and mass spectral characteristics to derivatized morphine and codeine. In the peak 1 studies, the only significant peak in the chromatogram had the same retention time (Fig. 17-1) and mass spectrum (Fig. 17-2) as authentic morphine. In the peak 4 studies the chromatogram from the biological extract contained several peaks, one of which had the retention time (Fig. 17-3) and mass spectrum of authentic codeine (Fig. 17-4).

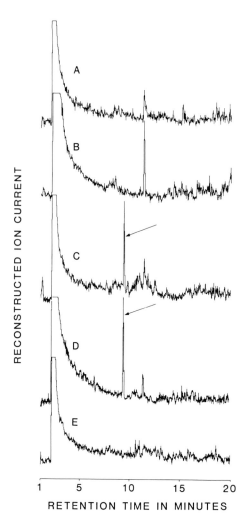

Figure 17-1. Reconstructed total ion chromatograms from the GC/MS analysis of peak 1: **A,** HPLC solvent blank (500 μl); **B,** sequential blank; **C,** immunoreactive material from tissue (peak 1, approx 1 nm of ir-morphine equivalents); **D,** morphine external standard (1 nm); **E,** GC solvent blank (5 μl heptane). The arrows indicate the two peaks, the mass spectra of which are shown in Figure 17-2. The peak at 11.25 minutes, variably present in all samples, is undoubtedly due to a plasticizer contaminant because of the abundant ions at m/z 149 and 167 in the mass spectra.

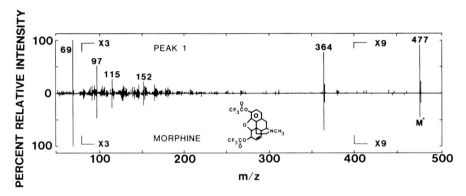

Figure 17-2. Comparison of the electron impact mass spectra of the trifluoroacetyl derivatives of peak 1 **(top)** and authentic morphine **(bottom,** presented as an inverted tracing).

Elemental composition of the molecular ion at m/z 477 and the major fragment ion at m/z 364 from peak 1 were found by high-resolution mass spectrometry to agree within experimental error with what would be expected for the same ions derived from the TFA derivative of morphine. The available quantity of peak 4 material was not sufficient for high-resolution mass spectrometric measurements.

Independent of this work, Spector's group has published a series of reports on the characterization of material extracted from rat, cat, and rabbit brain and from human lumbar and cisternal cerebrospinal fluid, that was recognized by antibodies generated against morphine (Donnerer et al., 1986; Gintzler et al., 1976; Shorr et al., 1978). These contributions eventually culminated in the mass spectrometric identification of morphine and codeine in extracted spinal cord from rats in which arthritis had been induced by intradermal injection of heat-killed *Mycobacterium butyricum* (Donnerer et al., 1987). Equally compelling evidence for the unequivocal identification of the immunoreactive peaks from untreated animals has yet to be provided by this group. However, the published data on the similarities between the endogenous compounds and morphine and codeine, on the basis of immunological, chromatographic, electrochemical oxidation, and bioactivity criteria, are persuasive if short of definitive.

Identification of 6-Acetylmorphine in Extracts of Mammalian Brain

In the large-scale purification of peaks 1 and 4, Weitz and Goldstein observed the disappearance of peak 5 during alkaline phase partition. A series of control experiments indicated that peak 5 was degraded to morphine in 1 M NH$_4$OH, 3.5 mM NaOH and 1 M HCl. Preparative purification of peak 5 was carried out from about 1750 bovine hypothalami (wet weight about 28 kg; Weitz et al., 1988), with care taken to avoid strongly acidic or basic conditions. In the final RPLC step, peak 5 eluted as a single peak of UV absorbance (15 nmol total, assuming a molar extinction coefficient equal to that of morphine) that corresponded to a peak of immunoreactivity (total of 16 nmol of immunoreactive morphine equivalents).

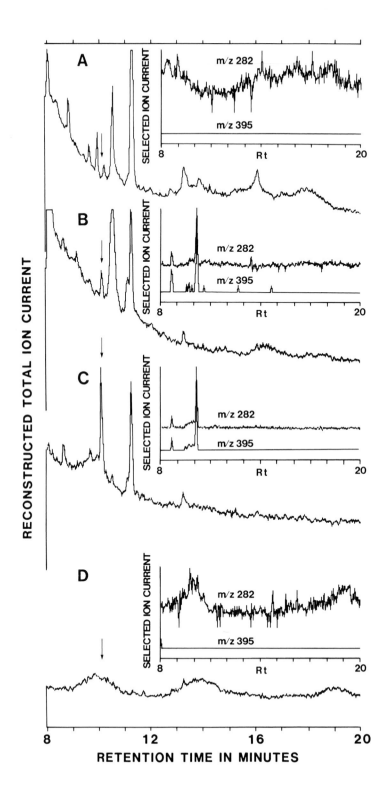

During GC/MS (TFA derivative) of the purified material, the reconstructed total ion chromatogram showed a predominant peak that was not present in the corresponding blank samples. The deduced molecular weight and elemental composition from high-resolution data and the fragmentation pattern for peak 5 were consistent with monoacetylmorphine. Some time after the GC/MS studies were complete, samples of authentic 3- and 6-acetylmorphine were obtained. The 6-acetyl standard had a GC retention time and mass spectra (Fig. 17-5) identical to that of peak 5, whereas the 3-acetyl standard had a longer retention time and different mass spectral fragmentation pattern. Weitz and Goldstein also showed from other experiments that added labeled morphine was not converted to peak 5 during extraction and purification.

Identification of Thebaine in Extracts of Mammalian Brain

Recently, Spector's group reported the isolation and identification of thebaine from extracts of sheep brain. Thebaine is a precursor of morphine in the poppy biosynthetic pathway. By virtue of the fact that their antibody raised against morphine had about 10% cross-reactivity with thebaine, Kodaira et al. (1989) were able to purify approximately 45 pmol of material from 2 kg of lyophilized sheep brain using a combination of gel filtration and RPLC. The peak of immunoreactivity behaved identically to authentic thebaine in two RPLC systems and was confirmed to be thebaine by combined gas chromatography/mass spectrometry.

MORPHINAN BIOSYNTHESIS IN MAMMALS

The biosynthetic pathway for morphine in the opium poppy (Fig. 17-6) involves tetrahydropapaveroline (THP) formation from tyrosine and dopamine. THP is then sequentially converted via a series of reactions to reticuline, salutaridine, thebaine, codeine, and morphine (Barton et al., 1965; Battersby et al., 1964; Borkowski et al., 1978). Of particular interest has been the critical step involving intramolecular oxidative coupling of reticuline to form salutaridine (Hodges & Rapoport, 1982) that generates the morphinan skeleton and the stereochemistry of the series (Kirby, 1967).

Figure 17-3. Reconstructed total ion chromatograms from the analysis of peak 4. **A,** sequential blank; **B,** immunoreactive material from tissue (peak 4, approx 750 pmol of ir-morphine equivalents); **C,** codeine external standard (1 nm); **D,** GC solvent blank (5 μl heptane). The arrows correspond to the peak for trifluoroacetyl-codeine in **C** and the corresponding positions in the other chromatograms. The inserts represent the tracings of the relative intensity of the ions at m/z 282 and 395 in each chromatogram. The mass spectra of the peaks indicated by arrows in **B** and **C** are shown in Figure 17-4.

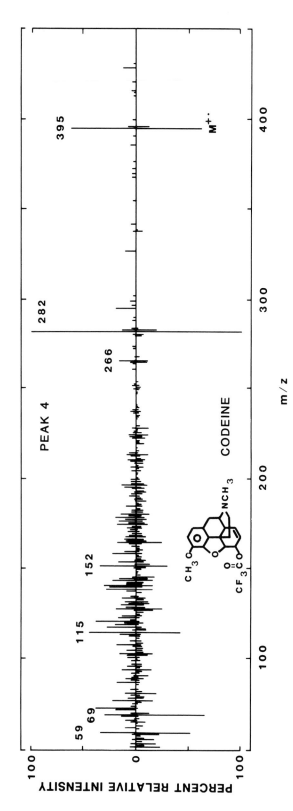

Figure 17-4. Comparison of the electron impact mass spectra of the trifluoroacetyl derivatives of peak 4 (**top**) and authentic codeine (**bottom,** presented as an inverted tracing).

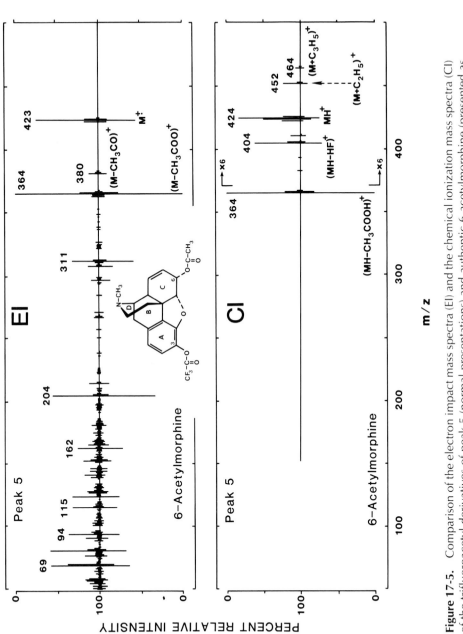

Figure 17-5. Comparison of the electron impact mass spectra (EI) and the chemical ionization mass spectra (CI) of the trifluoroacetyl derivatives of peak 5 (normal presentations) and authentic 6-acetylmorphine (presented as inverted tracings).

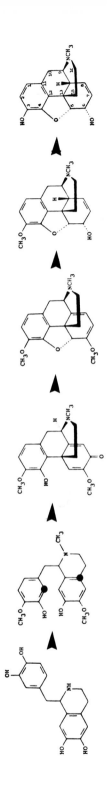

Figure 17-6. Biosynthetic pathway for morphine in the opium poppy. Tetrahydropapaveroline is derived from tyrosine and dopamine. The marked carbon atoms in reticuline participate in oxidative coupling to generate salutaridine, the earliest intermediate with the chiral four-ring arrangement defined as the morphinan structure.

Conversion of Reticuline to Salutaridine by Mammals

Weitz and Goldstein had observed the in vivo and in vitro conversion by rat liver of tritiated reticuline to a peak with the same RPLC retention time as salutaridine. Unequivocal identification of the product was achieved by GC/MS. By the addition of an excess of unlabeled reticuline to liver homogenate containing tritiated reticuline, sufficient unlabeled product was co-purified for GC/MS analysis. This necessitated the development of a procedure for gas chromatographic and mass spectrometric analysis of salutaridine with sensitivity down to a few pmol. Attempts to do gas chromatography of underivatized salutaridine (free base) were unsuccessful, presumably because it decomposed during passage through the column. This decomposition occurred despite the fact that underivatized morphine and codeine (free bases) eluted from the same column with reasonable retention times and peak shapes. Attempts to derivatize salutaridine on the hydroxyl function by treatment with silylating reagents and perfluoroacid anhydrides were also unsuccessful, presumably because of steric restrictions. However, salutaridine was successfully derivatized by treatment with O-[pentafluorobenzyl]hydroxylamine HCl in pyridine. The resulting oxime derivative gave the expected mass spectra and under electron capture conditions had abundant high mass ions suitable for selected ion monitoring. The sensitivity obtained for the molecular ion under electron capture conditions exceeded that obtained under electron impact conditions by approximately 200-fold. At the 30 pmol level, with electron capture and selected ion monitoring, the four predominant ions (m/z 522 (M^-), 492, 341 ([M-$C_6F_5CH_2$]$^-$), and 324) yielded relatively intense peaks with signal : noise ratios between 23 : 1 and 33 : 1.

Analysis of the biosynthetic product obtained from in vitro incubations of reticuline with rat liver homogenate found that the biosynthetic product and salutaridine standard yielded ion currents with retention times and relative peak areas that were essentially the same (Weitz et al., 1987; Fig. 17-7). A preboiled control homogenate did not generate selected ion currents at the retention time of interest.

These results demonstrate the in vivo and in vitro conversion of reticuline to salutaridine by rat liver. Although the conversion was not detectable in rat brain or bovine adrenal, the ability of mammalian liver to catalyze the same critical step in morphine biosynthesis as in the opium poppy has attracted comment (Kosterlitz, 1987). This is primarily because it would seem unlikely that the unusual features of this complex intramolecular coupling reaction could be supported by a nonspecific enzyme: The more likely possibility that a specific enzyme is involved has prompted speculation about morphinan biosynthesis by mammals.

Other Aspects of Morphinan Metabolism by Mammals

Misra and colleagues (1973, 1974) had earlier observed that subcutaneous injections of tritiated thebaine resulted in the formation of a series of labeled metabolites in the rat, of which norcodeine, normorphine, morphine, and codeine were identified on the basis of ion exchange and silica gel thin layer chromato-

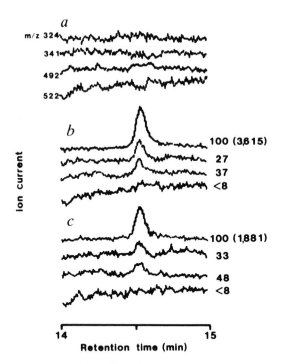

Figure 17-7. Gas chromatography-selected ion monitoring mass spectrometric (electron capture ionization, negative ion mode) comparison of the putative salutaridine synthesized in a liver homogenate and authentic salutaridine (O-pentafluoro-benzyl oxime derivatives). **a,** preboiled control; **b,** putative salutaridine biosynthetic product; **c,** salutaridine standard. Equivalent amounts of **b** and **c** were injected (about 20 pmol). Relative peak areas given on the right.

graphic behavior in brain 45 minutes after injection. More recently, Kodaira and Spector (1988) have independently shown using RPLC that rat liver, kidney, and brain microsomes carry out similar metabolic transformations of thebaine to oripavine, codeine, and morphine.

Mention should be made of findings concerning tetrahydropapaveroline (THP), which are obviously relevant. THP is a 16-carbon alkaloid that is the first heterocyclic intermediate in the biosynthesis of morphine in the opium poppy. In vitro experiments have shown that homogenates of mammalian brain and liver can convert dopamine to THP (Davis & Walsh, 1970; Turner et al., 1974; Walsh et al., 1970). Furthermore, in vivo experiments have shown that L-3,4-dihydroxyphenylalanine (L-DOPA) administration, either alone or in combination with ethanol, results in the formation of THP in rat brain (Turner et al., 1974).

More recently, Matsubara et al. (1992) have reported on the concentrations of THP, and morphine and codeine, in urine collected from normal subjects and parkinsonian subjects receiving L-DOPA therapy. They identified these three alkaloids in human urine using GC/MS of the TFA derivatives, and made quantitative measurements of the urinary concentrations using selected ion monitoring with deuterated internal standards. The morphine, codeine and THP levels they found in urine from healthy non-drinker controls were 2.93, 2.01 and 6.70 pmol/ml, respectively. The codeine and THP concentrations they found in urine from L-DOPA-treated parkinsonian patients were significantly elevated to 62.2 and 31.04 pmol/ml, respectively. They also found that some of the parkinsonian patients showed high urinary morphine concentrations.

SUMMARY

On the basis of multiple criteria, including immunological recognition, liquid and gas chromatographic retention times, and mass spectrometry, morphine, codeine, 6-acetylmorphine, and thebaine have been identified in extracts of mammalian brain. Immunoreactivity for morphine and codeine has also been detected in adrenal extracts by Goldstein's group (Weitz et al., 1986).

Many of the main steps in the poppy biosynthetic pathway for morphine have been shown to occur in mammals, including the critical conversion of reticuline to salutaridine. The steps that have yet to be documented in mammals are the formation of reticuline and the conversion of salutaridine to thebaine (see Fig. 17-6). Thus, the principal components for a postulated mammalian biosynthetic capability are already in place.

If endogenous morphine alkaloids have a neuroregulatory or hormonal role in mammalian physiology, one would expect them to show certain characteristics of these types of agents. First, the endogenous concentrations must be sufficiently high to have effects at the appropriate receptor. There are as yet little available precise data on the tissue concentrations in which morphinans occur in mammals. Donnerer et al. (1986) have reported concentrations for codeine and morphine in rat whole brain, intestine, liver, kidney, and blood that range between 2-79 and 2-26 fmol/g of tissue, respectively. Weitz et al. (1986) report that the total immunoreactive morphine content of bovine hypothalamus varies between 5-25 pmol/g wet weight of tissue. More recently, Lee and Spector (1991) reported on the concentrations of morphine and codeine, measured by radioimmunoassay following high pressure liquid chromatography, in various brain regions and peripheral tissues in the fasting rat. They found that in the cortex, midbrain, cerebellum and pons/medulla the morphine and codeine concentrations varied between 0.50-0.37 and 0.63-0.38 pmol/gm of tissue, respectively. They also found that the concentrations of these two alkaloids were low in pancreas (0.12 and 0.06 pmol/gm, respectively), but were considerably higher in adrenal (4.21 and 6.21 pmol/gm, respectively), and that the tissue concentrations tended to increase in the 4-day experimental fasting condition they used although there was a considerable fluctuation in the measured concentrations between the various groups of animals they tested. Although there is clearly a need for more work to define better the regional concentrations of these compounds in brain and elsewhere, the reported values in hypothalamus are in the same range as the Kd of morphine at the mu opioid receptor in binding assays (Chang & Cuatrecasas, 1979).

However, measurements of bulk tissue concentrations of morphinans do not reflect localized concentrations, either inter- or intracellular. Gintzler et al. (1978) have reported evidence for intraneuronal localization of morphine immunoreactivity in perikarya and neuronal processes in mouse brain nuclei related to the vestibular, cerebellar, and raphe systems. No reactive neurons or processes were seen in adjacent sections treated with nonimmune serum or with antimorphine antiserum from which specific antibodies had been removed by passage over an affinity column containing immobilized morphine. Although an independent replication of this important result has yet to be reported for mammalian systems, Hathaway and Epple (1990) recently reported immunohistochemical evidence for the presence of morphine immunoreactivity in chromaffin cells of the American eel using the same techniques as used by the Spector group.

Finally and possibly most importantly, a physiological role as either a hormone or a neurotransmitter can only be considered when it has been demonstrated that the release of these compounds is under some type of control and that it can be regulated in the expected fashion by appropriate pharmacological and behavioral conditions. This demonstration has yet to be made for the mammalian morphinans. Nevertheless, the identification of the compounds in brain and evidence of the activity of critical steps in the biosynthetic pathway warrant further investigation along these lines.

ACKNOWLEDGMENTS

The assistance of Dr. Charles Weitz in preparing this manuscript is gratefully acknowledged. With permission of the authors, Figures 2 and 4 are reproduced from Weitz et al. (1986), and Figure 5 is reproduced from Weitz et al. (1988). Figures 6 and 7 are reproduced from Weitz et al. (1988) with permission of the authors and publisher.

REFERENCES

Akil, H., Watson, S.J., Young, E., Lewis, M.E., Khachaturian, H., & Walker, J.M. (1984). Endogenous opioids: Biology and function. *Annu. Rev. Neurosci., 7,* 223-255.

Barton, D.H.R., Kirby, G.W., Steglich, W., Thomas, G.M., Battersby, A.R., Dobson, T.A., & Ramuz, H. (1965). Investigations on the biosynthesis of morphine alkaloids. *J. Chem. Soc.,* 2423-2438.

Battersby, A.R., Binks, R., Francis, R.J., McCaldin, D.J., & Ramuz, H. (1964). Alkaloid biosynthesis. Part IV. 1-Benzylisoquinolines as precursors of thebaine, codeine and morphine. *J. Chem. Soc.,* 3600-3610.

Borkowski, P.R., Horn, J.S., & Rapoport, H. (1978). Role of 1,2-dehydroreticulinium ion in the biosynthetic conversion of reticuline to thebaine. *J. Am. Chem. Soc., 100,* 276-281.

Chang, K.-J., & Cuatrecasas, P. (1979). Multiple opiate receptors: Enkephalins and morphine bind to receptors of different specificity. *J. Biol. Chem., 254,* 2610-2618.

Chein, I., Gerard, D.L., Lee, R.S., & Rosenfeld, E. (1964). *The road to H: Narcotics, delinquency and social policy*. New York: Basic Books Inc.

Davis, V.E., & Walsh, M.J. (1970). Alcohol, amines and alkaloids: A possible biochemical basis for alcohol addiction. *Science, 167*, 1005-1007.

De Weid, D. (Ed.). (1990). *Neuropeptides: Basics and perspectives*. New York: Elsevier Science.

Donnerer, J., Oka, K., Brossi, A., Rice, K.C., & Spector, S. (1986). Presence and formation of codeine and morphine in the rat. *Proc. Natl. Acad. Sci. USA., 83*, 4566-4567.

Donnerer, J., Cardinale, G., Coffey, J., Lisek, C.A., Jardine, J., & Spector, S. (1987). Chemical characterization and regulation of endogenous morphine and codeine in the rat. *J. Pharmacol. Exp. Ther., 242*, 583-587.

Douglass, J., Civelli, O. & Herbert, E. (1984). Polyprotein gene expression: Generation of diversity of neuroendocrine peptides. *Annu. Rev. Biochem., 53*, 665-715.

Eddy, E.B., & May, E.L. (1973). The search for a better analgesic. *Science, 181*, 407-414.

Evans, C.J., Erdelyi, E., Hunter, J., & Barchas, J.D. (1985). Co-localization and characterization of immunoreactive peptides derived from two opioid precursors in guinea pig adrenal glands. *J. Neurosci., 5*, 3423-3427.

Evans, C.J., Hammond, D.L., & Frederickson, R.C.A. (1988). The opioid peptides. In G.W. Pasternak (Ed.), *The opiate receptors* (pp. 23-71). Clifton, NJ: The Humana Press.

Gintzler, A.R., Mohacsi, E. & Spector, S. (1976). Radioimmunoassay for the simultaneous determination of morphine and codeine. *Eur. J. Pharmacol., 38*, 149-156.

Gintzler, A.R., Gershon, M.D., & Spector, S. (1978). A nonpeptide morphine-like compound: Immunocytochemical localization in the mouse brain. *Science, 199*, 447-448.

Goldstein, A. (1973). Are opiate tolerance and dependence reversible? Implications for the treatment of heroin addiction. In A. Cappell & A.E. LeBlanc (Eds.), *Biological & behavioral approaches to drug dependence* (pp. 27-41). Proceedings International Symposium on Alcohol and Drug Research. Toronto: Addiction Research Foundation.

Goldstein, A., & James, I.F. (1984a). Multiple opioid receptors: Criteria for identification and classification. *Trends Pharmacol. Sci., 5*, 503-505.

Goldstein, A., & James, I.F. (1984b). Site-directed alkylation of multiple opioid receptors. II. Pharmacological selectivity. *Mol. Pharmacol., 25*, 343-348.

Goldstein, A., & Kalant, H. (1990). Drug policy: Striking the right balance. *Science, 249*, 513-521.

Goldstein, A., Lowney, L.I., & Pal, B.K. (1971). Stereo-specific and non-specific interactions of the morphine congener levorphanol in subcellular fractions of mouse brain. *Proc. Natl. Acad. Sci. USA., 68*, 1742-1747.

Goldstein, A., Barrett, R.W., James, I.F., Lowney, L.I., Weitz, C.J., Knipmeyer, L., & Rapoport, H. (1985). Morphine and other opiates from beef brain and adrenal. *Proc. Natl. Acad. Sci. USA., 82*, 5203-5207.

Hathaway, C.B., & Epple, A. (1990). Catecholamines, opioid peptides, and true opiates in the chromaffin cells of the eel: immunohistochemical evidence. *Gen. Comp. Endocrinol., 79*, 393-405.

Hazum, E., Sabatka, J., Chang, K.-J., Brent, D.A., Findlay, J.W.A., & Cuatrecasas, P. (1981). Morphine in cow and human milk: Could dietary morphine constitute a ligand for specific morphine (u) receptors? *Science, 213*, 1010-1012.

Hodges, C.H., & Rapoport, H. (1982). Enzymatic conversion of reticuline to salutaridine by cell-free systems from *Papaver somniferum. Biochem. J., 21,* 3729-3734.

Hollt, V. (1986). Opioid peptide processing and receptor selectivity. *Annu. Rev. Pharmacol. Toxicol., 26,* 59-77.

Hughes, J., Smith, T.W., Kosterlitz, H.W., Fothergill, L.A., Morgan, B.A., & Morris, H.R. (1975). Identification of two related pentapeptides from the brain with potent opiate agonist activity. *Nature, 258,* 577-579.

Itzhak, Y. (1988). Multiple opioid binding sites. In G.W. Pasternak (Ed.), *The opiate receptors* (pp. 95-142). Clifton, NJ: The Humana Press.

James, I.F., & Goldstein, A. (1984). Site-directed alkylation of multiple opioid receptors. I. Binding selectivity. *Mol. Pharmacol., 25,* 337-342.

James, I.F., Fischli, W., & Goldstein, A. (1984). Opioid receptor selectivity of dynorphin gene products. *J. Pharmacol. Exp. Ther., 228,* 88-93.

Jarvic, M. (1990). The drug dilemma: Manipulating the demand. *Science, 250,* 387-391.

Killian, A., Schuster, C.R., House, J.T., Sholl, S., Connors, M., & Wainer, B.H. (1981). *Life Sci., 28,* 811–817.

Kirby, G.W. (1967). Biosynthesis of the morphine alkaloids. *Science, 155,* 170-173.

Kodaira, H., & Spector, S. (1988). Transformation of thebaine to oripavine, codeine, and morphine by rat liver, kidney, and brain microsomes. *Proc. Natl. Acad. Sci. USA., 85,* 1267-1271.

Kodaira, H., Lisek, C.A., Jardine, I., Arimura, A., & Spector, S. (1989). Identification of the convulsant opiate thebaine in mammalian brain. *Proc. Natl. Acad. Sci. USA., 86,* 716-719.

Kosterlitz, H.W. (1985). Has morphine a physiological function in the animal kingdom? *Nature, 317,* 671.

Kosterlitz, H.W. (1987). Bionsynthesis of morphine in the animal kingdom. *Nature, 330,* 606.

Lee, C.S., & Spector, S. (1991). Changes of endogenous morphine and codeine contents in the fasting rat. *J. Pharmacol. Exp. Ther. 257,* 647-650.

Lord, J.A.H., Waterfield, A.A., Hughes, J., & Kosterlitz, H.W. (1977). Endogenous opioid peptides: Multiple agonists and receptors. *Nature, 267,* 495-499.

Martin, W.R., Eades, C.G., Thompson, J.A., Huppler, R.E., & Gilbert, P.E. (1976). The effects of morphine and nalorphine-like drugs in the nondependent and morphine-dependent chronic spinal dog. *J. Pharmacol. Exp. Ther., 197,* 517-532.

Matsubara, K., Fukushima, S., Akane, A., Kobayashi, S., & Shiono, H. (1992). Increased urinary morphine, codeine and tetrahydropapaveroline in Parkinsonian patient undergoing L-3,4-dihydroxyphenylalanine therapy: a possible biosynthetic pathway of morphine from L-3,4-dihydroxyphenylalanine in humans. *J. Pharmacol. Exp. Ther., 260,* 974-978.

McCubbin, J.A., Kaufmann, P.G., & Nemeroff, C.B. (Eds.). (1991). *Stress, neuropeptides, and systemic disease.* San Diego: Academic Press.

Misra, A.L., Pontani, R.B., & Mule, S.J. (1973). Relationship of pharmacokinetic and metabolic parameters to the absence of physical: dependence liability with thebaine-^{3}H. *Experientia, 29,* 1108-1110.

Misra, A.L., Pontani, R.B., & Mule, S.J. (1974). Pharmacokinetics and metabolism of [^{3}H]Thebaine. *Xenobiotica, 4,* 17-32.

Pasternak, G. (Ed.). (1988). *The opiate receptors.* Clifton, NJ: The Humana Press.

Patey, G., Liston, D., & Rossier, J. (1984). Characterization of new enkephalin-containing peptides in the adrenal medulla by immunoblotting. *FEBS Lett., 172,* 303-308.

Pert, C.B., & Snyder, S.H. (1973). Opiate receptor: Demonstration in nervous tissue. *Science, 179,* 1011-1014.

Pert, C.B., Pert, A., & Tallman, J. (1976). Isolation of a novel endogenous opiate analgesic from human blood. *Proc. Natl. Acad. Sci. USA, 73,* 2226-2230.

Schulz, R., Wuster, M., & Herz, A. (1977). Detection of a long acting endogenous opioid in blood and small intestine. *Life Sci., 21,* 105-115.

Seizinger, B., Hollt, V., & Herz, A. (1984). Proenkephalin B (prodynorphin)-derived opioid peptides: Evidence for a differential processing in lobes of the pituitary. *Endocrinology, 115,* 662-671.

Shorr, J., Foley, K., & Spector, S. (1978). Presence of a non-peptide morphine-like compound in human cerebrospinal fluid. *Life Sci., 23,* 2057-2062.

Simon, E.J., Hiller, J.M., & Edelman, I. (1973). Stereo-specific binding of the potent narcotic analgesic [^{3}H]etorphine to rat brain homogenate. *Proc. Natl. Acad. Sci. USA., 70,* 1947-1949.

Terenius, L. (1973). Characteristics of the "receptor" for narcotic analgesics in synaptic plasma membrane fraction from rat brain. *Acta Pharmacol. Toxicol., 33,* 377-384.

Terry, C.E., & Pellens, M. (1928). *The opium problem.* New York: Bureau of Social Hygiene Inc.

Turner, A., Baker, K., Algeri, S., Frigerio, A., & Garattini, S. (1974). Tetrahydropapaveroline: Formation in vivo and in vitro in rat brain. *Life Sci., 14,* 2247-2257.

Walsh, M.J., Davis, V.E., & Yamomaka, Y. (1970). Tetrahydropapaveroline: An alkaloid metabolite of dopamine in vitro. *J. Pharmacol. Exp. Ther., 174,* 388-400.

Weber, E., Evans, C.J., & Barchas, J.D. (1983). Multiple endogenous ligands for opioid receptors. *Trends Neurosci., 6,* 333-336.

Weitz, C.J. (1988). *Morphinans from mammalian brain.* Unpublished doctoral dissertation, Stanford University, Palo Alto, CA.

Weitz, C.J., Lowney, L.I., Faull, K.F., Feistner, G., & Goldstein, A. (1986). Morphine and codeine from mammalian brain. *Proc. Natl. Acad. Sci. USA., 83,* 9784-9788.

Weitz, C.J., Faull, K.F., & Goldstein, A. (1987). Synthesis of the skeleton of the morphine molecule by mammalian liver. *Nature, 330,* 674-677.

Weitz, C.J., Lowney, L.I., Faull, K.F., Feistner, G., & Goldstein, A. (1988). 6-Acetylmorphine: A natural product present in mammalian brain. *Proc. Natl. Acad. Sci. USA., 85,* 5335-5338.

Wright, C.R.A. (1874). On the action of organic acids and their anhydrides on the natural alkaloids. Part 1. *J. Chem. Soc., 27,* 1031-1043.

Xie, G.-X., & Goldstein, A. (1987). Characterization of big dynorphins from rat brain and spinal cord. *J. Neurosci., 7,* 2049-2055.

18

Neurochemical Substrates Underlying the Mechanism of Action of Phencyclidine (PCP)

ROBERT N. PECHNICK

Phencyclidine (PCP), also known as angel dust, was first developed in the late 1950s for use as a general anesthetic (Maddox, 1981). At subanesthetic doses, PCP has a unique pharmacological profile, producing a feeling of depersonalization, a sense of unreality, delusional thinking, loosened associations, disorganized thought processes, and a reduction in the user's ability to distinguish self from surroundings (Domino, 1964; Pradhan, 1984). At higher doses it produces an unusual form of anesthesia known as dissociative anesthesia; subjects become analgesic, many of their reflexes remain intact, and they may keep their eyes open even though they are completely unresponsive to outside stimuli and do not remember what has taken place. Although PCP has some characteristics that are highly useful in an anesthetic, subjects emerging from PCP-induced anesthesia experience confusional states manifested by disorientation, hallucinations, and bizarre and frightening dreams, and in some cases these effects last for hours.

Some of the acute effects of PCP are very similar to the manifestations of schizophrenia (Domino et al., 1964; Luby et al., 1962; Pradhan, 1984), which has led to the suggestion that PCP-induced psychosis may be the best model of schizophrenia. For example, in a blind study, only 2 of 54 symptoms were significantly different between patients with schizophrenia and those with PCP-induced psychosis. This overlap of symptomatology has caused psychiatrists to frequently misdiagnose PCP users as schizophrenics; in two studies more than 40% of newly admitted psychiatric patients were found to be positive for PCP on toxicological screens (Gorelick et al., 1984; Yago et al., 1981). The signs and symptoms of PCP-induced psychosis are clearly different from the psychotic reactions produced in normal individuals by psychotomimetic agents, such as lysergic acid diethylamide (LSD), or by the repeated administration of such psychostimulants as amphetamine. In addition, whereas LSD produces effects in schizophrenics that are no more severe than those found in normals, schizo-

This work was supported by NIDA grants (DA 04113 and DA 05448).

phrenics in remission can develop severe and prolonged relapses of acute symptomatology after PCP administration. Moreover, PCP-induced psychosis in nonschizophrenics can last as long as 4 weeks, far longer than the sojourn of the drug in the body. Thus, ingestion of a single dose of PCP seems to be able to activate events in the brain that far outlast its acute pharmacological effect.

Although the side effects of PCP precluded its use as a general anesthetic, it soon became a much sought-after drug of abuse. Despite the media's focus on other drugs, PCP abuse remains a widespread and important problem in the United States, with the Drug Abuse Warning Network (DAWN) reporting increases in seven metropolitan areas from 1984 to 1986. In St. Louis between 1983 and 1986, 47% of individuals arrested for driving under the influence of drugs were found to be PCP-positive (Poklis et al., 1987). From 1981 to 1983, the monthly total number of PCP-related cases appearing in emergency rooms in the United States was estimated to be 12,500 (Pradhan, 1984), but this figure may underestimate the actual prevalence. PCP abuse is especially important in that it has proved to be associated with aggressive and violent offenses against other people (Simonds & Kashani, 1980): In 1986 the percentage of black homicide victims with detectable PCP levels in New Orleans was 13.9% (Lowrey et al., 1988), and in a screening study at a San Diego medical center, 47% of those found to be PCP-positive were trauma unit patients (Baily, 1987).

PCP is readily available because it can be made easily and cheaply by "garage" chemists without the risks of illegal importation; at least six "designer drug" analogs of PCP are sold on the street. Therefore, PCP represents a class of abused drugs, rather than a single entity. PCP is a classical "dirty drug," meaning that it has multiple effects on many different neurotransmitter systems. There have been many excellent reviews of the mechanisms of action and effects of PCP (Balster, 1987; Itzhak & Stein, 1990; Johnson & Jones, 1990; Lodge & Johnson, 1990; Musacchio, 1990; Sonders et al., 1988; Walker et al., 1990; Willetts et al., 1990). This chapter highlights some of the current knowledge about the mechanisms of action of PCP and defines some of the key research questions.

EFFECTS OF PCP ON CHOLINERGIC, SEROTONERGIC, AND CATECHOLAMINERGIC SYSTEMS

At one time it was thought that PCP produced its various effects by acting directly on certain neurotransmitter systems. Because PCP was originally (and inappropriately) classified as a hallucinogen, some of the early studies of the drug focused on putative neurochemical substrates for other hallucinogens. It had been suggested that the psychotropic effects of some drugs could be due to their anticholinergic properties (Abood & Biel, 1962), and it was later found that PCP had antagonist activity at muscarinic-cholinergic synapses. For example, it was shown that PCP can inhibit the contractile responses produced by muscarinic agonists in the guinea pig ileum (Kloog et al., 1977; Maayani et al., 1973; Vargas & Pechnick, 1991; Vincent et al., 1978), as well as bind to muscarinic receptors in brain (Kloog et al., 1977; Vargas & Pechnick, 1991; Vincent et al., 1978). PCP has other effects on cholinergic systems: It can block the ion channel associated with nicotinic-cholinergic receptors (Albuquerque et al., 1980), and it is a weak inhibitor of acetylcholinesterase (Kloog et al., 1977). However, the behavioral effects of PCP do not seem to be a direct consequence of its effects on cholinergic neurotransmission.

Other hallucinogens have been hypothesized to mediate their effects by interacting with serotonergic neurons, and early experiments showed that the acute administration of PCP increased brain levels of serotonin (Tonge & Leonard, 1969). Later, PCP was found to inhibit the reuptake and decrease the turnover of serotonin (for review, see Johnson & Jones, 1990) and to increase extracellular levels of serotonin (Hernandez et al. 1988). Other studies supported a role for the involvement of serotonergic systems in some of the behavioral effects of PCP as certain behaviors were reduced by producing electrolytic lesions of areas containing serotonergic cell bodies, using selective serotonergic neurotoxins, or by pretreating the animals with serotonergic antagonists (Nabeshima et al., 1984). There is also evidence that PCP may act directly with the 5-HT$_2$ serotonin receptor subtype (Nabeshima et al., 1988). However, the exact role of serotonergic systems in the effects of PCP remains unclear.

PCP also has major effects on catecholaminergic neurotransmission, notably on dopaminergic neurons (Johnson, 1983; Johnson & Jones, 1990). PCP is an indirectly acting dopamine agonist; at low doses it inhibits the reuptake of dopamine and at higher doses causes its release. Structure-activity studies have shown that the ability to inhibit dopamine reuptake and bind to the PCP/NMDA receptor can be dissociated, indicating that the PCP-induced inhibition of dopamine reuptake is not mediated by the PCP/NMDA receptor complex. For example, analogs of PCP have been developed that are very potent inhibitors of dopamine reuptake but have low affinity for the PCP/NMDA receptor (Chaudieu et al., 1989), and (+)-5-methyl-10,11-dihydro-5H-dibenzo-[a,d]-cyclohepten-5,10-imine maleate (MK-801), a drug with high affinity and a high degree of selectivity for the PCP/NMDA receptor, is only a weak inhibitor of dopamine reuptake (Snell et al., 1988). PCP increases levels of dopamine in dialysates obtained from areas of the striatum and nucleus accumbens in freely moving animals (Hernandez et al., 1988), and some but not all of the behavioral effects of PCP can be altered by manipulating dopaminergic systems (Balster, 1987; Johnson, 1983). PCP also inhibits the reuptake of norepinephrine, but the exact involvement of noradrenergic systems in the effects of PCP is unclear.

THE CONCEPT OF A PCP RECEPTOR

None of the effects of PCP described above seems to be mediated by a specific PCP receptor. In 1979 two groups (Vincent et al., 1979; Zukin & Zukin, 1979) found that ³H-PCP bound with high affinity and in a saturable and selective manner to membrane homogenates from rat brain. This finding suggested the existence of a specific PCP binding site or receptor in brain. In addition, Zukin and Zukin (1979) found that (±)-N-allylnormetazocine [(±)-SKF 10,047], a structurally unrelated opiate that had psychotomimetic activity, also inhibited the binding of ³H-PCP. Quirion et al. (1981) found that other opiates and opiate analogs with psychotomimetic properties displaced the binding of labeled PCP, and Zukin and Zukin (1981) reported that PCP and PCP analogs could inhibit the binding of ³H-cyclazocine, another psychotomimetic opiate. Previously, Martin et al. (1976), based upon in vivo experiments, classified (±)-SKF 10,047 as the prototypic agonist at a receptor that they had termed the sigma opiate receptor, and it was hypothesized that the psychotomimetic activity of some opiates was due to interactions with this receptor. Taken together, these data led Zukin and Zukin (1981) to suggest that the PCP receptor and the sigma receptor might be the same site, and that this single receptor could mediate the behavioral effect of PCP and the "sigma opiates." This common binding site came to be known as the sigma/PCP receptor.

Later, it became apparent that PCP interacts with at least two separate and distinct entities: the *PCP binding site* and the *sigma binding site* (Quirion et al., 1987). This terminology can be confusing because PCP binds to *both* sites. Because haloperidol binds with high affinity to the sigma binding site but with very low affinity to the PCP site, the sigma binding site also has been called the haloperidol-sensitive sigma binding site. The PCP and sigma binding sites can be differentiated on the basis of ligand selectivity (Largent et al., 1986; Wong et al., 1988), regional localization (Largent et al., 1986), and differences in ontogeny (Majewska et al., 1989; Paleos et al., 1990). Compounds that have a high degree of selectivity for the PCP over the sigma binding site include MK-801 and N-(1-(2-thienyl) cyclohexyl) piperidine (TCP) (Largent et al., 1986; Wong et al., 1988), whereas haloperidol, (+)-SKF 10,047, (+)-3-(3-hydroxyphenyl)-N-(1-propyl) piperidine [(+)-3-PPP], (+)-pentazocine, and 1,3-di-o-tolyl-guanidine (DTG) have selectivity for the sigma binding site as opposed to the PCP binding site (Sonders et al., 1988; Steinfels et al., 1988). It should be pointed out that, although haloperidol also has high affinity for dopaminergic receptors, the sigma binding site is not a dopamine receptor. The binding of drugs to either site is unaffected by opiate antagonists, such as naloxone; thus, neither site is an opiate receptor as classically defined. Supporting this conclusion, the effects of PCP on body temperature and neuroendocrine function are not altered by pretreatment with opiate antagonists (Pechnick & George, 1989; Pechnick et al., 1989a). The PCP binding sites are most abundant in the CA1 region of the hippocampus, cerebral cortex, striatum, thalamus, and amygdala, but highest densities of sigma binding sites are found in the hypothalamus, brainstem, and cerebellum (Largent et al., 1986; Sonders et al., 1988).

PCP/NMDA RECEPTOR IONOPHORE COMPLEX

Over the last several years, major advances in the characterization of the PCP binding site have been made. There are several subtypes of receptors for the excitatory amino acid glutamate in the central nervous system; one of these receptors is known as the N-methyl-D-aspartate (NMDA) receptor. The NMDA receptor is a member of the ligand-gated ion channel class of receptors; the binding of agonists to the NMDA receptor causes neuronal excitation by increasing the flux of cations (Na^+, K^+ and Ca^{++}) through the ion channel. In 1983 Lodge and colleagues (Anis et al., 1983) reported a key finding—PCP could selectively antagonize the excitatory effects mediated by NMDA receptors. Further studies demonstrated that the antagonism was noncompetitive in nature; that is, PCP does not inhibit the effects of glutamate by competing for the same binding site, but binds to a separate site and inhibits the glutamate-stimulated flux in cations. PCP is thought to bind near or possibly within the ion channel of the NMDA receptor (MacDonald & Nowak, 1990), so access to the site is limited unless the channel is open. Therefore, any treatment that increases the level of channel activation will increase the ability of PCP to reach its binding site, and the inhibitory effects of PCP are both voltage- and use-dependent (Johnson & Jones, 1990; Lodge & Johnson, 1990; MacDonald & Nowak, 1990). Because the PCP binding site is associated with the NMDA receptor-channel complex, this site has come to be known as the PCP/NMDA receptor.

The NMDA receptor has turned out to be a very complicated entity, and it is sometimes referred to as the NMDA receptor-channel complex (Fig. 18-1). It is not coupled to G-proteins as are some other neurotransmitter receptors. In addition to binding sites for glutamate and PCP, the NMDA receptor has other separate binding sites for such diverse endogenous substances as Mg^{++}, Zn^{++}, glycine, and polyamines. The binding of glycine to the NMDA receptor complex is not inhibited by strychnine, indicating that this receptor is different from the previously characterized strychnine-sensitive glycine receptor that is involved in neuronal inhibition. The binding of these endogenous substances to their respective binding sites on the NMDA receptor-channel complex is able to affect the binding of the other endogenous factors and also to modulate glutamate-induced receptor activation (Johnson & Jones, 1990; Lodge & John-

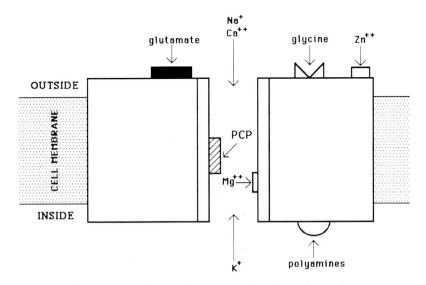

Figure 18-1. The NMDA receptor-ion channel complex.

son, 1990; Reynolds, 1990). For example, glycine increases the effects of NMDA and stimulates the binding of PCP to the PCP/NMDA receptor, leading to the suggestion that glycine might be a "cotransmitter" at the NMDA receptor. Some polyamines stimulate the binding of PCP to the PCP/NMDA receptor, whereas other polyamines inhibit its binding. Both Mg^{++} and Zn^{++} can inhibit the binding of PCP, but Mg^{++} can also stimulate binding at certain concentrations. Because the NMDA receptor has not yet been cloned or its structure defined, the exact relationships among the various binding sites on the receptor complex remain unknown. Moreover, it is not known whether all NMDA receptors possess all of these binding sites or if they are differentially expressed in subtypes of NMDA receptors.

Some of the behavioral effects of PCP and compounds with PCP-like activity, such as their discriminative stimulus effects and their ability to produce ataxia, are highly correlated with their affinity for PCP/NMDA receptors (Johnson & Jones, 1990; McCann et al., 1989; Willetts et al., 1990; Zukin & Zukin, 1988). Moreover, competitive antagonists at the NMDA receptor can produce some PCP-like behavioral effects, and drugs that interact with other binding sites on the NMDA receptor complex can affect some of the behavioral responses produced by PCP. These findings provide strong evidence that some of the effects of PCP and PCP-like drugs are mediated by the PCP/NMDA receptor.

SIGMA BINDING SITE

Research involving the sigma binding site has generated intense controversy; in fact, a review of a symposium devoted to this topic described it as "the sigma enigma" (Chavkin, 1990). The concept of the "sigma opiate receptor" was first developed by Martin et al. (1976) based upon the in vivo effects of certain opiates; namely, nalorphine, (±)-cyclazocine, (±)-pentazocine, and (±)-SKF 10,047. In the experiments that led Martin et al. (1976) to introduce the term "sigma opiate receptor," the psychotomimetic effects that these compounds produced in humans and the delirium elicited in dogs could be antagonized by opiate antagonists, such as naltrexone, indicating that these effects were mediated by some type of opiate receptor. However, the current definition of the sigma binding site is based on in vitro binding studies, and binding of ligands to the sigma binding site is not inhibited by opiate antagonists. Because this critical criterion for the involvement of opiate receptors is not met, the sigma binding site is not an opiate receptor, and the term "sigma opiate receptor" is incorrect. Thus, the "sigma opiate receptor" defined by Martin et al. (1976) is a different entity than the sigma binding site as currently defined.

Originally, it was thought that the psychotomimetic effects of some of the opiates and opiate analogs, and possibly PCP, were mediated by interactions with sigma receptors. At that time, this conclusion was supported by the following assumptions: (1) PCP and the sigma opiates were hypothesized to bind to a single receptor that mediated their psychotomimetic activity; (2) the psychotomimetic activity of the sigma opiates in humans and the delirium induced in dogs were thought to be produced by the (+)-enantiomers rather than by the (−)-enantiomers; (3) these (+)-enantiomers were known to bind to the sigma binding site; and (4) the antipsychotic agent haloperidol has high affinity for the sigma binding site, where it was suggested to be a sigma receptor antagonist. However, it is now known that the first assumption is incorrect, and the second conclusion is also probably erroneous; the work of Martin et al. (1976) utilized racemic mixtures, so it cannot be concluded which of the enantiomers produced the psychotomimetic activity. Moreover, on re-examination on the older clinical literature, it is not clear whether the psychotomimetic effects of some of these opiates and opiate analogs were mediated by the (−)-or (+)-enantiomers. This discrepancy has been reviewed by Musacchio (1990). Thus, it has not been proven that the sigma binding site has any role in the production of psychotomimetic activity.

Although it is generally accepted that the sigma binding site is separate and distinct from the PCP/NMDA receptor, it is not clear whether it is a neurotransmitter (or drug) receptor or some other entity. Whereas there is some degree of structure-binding activity relationships within certain series of sigma ligands, a wide range of structurally and pharmacologically diverse drugs bind to the sigma site, including steroids, neuroleptics, antidepressants, antihistamines, monoamine oxidase inhibitors, some opiates, antianxiety and antimuscarinic agents, and cocaine (Itzhak & Stein, 1990; Klein et al., 1991; McCann et al., 1989; Sharkey, 1988; Su et al., 1988; Walker et al., 1990). Whereas most neurotransmitter receptors are found on cell membranes, subcellular localization studies have found that sigma binding sites are found in the microsomal, as well as the synaptosomal fraction (McCann et al., 1989). Sigma binding sites are found outside the CNS within endocrine glands (pituitary, adrenals, testis, and ovary) (Blades et al., 1989; Wolfe et al., 1989), spleen (Su et al., 1988), on leukocytes (Wolfe et al., 1988), and in liver (Samovilova et al., 1988). These characteristics have led some investigators to conclude that the sigma binding site is not a functional receptor, but might be a microsomal membrane-bound enzyme, such as a member of the cytochrome P450 superfamily of isoenzymes (Klein et al., 1991). However, there may be subtypes of sigma binding sites (Musacchio et al., 1989; Rothman et al., 1991), one or more of which could be an enzyme. Perhaps the most crucial weakness in classifying the sigma binding site as a receptor is that no unique physiological or functional response has been shown unequivocally to be elicited by a sigma ligand binding to the sigma binding site. Therefore, at this time it is inappropriate to term this site a receptor, using the classical definition of a receptor.

SEARCH FOR A SIGMA RECEPTOR-MEDIATED EFFECT

Although some drugs that bind to the sigma binding sites can produce certain responses after administration in vivo, it has not been proven that these effects are specifically mediated by sigma receptors. For example, it has been reported that sigma ligands can inhibit carbachol-induced phosphatidylinositol turnover in rat brain (Bowen et al., 1988), but we have found that many sigma ligands have substantial antimuscarinic activity (Vargas & Pechnick, 1991). Thus, the inhibition of carbachol-induced phosphatidylinositol turnover could be due to the antimuscarinic properties of the sigma ligands. Using functional assays both in vivo and in vitro to determine the differential involvement of PCP/ NMDA receptors and sigma binding sites in some of the effects of PCP and drugs with PCP-like activity, we have found that PCP stimulates the pituitary-adrenal axis in the rat, causing the rapid and long-lasting release of ACTH and corticosterone (Pechnick et al., 1986, 1989b, 1990). The effects of PCP occur at doses lower than those required to produce behavioral effects, indicating that the neuroendocrine responses are a more sensitive measure of drug action. Because this effect could be mediated by either the PCP/NMDA receptor or the sigma binding site, we have tested the effects of more selective compounds. (+)-SKF 10,047, a compound that also binds to both sites, and MK-801, a compound that is highly selective for the PCP/NMDA receptor, both stimulated the release of ACTH and corticosterone (Pechnick et al., 1989c and unpublished data). We have also studied dexoxadrol and levoxadrol; the two enantiomers have relatively equal binding affinities at the sigma binding site, but dexoxadrol has a much higher affinity for the PCP/NMDA site than levoxadrol. Dexoxadrol was a far more potent stimulator of the pituitary-adrenal axis than levoxadrol (Pechnick et al., unpublished data). In addition, (+)-pentazocine, which is highly selective for the sigma binding site, is a very weak stimulator of the pituitary-adrenal axis (Pechnick et al., unpublished data). Taken together, these results suggest that the PCP-induced stimulation of the pituitary-adrenal axis probably is mediated by PCP/NMDA receptors rather than by the sigma site.

We also studied the direct effects of PCP on the ACTH-induced release of corticosterone from dispersed adrenal cells (Pechnick et al., 1990) and made a very unexpected finding; in contrast to the effects seen after in vivo administration, PCP produces dose-dependent inhibition of the ACTH-induced release of corticosterone in vitro. The finding of a PCP-mediated effect outside the CNS was surprising. It has been shown that the binding sites in the adrenal show the ligand binding selectivity indicative of sigma binding sites (Blades et al., 1989; Wolfe et al., 1989), and autoradiographic studies revealed that these sigma binding sites were highly localized in the adrenal cortex (Wolfe et al., 1989; E.H.F. Wong, personal communication). It has not been determined whether the inhibitory effects of PCP on the ACTH-induced release of corticosterone in vitro are mediated by these sigma binding sites or are due to other mechanisms.

We have characterized the effects of PCP and sigma ligands on body temperature to attempt to find a sigma-mediated effect. The acute administration of PCP causes dose-dependent hypothermia in the rat (Pechnick & George, 1989). Hypothermia also is produced by the acute administration of (+)-SKF 10,047 (Bejanian et al., 1990), as well as by the systemic and intracerebroventricular administration of the sigma-selective compound DTG (Bejanian et al., 1991). The mechanism underlying the hypothermia could be mediated by the sigma binding site; however, two purported sigma "antagonists," BMY-14802 and rimcazole, failed to affect the DTG-induced hypothermia (Bejanian et al., 1991). Thus, the mechanism of the hypothermia produced by PCP, (+)-SKF

10,047 and DTG remains unknown. In contrast, the acute administration of drugs that have selectivity for PCP/NMDA receptors over the sigma binding site, such as MK-801, causes hyperthermia (Pechnick et al., 1989d). Hyperthermia also is produced by the acute administration of dexoxadrol, but levoxadrol, the enantiomer that has far lower affinity for the PCP/NMDA receptor, fails to alter body temperature (Pechnick et al., 1989d). Thus, the hyperthermia produced by MK-801 and dexoxadrol may be mediated by the PCP/NMDA receptor.

CURRENT RESEARCH ISSUES

Although much is known about the underlying molecular mechanisms of action of PCP, the specific systems involved in manifesting its various effects remain unclear. How does PCP produce its reinforcing effects, and why do only some individuals find the effects of PCP to be pleasurable? How does PCP produce psychotomimetic effects, and is this mechanism of action related to the neurochemical substrates underlying schizophrenia? Does PCP produce its psychotomimetic effects via its interactions with the NMDA receptor, by modifying dopaminergic neurotransmission, through other mechanisms, or by a combination of its effects on different neurochemical systems? Because PCP affects multiple neurotransmitter systems, these questions are very difficult to answer. However, as drugs only modify ongoing processes, understanding the mechanism of action of PCP may provide important information on the etiology of some forms of psychosis. The finding of specific receptors in the CNS at which PCP binds suggests that there might be an endogenous substance or substances in the brain that interact with these receptors. In agreement with such a hypothesis, endogenous PCP-like ligands obtained from brain extracts have been reported (Quirion et al., 1984; Su et al., 1986; Zukin & Zukin, 1988). A question of major importance is whether these endogenous PCP-like substances are involved in the etiology of some forms of schizophrenia; PCP might produce psychosis in normals and exacerbate symptoms in schizophrenics by mimicking the action of these endogenous factors. If these endogenous factors do exist and have pharmacological characteristics similar to PCP, hyperactivity in these systems would be expected to produce extreme behavioral disruption. Thus, a PCP antagonist could have major utility in the treatment of some forms of psychosis. Can such antagonists be developed? As Mg^{++}, Zn^{++}, glycine, and polyamines can affect neurotransmission at the NMDA receptor-channel complex, perhaps these other ''modulators'' or analogs of these substances may be useful in the treatment of some forms of psychosis.

Another area of active research centers around the NMDA receptor. There is increasing evidence that excitatory amino acids play an important role in the etiology of certain pathophysiological processes, so called ''excitotoxicity'' (Meldrum & Garthwaite, 1990; Olney, 1989). For example, high concentrations of glutamate are neurotoxic, and the excessive release of endogenous glutamate during traumatic head injury, hypoxia, seizures, or ischemic conditions, such as stroke, could lead to neuronal death. Moreover, abnormal regulation of glutaminergic systems had been hypothesized in such neurodegenerative conditions as Huntington's and Parkinson's diseases. In experimental models, pretreatment with drugs with NMDA antagonist activity, such as PCP or MK-801, have been shown to block neurodegeneration in response to ischemia. In some cases the NMDA antagonist can be given after the ischemic insult and still provide neuroprotection. Thus, these NMDA antagonists may have tremendous therapeutic potential in the treatment of stroke and neurodegenerative conditions involving excitatory amino acids. Although PCP has NMDA antagonist activity, its psychotomimetic activity would preclude its use as a neuroprotective agent. MK-801 also has been shown to have profound neuroprotective activity, but it is not known whether MK-801, like PCP, is psychotomimetic. Are there subtypes of NMDA receptors or different subunits that are differentially expressed in the brain, analogous to the $GABA_A$ receptor? Does a specific subtype of NMDA receptor mediate the psychotomimetic activity, perhaps allowing the development of subtype-selective, nonpsychotomimetic analogs? Because the behavioral and neuroprotective attributes of these compounds must be separated in order to develop useful therapeutic agents, the issue of determining the mechanism of action of the psychotomimetic activity of PCP assumes a very practical purpose.

Research on the mechanism of action of PCP has demonstrated that molecular studies must be coupled with approaches involving the entire organism. There are over 100 papers describing sigma receptor binding, yet it is still not clear which drugs are sigma agonists and which are sigma antagonists, whether the sigma binding site is a functional receptor, or whether it is only a binding site with no function or even an enzyme that can bind certain drugs. It is obvious that new clinical studies could help determine the mechanisms underlying the psychotomimetic activity of PCP and drugs with PCP-like activity, but subjecting volunteers to drug-induced dysphoria is not ethically sound. Although PCP has the potential to be an important "pharmacological bridge" to understanding the etiology of some forms of mental illness, the distance between basic molecular approaches and clinical relevance is ever increasing, and there must be a middle ground to bridge these disciplines. Understanding the mechanism of action of abused drugs can have far-ranging implications outside the arena of drug abuse. Studying the mechanisms of action of PCP, a drug that was introduced as a general anesthetic but is now a major drug of abuse, may lead to new and important discoveries in understanding the etiology and treatment of neurological and mental disorders.

REFERENCES

Abood, L.G., & Biel, J.H. (1962). Anticholinergic psychotomimetic agents. *Int. Rev. Neurobiol., 4*, 217-273.

Albuquerque, E.X., Tsai, M.C., Aronstam, R.S., Eldefrawi, A.T., & Eldefrawi, M.E. (1980). Sites of action of phencyclidine. II. Interaction with the ionic channel of the nicotinic receptor. *Mol. Pharmacol., 18*, 167-183.

Anis, N.A., Berry, S.C., Burton, N., & Lodge, D. (1983). The dissociative anesthetics ketamine and phencyclidine selectively reduce excitation of central mammalian neurons by N-methyl-aspartate. *Br. J. Pharmacol.*, *79*, 565-575.

Baily, D.N. (1987). Phencyclidine detection during toxicology testing of a university medical center patient population. *Clin. Toxicol.*, *25*, 517-526.

Balster, R.L. (1987). The behavioral pharmacology of phencyclidine. In H.Y. Meltzer (Ed.), *Psychopharmacology: The third generation of progress* (pp. 1573-1579). New York: Raven Press.

Bejanian, M., Pechnick, R.N., & George, R. (1990). Effects of acute and chronic administration of (+)-SKF 10,047 on body temperature in the rat: Cross-sensitization with phencyclidine. *J. Pharmacol. Exp. Ther.*, *253*, 1253-1258.

Bejanian, M., Pechnick, R.N., Bova, M.P., & George, R. (1991). Effects of subcutaneous and intracerebroventricular administration of the sigma-selective compound, 1,3-Di-o-tolylguanidine (DTG) on body temperature in the rat: Interactions with BMY-14802 and Rimcazole. *J. Pharmacol. Exp. Ther.*, *258*, 88-93.

Blades, R.H., Knight, A.K., & Wong, E.H.F. (1989). Identification of a sigma site in guinea-pig adrenal gland. *Br. J. Pharmacol.*, *97*, 488P.

Bowen, W.D., Kirschner, B.N., Newman, A.H., & Rice, K.C. (1988). σ Receptors negatively modulate agonist-stimulated phosphoinositide metabolism in rat brain. *Eur. J. Pharmacol.*, *149*, 399-400.

Chaudieu, I., Vignon, J., Chicheportiche, M., Kamenka, J.-M., Trouiller, G., & Chicheportiche, R. (1989). Role of the aromatic group in the inhibition of phencyclidine binding and dopamine uptake by PCP analogs. *Pharmacol. Biochem. Behav.*, *32*, 699-705.

Chavkin, C. (1990). The sigma enigma: Biochemical and functional correlates emerge for the haloperidol-sensitive sigma binding site. *Trends Pharmacol. Sci.*, *11*, 213-215.

Domino, E.F. (1964). Neurobiology of phencyclidine (Sernyl), a drug with an unusual spectrum of pharmacological activity. *Int. Rev. Neurobiol.*, *6*, 303-347.

Gorelick, D.A., Wilkins, J.N., Smith, G.B., & Derrick, B.E. (1984). Clinical and pharmacokinetic aspects of phencyclidine (PCP) abuse. *Proc. Soc. Neurosci.*, *10*, 1206.

Hernandez, A., Aurbach, S., & Hoebel, B.G. (1988). Phencyclidine (PCP) injected in the nucleus accumbens increases extracellular dopamine and serotonin as measured by microdialysis. *Life Sci.*, *42*, 1713-1723.

Itzhak, Y., & Stein, I. (1990). Sigma binding sites in the brain: An emerging concept for multiple sites and their relevance for psychiatric disorders. *Life Sci.*, *47*, 1073-1081.

Johnson, K.M. (1983). Phencyclidine: Behavioral and biochemical evidence supporting a role for dopamine. *Fed. Proc.*, *42*, 2579-2583.

Johnson, K.M., & Jones, S.M. (1990). Neuropharmacology of phencyclidine: Basic mechanisms and therapeutic potential. *Annu. Rev. Pharmacol. Toxicol.*, *30*, 707-750.

Klein, M., Canoll, P.D., & Musacchio, J.M. (1991). SKF 525-A and cytochrome P-450 ligands inhibit with high affinity the binding of [3H]dextromethorphan and σ ligands to guinea pig brain. *Life Sci.*, *48*, 543-550.

Kloog, Y., Rehavi, M., Maayani S., and Sokolovsky, M. (1977). Anticholinesterase and antiacetylcholine activity of 1-phenyl-cyclohexylamine derivatives. *Eur. J. Pharmacol.*, *45*, 221-227.

Largent, B.L., Gundlach, A.L., & Snyder, S.H. (1986). Pharmacologic and autoradiographic discrimination of sigma and phencyclidine receptor binding sites in brain with (+)-[3H]SKF 10,047, (+)-[3H]-3-[Hydroxyphenyl]-N-(1-Propyl)Piperidine and [^{3}H]-1-[1-(2-Thienyl)Cyclohexyl]Piperidine. *J. Pharmacol. Exp. Ther., 238,* 739-748.

Lodge, D., & Johnson, K.M. (1990). Noncompetitive excitatory amino acid receptor antagonists. *Trends Pharmacol. Sci., 11,* 81-86.

Lowrey, P.W., Hassig, S.E., Gunn, R.A., & Mathison, J.B. (1988). Homicide victims in New Orleans: Recent trends. *Am. J. Epidemiol., 128,* 1130-1136.

Luby, E.D., Gottlieb, J.S., Cohen, B.D., Rosenbaum, G., & Domino, E.F. (1962). Model psychosis and schizophrenia. *Am. J. Psychiat., 119,* 61-67.

Maayani, S., Weinstein, H., Cohen, S., & Sokolovsky, M. (1973). Acetylcholine-like molecular arrangement in psychotomimetic anticholinergic drugs. *Proc. Nat. Acad. Sci. USA., 70,* 3103-3107.

MacDonald, J.F., & Nowak, L.M. (1990). Mechanisms of blockade of excitatory amino acid receptor channels. *Trends Pharmacol. Sci., 11,* 167-172.

Maddox, V.H. (1981). The historical development of phencyclidine. In E.F. Domino (Ed.), *PCP (phencyclidine): Historical and current perspectives* (pp. 1-8) Ann Arbor, MI: NPP Books.

Majewska, M.D., Parameswaran, S., Vu, T., & London, E.D. (1989). Divergent ontogeny of sigma and phencyclidine binding sites in rat brain. *Dev. Brain Res., 47,* 13-18.

Martin, W.R., Eades, C.G., Thompson, J.A., Huppler, R.E., & Gilbert, P.E. (1976). The effects of morphine- and nalorphine-like drugs in the nondependent and morphine-dependent chronic spinal dog. *J. Pharmacol. Exp. Ther., 197,* 517-532.

McCann, D.J., Rabin, R.A., Rens-Domiano, S., & Winter, J.C. (1989). Phencyclidine/ SKF-10,047 binding sites: Evaluation of function. *Pharmacol. Biochem. Behav., 32,* 87-94.

Meldrum, B., & Garthwaite, J. (1990). Excitatory amino acid neurotoxicity and neurodegenerative disease. *Trends Pharmacol. Sci., 11,* 379-387.

Musacchio, J.M. (1990). The psychotomimetic effects of opiates and σ receptor. *Neuropsychopharmacology, 3,* 191-200.

Musacchio, J.M., Klein, M., & Canoll, P.D. (1989). Dextromethorphan and sigma ligands: Common sites but diverse effects. *Life Sci., 45,* 1721-1732.

Nabeshima, T., Yamaguchi, K., Hiramatsu, M., Amano, M., Furukawa, H., & Kameyama, T. (1984). Serotonergic involvement in phencyclidine-induced behaviors. *Pharmacol. Biochem. Behav., 21,* 401-408.

Nabeshima, T., Ishikawa, K., Yamaguchi, K., Furukawa, H., & Kameyama, T. (1988). Property of phencyclidine as a 5-HT$_2$ receptor agonist. In E.F. Domino & J.-M. Kamenka (Eds.), *Sigma and phencyclidine-like compounds as molecular probes in biology* (pp. 439-450). Ann Arbor, MI: NPP Books.

Olney, J.W. (1989). Excitatory amino acids and neuropsychiatric disorders. *Biol. Psychiat. 26,* 505-525.

Paleos, G.A., Yang, Z.W., & Byrd, J.C. (1990). Ontogeny of PCP and sigma receptors in rat brain. *Brain Res., 51,* 147-152.

Pechnick, R.N., & George, R. (1989). Characterization of the effects of the acute and chronic administration of phencyclidine on body temperature in the rat: Lack of evidence for the involvement of opiate receptors. *J. Pharmacol. Exp. Ther., 248,* 900-909.

Pechnick, R.N., George, R., Poland, R.E., & Lee, R.J. (1986). The effects of the acute administration of phencyclidine hydrochloride (PCP) on the release of corticosterone, growth hormone and prolactin in the rat. *Life Sci., 38,* 291-296.

Pechnick, R.N., George, R., & Poland, R.E. (1989a). Naloxone does not antagonize

PCP-induced stimulation of the pituitary-adrenal axis in the rat. *Life Sci., 44,* 143-147.

Pechnick, R.N., George, R., Poland, R.E., Hiramatsu, M., & Cho, A.K. (1989b). Characterization of the effects of the acute and chronic administration of phencyclidine on the release of adrenocorticotropin, corticosterone and prolactin: Evidence for the differential development of tolerance. *J. Pharmacol. Exp. Ther., 250,* 534-540.

Pechnick, R.N., George, R., & Poland, R.E. (1989c). Characterization of the effects of the acute and repeated administration of MK-801 on the release of adrenocorticotropin, corticosterone and prolactin in the rat. *Eur. J. Pharmacol., 164,* 257-263.

Pechnick, R.N., Wong, C.A., George, R., Thurkauf, A., Jacobson, A.E., & Rice, K.C. (1989d). Comparison of the effects of the acute administration of dexoxadrol, levoxadrol, MK-801 and phencyclidine on body temperature in the rat. *Neuropharmacology, 28,* 829-835.

Pechnick, R.N., Chun, B.M., George, R., Hanada, K., & Poland, R.E. (1990). Determination of the loci of action of phencyclidine on the CNS-pituitary-adrenal axis. *J. Pharmacol. Exp. Ther., 254,* 344-349.

Poklis, A., Maginn, D., & Barr, J.L. (1987). Drug findings in "driving under the influence of drugs" cases: A problem of illicit drug use. *Drug Alcohol Depend., 20,* 57-62.

Pradhan, S.N. (1984). Phencyclidine (PCP): Some human studies. *Neurosci. Biobehav. Rev., 8,* 493-501.

Quirion, R., Hammer, R.P. Jr., Herkenham, M., & Pert, C.B. (1981). Phencyclidine (angel dust)/σ "opiate" receptor: Visualization by tritium-sensitive film. *Proc. Nat. Acad. Sci. USA., 78,* 5881-5885.

Quirion, R., DiMaggio, D.A., French, E.D., Contreras, P.C., Shiloach, J., Pert, C.B., Everist, H., Pert, A., & O'Donohue, T.L. (1984). Evidence for an endogenous peptide ligand for the phencyclidine receptor. *Peptides, 5,* 967-973.

Quirion, R., Chicheportiche, R., Contreras, P.C., Johnson, K.M., Lodge, D., Tam, S.W., Woods, J.H., & Zukin, S.R. (1987). Classification and nomenclature of phencyclidine and sigma receptor sites. *Trends Neurosci., 10,* 444-446.

Reynolds, I.J. (1990). Modulation of NMDA receptor responsiveness by neurotransmitters, drugs and chemical modification. *Life Sci., 47,* 1785-1792.

Rothman, R.B., Reid, A., Mahoubi, A., Kim, C.-H., De Costa, B., Jacobson, A.E., & Rice, K.C. (1991). Labeling of [³H]1,3-di(2-tolyl)guanidine of two high affinity binding sites in guinea pig brain: Evidence for allosteric regulation by calcium channel antagonists and pseudoallosteric modulation by σ ligands. *Mol. Pharmacol., 39,* 222-232.

Samovilova, N.N., Nagornaya, L.V., & Vinogradov, V.A. (1988). (+)-[³H]SK&F 10,047 binding sites in rat liver. *Eur. J. Pharmacol., 147,* 259-264.

Sharkey, J., Glen, K.A., Wolfe, S., & Kuhar, M.J. (1988). Cocaine binding at σ receptors. *Eur. J. Pharmacol., 149,* 171-174.

Simonds, J.F., & Kashani, J. (1980). Specific drug use and violence in delinquent boys. *Am. J. Drug Alcohol Abuse, 7,* 305-322.

Snell, L.D., Yi, S.-J., & Johnson, K.M. (1988). Comparison of the effects of MK-801 and phencyclidine on catecholamine uptake and NMDA-induced norepinephrine release. *Eur. J. Pharmacol., 145,* 223-226.

Sonders, M.S., Keana, J.F.W., & Weber, E. (1988). Phencyclidine and psychotomimetic opiates: Recent insights into their biochemical and physiological sites of action. *Trends Neurosci., 11,* 37-40.

Steinfels, G.F., Alberici, G.P., Tam, S.W., & Cook, L. (1988). Biochemical, behavioral and electrophysiologic actions of the selective sigma receptor ligand (+)-penta-zocine. *Neuropsychopharmacology, 1*, 321-327.

Su, T.-P., Weissman, A.D., & Yeh, S.-Y. (1986). Endogenous ligands for sigma opioid receptors in the brain ("sigmaphin"): Evidence from binding assays. *Life Sci., 38*, 2199-2210.

Su, T.-P., London, E.D., & Jaffe, J.H. (1988). Steroid binding at σ receptors suggests a link between endocrine, nervous and immune systems. *Science, 240*, 219-221.

Tonge, S.R., and Leonard, B.E. (1969). The effects of some hallucinogenic drugs on the metabolism of 5-hydroxytryptamine in the brain. *Life Sci., 8*, 805-814.

Vargas, H.M., & Pechnick, R.N. (1991). Binding affinity and antimuscarinic activity of σ and phencyclidine receptor ligands. *Eur. J. Pharmacol., 195*, 151-156.

Vincent, J.P., Cavey, D., Kamenka, J.M., Geneste, P., & Lazdunski, M. (1978). Inter-action of phencyclidines with the muscarinic and opiate receptors in the central nervous system. *Brain Res., 152*, 176-182.

Vincent, J.P., Kartalovski, B., Geneste, P., Kamenka, J.M., & Lazdunski, M. (1979). Interaction of phencyclidine ("angel dust") with a specific receptor in rat brain membranes. *Proc. Nat. Acad. Sci. USA., 76*, 4678-4682.

Walker, J.M., Bowen, W.D., Walker, F.O., Matsumoto, R.R., De Costa, B., & Rice, K.C. (1990). Sigma receptors: Biology and function. *Pharmacol. Rev., 42*, 355-403.

Willetts, J., Balster, R.L., & Leander, J.D. (1990). The behavioral pharmacology of NMDA receptor antagonists. *Trends Pharmacol. Sci., 11*, 423-428.

Wolfe, S.A. Jr., Kulsakdinun, C., Battaglia, G., Jaffe, J.H., & De Souza, E.B. (1988). Initial identification and characterization of sigma receptors on human peripheral blood leukocytes. *J. Pharmacol. Exp. Ther., 247*, 1114-1119.

Wolfe, S.A. Jr., Culp, S.G., & De Souza, E.B. (1989). σ-Receptors in endocrine organs: Identification, characterization, and autoradiographic localization in rat pitui-tary, adrenal testis and ovary. *Endocrinology, 124*, 1160-1172.

Wong, E.H.F., Knight, A.R., & Woodruff, G.N. (1988). [³H]MK-801 labels a site on the N-methyl-D-aspartate receptor channel complex in rat brain membranes. *J. Neurochem., 50*, 274-281.

Yago, K.B., Pitts, F.N. Jr., Burgoyne, R.W., Aniline, O., Yago, L.S., & Pitts, A.F. (1981). The urban epidemic of phencyclidine (PCP) use: Clinical and laboratory evidence from a public psychiatric hospital emergency service. *J. Clin. Psy-chiat., 42*, 193-196.

Zukin, S.R., & Zukin, R.S. (1979). Specific [³H]phencyclidine binding in rat central nervous system. *Proc. Nat. Acad. Sci. USA., 76*, 5372-5376.

Zukin, R.S., & Zukin, S.R. (1981). Demonstration of [³H]cyclazocine binding to multi-ple opiate receptor sites. *Mol. Pharmacol., 20*, 246-254.

Zukin, R.S., & Zukin, S.R. (1988). Phencyclidine, σ and NMDA receptors: Emerging concepts. In E.F. Domino & J.-M. Kalenka (Eds.), *Sigma and phencyclidine-like compounds as molecular probes in biology* (pp. 407-424). Ann Arbor, MI: NPP Books.

19

Ice: d-Methamphetamine Hydrochloride

ARTHUR K. CHO

Ice is one of the street names for methamphetamine hydrochloride, an amphetamine analog that has been abused for several decades. This and its other name, crystal, are based on the ice-like crystal structure of the drug. In the late 1980s, there was a resurgence of its abuse in Hawaii and Japan, which led to the concern that ice would be the "drug of the 1990s". Fortunately, that concern does not seem to have materialized in the continental United States, but methamphetamine abuse in Hawaii is serious enough to be considered its major drug problem. This chapter reviews the pharmacology, pharmacokinetics, and chemistry of the amphetamines in general, with particular emphasis on methamphetamine.

Amphetamine is phenyl isopropylamine (1), a lipophilic substance with sympathomimetic properties. Its lipophilicity allows it free access to the brain, and its isopropyl amine structure renders it resistant to the actions of monoamine oxidase. Amphetamine was used therapeutically as a nasal decongestant and as an anorexic agent before its use as a drug of abuse. These applications resulted in the generation of a series of related compounds that were also sold as anorexics or as decongestants. The structures of some of these compounds are shown in Figure 19-1. Methamphetamine (2) is an N-methyl derivative with reduced polarity, giving it more potent CNS actions. The isopropylamines all contain a chiral center adjacent to the amine function, and the compounds exhibit an enantioselectivity with respect to this center. The S (+) configuration for amphetamine is the more potent one, and many of the commercial preparations are enantiometrically pure. Ephedrine (3) differs from methamphetamine in its benzylic hydroxyl group. This compound is a natural product extracted from plants as a pure enantiomer. It is also a sympathomimetic, but because of its greater polarity, has weaker CNS effects. It is currently available as a bronchodilator and nasal decongestant.

One of the properties of methamphetamine hydrochloride that is of interest from the perspective of abuse is its volatility. Although most amine salts are not volatile and decompose at high temperatures, the hydrochloride salt of methamphetamine is sufficiently volatile that it can be smoked (Chiang & Hawks, 1990). Thus, abusers can use this compound in a manner similar to the crack

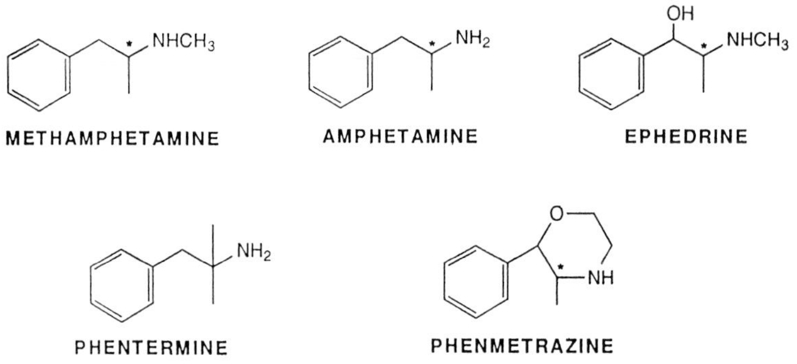

METHAMPHETAMINE   AMPHETAMINE   EPHEDRINE

PHENTERMINE   PHENMETRAZINE

Figure 19-1. Structures of phenylisopropylamines related to amphetamine. The asterisks are adjacent to chiral centers.

form of cocaine, with similar pharmacological and toxicological consequences. When inhaled in the vapor state, these drugs enter the plasma compartment almost as rapidly as they do after intravenous administration (Jeffcoat et al., 1989). The resulting rapid rise in brain levels causes the "rush" or intense euphoria that is sought by abusers.

PHARMACOLOGY

Amphetamine and its congeners are indirectly acting sympathomimetic agents. They have little or no action on sympathetic receptors and stimulate the sympathetic nervous system indirectly by increasing synaptic neurotransmitter concentration. This action occurs both in the central and peripheral nervous systems, but different derivatives seem to vary in their selectivities. For example, methamphetamine seems to be more potent than amphetamine in its central actions (Weiner, 1985). In their central actions, the amphetamines are stimulants; they increase general awakeness, give an increased sense of energy and self-confidence, and permit the individual to perform repetitive tasks with minimal boredom. These actions have led to their abuse by truck drivers, combat pilots during World War II, and students studying for exams. The compounds also cause anorexia and have been used to control appetite. In addition, the amphetamines induce a sense of euphoria that is sought by abusers. In the periphery, the sympathomimetic actions increase heart rate and blood pressure and cause vasoconstriction. The ability to cause vasoconstriction is the basis for its use as a nasal decongestant. When amphetamine was sold over the counter as a decongestant in nasal inhalers, abusers were known to extract the matrix containing the drug to obtain it.

The actions of amphetamine on the CNS are thought to be dominated by dopamine systems, whereas the peripheral actions are primarily on the norepinephrine system. The neurochemical basis for these actions is an exchange diffusion process (Fischer & Cho, 1979; Raiteri et al., 1979; Rutledge, 1978) involving components of the presynaptic catecholamine terminals (Fig. 19-2).

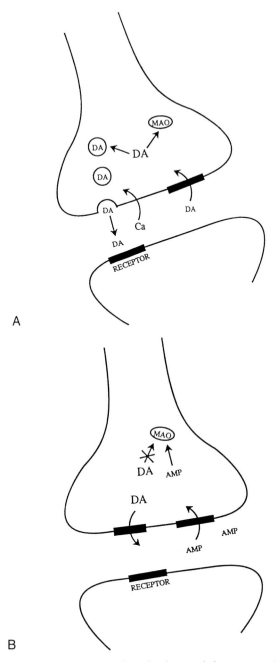

Figure 19-2. **A,** Depolarization-induced release of dopamine. The neurotransmitter is stored in vesicles that fuse with the plasma membrane and release their contents by a calcium-dependent process. The cytoplasmic concentration of dopamine (DA) is normally controlled by the uptake into vesicles and by degradation by monoamine oxidase (MAO). **B,** Amphetamine-induced release. Amphetamine (AMP) is taken up into the terminal by the carrier where it inhibits monoamine oxidase and increases cytoplasmic dopamine. The cytoplasmic dopamine is transported out into the synapse by the transporter.

In normal depolarization-induced stimulation of catecholamine neurons, the storage vesicles that contain neurotransmitter attach to the neuronal membrane and release their contents into the synapse by exocytosis through a calcium ion-dependent mechanism. However, amphetamine and other indirect agents act by a different mechanism as they do not require calcium ion to effect their release action (Katz & Kopin, 1969; Paton, 1973). These compounds are substrates for the neuronal uptake transporter and bind to the carrier, causing it to translocate to the interior of the terminal where it releases the bound drug. Amphetamine is a competitive inhibitor of monoamine oxidase (Arai et al., 1990; Miller et al., 1980) and thereby increases cytoplasmic catecholamine. This cytoplasmic catecholamine binds to the inward facing carrier and is transported into the synapse. Once outside, the catecholamine activates the postsynaptic receptor, but is not taken back up because of the presence of amphetamine. Amphetamines have minimal activity at the postsynaptic receptor, and all of the response is due to released neurotransmitter. Thus, there is an increase in synaptic neurotransmitter concentration by a process that is independent of calcium ion and that is sensitive to inhibitors of neuronal uptake. This mechanism of amphetamine action was proposed on the basis of in vitro experiments with peripheral (Paton, 1973) and brain tissue (Fischer & Cho, 1979; Raiteri, 1979; Rutledge, 1978). Brain tissue release studies wth synaptosomes preloaded with 3Hdopamine showed that d-amphetamine was about four times more potent than 1-amphetamine and that methamphetamine was slightly more active than d-amphetamine (Fischer & Cho, 1979). Although this exchange diffusion model was consistent with in vitro observations, it was only recently that investigators demonstrated its validity in vivo. In separate studies, Butcher et al. (1990) and Hurd and Ungerstedt (1989), using in vivo microdialysis techniques, demonstrated that the increase in extracellular dopamine in the striatum of cats caused by amphetamine was unaffected by calcium ion removal from the perfusing fluid and that the actions of amphetamine could be inhibited by nomifensine, an inhibitor of the dopamine transporter. In contrast, cocaine-induced increase in extracellular dopamine, which is thought to be only due to inhibition of reuptake, was reduced with calcium ion reduction.

A severe form of abuse is the so-called speed run, during which the abuser self-administers the drug repeatedly over a period of as long as 10 days (Kramer et al., 1967). During this time the subject is seeking the flash or euphoria associated with the rapid change in brain levels of the drug, and in the past the drug was administered intravenously. In the course of a run, a tolerance develops, and the dose steadily increases to as high as 1-5 grams per injection. Toward the end of a run, dysphoria and in some instances a psychosis develops. At this stage, these individuals can also become violent and dangerous. Tolerance to the peripheral sympathomimetic effects has been attributed to the formation of p-hydroxynorephedrine during metabolism (Brodie et al., 1970; Clay et al., 1971; Thoa et al., 1975). This compound can act as a false transmitter and be accumulated by norepinephrine (and possibly dopamine) nerve endings. When amphetamine exerts it action on the nerve terminal, the p-hydroxynorephedrine is released, and as it is a much weaker agonist than norepinephrine, its actions on the terminal are substantially weaker. Although the peripheral tolerance may be consistent with this mechanism, the central tolerance is not yet explained (Lewander, 1977). In fact, the stereotypy response, one of the behavioral paradigms of amphetamine action, is enhanced after repeated administration (Segal & Schuckit, 1983).

PHARMACOKINETICS AND METABOLISM

Amphetamine and methamphetamine have half-lives of about 10-15 hours (Davis et al., 1971; Vree & Van Rossum, 1970) in humans. Significant levels (approximately 30%) of unchanged drug are eliminated in the urine of human subjects given small doses of the drug (Dring et al., 1970), and changes in urine pH alter the plasma half-life of the drug as would be expected (Davis et al., 1971). The volume of distribution has been estimated to be in the range of 3 to 14 L/kg (Vree & Van Rossum, 1970). Studies with rats in our laboratories have generated the pharmacokinetics shown in Figure 19-3, and as can be seen, methamphetamine and amphetamine have very similar pharmacokinetic properties in this species.

Metabolism of the amphetamines follows three major routes—oxidation of the carbon attached to the nitrogen or deamination, oxidation of the nitrogen, and oxidation of the aromatic ring (Fig. 19-4). Because the ring oxidation pathway is the more relevant from a pharmacological perspective, this chapter focuses on it. More general reviews of amphetamine metabolism have been published (Cho & Wright, 1978; Yamada & Yoshimura, 1989). p-Hydroxylation of the aromatic ring to p-hydroxyamphetamine (5) generates a pharmacologi-

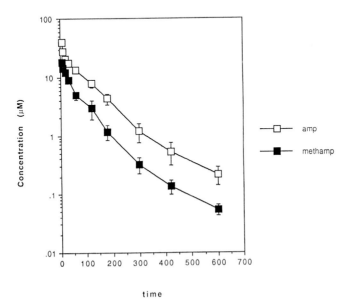

Figure 19-3. Plasma concentration of amphetamine (□) and methamphetamine (■) after intravenous administration of equimolar doses (~10 mg/kg) to separate groups of rats.

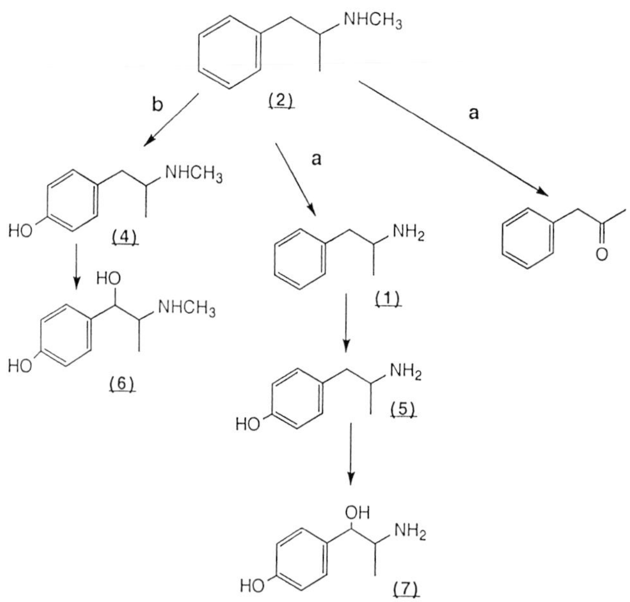

Figure 19-4. Metabolism of methamphetamine. Three pathways are shown. Two reactions involve oxidation of the carbon atom attached to nitrogen (a), and one involves hydroxylation of the aromatic ring. N-hydroxylation also occurs, but is not shown.

cally active species. This compound and its beta hydroxylated derivative, p-hydroxynorephedrine (7), can deplete catecholamines from peripheral tissue (Clay et al., 1971; Katz & Kopin, 1969) and have been proposed as the false transmitters involved in the tolerance associated with repeated amphetamine administration (Brodie et al., 1970; Katz & Kopin, 1969). p-Hydroxyamphetamine also releases dopamine from synaptosomes prepared from cortex and striatum of rats (Cho et al., 1977) so that if significant levels are in the brain, it could contribute to the pharmacology of the parent compound. The p-hydroxylation pathway is a major pathway in rats but only a minor one in humans (Caldwell et al., 1972; Dring et al., 1970). p-Hydroxy-methamphetamine and amphetamine, however, have relatively short half-lives when given directly (Hiramatsu et al., unpublished observations). p-Hydroxylation of amphetamine is a somewhat unusual metabolic reaction as it exhibits substrate inhibition when examined in vitro (Jonsson, 1974). More recent studies on this reaction have confirmed its formation by a constitutive cytochrome P450 (Baba, 1988) that is not inducible. There are significant species differences in the metabolism of amphetamine (Caldwell et al., 1972; Dring et al., 1970) so that the importance of the different pathways varies with species. In the rat, p-hydroxy metabolites are the major urinary metabolites after amphetamine and methamphetamine injection (Fig. 19-5), whereas in humans, pathways leading to benzoic acid seem to dominate. Plasma amphetamine concentrations are approximately two times those of methamphetamine when the amines are given to rats. The lower

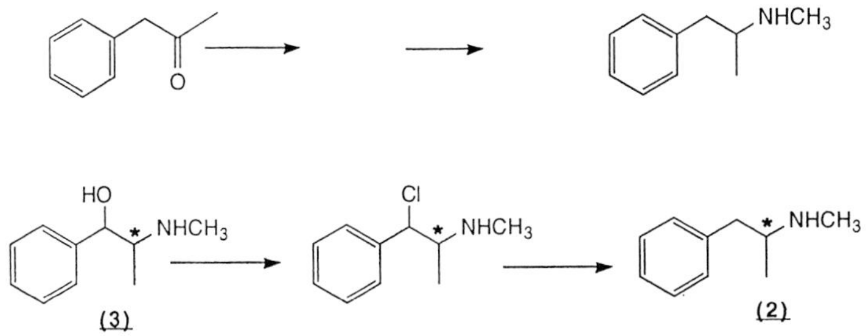

Figure 19-5. Synthesis of methamphetamine. The first reaction involves a condensation between phenyl acetone and methyl amine. The second reaction is a reduction of ephedrine. Note that the second reaction retains the stereochemistry of the alpha carbon.

methamphetamine concentration probably reflects the greater distribution of this more lipophilic derivative.

CHEMICAL PROPERTIES

Unlike cocaine, which is obtained only from plants, amphetamines can be readily synthesized from available chemicals. However, the synthesis of (+)methamphetamine seems to utilize ephedrine, a natural product. Thus, there are two general pathways for methamphetamine synthesis (Soine, 1986). One pathway also can be used to synthesize amphetamine and is based on condensation reactions with phenylacetone or phenylacetic acid, compounds that are readily available. These reactions, however, involve the carbon adjacent to the nitrogen and result in the preparation of the racemic mixture of the drug that is less potent than the pure enantiomer. In addition, because of the nature of the reactions, there is a greater possibility for contamination (Kramm & Kruegel, 1977). This pathway seems to be the more common one used by illicit manufacturers in the continental United States, and the samples confiscated have varied in purity from 20 to 80%. The preparation of ice that is abused in Hawaii and in Japan seems to be synthesized from ephedrine obtained from its plant source as the enantiomerically pure form and is converted to S (+)methamphetamine by reduction of the benzylic hydroxyl function. This reaction does not involve a condensation and yields a much purer product. The synthesis of the material entering Hawaii is thought to take place in the Far East, notably Taiwan and Korea. Thus, the methamphetamine abused as ice is a purer form of the drug and consists of the more active enantiomer.

SUMMARY

The abuse of amphetamines has a long history. The drugs are sought for their stimulant actions and for their euphoric effects. The recent surge in their abuse includes a novel route of administration that, from a drug abuse perspective, could be potentially worse than crack. When inhaled in the vapor state, the drug enters the bloodstream and the brain rapidly and at high concentrations in a manner analogous to inhaled cocaine. The CNS effects of cocaine and amphetamine are so similar that subjects are unable to distinguish them after intravenous dosage. The major difference between the two compounds is the substantially longer half-life of amphetamine. With a longer half-life, the possibility of toxicity is greater, and the incidence of amphetamine psychoses associated with a "speed run" is also greater. Although amphetamine has not replaced cocaine, the possibility exists that if cocaine interdiction becomes more successful, the ease of amphetamine synthesis will result in its increased abuse.

REFERENCES

Arai, Y., Kim, S.K., Kinemuchi, H., Tadano, T., Satoh, S.E., Satoh, N., & Kisara, K. (1990). Inhibition of brain type A monoamine oxidase and 5-hydroxytryptamine uptake by two amphetamine metabolites, p-hydroxyamphetamine and p-hydroxynorephedrine. *J. Neurochem., 55*, 403-408.

Baba, T., Yamada, H., Oguri, K., & Yoshimura, H. (1988). Participation of cytochrome P450 isozymes in N-demethylation, N-hydroxylation, and aromatic hydroxylation of methamphetamine. *Xenobiotica, 18*, 475-484.

Butcher, S.P., Fairbrother, I.S., Kelly, J.S., & Arbuthnott, G.W. (1990). Effects of selective monoamine oxidase inhibitors on the in vivo release and metabolism of dopamine in the rat striatum. *J. Neurochem., 55*, 981-988.

Brodie, B.B., Cho, A.K., & Gessa, G.L. (1970). Possible role of p-hydroxynorephedrine in the depletion of norephedrine induced by d-amphetamine in tolerance to this drug. In E. Costa & S. Garranti (Eds.), *Amphetamines and related compounds* (pp. 217-230). New York: Raven Press.

Caldwell, J., Dring, L.G., & Williams, R.T. (1972). Metabolism of 14c methamphetamine in man, the guinea pig, and the rat. *Biochem. J., 129*, 11-22.

Chiang, N., Hawks, R.L. (1990). *Pyrolysis studies–cocaine, phencycline, heroin and methamphetamine*. Technical Review Brief, NIDA.

Cho, A.K., & Wright, J. (1978). Minireview: Pathways of metabolism of amphetamine and related compounds. *Life Sci., 22*, 363-372.

Cho, A.K., Fischer, J.F., & Schaeffer, J.C. (1977). The accumulation of p-hydroxyamphetamine by brain homogenates and its role in release of catecholamines. *Biochem. Pharmacol., 26*, 1367-1372.

Clay, G.A., Cho, A.K., & Roberfroid, M. (1971). Effect of diethylaminoethyl diphenylpropylacetate hydrochloride (SKF-525A) on the norepinephrine-depleting actions of d-amphetamine. *Biochem. Pharmacol., 20*, 1821-1831.

Davis, J.M., Kopin, I.J., Lemberger, L., & Axelrod, J. (1971). Effects of urinary pH on amphetamine metabolism. *Ann. N.Y. Acad. Sci.*, 493-501.

Dring, L.G., Smith, R.L., & Williams, R.T. (1970). The metabolic fate of amphetamine in man and other species. *Biochem. J., 116*, 425-435.

Fischer, J.F., & Cho, A.K. (1979). Chemical release of dopamine from striatal homogenates: Evidence for an exchange diffusion model. *J. Pharmacol. Exp. Ther., 208*, 203-209.

Griffith, J.D. (1977). Amphetamine dependence; Clinical features. In W. R. Martin (Ed.), *Drug addiction II: Amphetamine, psychotogen and marihuana dependence*. (pp. 277-296). Berlin: Springer-Verlag.

Hurd, Y.L., & Ungerstedt, U. (1989). Cocaine: An in vivo microdialysis evaluation of its acute action on dopamine transmission in rat striatum. *Syanapse, 3*, 48-54.

Jeffcoat, A.R., Perez-Reyes, M., Hill, J.M., Sadler, B.M., & Cook, C.E. (1989). Cocaine disposition in humans after intravenous injection, nasal insufflation (snorting) or smoking. *Drug. Metab. Disp., 17*, 153-159.

Jonsson, J.A. (1974). Hydroxylation of amphetamine to prahydroxyamphetamine by rat liver microsomes. *Biochem. Pharmacol., 23*, 3191-3197.

Katz, R.I., & Kopin, I.J. (1969). Release of norepinephrine-^{3}H and serotonin-^{3}H evoked from brain slices by electrical field stimulation, calcium dependency and the effects of lithium, ouabain and tetrodotoxin. *Biochem. Pharmacol., 18*, 1935-1939.

Kramer, J.C., Fischman, V.S., & Littlefield, D.C. (1967). Amphetamine abuse: Pattern effects of high doses taken intravenously. *JAMA, 201*, 305.

Kramm, T.C., & Kruegel, A.V. (1977). The identification of impurities in illicit methamphetamine exhibits by gas chromatography/mass spectroscopy and nuclear magnetic resonance spectroscopy. *J. Forensic Sci., 22*, 40, 1977.

Lewander, T. (1977). Effects of amphetamine in animals. In W.R. Martin (Ed.), *Drug addiction II: Amphetamine, psychotogen and marihuana dependence* (pp. 33-181). Berlin: Springer-Verlag.

Miller, H.H., Parkhurst, A., Shore, A., Clark, D.E. (1980). In vivo monoamine oxidase inhibition by d-amphetamine. *Biochem. Pharmacol., 29*, 1347-1354.

Paton, D.M. (1973). Mechanisms of efflux of noradrenaline from adrenergic nerves in rabbit atria. *Br. J. Pharmacol., 49*, 614-627.

Raiteri, M., Cerrito, F., Cervoni, A.M., & Levi, G. (1979). Dopamine can be released by two mechanisms differentially affected by the dopamine transport inhibitor nomifensine. *J. Pharmacol. Exp. Ther., 208*, 195-0227.

Rutledge, C.O. (1978). Effect of metabolic inhibitors and ouabain on amphetamine- and potassium-induced release of biogenic amines from isolated brain tissue. *Biochem. Pharmacol., 27*, 511-516.

Segal, D.S., & Schuckit, M.A. (1983). Animal models of stimulant-induced psychosis. In I. Creese (Ed.), *Stimulants: Neurochemical, behavioral, and clinical perspectives* (pp. 131-168). New York: Raven Press.

Soine, W.H. (1986). Clandestine drug synthesis. *Med. Res. Rev., 6*, 41-74.

Thoa, N.B., Wooten, G.F., Axelrod, J., & Kopin, I.J. (1975). On the mechanism of release of norepinephrine from sympathetic nerves induced by depolarizing agents and sympathomimetic drugs. *Mol. Pharmacol., 11*, 10-18.

Vree, T.B., & Van Rossum, J.M. (1970). Kinetics of metabolism and excretion of amphetamines in man. In E. Costa & S. Garattini (Eds.), *Amphetamines and related compounds* (pp. 165-170). New York: Raven Press.

Weiner, N. (1985). Norepinephrine, epinephrine, and the sympathomimetic amines. In A.G. Gilman, L.S. Goodman, T.W. Rall, & F. Murad (Eds.), *The pharmacological basis of therapeutics*. (pp. 145-180). New York: Macmillan Publishing Company.

Yamada, H., & Yoshimura, H. (1989). Metabolism of amphetamine, methamphetamine and the related compounds. *Biochem. Aspects-Eisei Kagaku, 35*, 383-396.

20

Neuropharmacology of Ethanol

STEVEN J. HENRIKSEN

The cellular mechanisms of ethanol intoxication, reinforcement, and abuse remain obscure despite several decades of research on the pharmacological actions of ethanol in the CNS (for review, see Bloom, 1987; Galanter, 1987; Goldstein, 1983; Klemm, 1990; Rabin et al., 1987; Shefner, 1990; Siggins et al., 1987a). A view is emerging that the intoxicating effects of ethanol, including its behavioral reinforcing properties, reflect actions on a variety of neural circuits harboring numerous transmitters (see Chapter 1). This conceptualization coincides with a growing appreciation that ethanol does not have any single dominant pharmacological action, as comparisons of its biochemical and electrophysiological effects indicate.

Indeed, ethanol differs from most abusable drugs in several ways. First, it does not seem to interact selectively with any specific CNS macromolecule (protein or lipid) that would imbue it with pharmacological specificity. Second, ethanol is not derived from an organic alkaloid precursor and does not employ classical ligand-receptor interactions for its pharmacological effects. Third, ethanol's low pharmacological potency and diverse pharmacological profile suggest that its acute behavioral effects result from perturbations of several transmitter systems. Nevertheless, ethanol has surprisingly specific effects on behavior. Electrophysiological analyses of brain areas sensitive to intoxicating doses of ethanol (in the range of 100-200 mg% blood ethanol levels) suggest that transmitter hierarchies in ethanol-sensitive brain areas may give specificity to ethanol pharmacology. In addition, the actions of ethanol are likely to vary as a function of the regional neuronal template.

ETHANOL NEUROPHARMACOLOGY: AN UPDATE

Ethanol stands out as the drug of abuse for which least is known about the pharmacological mechanisms responsible for its intoxicating effects. Histori-

This work was supported by grants from the NIAAA (AA 07365) and NIDA (DA 00131) S.J.H.

cally classed as a general anesthetic, ethanol is generally regarded as exerting its major effects on behavior through its actions on biophysical processes in the brain (Goldstein, 1987). No specific neuronal "recognition site" is thought to mediate ethanol's pharmacological effects. Yet, dose-dependent effects of ethanol are observed on neurochemical (Gonzales & Hoffman, 1991), electrophysiological (Shefner, 1990), and behavioral measures (Koob and Bloom, 1988), similar to the presumed receptor-mediated effects of other drugs of abuse.

These observations reinforce the view that behaviorally active doses of ethanol exert their effects by altering neuronal synaptic efficacy. However, controversy surrounds the interpretation of studies of the interaction between ethanol and the numerous possible neurotransmitters in the brain (see Chapter 1). Recently, three neurotransmitters have received considerable attention as candidates for mediating the acute intoxicating effects of ethanol assessed by either behavioral or electrophysiological techniques. These are gamma-amino butyric acid (GABA), glutamate (via the N-methyl-d-aspartate receptor), and dopamine. Although this list is not likely to be inclusive, these substances serve to illustrate some recent advances in ethanol neuropharmacology. For a more comprehensive discussion of the effects of ethanol on central neurotransmission, the reader is directed to other reviews (e.g., Shefner, 1990).

GABA and Ethanol

For many years, GABA-mediated processes have been thought to underlie the acute sedating and anesthetic actions of ethanol (Allan & Harris, 1987; Hunt, 1985; Liljequist & Engel, 1982; Martz et al., 1983). Some recent neurochemical and behavioral studies support this contention. For example, ethanol has been reported to enhance GABA-stimulated chloride flux in subfractionated brain homogenates called synaptoneurosomes (Suzdak et al., 1986a, 1986b, 1988) and in cultured spinal neurons (Celentano et al., 1988; Mehta & Ticku, 1988; Ticku et al., 1986). Evidence that most of these effects could be mimicked or enhanced by GABA$_A$ agonists and reversed by GABA$_A$-selective antagonists suggested that the effect of ethanol on GABA receptors was mediated through the GABA$_A$-benzodiazepine receptor complex (Mehta & Ticku, 1988, 1990). However, because behavioral studies are indirect measures of ethanol neuropharmacology and because other neurochemical studies failed to show ethanol-induced enhancements in chloride conductance in the absence of GABA or GABA analogs (Allan & Harris, 1987; Shefner, 1990), neuropharmacologists turned to electrophysiological models to analyze the central actions of ethanol.

In Vitro Electrophysiological Studies

Most in vitro electrophysiological investigations of the acute effects of ethanol have not strongly implicated GABA mechanisms. Although ethanol increases responses of putative GABA circuits and/or to local application of GABA in spinal cord (Celentano et al., 1988; Davidoff, 1973; Gruol, 1982) and in dorsal root ganglion neurons (Nishio & Narahashi, 1990), most studies using in vitro preparations of CNS system tissue, including the nucleus locus ceruleus (Osmanovic & Shefner, 1990), have failed to show such enhancement of GABA transmission (Bloom & Siggins, 1987, Shefner, 1990). Studies focusing on GABA neuropharmacology after ethanol application in the hippocampal slice or cultured neuron preparation have failed uniformly to document an augmentation of GABAergic function (Carlen et al., 1982; Harrison et al., 1987; Siggins et al., 1987a; Takada et al., 1987). These in vitro results were obtained despite the known sensitivity of the hippocampus to the effects of ethanol in behavioral and electrophysiological studies in the intact brain (Dolce & Decker, 1972; Grupp, 1980; Grupp & Perlanski, 1979; Klemm, 1980; Klemm et al., 1976).

In Vivo Electrophysiological Studies

Although ethanol has been shown to enhance electrophoretically applied GABA in neocortical neurons of the anesthetized cat (Nestoros, 1980), other studies in the anesthetized rat employing electrophoresis of GABA in hippocampal neurons (Bloom & Siggins, 1987; Mancillas et al., 1986) or cerebellar Purkinje cells (Harris & Sinclair, 1984; Palmer and Hoffer, 1990; Siggins et al., 1987a, 1987b) have not demonstrated a consistent enhancement of GABAergic function.

Yet, other in vivo studies have pointed to a link between GABA processes and the acute effects of ethanol in low doses. Early studies of presynaptic inhibitory processes assessed in the feline spinal cord and gracilus and cuneatus nuclei indicated ethanol-induced enhancement of this GABA-mediated process (Banna, 1969; Miyahara et al., 1966). Ethanol has also been shown to increase recurrent inhibition of dorsal motor neurons mediated by GABAergic recurrent pathways (Meyer-Lohman et al., 1972). Ethanol potentiated the inhibitory effects of electrophoretically applied GABA, but not of serotonin, dopamine, or glycine in feline cortical neurons (Nestoros, 1980).

Thus, for both in vitro and in vivo preparations, tests of the hypothesis that the effect of intoxicating doses of ethanol is to enhance, selectively, the action of GABA at central synapses have produced mixed results. However, data recently obtained in my laboratory may partially resolve these divergent results. Using lightly halothane-anesthetized rats, we observed that intoxicating doses of ethanol (75-150 mg% Blood Alcohol Level) resulted in an early and selective enhancement of GABA-mediated, recurrent neuron-induced inhibition elicited in the dentate gyrus of the hippocampus (Wiesner & Henriksen, 1987). These studies evaluated the effects of systemically administered ethanol on afferent stimulation to the dentate gyrus that would evoke field population spikes. These evoked "field" events are believed to be the synchronous discharge of a number of individual neurons due to their simultaneous activation by common afferents. Using a condition-test stimulation paradigm, we were able to pair stimuli so that the second stimulus of the pair (delivered from 10-40 ms after the first stimulus) would evoke a population spike much smaller than the first stimulus (Fig. 20.1).

This so-called paired-pulse inhibition is produced by recurrent GABAergic neurons activated by the afferent stimulation of granule cells (Andersen et al., 1964a & b). In the dentate gyrus, glutamate decarboxylase immunoreactivity

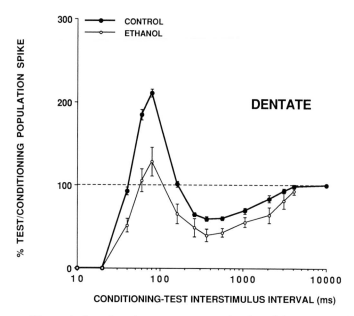

Figure 20-1. Effects of ethanol on dentate gyrus paired-pulse inhibition. Paired-pulse (PP) responses are expressed as percent test/conditioning population spike amplitudes (at 0.5 maximum stimulus level) as a function of interstimulus interval. Dentate control PP responses revealed a triphasic oscillation of inhibition/potentiation/inhibition. Intraperitoneal increased early PP inhibition, and ethanol produced a small but significant increase in late PP inhibition. CA1 control PP responses (data not shown) revealed a biphasic oscillation of inhibition/potentiation. The inhibitory phase was more prolonged and the potentiation phase less robust than corresponding phases observed in the dentate. Points on dentate control, ethanol curves represent n = 14.

found in neurons in a distinct band adjacent to the granule cell layer provides evidence that many of these cells are also GABAergic inhibitory interneurons (Ribak et al., 1978; Seress & Ribak, 1983; Storm-Mathisen, 1977). Anatomical studies have revealed numerous cell types in the hilar region of the dentate (Amaral, 1978; Ramon y Cajal, 1911), and electrophysiological studies have demonstrated at least two interneuron types distinguished by their location and by their response to afferent input (Kawaguchi & Hama, 1987; Misgeld & Frotscher, 1986; Sharfman et al., 1988; Steffensen & Henriksen, 1992).

We recently investigated the action of systemically administered ethanol on the spontaneous and evoked extracellular activity of these putative GABA interneurons. Using rigorous selection criteria (Lee et al., 1979), we recorded from individual putative interneurons of the dentate gyrus before and after the administration of intoxicating doses of ethanol. The most significant action of ethanol on these interneurons was to enhance the excitability of the recorded cell to afferent stimulation during the rising phase of blood ethanol. This altered excitability resulted in a greater number of unit discharges per stimulus. It was during this time that the greatest enhancement of paired-pulse inhibition was observed (Fig. 20-2).

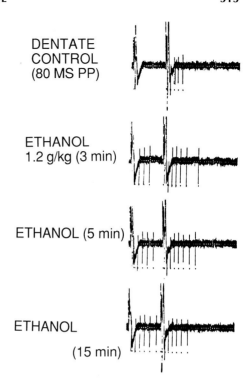

DENTATE
CONTROL
(80 MS PP)

ETHANOL
1.2 g/kg (3 min)

ETHANOL (5 min)

ETHANOL
(15 min)

Figure 20-2. Interneurons in the dentate: selective actions of ethanol. Effects of ethanol on dentate post-field potential evoked interneuron discharges. In this representative cell, four interneuron discharges are seen in the control trace after the second of paired shocks to the perforant path (80 ms interstimulus interval). After 1.2 g/kg of intraperitoneal ethanol, single-unit discharges appeared after the first shock and increased in number after the second shock. The time to onset of effect was 3-5 minutes, with the peak effect occurring at 20-30 minutes and with recovery after 2 hours.

Similar studies of the dorsal hippocampus (area CA1) demonstrated virtually identical effects of ethanol. These studies confirm and extend the reported action of prototypical benzodiazepines on CA1 interneurons previously studied by Lee, Dunwiddie, and Hoffer (1979). However, paired-pulse field potential curves obtained in CA1 after afferent stimulation (Schaffer collateral or commissural inputs) are not enhanced by ethanol, perhaps suggesting important regional differences in the effect of ethanol that are reflected in the in vitro data discussed above. Significantly, at optimal stimulation currents, dentate gyrus inhibition of the test population spike is at its maximum for only 20-30 ms, whereas in the dorsal hippocampus, maximal inhibition has a duration of over 100 ms, well beyond the effective range of $GABA_A$-mediated events. This finding suggests that, even though the dentate gyrus and dorsal hippocampus may have the same recurrent GABAergic circuitry, intrinsic membrane properties, as well as the non-GABA circuitry of the neurons in each area, dictate different responses to ethanol as a function of the exact level of cellular analysis.

Our data serve to clarify some of the contradictory evidence of GABAergic involvement in the action of ethanol, at least in the hippocampus. If GABA interneurons are selectively enhanced in their excitability after acute, intoxicating doses of ethanol as our data suggest, then one might not find an ethanol-induced increased sensitivity of postsynaptic GABA receptors to exogenously applied GABA as previously discussed (Mancillas et al., 1986; Shefner, 1990). Conversely, our studies support the strong, albeit indirect, behavioral and neurochemical data suggesting GABA involvement in the intoxicating pharmacology of ethanol. Our ethanol-induced, selective increase in interneuron excitability in both hippocampal areas studied is likely to give rise to a stimulus-induced, axon potential-dependent increase in the amount of GABA released by these interneurons. Thus, one would observe a stimulus-dependent, time-locked increase in endogenously released GABA, the postsynaptic effect of which would be greater than before the ethanol administration. These interneuron-derived events would give rise to an increase in poststimulus inhibition, which is exactly what we have observed in the dentate gyrus after low doses of ethanol in both the freely moving and anesthetized rat (Steffensen & Henriksen, 1992).

The data we obtained from the CA1 region interneurons illustrate another important point. Although the effect of ethanol on interneuron excitability in this area is qualitatively similar to what we observed in the dentate, the resulting effect on principal cell (the CA1 pyramidal cell) excitability is apparently masked by other factors, either intrinsic properties of the CA1 neuron or local circuitry perhaps involving other transmitters. For example, acute ethanol has been found to enhance the postsynaptic action of iontophoretically applied acetylcholine and somatostatin in the CA1 area of the hippocampus (Mancillas et al., 1986). Therefore, although ethanol may have a common action on all GABA interneurons—increasing their excitability to afferent stimulation—one would also predict that only those neuronal circuits highly and selectively regulated by these cells would be most sensitive to the effects of ethanol. This is what is generally observed, e.g., highly GABA-regulated spinal, cortical, hippocampal, and cerebellar neurons have been consistently observed to be most sensitive to the effects of ethanol in the intact subject (Grupp & Perlanski, 1979; Klemm et al., 1976; Miyahara et al., 1966; Nestoros, 1980).

Although our data suggest a primary role for GABA in some aspects of ethanol pharmacology, it must be acknowledged that most of this work has been done in halothane-anesthetized rats, and it has been shown previously that different anesthetics can alter the response of specific cell types to ethanol (Rogers et al., 1986; Siggins et al., 1987a). The data suggest two other significant points about the role of GABA in ethanol intoxication. First, regional differences in GABAergic control exist in brain areas as well as in individual cell types which could explain some of the diversity in the potential role of GABA in ethanol intoxication. Second, as ethanol is ubiquitously distributed after systemic administration, it is important to appreciate that some model systems (e.g., in vitro hippocampal slice), although providing far better pharmacological control and the ability to discern precise mechanisms of action of certain drugs, may not retain the critical neuronal elements needed to demonstrate a selective action of ethanol on any specific transmitter candidate or circuit.

Ethanol, Memory and the NMDA Receptor

Studies of the effects of prolonged ethanol use on brain and behavior far outnumber those dealing with the acute effects of the drug. This emphasis can be attributed in part to societal demands for understanding the processes underlying the devastating effects of the chronic abuse of ethanol. Neuropsychological, neuropathological, endocrinological, biochemical, and electrophysiological abnormalities attend abuse of the drug (for review, see Birnbaum & Platz, 1977; Porjesz et al., 1980; Tarter & Van Thiel, 1985). Chronic and excessive use of alcohol may give rise to major cognitive deficits, including a wide range of specific decrements in perception, abstracting ability, motor performance, and memory. Even more disturbing is evidence that those same capacities in non-abusing or "social drinkers" may be altered by the amount and duration of drinking (Parker & Noble, 1980; Porjesz & Begleiter, 1985).

Clinical studies of acute alcohol abuse have primarily focused on the effects of ethanol intoxication on human performance, cognition, and measures of intoxication (Begleiter & Platz, 1977; Birnbaum & Parker, 1977; Goldstein, 1983; Porjesz & Begleiter, 1985). Although it was recognized early that acute intoxication may provoke disturbances in information processing (Birnbaum & Parker, 1977), it is becoming increasingly clear that the deficits observed are dose and task dependent (Devenport et al., 1983; Melia & Ehlers, 1986). In general, memory tasks most affected by intoxicating doses of ethanol are those requiring decision making and response flexibility (Birnbaum & Parker, 1977; Melia & Ehlers, 1986). Memory tasks least affected are those involving stereotyped responses. Moreover, acute intoxication seems to interfere with the ability to store newly presented information, rather than the retrieval of recently stored events (Birnbaum & Parker, 1977). Accordingly, there seems to be a haunting similarity between the types of cognitive impairment seen in acute and chronic ethanol exposure (Cermak & Butters, 1973). This similarity lends strong support to the hypothesis that there may be a continuum of memory deficits associated with acute intoxication and the chronic amnesia of major alcohol abuse (Ryback, 1971).

Recent clinical evidence strongly confirms basic experimental data implicating the hippocampal formation in mnemonic mechanisms. A unique case report of brain pathology limited exclusively to the CA1 field of the human hippocampus (unrelated to alcohol usage) described a clinical picture of memory impairment identical to that observed after chronic and excessive ethanol abuse (Squire, 1986; Zola-Morgan et al., 1986). In addition, animal studies have shown an identity between the behavioral deficits elicited by hippocampal lesions and those of acute ethanol intoxication in rats (Devenport et al., 1981). These studies implicate the cellular fields of the hippocampus as a primary site of ethanol's effect on memory processes. Moreover, these studies suggest that the acute cognitive effects of ethanol, although transient, become chronic during continued perturbations of hippocampal physiology.

Recently, a specific receptor subtype for excitatory amino acid transmitters has been tied to the induction of model memory processes (long-term potentiation; LTP) in the hippocampus. This receptor, selectively sensitive to N-methyl-D-aspartate (NMDA), is one of a family of receptors whose endogenous ligand is glutamate or aspartate (Johnson & Koerner, 1988). Long-term potentiation (also termed enhancement) can be generated by patterned stimulation of hippocampal afferents, resulting in the lasting increase of the postsynaptic response. Because our earlier studies indicated that ethanol could enhance hippocampal inhibition (Wiesner & Henriksen, 1987), which could then potentially alter the ability to elicit LPT, we have evaluated the effect of acute ethanol on this phenomenon. Systemic doses of ethanol (0.5-1.5 g/kg) blocked, but did not reverse, the development of LTP in the dentate of both halothane-anesthetized and unrestrained rats (Fig. 20-3). A similar finding has been reported during elicitation of LTP in the CA1 field of an in vitro preparation of the hippocampus (Durand et al., 1981). Taken together, these findings support the hypothesis that ethanol may block the induction of LTP by the mechanism described above; that is, by selectively enhancing excitability of local interneurons.

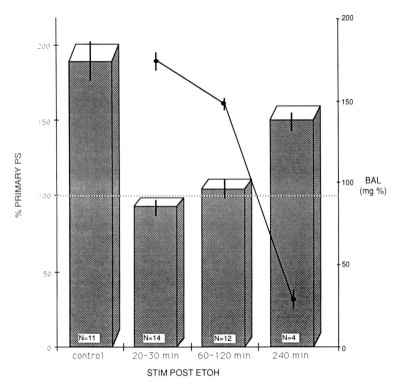

Figure 20-3. Effect of acute ethanol on the generation of long-term potentiation (LTP). Comparison of the ability to elicit LTP in untreated (control) and ethanol-treated rats. LTP induction in control subjects (*left column*) resulted in a mean increase of 190% in the dentate-evoked population spike as compared to pretetanus baseline. The effect of acute ethanol (2 g/kg) given at various times (20-30 minutes, 60-120 minutes, or 240 minutes) before tetanizing stimuli is illustrated in the columns to the right. Ethanol was able to prevent the development of LTP when given between 20-120 minutes before LTP tetani stimuli. When ethanol was given 240 minutes before LTP-inducing stimuli, partial recovery was observed. In all cases, LTP was assessed 60 minutes after the tetanizing stimulation. Blood ethanol levels for the representative latencies after ethanol injection are illustrated as a superimposed curve.

However, some recent in vitro investigations have called into question a major GABA-related component for ethanol's blockade of LTP (Lovinger & Weight, 1988; Lovinger et al., 1989, 1990). Using in vitro preparations of cultured neurons and the hippocampal slice preparation, these authors demonstrated that low doses of ethanol effectively block NMDA currents and excitatory postsynaptic potentials measured using intracellular voltage/current-clamp techniques. These elegant electrophysiological investigations coincided with reports of other studies in several in vitro model systems that suggested a related ethanol-induced decrease in NMDA receptor-coupled ion fluxes (Hoffman et al., 1989; Lima-Landman & Albuquerque, 1989; White et al., 1990).

It is well established that the opening and functionality of these NMDA receptors are both ion and voltage sensitive and can be blocked by both competitive and noncompetitive selective antagonists, including 2-amino-5-phosphopentanoate (AP-5) and MK-801 (Lodge & Collingridge, 1990). These antagonists are also capable of effectively blocking the induction of LTP in both in vivo and in vitro models. We surmised that, if a similar antagonism of the NMDA receptor complex was important for the effects of acute alcohol in our in vivo hippocampal model, NMDA antagonists should have the same effect as low doses of ethanol on dentate paired-pulse population spike curves. Using a series of low to high doses (0.1-0.5 mg/kg) of systemically administered MK-801, a noncompetitive NMDA antagonist, we failed to observe the same increase in paired-pulse inhibition as occurred with ethanol in either the intact or anesthetized rat. In fact, at moderate doses (0.25 mg/kg) that were effective in blocking the development of LTP in the same rat, a *decrease* in paired-pulse inhibition was observed (Fig. 20-4). Identical results were obtained with electrophoretic application of AP-5 locally into the dentate while assessing granule cell population responses. This effect was opposite to the effect of ethanol on the same measures.

Therefore, it seems that NMDA receptor blockade in the intact rat does not result in the same change in synaptic excitability in the dentate gyrus as do low doses of ethanol. At the present time, it is difficult to reconcile the differences between the in vivo and in vitro role of the NMDA receptor in ethanol intoxication. It would seem that in vitro systems have an abundant expression of functional NMDA receptors, which, for reasons that may lie in the local circuitry, remain dormant or less dominant in the intact dentate gyrus and perhaps other neuronal circuits. Further studies in other brain areas known to be sensitive to ethanol in the intact brain must pursue the role of NMDA receptors in ethanol pharmacology.

Ethanol, Dopamine, and Reinforcement

There is a growing consensus that the nucleus accumbens neuronal complex located in the basal forebrain of mammals may be part of the final common pathway resulting in drug reinforcement (Koob & Bloom, 1988; see Chapter 1). Through both direct and indirect actions, drugs of abuse including cocaine, amphetamines, and opiates are thought to alter as yet obscure processes in this

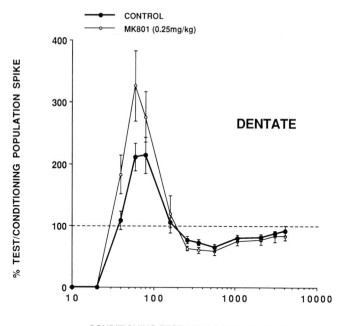

Figure 20-4. Effect of NMDA receptor antagonism by MK-801 on paired-pulse inhibition in the dentate gyrus. Paired-pulse curves generated in the hippocampal dentate gyrus before and after the systemic administration of 0.25 mg/kg MK-801, a potent, noncompetitive inhibitor of the NMDA receptor. Unlike ethanol, which increases early inhibition (see Fig. 20-1), MK-801 produces disinhibition and increases potentiation at this dose. However, when LTP was attempted in the same rats after the generation of these curves it was blocked.

structure, resulting in the increased probability of self-administration of these drugs. What is the evidence that ethanol's reinforcing effects are potentially mediated by this same neuronal circuit? Our own investigations, although preliminary, have shown no consistent mode of action of systemically administered ethanol on individually recorded nucleus accumbens neurons in the anesthetized rat. Yet, a considerable amount of evidence suggests that a major afferent system projecting to the nucleus accumbens, the dopamine-containing neurons of the ventral tegmental area of Tsai (VTA) in the midbrain, have increased discharge rates after systemic ethanol similar to what has been observed for many other drugs of abuse (Gessa et al., 1985; Gysling & Wang, 1983; Mereu et al., 1984, 1987). Similarly, in a recent in vitro investigation of the VTA, ethanol was found to produce a concentration-dependent increase in the activity of presumed dopamine-containing projection cells (Brodie et al., 1990). These authors thought that ethanol's effect on these neurons was a direct excitatory action, because it was obtained under perfusion conditions that they believed precluded indirect effects. However, in studies done in vivo, Mereu and Gessa (1985) recorded from GABA-containing neurons of the pars reticulata of the adjacent substantia nigra and demonstrated an inhibition of these neurons that resulted indirectly in activation of the dopamine neurons of the substantia nigra compacta. It is possible that this ethanol-induced disinhibition is in fact driven by increased excitability of recurrent GABAergic neurons originating in the caudate nucleus and impinging on these GABA interneurons of the pars reticulata. An identical neurochemical and anatomical pathway exists for the accumbens and the VTA. That is, GABAergic accumbens neurons send long projections to VTA reticulata interneurons (GABA containing) that regulate VTA dopamine neurons. Could ethanol produce increased VTA dopamine neuron activity by indirect GABA-induced disinhibition originating from increased accumbens excitability? This observation would be missed in an in vitro study in which these connections certainly had been severed. Much more work needs to be done to resolve these complicated neuropharmacological issues, but it is intriguing that in this structure as in the dentate gyrus, it seems that GABA mechanisms may be involved in some way in the acute effects of ethanol.

SUMMARY

The findings on the neuropharmacology of ethanol presented in this chapter are controversial, partly because of the diverse preparations used and partly because of the diverse brain areas studied. Although all of these findings are scientifically valid, their interpretation remains under debate. There is evidence that in some brain regions GABA mechanisms may be a strong candidate for a low-threshold system sensitive to acute actions of ethanol. However, the local circuitry, or neuronal template, in which GABA neurons may be embedded is the final arbiter of ethanol's effect. The responses of local brain regions will doubtless involve other hierarchically stationed neurotransmitter systems as well as biophysical processes.

ACKNOWLEDGMENTS

I thank Drs. Scott Steffensen, G.R. Siggins, and James Wiesner for allowing me to summarize portions of our collaborative work and Greta Berg, Dawn Miller, and Floriska Chizer for superior technical assistance.

REFERENCES

Allan, A.M., & Harris, R.A. (1987). Involvement of neuronal chloride channels in ethanol intoxication, tolerance and dependence. In M. Galandter (Ed.), *Recent developments in alcoholism*, Vol. 5. (pp. 313-322). New York: Plenum Press.

Amaral, D.G. (1978). A golgi study of cell types in the hilar region of the hippocampus in the rat. *J. Comp. Neurol., 182*, 851-914.

Andersen, P., Eccles, J.C., & Loyning, Y. (1964a). Location of presynaptic inhibitory synapses on hippocampus pyramids. *J. Neurophysiol., 27*, 592-607.

Andersen, P., Eccles, J.C., & Loyning, Y. (1964b). Pathway of postsynaptic inhibition in the hippocampus. *J. Neurophysiol., 27*, 608-619.

Banna, N.R. (1969). Potentiation of cutaneous inhibition by alcohol. *Experientia, 25*, 619-620.

Begleiter, H., & Platz, A. (1972). *The biology of alcoholism.* New York: Plenum Press.

Birnbaum, I., & Parker, E.S. (1977). *Alcohol and human memory.* New York: John Wiley and Sons.

Bloom, F.E. (1987). The emerging pharmacology of ethanol. *J. Psychopharmacol., 1*, 227-236.

Bloom, F.E., & Siggins, G.R. (1987). Electrophysiological action of ethanol at the cellular level. *Alcohol, 4*, 331-337.

Brodie, M.S., Shefner, S.A., & Dunwiddie, T.V. (1990). Ethanol increases the firing of dopamine neurons of the ventral tegmental area in vitro. *Brain Res., 508*, 65-69.

Carlen, P., Gurevich, N. & Durand, D. (1982). Ethanol in low doses augments calcium-mediated mechanisms measured intracellularly in hippocampal neurons. *Science, 215*, 306-309.

Celentano, J.J., Gibbs, T.T., and Farb, D.H. (1988). Ethanol potentiates GABA- and glycine-induced chloride currents in check spinal cord neurons. *Brain Res., 455*, 377-380.

Cermak, L., & Butters, N. (1973). Information processing deficits of alcoholic Korsakoff patients. *Q. J. Stud. Alcohol., 34*, 1110-1132.

Davidoff, R.A. (1973). Alcohol and presynaptic inhibition in an isolated spinal cord preparation. *Arch. Neurol., 28*, 60-63.

Devenport, L., Devenport, J., and Holloway, F. (1981). Alcohol and the hippocampus: Mutual antagonism on performance. *Alcoholism Clin. Exp. Res., 5*, 147.

Devenport, L., Merriman, V., & Devenport, J. (1983). Effects of ethanol on enforced spatial variability in the 8-arm radial maze. *J. Pharmacol. Biochem. Behav., 18*, 55-59.

Dolce, G., & Decker, H. (1972). The effects of ethanol on cortical and sub-cortical electrical activity in cats. *Res. Comm. Chem. Pathol. Pharmacol., 3*, 523-524.

Durand, D., Corrigal, W., Kujtan, P., & Carlen, P. (1981). Effects of low concentrations of ethanol on CA1 hippocampal neurons in vitro. *Canadian J. Physiol. Pharmacol., 59*, 979-984.

Galanter, M. (1987). *Recent developments in alcoholism.* New York: Plenum Press.

Gessa, G., Muntoni, F., Collu, M., Vargiu, L., & Mereu, G. (1985). Low doses of ethanol activate dopaminergic neurons in the ventral tegmental area. *Brain Res., 348*, 201-203.

Goldstein, D.B. (1983). *Pharmacology of alcohol.* New York: Oxford University Press.

Goldstein, D.B. (1987). Ethanol-induced adaptation in biological membranes. *Ann. NY. Acad. Sci., 492*, 103-115.

Gonzales, R., & Hoffman, P. (1991). Receptor-gated ion channels may be selective CNS targets for ethanol. *Trends Neurosci., 12*, 1-3.

Gruol, D.L. (1982). Ethanol alters synaptic activity in cultured spinal cord neurons. *Brain Res., 243*, 25-33.

Grupp, L.A. (1980). Biphasic action of ethanol on single units of the dorsal hippocampus and the relationship to the cortical EEG. *Psychopharmacology, 70*, 95-103.

Grupp, L., & Perlanski, E. (1979). Ethanol-induced changes in the spontaneous activity of single units in the hippocampus of the awake rat: A dose-response study. *Neuropharmacology, 18*, 62-70.

Gysling, K., & Wang, R.Y. (1983). Morphine-induced activation of A10 dopamine neurons in the rat. *Brain Res., 277*, 119-127.

Harris, D.P., & Sinclair, J.G. (1984). Ethanol-GABA interaction at the rat Purkinje cell. *Gen. Pharmacol., 15*, 449-454.

Harrison, N., Majewska, M., Harrington, J., & Barker, J. (1987). Structure-activity relationships for steroid interactions with the γ-aminobutyric acid$_A$ receptor complex. *J. Pharmacol. Exp. Ther., 241*, 346-353.

Hoffman, P., Rabe, C.S., Moses, F., & Tabakoff, B. (1989). N-methyl-D-aspartate receptors and ethanol: Inhibition of calcium flux and cyclic GMP production. *J. Neurochem., 52*, 1937-1940.

Hunt, W.A. (1985). Alcohol and biological membranes. In H. Bland & D. Goodwin (Eds.), *The Guilford alcohol studies series*. New York: The Guilford Press.

Johnson, R., & Koerner, J. (1988). Excitatory amino acid neurotransmission. *J. Med. Chem., 31*, 2057.

Kawaguchi, Y., & Hama, K. (1987). Fast spiking non-pyramidal cells in the hippocampal CA 3 region, dentate gyrus, and subiculum of rats. *Brain Res., 425*, 351-355.

Klemm, W.R. (1980). Effects of ethanol on nerve impulse activity. *Biochem. Pharmacol. Ethanol, 2*, 243-267.

Klemm, W.R. (1990). Dehydration: A new alcohol theory. *Alcohol, 7*, 49-59.

Klemm, W.R., Mallari, C.G., Dreyfus, L.R., Fiske, J.C., Forney, E., & Mikeska, J.A. (1976). Ethanol-induced regional and dose-response differences in multiple unit activity in rabbits. *Psychopharmacology, 49*, 235-244.

Koob, G.F., & Bloom, F.E. (1988). Cellular and molecular mechanisms of drug dependence. *Science, 242*, 715-723.

Lee, H.K., Dunwiddie, T.V., & Hoffer, B.J. (1979). Interaction of diazepam with synaptic transmission in the in vitro rat hippocampus. *Naunyn-Schmiedeberg's Arch. Pharmacol., 309*, 131-136.

Liljequist, S., & Engel, J. (1982). Effects of GABAergic agonists and antagonists on various ethanol-induced behavioral changes. *Psychopharmacology, 78*, 71-75.

Lima-Landman, M.T.R., & Albuquerque, E. (1989). Ethanol potentiates and blocks NMDA-activated single channel currents in rat hippocampal pyramidal cells. *FEBS Lett., 247*, 61-67.

Lodge, D., & Collingridge, G. (1990). Les agents provocateurs: A series on the pharmacology of excitatory amino acids. *Trends in Pharmacological Science, 11*, 22-24.

Lovinger, D.M., & Weight, F.F. (1988). Glutamate induces a depolarization of adult dorsal root ganglion neurons that is mediated predominantly by NMDA receptors. *Neurosci. Lett., 94*, 314-320.

Lovinger, D.M., White, G., & Weight, F.F. (1989). Ethanol inhibits NMDA activated ion current in hippocampal neurons. *Science, 243*, 1721-1724.

Lovinger, D.M., White, G., & Weight, F.F. (1990). NMDA receptor-mediated synaptic excitation selectively inhibited by ethanol in hippocampal slice from adult rat. *J. Neurosci., 10*, 1372-1379.

Mancillas, J., Siggins, G.R., and Bloom, F.E. (1986). Systemic ethanol: Selective enhancement of responses to acetylcholine and somatostatin in the rat hippocampus. *Science, 231*, 161-163.

Martz, A., Deitrich, R.A., and Harris, R.A. (1983). Behavioral evidence for the involvement of gamma-aminobutyric acid in the actions of ethanol. *Eur. J. Pharmacol., 89*, 53-62.

Mehta, A.K., & Ticku, M.K. (1988). Ethanol potentiation of GABAergic transmission in cultured spinal cord neurons involves gamma-aminobutyric acid a-gated chloride channels. *J. Pharmacol. Exp. Ther., 246*, 558-564.

Mehta, A.K., & Ticku, M.K. (1990). Are GABA B receptors involved in the pharmacological effects of ethanol? *Eur. J. Pharmacol., 182*, 473-480.

Melia, K., & Ehlers, C. (1986) Ethanol and monkey cognitive performance: A signal detection analysis. *Soc. Neurosci. Abstr., 192.*

Mereu, G., & Gessa, G.L. (1985). Low doses of ethanol inhibit the firing of neurons in the substantia nigra, pars reticulata: A GABAergic effect? *Brain Res., 348*, 201-203.

Mereu, G., Fadda, F., & Gessa, G.L. (1984). Ethanol stimulates the firing rate of nigral dopaminergic neurons in unanesthetized rats. *Brain Res., 292*, 63-69.

Mereu, G., Yoon, K., Boi, V, Gessa, G., Naes, L., & Westfall, T. (1987). Preferential stimulation of ventral tegmental area dopaminergic neurons by nicotine. *European J. Pharmacol., 141*, 395-399.

Meyer-Lohman, J., Hagenah, R., Hellweg, C., & Benecke, R. (1972). The action of ethyl alcohol on the activity of individual renshaw cells. *Naunyn-Schmiedeberg's Arch. Pharmacol., 272*, 131-142.

Misgeld, U., & Frotscher, M. (1986). Postsynaptic GABAergic inhibition of nonpyramidal neurons in the guinea pig hippocampus. *Neuroscience, 19*, 193-206.

Miyahara, J.T., Esplin, D.W., & Zablocka, B. (1966). Differential effects of depressant drugs on presynaptic inhibition. *J. Pharmacol. Exp. Ther., 154*, 119-127.

Nestoros, J.N. (1980). Ethanol specifically potentiates GABA-mediated neurotransmission in feline cerebral cortex. *Science, 209*, 708-710.

Nishio, M., & Narahashi, T. (1990). Ethanol enhancement of GABA-activated chloride currents in rat dorsal root ganglion neurons. *Brain Res., 518*, 283-286.

Osmanovic, S., & Shefner, S. (1990). Enhancement of current induced by superfusion of GABA in locus coeruleus neurons by pentobarbital, but not ethanol. *Brain Res., 517*, 324-329.

Palmer, M.R., & Hoffer, B.J. (1990). GABAergic mechanisms in the electrophysiological actions of ethanol on cerebellar neurons. *Neurochem. Res., 15*, 145-151.

Parker, E., & Noble, E. (1980). Alcohol and the aging process in social drinkers. *J. Stud. Alcohol, 41*, 170-178.

Porjesz, B., & Begleiter, H. (1985). Alcohol and the brain: *Chronic effects.* New York: Plenum Press.

Porjesz, B., Begleiter, H., & Garozzo, R. (1980). *Biological effects of alcohol.* New York: Plenum Press.

Rabin, R.A., Baker, R.C., & Dietrich, R.A. (1987). Specificity of the action of ethanol in the central nervous system: Behavioral effects. *Alcohol Alcohol, 1*, 133-138.

Ramon y Cajal, S. (1911). *Histologe du Systeme Nerveux de l'Homme et des Vertebres,* Paris: Maloine.

Ribak, C., Vaughn, J., & Saito, K. (1978). Immunocytological localization of glutamic acid decarboxylase in neuronal somata following colchicine inhibition of axonal transport. *Brain Res., 140*, 315-322.

Ryback, R.S. (1971). The continuum and specificity of the effects of alcohol on memory: A review. *Q. J. Studies Alcohol, 32*, 995-1016.

Rogers, J., Madamba, S.G., Staunton, D.A., & Siggins, G.R. (1986). Ethanol increases single unit activity in the inferior olivary nucleus. *Brain Res., 385*, 253-262.

Seress, L., & Ribak, C.E. (1983). GABAergic cells in the dentate gyrus appear to be local circuit and projection neurons. *Exp. Brain Res., 50*, 173-182.

Sharfman, H.E., & Schwartzkroin, P.A. (1988). Electrophysiology of morphologically identified mossy cells of the dentate hilus recorded in guinea pig hippocampal slices. *J. Neurosci., 8*, 3812-3821.

Shefner, S. (1990). Biochemistry and physiology of substance abuse—Electrophysiological effects of ethanol on brain neurons. Boca Raton, FL: CRC Press.

Siggins, G.R., Bloom, F.E., French, E.D., Madamba, S.G., Mancillas, J., Pittman,

Q.J., & Rogers, J. (1987a). Electrophysiology of ethanol on central neurons. *Ann. NY. Acad. Sci.*, *492*, 350-366.

Siggins, G.R., Pittman, Q.J., & French, E.D. (1987b). Effects of ethanol on CA1 and CA3 pyramidal cells in the hippocampal slice preparation: An intracellular study. *Brain Res.*, *414*, 22-34.

Squire, L. (1986). Mechanisms of memory. *Science, 232,* 1612-1619.

Steffensen, S., & Henrikson, S.J. (1992) Comparison of the effects of ethanol and chlordiazepoxide on electrophysiological activity in the fascia dentata and hippocampus regio superior. *Hippocampus, 2,* 201-212.

Storm-Mathisen, J. (1977). Localization of transmitter candidates in the brain: The hippocampal formation as model. *Prog. Neurobiol., 8,* 119-181.

Suzdak, P.D., & Schwartz, R.D. (1988). Alcohols stimulate gamma-aminobutyric acid receptor-mediated chloride uptake in brain vesicles: Correlation with intoxication potency. *Brain Res., 444,* 340-350.

Suzdak, P.D., Glowa, J.R., Crawley, J.N., Schwartz, R.D., Skolnick, P., & Paul, S.M. (1986a). A selective imidazobenzodiazepine antagonist of ethanol in the rat. *Science, 234,* 1243-1247.

Suzdak, P.D., Schwartz, R.D., Skolnick, P., & Paul, S.M. (1986b). Ethanol stimulates gamma-aminobutyric acid receptor-mediated chloride transport in rat brain synaptoneurosomes. *Proc. Natl. Acad. Sci. USA., 83,* 4071-4075.

Takada et al., 1987.

Tarter, R., & Van Thiel, D. (1985). *Alcohol and the brain: Chronic effects.* Plenum Press, NY.

Ticku, M.K., Lowrimore, P., & Lehoullier, P. (1986). Ethanol enhances GABA-induced Cl-influx in primary spinal cord cultured neurons. *Brain Res., 17,* 123-126.

White, G., Lovinger, D.M., & Weight, F.F. (1990). Ethanol inhibits NMDA activated current but does not alter GABA-activated current in an isolated adult mammalian neuron. *Brain Res., 507,* 332-336.

Wiesner, J.B., & Henriksen, S.J. (1987). Ethanol enhances recurrent inhibition in the dentate gyrus of the hippocampus. *Neurosci. Lett., 79,* 169-173.

Zola-Morgan, S., Squire, L., & Amaral, D.J. (1986). Human amnesia and the medial temporal region: Enduring memory impairment following a bilateral lesion limited to field CA1 of the hippocampus. *J. Neurosci., 6,* 2950-2967.

IV

BEHAVIORAL MECHANISMS

The behavioral effects of drugs can provide valuable insights into the drugs' actions. The discovery of neurobiological mechanisms of reward decades ago by Olds has proved to be critical to contemporary formulations of drug action and to understanding many forms of behavior. Two chapters deal with this topic. Dworkin and Smith consider the relationships of opioids to behavioral reinforcement, while Koob considers the relationship between the reward system and the actions of cocaine.

Drugs can have profound, long-lasting effects on behavior that alter neuronal processes in quantifiable ways. Continuous stimulant treatment can result in a pattern of behavioral changes as well as neurotoxicity in specific systems, as described by Ellison. Brain dopamine systems can be sensitized by drugs with subsequent effects on behavior, as noted by Robinson.

21

Opiates/Opioids and Reinforcement

STEVEN I. DWORKIN AND JAMES E. SMITH

Agonists for opioid receptors have been used for many centuries to produce a behavioral state of euphoria or feelings of well-being. These reinforcing effects are probably exerted through the neuronal pathways that mediate similar consequences of other pharmacological as well as nondrug reinforcers. The existence of neuronal circuits dedicated to mediating hedonic processes was hypothesized after the development of intracranial electrical self-stimulation (ICSS) (Olds & Milner, 1954). The notion that endogenous opioids are involved in the regulation of hedonic valence followed the observation that electrical stimulation of the midbrain central gray area suppressed pain through a naloxone-reversible process (Liebeskind & Paul, 1977). The reinforcing efficacy of opiates is significantly greater than that of most other environmental stimuli that function reliably as reinforcers. Opiates also seem to be more potent than most other environmental events in activating neural systems implicated in reinforcing mechanisms. Thus, it seems that at least a subset of opioid-releasing neurons participate in the biological substrates of reinforcement. This chapter reviews the biological basis of opiate reinforcement.

ACTIONS OF OPIATES ON BEHAVIOR

Opiate agonists and antagonists have a profound effect on a number of behaviors, suggesting an important role for their receptors in complex behavioral processes. Opiate receptor agonists increase food (Reid & Siviy, 1983) and water (Sanger & McCarthy, 1980) intake, whereas antagonists for these sites decrease consumption (Margules et al., 1978). Studies of the central mechanisms of feeding and satiety using several neurobiological procedures indicate that the paraventricular nucleus and the ventral medial hypothalamus are involved in the effects of opiates on food intake (for review, see Hoebel, 1988). Opiate receptor agonists also decrease mating behaviors (Meyerson & Terenius, 1977) and separation distress (Panksepp et al., 1983), whereas antagonists generally have the opposite consequences (Gessa et al., 1979; Panksepp et al., 1983). Opiate agonists also increase the reinforcing efficacy of ICSS (lower thresholds), whereas antagonists seem to have the opposite effect (Kornetsky & Bain, 1983). These findings collectively suggest the presence of opioid receptors on neurons that participate in complex behavioral processes or that innervate other neurons that do so. Opioid agonists generally heighten activity in neuronal systems mediating reinforcement, whereas antagonists decrease such activity.

OPIATE SELF-ADMINISTRATION

Animal models of drug self-administration have been developed within the past few decades for laboratory investigations of the actions of opiates (Headlee, 1955). Agonists for some opiate receptor subtypes will engender and maintain responses that result in their presentation whereas others will not (Tables 21-1 and 21-2). In general, agonists that have some action at mu or delta opioid receptor subtypes are self-administered, whereas those with actions at kappa receptor sites are not (Woods & Winger, 1987).

Table 21-1. Opiates that maintain intravenous self-administration

Compound	Species
Buprenorphine	Rhesus monkey
Codeine	Rat
	Rhesus monkey
D-Enkephalin	Rat
Enkephalin analog FK-33-824	Rhesus monkey
Ethyl ketocyclazocine	Rat
Etonitazene	Rat
Fentanyl	Rat
Heroin	Rat
	Rhesus monkey
Hydromorphone	Rat
Ketamine	Baboon
	Dog
	Rhesus monkey
Ketocyclazocine	Rat
Meperidine	Rat
Methadone	Rat
	Rhesus monkey
Morphine	Dog
	Mouse
	Rat
	Rhesus monkey
	Squirrel monkey
Nalbuphine	Rat
	Rhesus monkey
Nalorphine	Rat
Pentazocine	Rat
	Rhesus monkey
Butorphanol	Rhesus monkey

Table 21-2. Opiates that failed
to maintain intravenous
self-administration

Compound	Species
Cyclazocine	Rat
	Rhesus monkey
Levallorphan	Rhesus monkey
Nalorphine	Rhesus monkey
Naloxone	Rat
	Rhesus monkey
Cyclazocine	Rhesus monkey
Bremazocine	Rhesus monkey
Ketazocine	Rhesus monkey

The involvement of other neuronal systems in the central events underlying opiate self-administration have been investigated by pretreating with specific receptor antagonists. These pharmacological blockade experiments have demonstrated that cholinergic (Davis & Smith, 1975; Glick & Cox, 1975), dopaminergic (Glick & Cox, 1975; Pozuelo & Kerr, 1972; Smith & Davis, 1973), and noradrenergic (Davis et al., 1975) receptors are important to the processes responsible for intravenous opiate self-administration. Other studies have attempted to identify brain sites and innervations involved using either electrolytic or neurotoxin lesions of discrete brain regions or intracranial injections of opiate antagonists in animals intravenously self-administering opiates. Electrolytic lesions of the anterior cingulate (Trafton & Marques, 1971) or frontal cortex, hippocampus (Glick & Cox, 178), and medial raphe' nuclei (Glick & Cox, 1977) decrease intravenous self-administration, whereas similar lesions of the caudate nucleus (Glick et al., 1975), substantia nigra, and medial forebrain bundle (Glick & Cox, 1977) increase such intake. Lesions of the locus coeruleus (Glick & Cox, 1977), amygdala (Glick & Ross, 1983), nucleus accumbens, and olfactory tubercle (Glick & Cox, 1978) have no effect. These findings led Glick to propose that the intravenous self-administration of morphine depends on two neuronal circuits: a nigral-thalamic-striatal-cortical circuit and a medial raphe'-hippocampal-septal-cortical circuit (Glick & Ross, 1983).

Electrolytic lesions, however, are nonspecific. One cannot assess the role of an identified population of neurons because the destruction of discrete neuronal systems is impossible. More recently, intracranial injections of opiate receptor antagonists or neurotoxins that remove innervations or projections from discrete brain regions with some degree of specificity have been used to evaluate the brain mechanisms necessary to opiate self-administration. Injections of quaternary nalorphine into the ventral tegmental area attenuate intravenous heroin self-administration in rats, whereas similar injections into the nucleus accumbens have no effect (Britt & Wise, 1983). However, methyl naloxonium injected into the lateral ventricles, ventral tegmental area, or nucleus accumbens increases intravenous administration of heroin in a manner indicating the attenuation of reinforcing efficacy (Vaccarino et al., 1984). Injections of methyl naltrexone into the periaqueductal gray, nucleus accumbens

(Corrigall & Vaccarino, 1988), and lateral hypothalamus also decrease the reinforcing efficacy of intravenous heroin, whereas similar injections into the medial prefrontal cortex have no effect (Corrigall, 1987). These studies indicate that opiate receptors in the nucleus accumbens, ventral tegmental area, and periaqueductal gray are involved in the neuronal processes maintaining intravenous opiate self-administration.

The effects of these chemically induced lesions have been evaluated in rats that have been exposed to drug alone or to food, water, and drug on concurrent chained schedules. Bilateral 6-hydroxydopamine (6-OHDA) lesions of the nucleus accumbens increase drug intake and shift the dose intake relationship to the right in rats that are exposed to intravenous morphine self-administration (Smith et al., 1985). There is no change in intake, however, in rats with similar lesions that are exposed to heroin and cocaine self-administration on alternate days (Pettit et al., 1984) or to concurrent food, water, or intravenous morphine (Dworkin et al., 1988a). These findings suggest that the behavioral consequences of the removal of dopaminergic innervations of the nucleus accumbens depend on the behavioral history of the animal and/or the behavioral environment. Serotonergic innervations and either interneurons or efferents from the nucleus accumbens seem to be more important to the biological mechanisms of intravenous opiate self-administration. Bilateral 5,7-dihydroxytryptamine-(5,7-DHT) induced lesions of this structure decrease the reinforcing efficacy of intravenous morphine, resulting in a disruption of dose-related intake (Smith et al., 1987). Similar lesions in rats on concurrent food, water, and intravenous morphine result in a reduction in intake at the lower doses, suggesting a decrease in reinforcing efficacy (Dworkin et al., 1988b). Bilateral removal of the neurons of origin in the nucleus accumbens, with kainic acid-induced lesions of this structure in animals on concurrent schedules of food, water, and intravenous morphine presentation, has a similar effect in that intake at lower doses is decreased (Dworkin et al., 1988c). Kainate lesions of the ventral pallidum also decrease intravenous self-administration of heroin (Hubner & Koob, 1990). These data collectively suggest that serotonergic innervations of the nucleus accumbens and interneurons or efferents from the nucleus accumbens and ventral pallidum are important to the neuronal processes mediating intravenous opiate self-administration. This finding may seem to be somewhat in disagreement with the electrolytic lesion studies, which show that the ablation of the nucleus accumbens has no effect on intravenous morphine intake. However, as previously stated, electrolytic lesions destroy innervations, projections, interneurons, and fibers in passage indiscriminately, which is very different than the selective chemical removal of small subpopulations of neurons. This different finding could result from the removal of both an excitatory and inhibitory influence on the behavior or from procedural differences between these studies.

NEUROCHEMICAL STUDIES OF OPIATE SELF-ADMINISTRATION

Several studies have addressed the biological mechanisms of opiate self-administration by assessing neurochemical indices in animals that are self-administering these drugs. Using liquid scintillation spectrometry, one experiment evaluated the distribution of radioactive 2-deoxyglucose (2-DG) into various brain areas of rats either intravenously self-administering morphine or receiving yoked infusions of morphine or vehicle (Glick et al., 1980). Glucose uptake and utilization by neurons are thought to be related directly to neuronal activity. 2-DG is transported into neurons through the same uptake system as glucose and is phosphorylated, but metabolized no further. The phosphorylated polar product remains in the cell and represents the level of glucose uptake. Therefore, the distribution of 2-DG is thought to represent rates of glucose utilization, which is directly related to neuronal activity since nerve cells do not have stored energy sources. This experiment found a difference in the uptake of 2-DG in the striatum between the self-administering animals and the vehicle-infused group; however, there were no differences between the yoked morphine and self-administering rats. These data suggest that there are no differences in neuronal activity in the brains of animals receiving contingent and noncontingent administration of morphine. However, these data merely indicate that there is no *net* difference in total neuronal activity, which would not differentiate increases and decreases in the activity of subsets of neurons in the same region.

The activity of subsets of neurons in discrete brain regions of rats that are self-administering morphine has been assessed using neurotransmitter turnover rate measures and receptor binding techniques. One experiment measured the turnover rates of dopamine, norepinephrine, serotonin, aspartate, glutamate, and gamma-aminobutyric acid in small brain regions of rats either intravenously self-administering morphine or receiving yoked infusions of morphine or vehicle (Smith et al., 1982). A second experiment measured the turnover rates of acetylcholine (Smith et al., 1984a) and the cholinergic muscarinic receptor densities (Smith et al., 1984b) in brain regions of similarly treated animals. The triad design permitted assessment of the neurochemical effects of response-independent morphine, which should reflect the pharmacological actions of the drug, by comparing neurotransmitter turnover rates in the yoked vehicle and yoked morphine-infused rats. The effects of response-dependent presentation of morphine, which should reflect the reinforcing actions of the drug, were estimated by comparing the neurotransmitter turnover rates in the self-administering rats with the yoked morphine-infused rats.

The differences in the turnover rates of these neurotransmitters were generally more numerous and of a greater magnitude between the self-administering and yoked morphine-infused rats than between the yoked vehicle and yoked morphine-infused rats. In the second experiment the binding densities of quinuclidinyl benzilate (QNB) were determined as another measure of cholinergic neuronal activity. The self-administering animals had significant decrease in QNB binding in the frontal cortex and entorhinal-subicular cortex and a significant increase in binding in the amygdala (Smith et al., 1984b). These data collectively suggest that the neurochemical consequences of the control over drug presentation (primarily representing reinforcement) are greater than those of the other pharmacological actions of the drug. Clearly, intravenous morphine alone has significant effects on brain neurotransmitter systems (Clouet &

Iwatsubo, 1975). However, the ability to control drug presentation has even greater effects on brain neuronal systems.

Integration of the data from these turnover rate experiments and the neurotoxin lesion experiments in self-administering rats with current knowledge of neurotransmitter-specific neuronal pathways has resulted in the identification of two neuronal circuits that may mediate some of the neuronal events underlying reinforcement processes. Although only eight neurotransmitters have been evaluated in from 13 to 22 brain regions, the results provided some crude estimate of the intricate neuronal processes that likely underlie these complex behaviors. As knowledge of the involvement of neuropeptides and other neurohumors in behavioral function evolves, the configuration and neuronal components of these circuits will be modified significantly. However, until then, the following section describes an initial organization of the neuronal pathways involved in morphine self-administration.

The identified circuits include a frontal cortex-striatum-frontal cortex circuit utilizing acetylcholine and glutamate-releasing neurons (Fig. 21-1). Activity in this circuit is modulated by biogenic amine pathways from the brainstem that innervate the caudate nucleus and the frontal cortex (Fig. 21-2) while the circuit sends feedback pathways to the ventral tegmental area utilizing GABA, which modulate activity in the biogenic amine nuclei in the brainstem (Fig. 21-3). The other circuit includes the nucleus accumbens-preoptic nucleus-amygdala-entorhinal cortex-hippocampus-septum and nucleus accumbens. This circuit utilizes acetylcholine, glutamate, GABA-releasing neurons and is modulated by biogenic amine feed-forward pathways from the brainstem utilizing dopamine, norepinephrine, and serotonin (Fig. 21-2). The circuit modulates activity in the brainstem biogenic amine nuclei through GABA and perhaps aspartate feedback pathways (Fig. 21-3). There are reciprocal pathways in some portions of each of these circuits. For example, the increased acetylcholine and glutamate turnover in the nucleus accumbens could result from inner-

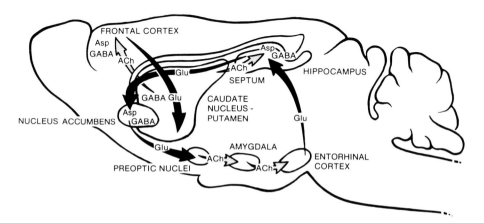

Figure 21-1. A frontal cortex-striatum-frontal cortex circuit using acetylcholine and glutamate-releasing neurons.

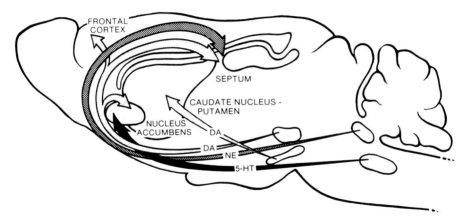

Figure 21-2. Biogenic amine pathways from the brainstem that innervate the caudate nucleus and the frontal cortex, thereby modulating the circuit shown in Figure 21-1.

vations not only from the hippocampus and frontal cortex but also from the amygdala. Therefore, the amygdala may receive input from the nucleus accumbens and in turn send innervations back to this structure. It is likely that there are extensive reciprocal connections in these networks. Also, these two circuits are not independent in that there seem to be pathways that interconnect the two at several points. These pathways include the GABA efferent pathway from the nucleus accumbens to the ventral pallidum and glutamate or aspartate efferents from the frontal cortex to the nucleus accumbens. These circuits should be seen as very preliminary representations of the neuronal networks that mediate these complex behavioral processes. It is likely that the configuration and neuronal pathways participating will change substantially as the roles of dozens of other neurohumors become better understood.

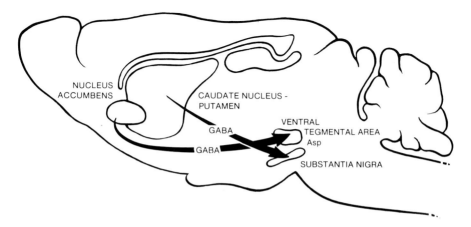

Figure 21-3. Feedback to the ventral tegmental area using GABA, which modulate activity in the biogenic amine nuclei in the brainstem.

There is a great deal of concordance between these two circuits and the brain regions that have shown increased glucose utilization with intracranial self-stimulation of the ventral tegmental region (Esposito et al., 1984), the substantia nigra (Porrino, 1987), and the medial forebrain bundle (Porrino et al., 1990). The distribution of 2-DG has been evaluated in brain regions of rats receiving either response-dependent or response-independent brain stimulation of the ventral tegmental area (Esposito et al., 1984). Increases in activity specific to response-contingent stimulation occurred bilaterally in the nucleus accumbens, bed nucleus of the stria terminalis, and medial brachial nucleus; ipsilaterally to the stimulating electrode in the medial prefrontal cortex, central amygdala, and basolateral amygdala; and contralaterally to the stimulating electrode in the lateral septum, mediodorsal thalamus, and CA3 area of the hippocampus. This same laboratory has also investigated brain glucose utilization in rats receiving contingent and noncontingent stimulation of the substantia nigra (Porrino, 1987). Rats receiving contingent stimulation showed significant increases in glucose utilization bilaterally in the prefrontal and anterior cingulate cortices, nucleus accumbens, ventral pallidum, mediodorsal thalamus, and lateral habenulae and significant increases contralaterally to the stimulating electrode in the caudate nucleus, lateral septum, and globus pallidus compared to response-independent stimulated controls. Recently, similar investigations of cerebral glucose utilization have been completed in rats receiving ICSS of the medial forebrain bundle at the level of the lateral hypothalamus (Porrino et al., 1990). The animals receiving response-contingent stimulation showed similar changes to those seen with ventral tegmental area stimulation, except that the increased utilization was greater in the olfactory tubercle.

In these three studies, some brain regions showed increased glucose utilization that was unique to the site of stimulation (Porrino, 1987). For substantia nigra stimulation, these areas included the caudate nucleus and the anterior cingulate cortex. For ventral tegmental area and medial forebrain bundle stimulation, these regions included the central and medial nuclei of the amygdala, the hippocampus, bed nucleus of the stria terminalis, and the olfactory tubercle. Increased glucose utilization with ICSS of all three brain sites was shown in nine brain regions: the prefrontal cortex, nucleus accumbens, lateral septum, globus pallidus, mediodorsal thalamus, entopeduncular nucleus, subthalamic nucleus, ventrolateral thalamus, and sensorimotor complex. These data suggest that reinforcement produced by brain stimulation may involve some shared or common components, as well as some unique elements. This would clearly argue for a complexity of systems involved in reinforcement processes.

Many of the brain regions activated with electrical intracranial self-stimulation also showed changes in neurotransmitter turnover rates specific to intravenous morphine self-administration. This finding suggests that the initial hypothesis—drugs produce positive effects through neuronal networks dedicated to reinforcement processes—may be correct. Thus, the neuronal circuits identified in the morphine self-administering rats may be part of the dedicated neuronal networks that mediate these complex processes. Opiates likely initiate activity in these circuits through receptor-mediated processes at specific brain sites. Therefore, the drug should initiate a reinforcing stimulus when directly delivered to a brain region where such receptors initiate activity in these neuronal networks dedicated to reinforcement. Two studies have addressed these issues. Rats have been demonstrated to self-administer morphine directly into the ventral tegmental area, but not into the caudate nucleus or nucleus accumbens (Bozarth & Wise, 1981). Methionine enkephalin is self-administered into the nucleus accumbens, and this intake can be attenuated with co-infusion of naloxone, suggesting receptor-mediated mechanisms (Goeders et al., 1984). These data may indicate that agonists for opiate receptor subtypes act in discrete brain regions to initiate activity in neuronal networks mediating reinforcement. It seems that agonists for delta receptors (but not mu receptors) will initiate such activity in the nucleus accumbens, whereas mu receptors seem to be important to these processes in the ventral tegmental area.

The intracranial administration studies demonstrate that opiate receptors in the nucleus accumbens and ventral tegmental area are important to the neuronal mechanisms for the initiation of reinforcing neuronal activity. Antagonists injected into these brain regions attenuate intravenous self-administration which suggests that opiate receptors in the periaqueductal gray and lateral hypothalamus have some role in these complex behaviors.

OPIOID INVOLVEMENT IN REINFORCEMENT OF NONOPIATE DRUGS

Other drugs of abuse likely produce positive effects through neuronal networks that are committed to these purposes. Data exist that suggest the involvement of opioid-releasing neurons in these neuronal networks that mediate reinforcement for other reinforcing stimuli. Opiate agonists decrease while opiate antagonists seem to increase thresholds for intracranial electrical self-stimulation (Kornetsky & Bain, 1983). These data are consistent with the hypothesis that neuronal circuits mediating opiate reinforcement are congruent with those mediating general reinforcement processes demonstrated by ICSS. Ethanol has been shown to inhibit ligand binding to delta opiate receptors (Goodwin et al., 1977). Delta opiate receptor blockade attenuates ethanol preference in ethanol-preferring rats (Froehlich et al., 1990), indicating a potential relationship in the neuronal mechanisms underlying the reinforcing actions of this drug. Opiate receptors may also be involved in the actions of cocaine since the ICSS threshold-lowering effect of cocaine can be antagonized with naloxone (Kornetsky & Esposito, 1981). Morphine injections into the ventral tegmental area also reinstate intravenous cocaine self-administration in rats with prior experience with cocaine (de Wit & Stewart, 1981). More recently, data suggest that buprenorphine will antagonize cocaine self-administration in nonhuman (Mello et al., 1989, 1990) and human primates. These data collectively support the involvement of opioid releasing neurons in the brain processes underlying the reinforcing actions of several reinforcing stimuli.

OPIOID-RELEASING NEURONS AND REINFORCEMENT

Opiate receptor agonists and antagonists modify several classes of complex behavior, including feeding, drinking, footshock reactivity, and separation distress. In addition, these substances differentially affect ICSS thresholds, suggesting a direct action on neuronal networks mediating reinforcement. This action is further supported by the concordance of the brain sites showing increased glucose utilization in animals receiving ICSS and the neuronal circuits identified with neurotransmitter turnover rate measures in intravenous morphine self-administering rats. Opiate receptors seem to be involved in the brain processes underlying ethanol preference and in those responsible for the self-administration of cocaine. It is likely that opioid-releasing neurons participate in the neuronal circuits and networks that mediate positive reinforcement processes.

REFERENCES

Bozarth, M., & Wise, R. (1981). Intracranial self-administration of morphine into the ventral tegmental area in rats. *Life Sci., 28*, 551-555.

Britt, M., & Wise, R. (1983). Ventral tegmental site of opiate reward: Antagonism by a hydrophilic opiate receptor blocker. *Brain Res., 258*, 105-108.

Clouet, D., & Iwatsubo, K. (1975). Mechanisms of tolerance to and dependence on narcotic analgesic drugs. *Annu. Rev. Pharmacol., 15*, 49-71.

Corrigall, W. (1987). Heroin self-administration: Effects of antagonist treatment in lateral hypothalamus. *Pharmacol. Biochem. Behav., 27*(4), 693-700.

Corrigall, W., & Vaccarino, F.J. (1988). Antagonist treatment in nucleus accumbens or periaqueductal grey affects heroin self-administration. *Pharmacol. Biochem. Behav., 30*, 443-450.

Davis, W., & Smith, S. (1975). Effect of haloperidol on ($\pm$)-amphetamine self-administration. *J. Pharmacol. Pharm., 27*, 540-542.

Davis, W., Smith, S., & Khalsa, J. (1975). Noradrenergic role in the self-administration of morphine or amphetamine. *Pharmacol. Biochem. Behav., 3*, 477-484.

de Wit, H., & Stewart, J. (1981). Reinstatement of cocaine-reinforced responding in the rat. *Psychopharmacology, 75*, 134-143.

Dworkin, S.I., Guerin, G.F., Co, C., Goeders, N.E., & Smith, J.E. (1988a). Lack of an effect of 6-hydroxydopamine lesions of the nucleus accumbens on intravenous morphine self-administration. *Pharmacol. Biochem. Behav., 30*, 1051-1057.

Dworkin, S., Goeders, N., Guerin, G., Co, C., & Smith, J. (1988b). Effects of 5,7-dihydroxytryptamine lesions of the nucleus accumbens in rats responding on a concurrent schedule of food, water and intravenous morphine self-administration. *NIDA Res. Monogr., 81*.

Dworkin, S., Guerin, G., Goeders, N., & Smith, J. (1988c). Kainic acid lesions of the nucleus accumbens selectively attenuate morphine self-administration. *Pharmacol. Biochem. Behav., 29*, 175-181.

Esposito, R., Porrino, L., Seeger, T., Crane, A., Everist, H., & Pert, A. (1984). Changes in local cerebral glucose utilization during rewarding brain stimulation. *Proc. Nat. Acad. Sci. USA., 81*, 635-639.

Froehlich, J., Zweifel, M., Kurtz, D., & Li, T. (1990, June). *Opioid antagonists selec-*

tively suppress ethanol intake. Abstract presented at the Fifth Congress of the International Society for Biomedical Research on Alcoholism held jointly with the Research Society on Alcoholism, Toronto.

Gessa, G., Paglietti, E., & Quarantotti, B. (1979). Induction of male copulatory behavior in sexually inactive rats by naloxone. *Science, 198*, 756-758.

Glick, S., & Cox, R. (1975). Dopaminergic and cholinergic influence on morphine self-administration in rats. *Res. Commun. Chem. Pathol. Pharmacol., 12*, 17-24.

Glick, S., & Cox, R. (1977). Changes in morphine self-administration after brainstem lesions in rats. *Psychopharmacology, 52*, 151-156.

Glick, S., & Cox, R. (1978). Changes in morphine self-administration after teldiencephalic lesions in rats. *Psychopharmacology, 57*, 283-288.

Glick, S., & Ross, D. (1983). Neuroanatomical substrates of opiate reinforcement—lateralized effects. In J. Smith & J. Lane (Eds.), *The neurobiology of opiate reward processes* (pp. 309-330). New York: Elsevier Biomedical Press.

Glick, S., Cox, R., & Crane, A. (1975). Changes in morphine self-administration and morphine dependence after lesions of the caudate nucleus in rats. *Psychopharmacologia, 41*, 219-224. Berlin.

Glick, S., Weaver, L., & Meibach, R. (1980). Lateralization of reward in rats: Differences in reinforcing thresholds. *Science, 207*, 1093-1095.

Goeders, N., Lane, J., & Smith, J. (1984). Intracranial self-administration of methionine enkephalin into the nucleus accumbens. *Pharmacol. Biochem. Behav., 20*, 451-455.

Goodwin, D., Schulsinger, F., Moller, N., Mednick, S., & Guze, S. (1977). Alcoholism and depression in adopted-out daughters of alcoholics. *Arch. Gen. Psychiat., 34*, 751-755.

Headlee, C. (1955). Apparatus and technique involved in a laboratory method of detecting the addictiveness of drugs. *J. Am. Pharm. Assoc., 44*, 229-231.

Hoebel, B.G. (1988). Neuroscience and motivation: Pathways and peptides that define motivational systems. In R. Atkinson, R. Herrnstein, G. Lindzey, & R. Luce (Eds.), *Perception and motivation* (2nd ed.) (pp. 547-625). New York: John Wiley & Sons, Inc.

Hubner, C., & Koob, G. (1990). Bromocriptine produces decreases in cocaine self-administration in the rat. *Neuropsychopharmacology, 3*(2), 101-108.

Kornetsky, C., & Bain, G. (1983). Effects of opiates on rewarding brain stimulation. In J.E. Smith & J.D. Lane (Eds.), *The neurobiology of opiate reward processes* (pp. 237-256). Amsterdam: Elsevier Biomedical Press.

Kornetsky, C., & Esposito, R. (1981). Reward and detection thresholds for brain stimulation: Dissociative effects of cocaine. *Brain Res., 209*, 496-500.

Liebeskind, J., & Paul, L. (1977). Psychological and physiological mechanisms of pain. *Annu. Rev. of Psychol., 28*, 41-60.

Margules, D., Moisset, B., Lewis, M., Shibuya, H., & Pert, C. (1978). Beta-endorphin is associated with overeating in genetically obese mice (ob/ob) and rats (fa/fa). *Science, 202*, 988-991.

Mello, N., Mendelson, J., Bree, M., & Lukas, S. (1989). Buprenorphine suppresses cocaine self-administration by rhesus monkeys. *Science, 245*(4920), 859-862.

Mello, N., Mendelson, J., Bree, M., & Lukas, S. (1990). Buprenorphine and naltrexone effects on cocaine self-administration by rhesus monkeys. *J. Pharmacol. Exp. Ther. 254*(3), 926-939.

Meyerson, B., & Terenius, L. (1977). Beta-endorphin and male sexual behavior. *Eur. J. Pharmacol. 42*, 191-192.

Olds, J., & Milner, P. (1954). Positive reinforcement produced by electrical stimulation of septal area and other regions of rat brain. *J. Comp. Physiol. Psychol. 47,* 419-427.

Panksepp, J. (1983). Hypothalamus integration of behavior: Rewards, punishments, and related psychological processes. In P.J. Morgane & J. Panksepp (Eds.), *Behavioral studies of the hypothalamus. Vol 3b: Handbook of the hypothalamus* (pp. 289-432). New York: Marcel Dekker, Inc.

Pettit, H., Ettenberg, A., Bloom, F., & Koob, G. (1984). Destruction of dopamine in the nucleus accumbens selectively attenuates cocaine but not heroin self-administration in rats. *Psychopharmacology* Berlin, *84,* 167-173.

Porrino, L. (1987). Cerebral metabolic changes associated with activation of reward systems. In J. Engel & L. Oreland (Eds.), *Brain reward systems* (pp. 51-60). New York: Raven Press.

Porrino, L., Huston-Lyons, D., Bain, G., Sokoloff, L., & Kornetsky, C. (1990). The distribution of changes in local cerebral energy metabolism associated with brain stimulation reward to the MFB in the rat. *Brain Res., 511,* 1-6.

Pozuelo, J., & Kerr, F. (1972). Suppression of craving and other signs of dependence in morphine-addicted monkeys by administration of alpha-methyl-para-tyrosine. *Mayo Clin. Proc., 47,* 621-638.

Reid, L.D., & Siviy, S.M. (1983). Administration of opiate antagonists reveal endorphinergic involvement in reinforcement processes. In J.E. Smith & J.D. Lane (Eds.), *The neurobiology of opiate reward processes* (pp. 257-279). Amsterdam: Elsevier Biomedical Press.

Sanger, D., & McCarthy, P. (1980). Differential effects of morphine on food and water intake in food deprived and freely feeding rat. *Psychopharmacology, 72,* 103-106.

Smith, J., Co, C., Freeman, M., & Lane, J. (1982). Brain neurotransmitter turnover correlated with morphine-seeking behavior in rats. *Pharmacol. Biochem. Behav. 16,* 509-519.

Smith, J., Co, C., & Lane, J. (1984a). Limbic acetylcholine turnover rates correlated with rat morphine-seeking behaviors. *Pharmacol. Biochem. Behav., 20,* 429-441.

Smith, J., Co, C., & Lane, J. (1984b). Limbic muscarinic cholinergic and benzodiazepine receptor changes with chronic intravenous morphine and self-administration. *Pharmacol. Biochem. Behav., 20,* 443-450.

Smith, J., Guerin, G., Co, C., Barr, T., & Lane, J. (1985). Effects of 6-OHDA lesions of the central medial nucleus accumbens on rat intravenous morphine self-administration. *Pharmacol. Biochem. Behav., 23,* 234-249.

Smith, J.E., Schultz, K., & Co, C. (1987). Effects of 5,7-dihydroxytryptamine lesions of the nucleus accumbens on rat intravenous morphine self-administration. *Pharmacol. Biochem. Behav., 26,* 607-611.

Smith, S., & Davis, W. (1973). Haloperidol affects morphine self-administration: testing for pharmacological modification of the primary reinforcement mechanisms. *Psychol. Rec., 23,* 215-221.

Trafton, C., & Marques, P. (1971). Effects of septal area and cingulate cortex lesions on opiate addiction behavior in rats. *J. Comp. Physiol. Psychol. 75*(2), 277-285.

Vaccarino, F., Pettit, H., Bloom, F., & Koob, G. (1984). Effects of intracerebroventricular administration of methylnaloxonium chloride on heroin self-administration in the rat. *Pharmacol. Biochem. Behav., 23,* 495-498.

Woods, J.H., & Winger, G. (1987). Opioids, receptors, and abuse liability. in H.Y. Meltzer (Ed.), *Psychopharmacology: The third generation of progress* (pp. 1555-1579). New York: Raven Press.

22

The Reward System and Cocaine Abuse

GEORGE F. KOOB

Dependence and addiction are characterized by two important phenomena: a compulsion to take the drug with a loss of control in limiting intake and a characteristic withdrawal syndrome that results in both physical and behavioral signs of discomfort when the drug is removed. The development of animal models, both for the acute reinforcing or rewarding effects of drugs and for the withdrawal syndromes associated with the removal of the drug after chronic access or administration, has significantly aided the search for neurobiological substrates of these phenomena.

This search for a neurobiological substrate of drug dependence has begun to focus on a particular site in the forebrain that integrates limbic function with the extrapyramidal motor system. The region of the nucleus accumbens in the anterior part of the basal forebrain with its connections to the medial forebrain bundle seems to play a critical role in mediating not only the acute reinforcing effects of drugs but also the motivational aspects of drug withdrawal. This chapter explores studies directed at elucidating the neurobiological substrates of reinforcing and dependence-inducing properties of cocaine. Further, a conceptual framework for the motivational aspects of drug dependence that is possibly common to all drugs of abuse is elaborated.

PSYCHOMOTOR STIMULANT EFFECTS OF COCAINE

Cocaine has stimulator-activating effects similar to many other drugs classified as psychomotor stimulants. For example, cocaine has been used for centuries to suppress hunger and fatigue (Angrist & Sudilovsky, 1976). Clinical studies assessing its subjective effects have demonstrated that cocaine produces euphoria (Fischman et al., 1983). In animals, cocaine acutely increases motor activity (Groppetti et al., 1973), decreases food intake (Groppetti et al., 1973), has psychomotor stimulant actions on operant behavior (Spealman et al.,

This work was supported by a grant from The NIDA (DA 04398) to G.F.K.

1977), enhances conditioned responding (Spealman et al., 1977), decreases the threshold for reinforcing brain stimulation (Kornetsky & Esposito, 1981), and readily acts as a reinforcer for drug self-administration (Pickens & Thompson, 1968). Cocaine as a psychomotor stimulant is shorter acting and less potent than amphetamine (Simon, 1973). At higher doses, cocaine produces the intense stereotypy associated with amphetamine or apomorphine, but is significantly less potent (Randrup & Munkvad, 1970) and may be less effective (Simon, 1973).

Cocaine is a local anesthetic that is still used clinically. It also has convulsant properties (Matsuzaki, 1978), and with chronic administration, these properties seem to become sensitized, as do the motor effects of cocaine (Post et al., 1976). This sensitization has been hypothesized as being analogous to "kindling" associated with repeated electrical brain stimulation.

COCAINE NEUROPHARMACOLOGY

Cocaine has important effects on monoamine metabolism. It blocks norepinephrine and dopamine reuptake and increases catecholamine turnover (Groppetti et al., 1973). Cocaine also blocks the uptake of serotonin, thereby presumably alternating serotonin synthesis (Knapp & Mandell, 1972) and turnover (Friedman et al., 1975). The local anesthetic properties of cocaine are not thought to be important for the production of its acute psychological effects since similar subjective effects cannot be observed with other local anesthetics (Fischman et al., 1983).

A critical role for dopamine in the psychomotor stimulant effects of cocaine was suggested by the observation that the locomotor activation produced by cocaine could be blocked by 6-hydroxydopamine (6-OHDA) lesions of the nucleus accumbens (Kelly & Iversen, 1976). In that study, the lesion effect was thought to be largely due to dopamine depletion, since when norepinephrine forebrain depletions were minimized by pretreatment with desmethylimipramine, the dopamine lesions remained effective in blocking cocaine's effect. Furthermore, similar nucleus accumbens 6-OHDA lesions block the locomotor stimulant effects of d-amphetamine, but not of caffeine or scopolamine (Joyce & Koob, 1981), heroin, or corticotropin-releasing factor (Swerdlow & Koob, 1985; Vaccarino et al., 1986).

NEUROBIOLOGICAL SUBSTRATES OF THE ACUTE REINFORCING EFFECTS OF COCAINE—INTRACRANIAL SELF-STIMULATION

Animal models for the acute reinforcing effects of psychomotor stimulants have included studies of the effects of these drugs on reward thresholds, measures of preference for the environment paired with drug administration, and direct self-administration of the drug. The discovery of intracranial self-stimulation (ICSS) suggested a "short-circuiting" of the reinforcement process and provided a unique means to assess the motivation to respond to hedonic stimuli

(Olds & Milner, 1954). ICSS is typically obtained from most regions of the limbic system, but electrodes placed in a midbrain-forebrain system (the medial forebrain bundle including the ventral tegmental area), which courses through the lateral hypothalamus, produce the highest rates of responding. ICSS, however, has also been produced in regions as far removed from the classical limbic system as the cerebellum and nucleus solitarius of the brainstem.

The potency of ICSS as a reinforcer not only led to its rapid use as a tool to measure activity in the brain reward systems but also created many problems of measurement and interpretation (Stellar & Stellar, 1985). One of the first measures of brain stimulation reward was the absolute rate of responding. To obtain that measure, an animal would be tested using a specified suprathreshold current intensity until response rates had stabilized from session to session. Any treatment that increased the rate of responding was thought to reflect a facilitation of reward or a lowering of threshold for reward. This phenomenon, in which the actual value of the reinforcer would be directly related to the output of the organism to obtain the reinforcer, has a theoretical basis in motivational theory (Herrnstein, 1971). Lever-pressing rates for ICSS increase after administration of amphetamine (Cassens & Mills, 1973; Goodall & Carey, 1975; Koob et al., 1977; Phillips & Fibiger, 1973; Stein, 1964; Stein & Ray, 1960; Wauquier & Niemegeers, 1974a). Cocaine also facilitates responding for brain stimulation reward (Crow, 1970; Wauquier & Niemegeers, 1974b).

A limited amount of work has explored site-specific effects for the facilitation of brain stimulation by psychomotor stimulants (Stellar & Rice, 1989). In a study using a choice procedure and continuous access to brain stimulation from three separate electrodes in the same animals, rats preferred to self-stimulate in the ventral tegmental area at moderate and high doses of d-amphetamine (Koob et al., 1977). In the same study, rats given a choice of self-stimulating in the septal area, anterior lateral hypothalamus, or posterior lateral hypothalamus chose the posterior lateral hypothalamus under the influence of d-amphetamine. When given a choice of self-stimulating in the posterior lateral hypothalamus, the ventral tegmental area, or the region of the locus coeruleus, the rats, under the influence of d-amphetamine, chose the ventral tegmental area. This pattern of preference choices under the influence of the drug paralleled the nondrug thresholds, and anatomically, it also parallels the course of the mesocorticolimbic dopamine system.

Alternative procedures have been developed to evaluate thresholds for brain stimulation directly by establishing within each test session a function rating current intensity or current frequency with behavioral output. When rats are systemically subjected to an ascending or descending series of rate-intensity functions, a sigmoidal function results, the slope of which increases the closer one approaches the low threshold areas of midbrain/lateral hypothalamus (Fig. 22-1). Shifts of this function to the right or left without changes in the maximal rate of responding have been hypothesized to reflect changes in threshold for rewarding brain stimulation. Using rate/intensity (R/I) functions, psychomotor stimulants, such as amphetamine and cocaine, cause a shift to the left (Phillips & LePiane, 1986; Steiner & Stokely, 1973), as can be seen in Figure 22-2.

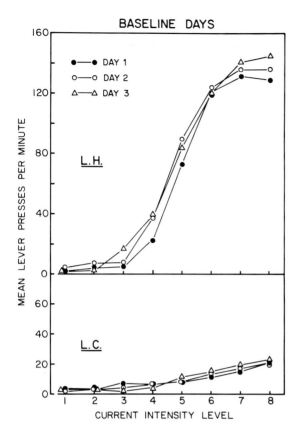

Figure 22-1. Rate versus intensity function for ICSS in rats. Eight rats had electrodes placed in the lateral hypothalamus (LH), and seven rats had electrodes aimed at the locus coeruleus (LC). Each curve represents one session with a descending sequence. Currents ranged from 5 to 40 μA (60 Herz AC RMS) for the LH and 15 to 50 μA for the LC.

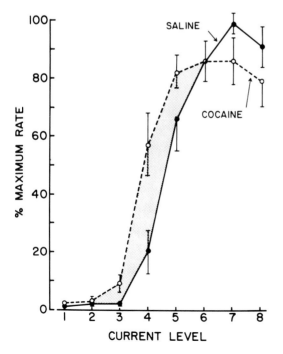

Figure 22-2. Effects of intraperitoneally injected cocaine (10 mg/kg) in rats lever-pressing for brain stimulation reward from electrodes in the lateral hypothalamus. Cocaine was injected intraperitoneally 15 minutes before the test session. Rats were tested for 5 minutes at each of eight current levels in a descending series. Data are expressed as mean ± SEM of the percent of maximal responding for each rat under the saline condition (n = 8).

The high-incentive, low-drive properties of ICSS have been exploited by Kornetsky and associates to develop a rate-independent measure of reward (Kornetsky & Esposito, 1979). Rate measures per se can be difficult to interpret when attempting to measure reinforcement threshold. For example, rats allowed a choice between brain stimulation in two different sites showed a preference for the site that maintained the lower rate of responding (Valenstein, 1964). Thus, threshold measures for a given reinforcer that are independent of the absolute rate of responding may be a more valid measure of the motivation to respond for a reinforcer.

In the Kornetsky threshold procedure, a series of trials begins with the delivery of a noncontingent 0.5-second stimulus of brain stimulation. If the animal responds by turning a wheel manipulandum one-quarter turn within 7.5 seconds of the onset of the "priming stimulus," a second stimulus is delivered that is identical to the first noncontingent stimulus. The intensity of the stimulus (magnitude of the reinforcer) is varied according to a psychophysical procedure in which stimuli are presented in an alternating descending and ascending series. Five trials are presented at each intensity level. The threshold value for each series is defined as the midpoint in current intensity between the current intensity at which the animal made three or more correct responses out of five stimulus presentations and the current intensity at which fewer than three correct responses were made (Marcus & Kornetsky, 1974). This discrete trial threshold measure of reward has proved sensitive to pharmacological manipulation, which is consistent with the hypothesis that it measures reward threshold reliably (Kornetsky & Esposito, 1979).

Amphetamine and cocaine also enhance reward in the "rate-independent" measures of ICSS threshold (Esposito et al., 1978; Kornetsky & Esposito, 1979; Liebman & Butcher, 1974). Using the threshold procedure (Kornetsky & Esposito, 1981), it was demonstrated that cocaine lowered the reward threshold at doses that actually increased the detection threshold (Fig. 22-3). For detection threshold measures, the initial noncontingent stimulus varied in intensity (at subreward levels) while the second or response-contingent stimulus was held constant at a rewarding intensity (above threshold) in order to maintain responding. Thus, the first stimulus acted as a discriminative stimulus indicating the availability of brain stimulation as a reward (Kornetsky & Esposito, 1981). This suggests that cocaine was having an effect on reward threshold

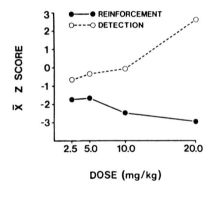

Figure 22-3. Mean effect of various doses of cocaine on the threshold for brain stimulation reward and on the threshold for brain stimulation detection. Data are expressed as Z scores based on the respective mean and standard deviation of the effects of saline (n = 4). (From Kornetsky & Bain, 1982, with permission.)

that was different from its effect on the ability of the animals to make a psychophysical discrimination of brain stimulation.

NEUROBIOLOGICAL SUBSTRATES OF THE ACUTE REINFORCING EFFECTS OF COCAINE—INTRAVENOUS SELF-ADMINISTRATION

In models involving direct self-administration of the drugs, rats with limited access (3 hours/day) show a stable and regular drug intake over each daily session (Fig. 22-4). In addition, after the loading dose, responding for cocaine within a session is remarkably regular. No obvious tolerance or dependence develops. Rats are generally maintained on a low-requirement, fixed-ratio (FR) schedule, such as an FR1 or FR5. A special aspect of this model using an FR schedule is that the rats seem to regulate the amount of drug self-administered. Lowering the dose from the training dose of 0.75 mg/kg per injection increases the number of cocaine infusions self-administered; increasing the dose decreases the number of self-administered cocaine infusions.

Studies using the intravenous self-administration model have strongly implicated dopamine in the reinforcing effects of cocaine. Low doses of dopamine receptor antagonists, when injected systemically, reliably increase cocaine self-administration (Davis & Smith, 1975; Ettenberg et al., 1982; Yokel & Wise, 1975, 1976; Fig. 22-5). Thus, rats seem to compensate for decreases in the magnitude of reinforcement with an increase in cocaine self-administration (or a decrease in the interinjection interval), a response similar to lowering the dose of cocaine. This finding suggests that a partial blockade of dopamine receptors produces a partial blockade of the reinforcing actions of cocaine.

In general, experiments investigating the effects of selective D_1 and D_2 antagonists on cocaine self-administration suggest that both D_1 (Caine et al., 1990; Hubner & Moreton, 1991; Kelven & Woolverton, 1990; Koob et al.,

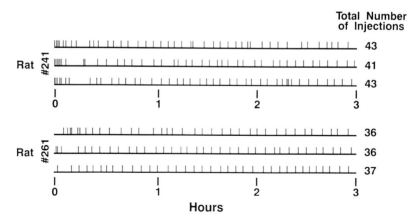

Figure 22-4. Representative response records for two rats self-administering cocaine. Test sessions were 3 hours in duration. Each mark represents a response/infusion of intravenous drug (0.75 mg/kg/injection).

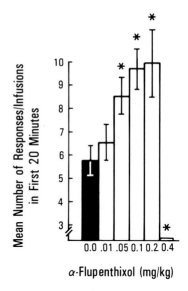

Figure 22-5. The effects of α-flupenthixol on the loading dose (infusions in the first 20 minutes of the 3-hour test sessions) in animals that are self-administering cocaine. A posteriori Newman-Keuls tests compared each treatment dose with the appropriate no-drug control. An asterisk in the base of histogram indicates that the treatment dose was reliably different from the no-drug saline condition ($P < 0.05$). (From Ettenberg et al., 1982, with permission.)

1987), and D_2 (Bergman et al., 1990; Creese and Iversen, 1974; De Wit & Wise, 1977; Woolverton & Virus, 1989) antagonists can decrease the reinforcing properties of cocaine. However, D_2 antagonists have been reported to decrease responding maintained by food, as well as responding maintained by cocaine (Caine et al., 1990; Nakajima & Baker, 1989; Woolverton & Virus, 1989), and recent studies suggest that D_2 antagonists can selectively block motor function (reaction time task) at low doses (Amalric et al., 1992). These results suggest that cocaine may act on D_1 receptors by a selective anatomical action on the mesocorticolimbic dopamine system.

A role for dopamine in the reinforcing properties of cocaine was extended by the observation that 6-hydroxydopamine (6-OHDA) lesions of the nucleus accumbens produce extinction-like responding and a significant and long-lasting decrease in self-administration of cocaine over days (Lyness et al., 1979; Roberts et al., 1977, 1980). Although these decreases in self-administration were interpreted as a reduction in the reinforcing efficacy of cocaine, not all rats showed a clear extinction-like pattern of responding, suggesting that factors other than the motivational aspects of cocaine reinforcement might be altered. To address this issue and to examine the anatomical specificity of this effect, rats trained to self-administer cocaine were subjected to a progressive ratio test in which the response requirement was increased by one step, then two steps, and then four steps, etc., until the rats stopped responding (termed the breaking point). Using this progressive ratio test, 6-OHDA lesions of the nucleus accumbens dramatically decreased the fixed ratio value for which rats would continue to work (Koob et al., 1987; Fig. 22-6). Similar lesions of the caudate nucleus failed to significantly alter performance on the progressive ratio test.

There are relatively little data regarding the efferent anatomical substrates through which the nucleus accumbens may process the stimulus of cocaine

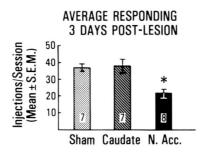

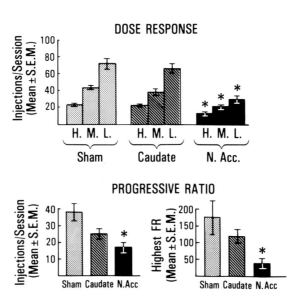

Figure 22-6. Effects of 6-hydroxydopamine (6-OHDA) lesions to the nucleus accumbens and corpus striatum on responding in rats self-administering cocaine. **Top,** Continuous reinforcement data averaged for the first 3 days postlesion (mean ± SEM). Sham, vehicle (0.1 mg/ml ascorbic acid in saline) injected controls; caudate, rats receiving 8 μg in 2 μl of 6-OHDA injected into the caudate nucleus; N.Acc., rats receiving 8 μg in 2 μl of 6-OHDA injected into the nucleus accumbens. **Middle,** Dose-effect functions for each group. H, two times the normal 0.75 mg/kg per injection dose; M, middle dose range, 0.75 mg/kg per injection; L, one-half of the 0.75 mg/kg per injection dose. **Bottom,** Mean rewards and mean highest ratio obtained by each group on the progressive ratio probe. *Significantly different from sham group, $P < 0.05$ Newman-Keuls test. (From Koob et al., 1987, with permission.)

reinforcement. However, there are established efferent connections between the nucleus accumbens and ventral pallidum, and previous work has established the substantia innominata-ventral pallidum as an important connection in the expression of behavioral stimulation produced by dopamine activation of the nucleus accumbens (Swerdlow et al., 1984). Thus, a logical hypothesis was that the region of the ventral pallidum may also be involved in the processing of the reinforcing properties of cocaine.

To test this hypothesis, rats were trained to intravenously self-administer cocaine and were then subjected to lesions of the substantia innominata-ventral pallidum. After establishment of a stable baseline (FR5 schedule), the rats received bilateral ibotenic acid lesions of the region of the substantia innominata-ventral pallidum (Hubner & Koob, 1990). The lesions significantly decreased baseline cocaine self-administration, and when the rats were subjected to a progressive ratio procedure, the rats with substantia innominata-ventral pallidum lesions produced a significant decrease in the highest ratio obtained for cocaine when compared to the control animals (Hubner & Koob, 1990). These results suggest that the region of the substantia innominata-ventral pallidum may be an important site in the processing of the reinforcing effects of cocaine. The precise component of the substantia innominata-ventral pallidum region critical for this functional output of the nucleus accumbens will need to be delineated in future studies.

NEUROBIOLOGICAL SUBSTRATES OF THE WITHDRAWAL ASSOCIATED WITH COCAINE DEPENDENCE

Cocaine dependence is not characterized by major opiate-like physical signs of withdrawal during abstinence. However, evidence exists to show that after a cocaine binge, abstinence is characterized by severe depressive symptoms combined with irritability and anxiety (Ellinwood & Petrie, 1977; Gawin & Kleber, 1986). These symptoms last several hours to several days and characterize the "crash" associated with the cocaine dependence cycle.

One of the more salient symptoms of the "crash" stage is anhedonia, which can be defined as the inability to derive pleasure from normally pleasurable stimuli. An animal model for anhedonia is an increase in reward thresholds as measured with ICSS. ICSS thresholds have been hypothesized to reflect the state of the reward systems in the brain of an animal because animals will readily self-administer the stimulations to their own brains, and ICSS is thought to activate the same neural substrates that mediate the reinforcing effects of natural reinforcers, e.g., water, food (Stellar & Stellar, 1985). As discussed above, cocaine, when injected acutely, has been well documented to lower self-stimulation thresholds in rats (Esposito et al., 1978).

To test the hypothesis that chronic self-administration of cocaine may result in the opposite effect on brain stimulation thresholds (i.e., an increase), animals were allowed to self-administer cocaine intravenously for long periods, and reward thresholds were monitored during the course of cocaine withdrawal. To accomplish this monitoring, rats were prepared with chronic indwelling brain stimulation electrodes aimed at the lateral hypothalamus. After establishment of stable measures of brain stimulation reward thresholds, the rats were implanted with jugular catheters and trained to self-administer cocaine on an FR5 schedule of reinforcement in daily 3-hour sessions until stable responding was achieved.

Subsequently, the rats in the experimental groups were allowed to self-administer cocaine for different time periods (3, 6, 12, 24, and 48 hours using a

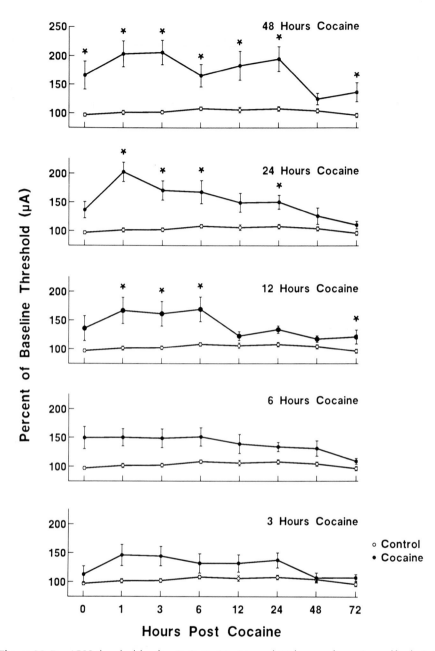

Figure 22-7. ICSS thresholds after 0, 3, 6, 12, 24, and 48 hours of cocaine self-administration at several time points postcocaine (0, 1, 3, 6, 12, 24, 48, and 72 hours). The results are expressed as percent change from baseline threshold levels. The mean ± SEM baseline threshold for the experimental group was 37.4 ± 2.5 μA and for the control group 35.9 ± 3.1 μA. The asterisks indicate statistically significant differences (P < 0.05) between control and experimental groups with Dunnett's tests, following a significant group × hours interaction in an analysis of variance. (From Markou & Koob, 1991, with permission.)

within-subject design). ICSS thresholds then were determined at varying times after the termination of the self-administration session (0, 1, 3, 6, 12, 24, 48, and 72 hours). Animals in the control group (repeated brain stimulation thresholds with no cocaine) were tested at these same time points.

Cocaine withdrawal produced an elevation in brain stimulation reward thresholds compared to predrug baseline levels and the thresholds of the control animals. The magnitude and duration of the elevation in reward thresholds were proportional to the amount of cocaine self-administered (duration of the self-administration session; Figure 22-7). This elevation in reward threshold has been hypothesized to reflect an "anhedonic" state, and as such it may be homologous to the anhedonia reported by human drug users after a cocaine binge (Markou & Koob, 1991). Another explanation for these results was that the elevation in reward thresholds reflects fatigue instead of a reward effect. However, this seems unlikely since the task used for brain stimulation (rotating a wheel) minimizes work output, and response latencies to respond to the priming stimulus were not significantly increased during cocaine withdrawal.

The effect of cocaine withdrawal on brain stimulation thresholds was the opposite of the effect of acute cocaine on brain stimulation reward (Esposito et al., 1978). These results suggest that cocaine, during the course of a cocaine self-administration bout and withdrawal, can dramatically alter the function of the substrates in the medial forebrain bundle that mediate brain stimulation reward.

To summarize, the acute reinforcing effects of cocaine seem to depend on the presynaptic release of dopamine within the region of the nucleus accumbens, in that destruction of this mesocorticolimbic dopamine system extinguishes cocaine responding and decreases the amount of work an animal will perform to obtain the drug. The dopamine receptor subtype important for this reinforcing effect may be the D_1 receptor. Chronic access to cocaine produces a withdrawal state as reflected in augmentation of brain stimulation reward thresholds, which seems to be opposite to the actions of the drug administered acutely. These results are thought to reflect a change in the activity of neural elements in the medial forebrain bundle and thus may be responsible for the negative reinforcing state associated with the anhedonia of cocaine withdrawal.

NEUROBIOLOGY OF COCAINE DEPENDENCE AND THE OPPONENT PROCESS THEORY OF MOTIVATION

The concept that drug tolerance and withdrawal may reflect neurobiological adaptation opposite to the acute effects of the drug itself has been elaborated at the behavioral level in opponent process theory (Solomon, 1980). In this theory it is hypothesized that reinforcers arouse positive affective and hedonic processes (termed a-processes) that are opposed by negative affective and hedonic processes (termed b-processes). In the case of drug dependence, the a-processes are hypothesized to be simple and stable and to follow the acute drug response closely in time. In contrast, the b-processes are of longer latency in time, are slow to build up strength, and are slow to decay. With such drugs as cocaine, the b-processes would follow an acute positive hedonic response of the drug (a-process). Thus for cocaine, the affective responses associated with intravenous self-administration, which in humans constitute the "high" or "rush," would reflect the a-process, and the aversive dysphoric effects of withdrawal (higher reward threshold) would reflect the opponent b-process. This b-process in humans would constitute the dysphoria associated with psychostimulant withdrawal.

One difficulty with this interpretation is that in the intravenous cocaine self-administration model there is little evidence of tolerance development. Even with 24- to 48-hour access to cocaine, rats continue to take the same amount of drug over time (Markou & Koob, 1991). However, a more careful microanalysis of the patterns of cocaine self-administration has shown that rats may develop a small local tolerance to the reinforcing effects of cocaine (Paulus, M.P., Markou, A., & Koob, G.F., unpublished data).

The results outlined above may provide a neurobiological basis for an opponent process as it relates to cocaine dependence. The region of the nucleus accumbens seems to be important for processing the cocaine-reinforcing stimulus. Dopamine receptors in the nucleus accumbens that connect through the region of the ventral pallidum may be critical for mediating the acute reinforcing properties of cocaine. This same circuitry may be involved in the aversive stimulus effects associated with cocaine withdrawal. Thus, the same neural elements responsible for "euphoria" may also be changed in the course of dependence to be responsible for the "dysphoria" associated with drug removal.

The cellular events that could mediate such plasticity remain to be discovered. However, two possible mechanisms have been hypothesized to exist at the molecular and cellular level to explain this neural adaptation: a "within-systems" adaptation and a "between-systems" adaptation (Koob & Bloom, 1988). In a within-systems opposing process, the primary molecular or cellular response to the drug would itself adapt to neutralize the effects of the drug. Persistence of this adaptation after the drug is removed would produce the aversive stimulus effects of withdrawal. In a between-systems opposing process, a different cellular system and separate molecular apparatus would be triggered by the changes in the primary drug response, and again removal of the drug would unmask the activity of this system to produce the aversive stimulus effects of withdrawal.

One possible neurochemical mechanism involved in the cocaine withdrawal state would be some alteration in dopamine function reflecting a dopamine depletion or hypofunction (Dackis & Gold, 1985). This would be an example of a within-systems adaptation (Koob & Bloom, 1988). At this time there is little evidence in direct support of this hypothesis. Alternatively, a separate neurochemical process may develop that opposes the acute action of the drug. This would be an example of a between-systems adaptation (Koob & Bloom, 1988). For example, there may be changes in one of the nucleus accumbens output systems that are augmented during the course of a cocaine self-administration bout, and this output system may overexpress its action during withdrawal.

Cocaine as a drug of abuse may be unique in that at both ends of the hedonic spectrum it may act mainly on motivational processes, with less extraneous effects. For example, the positive reinforcing actions of cocaine may be more intense than those of other drugs of abuse, and as a result the withdrawal effect may share not only the intensity but also the motivational selectivity. Identification of the cellular and molecular components of these adaptations may provide the keys to the understanding not only of cocaine addiction but also of the addiction process itself.

ACKNOWLEDGMENTS

I thank Molecular and Experimental Medicine's Word Processing for preparation of the manuscript. I thank also for their help and discussions C. Kornetsky, C. Hubner, A. Markou, A. Ettenberg, S.B. Caine, P. Robledo, R. Maldonado, F. Weiss, and F. Bloom whose work is represented in this chapter.

REFERENCES

Amalric, M., Berkow, M., Polis, I., & Koob, G.F. (1992). Selective effects of low dose D2 dopaminergic receptor antagonism in a reaction time task in rats. *Neuropsychopharmacology* (in press).

Angrist, B., & Sudilovsky, A. (1976). Central nervous system stimulants: Historical aspects and clinical effects. In L.L. Iversen, S.D. Iversen, & S.H. Snyder (Eds.), *Handbook of Psychopharmacology*, Vol. 11 (pp. 99-163). New York: Plenum Press.

Bergman, J., Kamien, J.B., & Spealman, R.D. (1990). Antagonism of cocaine self-administration by selective dopamine D1 and D2 antagonists. *Behav. Pharmacol., 1,* 355-363.

Caine, S.B., Berhow, M., Amalric, M., & Koob, G.F. (1990). The D1 antagonist SCH 23390 and the D2 antagonist raclopride selectively decrease behavior maintained by cocaine or food in the rat. *Neurosci. Abst. 16,* 252.

Cassens, G.P., & Mills, A.W. (1973). Lithium and amphetamine: Opposite effects on threshold of intracranial reinforcement. *Psychopharmacologia, 30,* 283-290.

Creese, I., & Iversen, S.D. (1974). A role of forebrain dopamine systems in amphetamine-induced stereotyped behavior in the rat. *Psychopharmacology, 39,* 345-347.

Crow, T.J. (1970). Enhancement of cocaine of intracranial self-stimulation in the rat. *Life Sci., 9,* 375-381.

Dackis, C.A., & Gold, M.S. (1985). New concepts in cocaine addiction: The dopamine depletion hypothesis. *Neurosci. Biobehav. Rev., 9,* 469-477.

Davis, W.M., & Smith, S.G. (1975). Effect of haloperidol on (+)-amphetamine self-administration. *J. Pharm. Pharmacol., 27,* 540-542.

De Wit, H., & Wise, R.A. (1977). Blockade of cocaine reinforcement in rats with the dopamine receptor blocker pimozide, but not with the noradrenergic blockers pentolamine and phenoxybenzamine. *Can. J. Psychol., 31,* 195-203.

Ellinwood, E.H., & Petrie, W.M. (1977). Dependence on amphetamine, cocaine and other stimulants. In S.N. Pradhan (Ed.), *Drug abuse: Clinical and basic aspects* (pp. 248-262). St. Louis: CV Mosby.

Esposito, R.U., Motola, A.H.D., & Kornetsky, C. (1978). Cocaine: Acute effects on reinforcement thresholds for self-stimulation behavior to the medial forebrain bundle. *Pharmacol. Biochem. Behav., 8,* 437-439.

Ettenberg, A., Pettit, H.O., Bloom, F.E., & Koob, G.F. (1982). Heroin and cocaine intravenous self-administration in rats: Mediation by separate neural systems. *Psychopharmacology, 78,* 204-209.

Fischman, M.W., Schuster, C.R., & Hatano, Y. (1983). A comparison of the subjective and cardiovascular effects of cocaine and lidocaine in humans. *Pharmacol. Biochem. Behav., 18,* 123-127.

Friedman, E., Gershon, S., & Rotrosen, J. (1975). Effects of active cocaine treatment on the turnover of 5-hydroxytryptamine in the rat brain. *Br. J. Pharmacol., 54,* 61-64.

Gawin, F.H., & Kleber, H.D. (1986). Abstinence symptomatology and psychiatric diagnosis in cocaine abusers. *Arch. Gen. Psychiat., 43,* 107-113.

Goodall, E.B., & Carey, R.J. (1975). Effects of d- versus l-amphetamine, food deprivation, and current intensity on self-stimulation of the lateral hypothalamus, substantia nigra, and medial frontal cortex of the rat. *J. Comp. Physiol. Psychol., 89,* 1029-1045.

Groppetti, A., Zambotti, F., Biazzi, A., & Mantegazza, P. (1973). Amphetamine and cocaine on amine turnover. In E. Usdin & S.H. Snyder (Eds.), *Frontiers in catecholamine research* (pp. 917-925). Oxford: Pergamon Press.

Herrnstein, R.J. (1971). Quantitative hedonism. *J. Psychiat. Res., 8,* 399-412.

Hubner, C.B., & Koob, G.F. (1990). The ventral pallidum plays a role in mediating cocaine and heroin self-administration in the rat. *Brain Res., 508,* 20-29.

Hubner, C.B., & Moreton, J.E. (1991). Effects of selective D1 and D2 receptor antagonists cocaine self-administration in the rat. *Psychopharmacology, 105,* 151-156.

Joyce, E.M., & Koob, G.F. (1981). Amphetamine-, scopolamine-, and caffiene-induced locomotor activity following 6-hydroxydopamine lesions of the mesolimbic dopamine system. *Psychopharmacology, 73,* 311-313.

Kelly, P.H., & Iversen, S.D. (1976). Selective 6-OHDA-induced destruction of mesolimbic dopamine neurons: Abolition of psychostimulant-induced locomotor activity in rats. *Eur. J. Pharmacol., 40,* 45-56.

Kleven, M.S., & Woolverton, W.L. (1990). Effects of continuous infusions of SCH 23390 on cocaine or food-maintained behavior in rhesus monkeys. *Behav. Pharmacol., 1,* 365-373.

Knapp, S., & Mandell, A.J. (1972). Narcotic drugs: Effects on the serotonin biosynthetic systems of the brain. *Science, 177,* 1209-1211.

Koob, G.F., & Bloom, F.E. (1988). Cellular and molecular mechanisms of drug dependence. *Science, 242,* 715-723.

Koob, G.F., Winger, G.D., Meyerhoff, J.L., & Annau, Z. (1977). Effects of d-amphetamine on concurrent self-stimulation of forebrain and brainstem loci. *Brain Res., 137,* 109-126.

Koob, G.F., Le, H.T., & Creese, I. (1987a). D-1 receptor antagonist SCH 23390 increases cocaine self-administration in the rat. *Neurosci. Lett., 79,* 315-321.

Koob, G.F., Vaccarino, F.J., Amalric, M., & Bloom, F.E. (1987b). Positive reinforcement properties of drugs: Search for neural substrates. In J. Engel & L. Oreland (Eds.), *Brain reward systems and abuse* (pp. 35-50). New York: Raven Press.

Kornetsky, C., & Bain, G. (1982). Biobehavioral bases of the reinforcing properties of opiate drugs. *Ann. NY. Acad. Sci., 398,* 240-259.

Kornetsky, C., & Esposito, R.U. (1979). Euphorigenic drugs: Effects on reward pathways of the brain. *Fed. Proc., 38,* 2473-2476.

Kornetsky, C., & Esposito, R.U. (1981). Reward and detection thresholds for brain stimulation: Dissociative effects of cocaine. *Brain Res., 209,* 496-500.

Liebman, J.M., & Butcher, L.L. (1974). Comparative involvement of dopamine and noradrenaline in rate-free self-stimulation in substantia nigra, lateral hypothalamus and mesencephalic central gray. *Nauny-Schmideberg's Arch. Pharmacol., 284,* 167-194.

Lyness, W.H., Friedle, N.M., & Moore, K.E. (1979). Destruction of dopaminergic nerve terminals in nucleus accumbens: Effect of d-amphetamine self-administration. *Pharmacol. Biochem. Behav., 11,* 663-666.

Marcus, R., & Kornetsky, C. (1974). Negative and positive intracranial reinforcement thresholds: Effects of morphine. *Psychopharmacologia, 38,* 1-14.

Markou, A., & Koob, G.F. (1991). Postcocaine anhedonia. An animal model of cocaine withdrawal. *Neuropharmacology, 4,* 17-26.

Matsuzaki, M. (1978). Alteration in pattern of EEG activities and convulsant effect of cocaine following chronic administration in the rhesus monkey. *Electroencephalogr. Clin. Neurophysiol., 45,* 1-15.

Nakajima, S., & Baker, J.D. (1989). Effects of D2 dopamine receptor blockade with raclopride on intracranial self-stimulation and food-reinforced operant behavior. *Psychopharmacology, 98,* 330-333.

Olds, J., & Milner, P. (1954). Positive reinforcement produced by electrical stimulation of septal area and other regions of rat brain. *J. Comp. Physiol. Psychol., 47,* 419-427.

Phillips, A.G., & Fibiger, H.C. (1973). Dopaminergic and noradrenergic substrates of positive reinforcement: Differential effects of d and l-amphetamine. *Science, 179,* 575-577.

Phillips, A.G., & LePiane, F.G. (1986). Effects of pimozide on and negative incentive contrast with rewarding brain stimulation. *Pharmacol. Biochem. Behav., 24,* 1577-1582.

Pickens, R., & Thompson, R. (1968). Cocaine-reinforced behavior in rats: effects of reinforcement magnitude and fixed ratio size. *J. Pharmacol. Exp. Ther., 161,* 122-129.

Post, R.M., Kopanda, R.T., & Black, K.E. (1976). Progressive effects of cocaine on behavior and central amine metabolism in rhesus monkeys: Relationship to kindling and psychoses. *Biol. Psychiatr., 11,* 405-419.

Randrup, A., & Munkvad, I. (1970). Biochemical, anatomical and psychological investigations of stereotyped behavior induced by amphetamines. In E. Costa & S. Garattini (Eds.), *Amphetamines and related compounds* (pp. 695-713). New York: Raven Press.

Roberts, D.C.S., Corcoran, M.E., & Fibiger, H.C. (1977). On the role of ascending catecholaminergic systems in intravenous self-administration of cocaine. *Pharmacol. Biochem. Behav., 6,* 615-620.

Roberts, D.C.S., Koob, G.F., Klonoff, P., & Fibiger, H.C. (1980). Extinction and recovery of cocaine self-administration following 6-hydroxydopamine lesions of the nucleus accumbens. *Pharmacol. Biochem. Behav., 12,* 781-787.

Simon, P. (1973). Psychopharmacological profile of cocaine. In E. Usdin & S.H. Snyder (Eds.), *Frontiers of catecholamine research* (pp. 1043-1044). Oxford: Pergamon Press.

Solomon, R.L. (1980). The opponent process theory of acquired motivation. *Am. Psychol., 35,* 691-712.

Spealman, R.D., Goldberg, S.R., Kelleher, R.T., Goldberg, D.M., & Charlton, J.P.

(1977). Some effects of cocaine and two cocaine analogs on schedule controlled behavior of squirrel monkeys. *J. Pharmacol. Exp. Ther., 202*, 500-509.

Stein, L. (1964). Self-stimulation of the brain and the central stimulant action of amphetamine. *Fed. Proc., 23*, 836-850.

Stein, L., & Ray, O.S. (1960). Brain stimulation reward "thresholds" self-determined in rat. *Psychopharmacologia, 1*, 251-256.

Steiner, S.S., & Stokely, S.N. (1973). Methamphetamine lowers self-stimulation thresholds. *Physiol. Psychol., 1*, 161-164.

Stellar, J.R., & Rice, M.B. (1989). Pharmacological basis of intracranial self-stimulation reward. In J.M. Liebman & S.J. Cooper (Eds.), *The neuropharmacological basis of reward* (p. 14-64). Oxford: Clarendon Press.

Stellar, J.R., & Stellar, E. (1985). *The neurobiology of reward and motivation.* New York: Springer-Verlag.

Swerdlow, N.R., & Koob, G.F. (1985). Separate neural substrates of the locomotor-activating properties of amphetamine, caffeine and corticotropin releasing factor (CRF) in the rat. *Pharmacol. Biochem. Behav., 23*, 303-307.

Swerdlow, N.R., Swanson, L.W., & Koob, G.F. (1984). Substantia innominata: Critical link in the behavioral expression of mesolimbic dopamine stimulation in the rat. *Neurosci. Lett., 50*, 19-24.

Vaccarino, F.J., Amalric, M., Swerdlow, N.R., & Koob, G.F. (1986). Blockade of amphetamine- but not opiate-induced locomotion following antagonism of dopamine function in the rat. *Pharmacol. Biochem. Behav., 24*, 61-65.

Valenstein, E.S. (1964). Problems of measurement and interpretation with reinforcing brain stimulation. *Psychol. Rep., 71*, 415-437.

Wauquier, A., & Niemegeers, C.J.E. (1974a). Intracranial self-stimulation in rats as a function of various stimulus parameters. IV. Influence of amphetamine on medial forebrain bundle stimulation with monopolar electrodes. *Psychopharmacologia, 34*, 265-274.

Wauquier, A., & Niemegeers, C.J.E. (1974b). Intracranial self-stimulation in rats as a function of various stimulus parameters. V. Influence of cocaine on medial forebrain bundle stimulation with monopolar electrodes. *Psychopharmacologia, 38*, 201-210.

Woolverton, W.L., & Virus, R.M. (1989). The effects of a D1 and a D2 dopamine antagonist on behavior maintained by cocaine or food, *Pharmacol. Biochem. Behav., 32*(3), 691-697.

Yokel, R.A., & Wise, R.A. (1975). Increased lever pressing for amphetamine after pimozide in rats. Implications for a dopamine theory of reward. *Science, 187*, 547-549.

Yokel, R.A., & Wise, R.A. (1976). Attenuation of intravenous amphetamine reinforcement by central dopamine blockade in rats. *Psychopharmacology, 48*, 311-318.

23

Paranoid Psychosis Following Continuous Amphetamine or Cocaine: Relationship to Selective Neurotoxicity

GAYLORD D. ELLISON

AMPHETAMINE PSYCHOSIS: STUDIES IN HUMANS

In schizophrenic patients, amphetamine (AMPH) worsens pre-existing psychotic symptoms. This effect implies an action on fundamental symptoms (Angrist et al., 1974) and suggests that AMPH psychosis may be a drug model of schizophrenia (Snyder et al., 1974). The classical description of AMPH psychosis is Connell's (1958) monograph reporting on 42 addicts who developed psychoses. Connell and others (Bell, 1965) concluded that AMPH psychosis, in the absence of physical signs, can manifest aberrant behaviors and ideations indistinguishable from paranoid schizophrenia, but others pointed to clear differences between schizophrenia and AMPH psychosis, i.e., auditory hallucinations were prominent in the former, in contrast to visual ones in the latter. How closely AMPH psychosis mimics schizophrenia seems to depend in part on the drug regimen used to precipitate the psychosis, for different types of AMPH-induced psychoses exist.

At one extreme are the rare but well-documented psychotic states that develop in certain drug-naive individuals shortly after they first ingest relatively low doses of AMPH. Although the resulting symptomatology can closely parallel schizophrenia, these acute low-dose cases are usually ascribed to a latent psychosis in the individual that has been triggered by the ingestion of the drug (Gold & Bowers, 1978). Presumably other drugs or events could have precipitated a developing psychosis in these vulnerable, borderline individuals. Most humans do not become psychotic on initial exposure to AMPH, but only after a chronic pattern of abuse has developed. This feature presents a problem in documenting the actual drug intake pattern, for such information can come only from the unreliable reports of the addicts themselves. Two less biased sources are reports from drug rehabilitation centers and observations during controlled studies on human volunteers. Ellinwood (1967) studied hospitalized addicts who reported well-formed delusions of persecution that grew out of an initial fear, suspiciousness, and an awareness of being watched. Over half of the patients had visual hallucinations (fleeting glimpses of just recognizable images converted into formed images of God, tormentors, etc.), auditory hallucinations (simple voices whispering the patient's name developing into voices with which the patient conversed), and tactile hallucinations (reports of infestations of microanimals and the presence of vermiform and encysted skin lesions that they felt, as well as saw). Three patients incurred punctuate scars when they attempted to dig out the imaginary encysted parasites (also described by Smith, 1969).

AMPH addicts develop a particular drug intake regimen. Kramer et al. (1967) reported that after initial phases of experimentation with AMPH, a pattern of usage emerges in which the abuser injects the drug about every 2 hours around the clock for a period of 3–6 days. The addict remains awake continuously, using the AMPH to ward off sleep and knowing full well that discontinuation of the drug would result in a rebound depression. During these "speed runs," behavior gradually becomes less organized as two alterations develop. First, the user pursues activities that progressively become less varied and more compulsive, eventually becoming perseverative hyperactivity that consists of repeatedly performing simple motor tasks, e.g., "motor stereotypies." The second alteration is a developing paranoia, the inevitability of which is accepted by the addicts. Early in the "speed run" the addict experiences suspicious thoughts that he or she recognizes as drug-induced, but as the run progresses, these thoughts intensify and begin to be accepted as real so that paranoid delusions develop (although experienced users sometimes become paranoid with a single dose of AMPH even after prolonged abstinence).

To reproduce these phenomena in a controlled hospital setting, Griffith et al. (1972) administered small doses of d-AMPH to volunteers hourly over a prolonged period. Within 1-5 days, eight of nine subjects developed a paranoid psychosis. During the course of the experiment the subjects gradually became hypochondriacal and dysphoric and were increasingly irritable. A distinct prepsychotic phase appeared, during which they confined themselves to their rooms and shut their doors. The onset of paranoia was usually abrupt. In an earlier study, Angrist and Gershon (1970) were able to elicit a greater variety of hallucinations, including auditory, cutaneous, olfactory, and visual, using higher doses than Griffith, but again administering the drug every few hours for several days. In both studies the patients spoke freely about their delusions. It may be that the symptomatology observed during these nearly continuous but relatively low-dose AMPH regimens is more similar to that of schizophrenia than symptoms produced by other schedules of drug administration, inasmuch as it combines progressive flattening of affect with well-formed delusions that are not predominantly visual (Ellison & Eison, 1983). A possible exception to this conclusion comes from a controlled experiment in which AMPH psychosis developed without prolonged drug intoxication. Bell (1973) was able to elicit a psychosis within an hour after injection of a single very large dose of methamphetamine administered intravenously to former addicts. Although this dose had a much greater effect on blood pressure than the small doses in Griffith's subjects, Bell's subjects for the most part concealed their psychosis rather well; most of them only admitted to having had hallucinations on later questioning. Emotional responsivity in such rapid, high-dose psychoses is usually brisk, often involving considerable anxiety (Bell, 1965; Slater, 1959), whereas schizophrenics and addicts towards the end of speed runs often exhibit a blunted affect. An even more important feature of such psychoses is that when Bell administered the methamphetamine, the former abusers, many of whom had been drug-free only a few days before testing, said that they experienced an immediate recurrence of the *identical paranoid delusions* they had previously experienced while taking AMPH. Indeed, whereas paranoia occurred in 12 of 14 patients who had previously experienced psychoses while taking AMPH, it did not develop in 2 patients who were eventually found not to have been previous regular users of AMPH nor to have had a previous episode of AMPH psychosis. In striking contrast, Griffith's study included five addicts who had no previous psychotic experiences with the drug, but who developed paranoid reactions when given the drug in frequent low doses. These findings lead to the conclusion that the relatively covert kinds of paranoid delusions studied by Bell may, in part, represent a conditioning phenomenon—the reinstatement of behavior learned under previous drug experiences (Ellinwood & Kilbey, 1977)— and that the most reliable way to induce a model paranoid psychosis in psychologically healthy individuals is by exposing them to frequent low doses of d-AMPH for several days. It may be that the continuous but low-level presence of psychoactive stimulants over an extended period of time is especially relevant to the study of schizophrenia because it results in a prolonged period of excitation similar to that which has been reported to occur during an acute psychotic episode (see Bowers, 1968).

CONTINUOUS AMPHETAMINES AND BEHAVIOR IN ANIMALS

Most animal studies on the effects of chronic AMPH administration involve only one or two daily intraperitoneal injections, rather than a continuous drug regimen. To enable the study of a continuous drug regimen, we developed slow-release, subcutaneous silicone pellets (Huberman et al., 1977) that produced an initial brain level of AMPH in rats equivalent to that produced by a 2.0 mg/kg d-AMPH sulfate injection (i.p.). Rats implanted with these AMPH pellets, like humans, showed clear stages of behavior (Ellison et al., 1978a). These stages were best seen when rats were raised in complex, social colonies for several months, and half were then implanted with AMPH pellets. On the first few hours after pellet implantation, the AMPH rats were hyperactive and exploratory. Gradually the space traversed by these animals decreased, and their behavior evolved over the next 24 hours into motor stereotypies of an increasingly more circumscribed nature that persisted for 2-3 days. During these 3 days the AMPH rats were out in the arena more than controls throughout the day and night. Motor stereotypies then disappeared, and the rats entered the next phase, during which the arousal and anorectic effects of AMPH waned and AMPH rats began to eat and retreated to the burrows for a day. They then

Table 23-1. Stages of effects of continuous amphetamine

	Human	Monkey	Rat
Initial stage, acute effects	Euphoria and exhilaration, except in low doses to addicts	Increased activity Fixated staring Motor stereotypy	Increased activity Motor stereotypy
Crash stage	Increased irritability Anhedonia, intellectual flattening Depression and self-isolation	General inactivity hunched posture Motor dyskinesias, including tongue protrusions, tremors	Retreat to burrows, heightened startle
Late stage	Paranoid delusions Parasitosis Hallucinations	Hallucinatory-like behaviors Parasitosis Sudden orient and fleeing "wet-dog" shakes	Parasitosis Hallucinogen-like behavior (limb flick "Wet-dog" shakes) Sudden startle Aberrant social behavior: fixations Fight or flight

began to show exaggerated startle responses, frequent vocalizations, and increased social behaviors. Whereas the AMPH rats had not engaged in social interactions during the initial stages of constant AMPH, during days 5-7 they showed heightened social behaviors, especially fight and flight responses. Stable pairs of implanted rats formed social bonds of aggressor-aggressee, so that the same pairs of implanted rats would seek each other out and fight, in a form of social stereotypy. This late and social phase of constant AMPH intoxication, which appeared after 4-7 days, represents an entirely different phenomenon from the earlier forms, and it has a number of similarities to AMPH psychosis in humans.

In comparable studies, we found that the stage of alterations in behavior after continuous AMPH administration in adult monkeys are similar to those in rats, but the forms of the behavior, particularly the late-stage behaviors, are much more complex and vivid (Ellison et al., 1981). After a brief period of heightened activity, each monkey either developed highly idiosyncratic episodes of extremely complex motor stereotypies or began to engage in prolonged bouts of staring at a distant, circumscribed spot on the wall. For higher organisms, such as a monkey, staring apparently can be an equivalent of motor stereotypies in rats. This phase was followed by a period of less focused activity when the monkeys were often inactive and seemed lethargic, although they did not sleep. On the fourth to sixth day several new behaviors developed, including sudden orienting responses; motor dyskinesias, such as limb tremors and oral protrusions; and discrete episodes of hallucinatory behaviors, including attack threats to the humans, sudden fleeing responses, capturing movements by the hands in midair, and excited grooming episodes suggestive of parasitosis. Some of these hallucinatory episodes were extraordinarily vivid.

Thus, monkeys also show stages of continuous AMPH intoxication, but the variety of behaviors are much more varied and the late-stage behaviors much more vivid than the rats, although the hallucinatory behaviors in the monkeys occurred at almost exactly the same point (4-5 days) as in the rats (Table 23-1).

The problem with studying these late-stage behaviors is that they have a very low rate of occurrence. Therefore, we developed a procedure in which rats primed with the AMPH pellet for 4½ days were given a brief drug-free period and then were "reactivated" with a low dose of AMPH. Using this paradigm, it was demonstrated that after several days of continuous administration, d-AMPH comes to have properties that are more like a hallucinogen than like acute d-AMPH (Nielsen et al., 1980a). After several days of pellet-pretreatment, the rats reinjected with AMPH showed increased "wet-dog shakes," episodes of parasitotic-like frantic grooming, and limb-flicks, a behavior normally suppressed by AMPH in drug-naive rats but observed after the administration of hallucinogens, such as LSD or mescaline. This finding is of theoretical importance, for it suggests that after several days of continuous AMPH the drug takes on properties that are in some ways more like a hallucinogen than AMPH. This syndrome then disappears relatively rapidly after removal of the pellet.

UNIQUE BIOCHEMICAL EFFECTS INDUCED BY CONTINUOUS AMPHETAMINES

In studies of catecholamine fluorescence in AMPH pellet rats (Ellison et al., 1978b), we found that in normal rats the caudate nucleus has a relatively diffuse fluorescence with extremely fine terminals and axons, whereas in rats sacrificed from 2 to 3 days after AMPH pellet implantation the caudate takes on a cloudy or filmy appearance as though much of the dopamine has diffused out into extracellular space. However, in rats sacrificed 5 days after pellet implantation, during the period of paranoid-like social disruptions, a highly unusual type of fluorescence is observed in the caudate nucleus. The background is less than in normals, and large, distinct axons with multiple and extremely large, swollen enlargements can be observed. These alterations persist long after the pellet is removed. Extremely large, stump-like objects can be observed, as can thick and long axons. These axons are larger in diameter than are observed in normal tissue in any brain area, and they sometimes have varicosities in them of an equally swollen nature. Similar swollen and enlarged fluorescent axons in the ventrolateral caudate have been observed after partial aspiration lesions of the caudate and are presumed to reflect an accumulation of amines in the remaining axons, implying that damage to dopamine terminals in the caudate can be produced by the continuous AMPH administration achieved through pellet implantation.

This implication was validated using regional assays of amines and tyrosine hydroxylase (TH) activity in several brain regions at various times after AMPH pellet implantation. The largest changes in TH activity during pellet implantation were in the caudate nucleus where it fell to 50% of control levels; dopamine content of the caudate was also significantly reduced, as were nore-pinephrine levels during pellet implantation in most brain regions. These results reflect the depletions produced by AMPH-stimulated release of catechol-amines. Yet, although catecholamine levels recovered to near-control levels in the rats sacrificed 110 days after pellet removal, caudate TH activity remained significantly less than in controls, although it was elevated in the other brain regions.

It was further found that these persisting decreases in caudate TH activity were due to the continuous nature of the AMPH release, rather than the total amount of AMPH released by the pellet in 7 days. One experimental group was implanted with AMPH pellets for 7 days and given a 60-day recovery period; a second was injected with an amount of AMPH equivalent to that released by the pellet in 7 days (25 mg), but given in seven daily injections of 3.7 mg AMPH each. TH activity in the caudate 60 days after the cessation of AMPH injections or pellet removal was again significantly reduced in the AMPH pellet rats relative to controls, but not in the injection groups. These results imply that continuous AMPH administration has a unique capability for inducing long-lasting structural and biochemical alterations in dopamine terminals in the cau-date nucleus. This conclusion has been validated in several other laboratories using different techniques, such as AMPH delivered by minipumps or very frequent injections (for example, Nwanze & Jonsson, 1981; Ricaurte et al., 1980; Steranka & Sanders-Bush, 1980). Fuller and Hemrick-Luecke (1980) found that AMPH administered in combination with drugs that slow its metabo-lism becomes neurotoxic to caudate dopamine terminals. There is also a downregulation of dopamine receptors after several days of continuous AMPH (Nielsen et al., 1980b).

Studies of rats injected with labeled 2-deoxyglucose (2-DG) and sacrificed at various times after AMPH pellet implantation (Eison et al., 1981a) showed that, as the caudate becomes depleted and damaged, the nucleus accumbens becomes more active. Whereas acute injections of AMPH induce increased 2-DG uptake in several brain regions (many of which were responsible for sensory functions), the "late-stage" pellet animal shows a distinctively differ-ent pattern of glucose uptake, characterized by an increased radioactivity in the nucleus accumbens and related mesolimbic structures. In a related study (Eison et al., 1981b), it was found that the regional distribution of 3-H-labeled AMPH-derived radioactivity is maximal in the accumbens of pellet rats. Simi-lar changes do not occur in 5-HT neurons (Ellison & Ratan, 1982).

CONTINUOUS AMPHETAMINES OR REPEATED INJECTIONS: WHICH MODELS PSYCHOSIS?

It has been repeatedly found that continuous AMPH has effects on behavior that are strikingly different from those of intermittent AMPH. When rats were pretreated with a 7-day AMPH pellet and then the pellet was removed and a drug-free period given, it was found that these rats then displayed a completely different reaction to injections of either AMPH or apomorphine, both just after drug treatment and 30 days after drug treatment, compared to rats given daily injections of AMPH (Nelson & Ellison, 1978). Whereas "daily injection" rats treated for 7 days (of strong injections) or 30 days (of weak injections) demonstrate *heightened* motor stereotypies compared to controls (showing the inverse tolerance effect), rats tested immediately after 7 days of the AMPH pellet conversely show *less* stereotypies to AMPH. This reflects the down regulation in dopamine D_2 receptors that occurs at this time (Nielsen et al., 1980a). Ellison and Morris (1981) found that 7-day pellet treatment induced changes opposite to daily injections of AMPH. A 28-day pellet group was included (continuous AMPH but at a much lower daily dose, one that we have found to be nontoxic to dopamine innervations of caudate). In this study it was also found that this pellet was quite different from the daily injections in its effects on behavior and in vivo spiroperidol accumulation. Intermittent (daily injections) of AMPH result in inverse tolerance for motor stereotypies, with little change in receptor number, whereas continuous AMPH initially leads to an "inverse tolerance" for motor stereotypies, but then to a late-stage tolerance of motor stereotypies and downregulation of receptors.

Robinson and Becker (1986) have a different interpretation of the effect of chronic AMPH administration, concluding that the "sensitization" produced by intermittent AMPH is the best model of AMPH psychosis, rather than the "neurotoxicity" produced by continuous AMPH. They argue that AMPH pellet experiments involve extreme drug doses—higher than addicts actually self-administer. Yet, the doses used by human addicts can become immense as bingeing progresses, the brain AMPH levels induced by pellets are not high, and one cannot compare human doses with rat doses in a simple manner and conclude that the dose required to produce AMPH neurotoxicity is higher than that required to produce an AMPH psychosis. Furthermore, the doses of continuous AMPH found sufficient in monkeys to induce a late stage were low and are close to the human range.

In addition, early stages of continuous AMPH actually do induce "inverse tolerance" or sensitization. If a rat is pretreated with a pellet for 24 hours, the pellet is removed, a 12-hour drug-free period is given, and then a probe injection of a low dose of d-AMPH is administered, a remarkable sensitization to motor stereotypies is observed, paralleled by increased in vivo accumulation of spiroperidol in caudate (Ellison & Morris, 1981). Robinson and Becker argue that former AMPH addicts show an enduring hypersensitivity to AMPH and cite our research on demonstrating that rats given continuous AMPH, withdrawn from AMPH, and later challenged with an acute injection are not supersensitive to AMPH. Yet, in fact, the published report of Ellison and Morris shows that rats do become hypersensitive to the drug, but that this supersensitivity develops over time. Most important is the clear fact that chronic AMPH (and cocaine) addicts *simply do not take the drug once or twice daily*. Such a regimen leads to a daily "crash" (which actually also sensitizes over time), far outlasting the action of the drug. An addict would not take the drug only once or twice daily in order to spend 18 hours a day depressed. Numerous studies of rats or monkeys allowed to self-administer AMPH or cocaine have also reported the development of "binge-like" patterns of intake.

Both effects seem to shed some light on schizophrenia and paranoia. The sensitization effect is clearly important, for motor stereotypies are present in schizophrenics and predominate in many. Yet, an animal in a motor stereotypy shows a complete inhibition of social behaviors and a suppression of the distinctive behaviors induced by hallucinogens, whereas these behaviors, particularly aberrant social interactions, are a hallmark of paranoid schizophrenia. Perhaps the sensitization effect models the early stages of addiction, when the drug is taken only sporadically. Then the binge or runs intake pattern would develop in some, with the ensuing paranoia and, eventually, neurotoxic effects in a minority of addicts.

COCAINE PSYCHOSIS

Fortunately, the argument that simple dopamine neurotoxicity is a hallmark of the late-stage behaviors can now be dismissed due to more recent developments. We recently began to extend our continuous drug model to the study of chronic cocaine administration. If similar late stages appeared with cocaine administration, this would be a highly significant finding, for it could permit one to dissociate the unique effects of these two drugs and to determine better what are the necessary and sufficient conditions for producing the late-stage paranoid-like effects.

On the one hand, it is quite remarkable that virtually every one of the above findings relating to paranoid psychosis from AMPH abuse have also been reported to be true for cocaine abuse. This same is true for the production of motor stereotypies. Thus, Post and Rose (1976) found that repeated cocaine injections in monkeys induced the development of a variety of stereotypic responses; in rats, they produced sensitization to the motor stereotypy-inducing effects, and seizure-inducing properties of cocaine have been reported in the 2-hour period after each of a series of daily injections of the same dose of cocaine (Kilbey & Ellinwood, 1977a; Post, 1975; Post & Rose, 1976; Stripling & Ellinwood, 1976). This increased sensitivity was still seen as long as 7 weeks after the end of chronic administration (Kilbey & Ellinwood, 1977b).

It is also clear that cocaine addicts binge and become paranoid, especially freebase addicts (Manschreck et al., 1988). In fact, cocaine is noted for inducing paranoid reactions that can be quite similar to those induced by AMPH (Lesko et al., 1982), and humans who abuse cocaine for prolonged periods of time often show increased irritability, difficulty in concentration, disruption of eating and sleeping habits, perceptual disturbances (pseudohallucinations), paranoid thinking, and, occasionally, overt psychosis (Siegal, 1978; Waldorf et al., 1977; Wesson & Smith, 1977). As with AMPH, this psychosis is treated with neuroleptics (Gawin, 1986).

It is also clear that cocaine, like AMPH, has important effects on the dopamine system. The question is whether, like AMPH, continuous cocaine also induces a destruction of dopamine terminals, for this could lead to an important test of the continuous AMPH-paranoid model. Some of this research has already been performed. Several investigators have studied whether cocaine, when administered continuously, has the same neurotoxic properties of d-AMPH. Although Trulson et al. (1986) reported that 10 mg/kg of cocaine administered every 12 hours for 10 consecutive days induced decreased tyrosine hydroxylase-staining axons and decreased TH activity in caudate when the rats were studied 60 days later, this report has not been replicated by many other laboratories. Kleven et al. (1988) administered this same dose and also two extremely large doses (12.5 mg/kg eight times daily for 10 days or 100 mg/kg/day for 21 days) and reported no long-lasting changes in DA, 5-HT, or their major metabolites in striatum, hippocampus, hypothalamus, or cortex. Ryan et al. (1988), administered cocaine continuously at doses of 50-450 mg/kg/day and failed to detect axonal degeneration in neostriatum using silver stain or TH immunolabeling. In contrast, the AMPH-induced degeneration was readily apparent. Indeed, Hanson et al. (1987) reported that cocaine co-administration could *block* the neurotoxic actions of multiple methamphetamine injections. This is presumably because, as has been well established (Scheel-Kruger, 1971), one of the primary effects of cocaine is to block presynaptic reuptake of DA. The vast majority of studies, then, indicate that cocaine does not have the same neurotoxic effect on caudate dopamine terminals that d-AMPH and methamphetamine have and that it even protects against these neurotoxic effects.

COCAINE PSYCHOSIS IN RATS: THE LATE STAGE

We have recently developed a slow-release cocaine pellet for rats that is similar in design to the AMPH pellet, it holds 125 mg of cocaine base, over 50% of which is released during the first 5 days after implantation. This is an extremely simple pellet to construct (Lipton et al., 1991), and it eliminates almost all of the extreme skin lesions that prevent the use of minipumps to administer cocaine. Rats implanted with these pellets are also initially hyperexploratory and then enter motor stereotypies, but the stereotypies are much less intense than with AMPH, involving less biting and more sniffing and head-bobbing. As the rats enter the late stage after several days, the two drugs become even more distinct. The cocaine rats are much more vividly "hallucinatory" than AMPH rats. Although these late-stage cocaine rats eventually develop an extremely strong syndrome of limb-flicks and wet-dog shakes, the other behaviors they exhibit are also particularly interesting. "Panic attacks" are seen, in which the rats suddenly explosively bounce off the sides of the cage, as though fleeing an invisible enemy. These sudden spontaneous startle attacks, which can be elicited by a slight noise but which also occur in the absolute absence of any obvious eliciting stimulus, are reminiscent of the explosive fleeing episodes observed in monkeys given continuous AMPH and the spontaneous startle responses shown by the AMPH rats in the colony and in activity cages. The cocaine rats have also been observed showing a variety of other behaviors that are very suggestive of hallucinatory behaviors. Some are observed reaching out repeatedly with the paws to grasp invisible objects in space; others also show much more parasitotic grooming than controls. It is clear that this cocaine pellet is an extraordinary tool for the elicitation of late-stage behaviors.

Until very recently we thought that these findings showed that our previous hypothesis linking dopamine neurotoxicity to the late stage of hallucinatory behaviors was incorrect. Yet, although the cocaine pellet clearly does not produce the dopamine neurotoxicity of the AMPH pellet, it does induce another and possibly related neurotoxicity. Various groups of rats were implanted with AMPH pellets, or cocaine pellets, or given intermittent injections of cocaine for 5 days, or given control injections (Zeigler et al., 1991). All rats were then given a prolonged recovery period and tested in open field. A clear dissociation between the groups was obtained. In open field, the cocaine injection rats were hyperactive, showing the well-known inverse tolerance effect, whereas the cocaine pellet rats behaved very differently, acting as though they were extremely frightened.

In vivo autoradiography was then used to examine whether there were persisting changes in receptor binding for D_2 ([³H]spiperone), D_1 ([³H]SCH23390), benzodiazepine ([³H]flunitrazepam), 5-HT-1 ([³H]5HT), 5-HT-2 ([³H]ketanserin), and muscarinic ACh receptors ([³H]QNB). The AMPH pellet rats showed large, persisting changes in D_1 and D_2 receptors, replicating the dopamine neurotoxicity effect; these changes were not present with chronic cocaine, either when administered intermittently or continuously (Fig. 23-1).

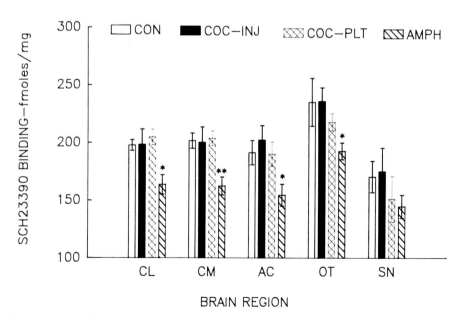

Figure 23-1. SCH23390-specific binding in five brain regions. Binding was significantly decreased (*$P <.05$) in the amphetamine pellet rats in all brain regions except substantia nigra; none of the other groups was significantly different from controls for any brain region. CL and CM, lateral and medial caudate; AC, nucleus accumbens; OT, olfactory tubercele; SN, substantia nigra.

This finding was as expected. Yet, the continuous cocaine (pellet) rats showed a completely different pattern of brain neurotoxicity, with appreciable increases in [³H]flunitrazepam binding in dopamine-rich areas, cortex, and amygdala (Fig. 23-2) but decreased [³H]QNB binding in dopamine-rich areas, hippocampus, and amygdala (Fig. 23-3). This means that continuous cocaine has enduring effects on completely different neurochemical systems from continuous AMPH: continuous cocaine alters acetylcholine and GABA systems in dopamine-rich areas. It seems that the uptake blockade of dopamine produced by the cocaine protected dopamine terminals from neurotoxicity, but resulted in persisting effects on those cells receiving dopamine input. We thought this might indicate that a functionally related kind of neurotoxicity occurs with both continuous AMPH and continuous cocaine.

To test for this possibility, patterns of degeneration following five days of continuous amphetamine or cocaine were studied using the cupric silver stain (Ellison, 1992). The caudate nucleus of the amphetamine pellet animals showed a pattern of alterations similar to those reported by Ryan et al. (1988), with a diffuse background in cell body regions of scattered silver grains which was considerably elevated over that of the controls and with some short axons densely labeled. None of this labeling was present in either cocaine group. This lack of evidence of neurotoxicity in caudate meant the persisting receptor changes in these animals were clearly not due to neurotoxicity in caudate. However, there was a strikingly consistent pattern of degeneration present in

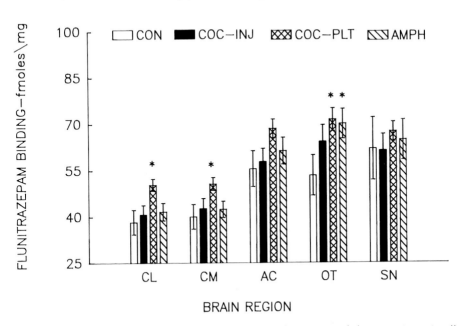

Figure 23-2. Flunitrazepam-specific binding in five dopamine-rich brain regions. In all brain regions depicted the cocaine pellet rats showed the lowest QNB binding and were significantly less than controls in both medial and lateral caudate, olfactory tubercle, and also in cortex and amygdala. None of the other drug groups showed significant alterations in QNB binding.

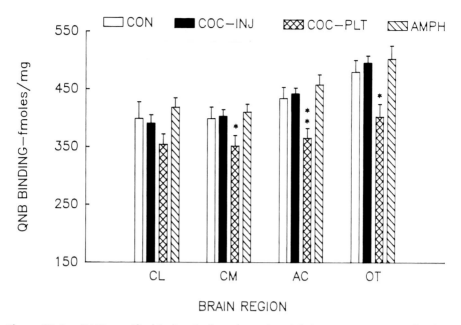

Figure 23-3. QNB-specific binding in four dopamine-rich brain regions. QNB binding was significantly decreased (**P <.01) in the cocaine pellet rats in medial caudate, accumbens, and olfactory tubercle, as well as in dorsal hippocampus and amygdala (data not shown).

both drug groups at the junction between diencephalon and midbrain. Figure 23-4 shows a section through fasciculus retroflexus from a cocaine pellet animal 24 hours after pellet removal. This demonstrates the dense staining in lateral habenula and fasciculus retroflexus which was present in every one of the amphetamine and cocaine animals. In each case long-labeled axons extended ventrally in the fasciculus retroflexus towards the ventral tegmentum. These axons could be traced in more caudal sections to extend along the fasciculus retroflexus ventrally. This pattern was still present, although somewhat less intense, in the animals sacrificed 5 days after pellet implantation, when the densely labeled and swollen axons could be observed beginning to disintegrate.

These results indicate that while continuous d-amphetamine and cocaine have very different long-lasting effects in caudate, they share a remarkably similar neurotoxic action on this tract interconnecting the habenula and the ventral midbrain. The lateral habenula receives, through the stria medularis, a significant input from dopamine-rich forebrain regions including the nucleus accumbens, and, through the fasciculus retroflexus, it interconnects with dopamine neurons in substantia nigra and other nuclei in the ventral tegmental area. The nucleus accumbens and ventral tegmental area are both known to play an important role in the behaviorally activating and rewarding actions of amphetamines and cocaine. 2DG studies have found that the lateral habenular nucleus shows substantial alterations in glucose metabolism during rewarding

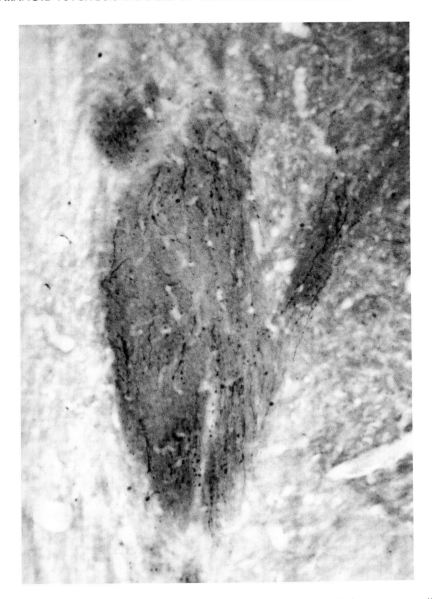

Figure 23-4. Photomicrograph of the fasciculus retroflexus in a 5-day cocaine pellet animal one day after pellet removal. The multiple degenerating axons are visible as dark axons with multiple varicosities. This figure shows both the extent of degeneration and the remarkable confinement of fasciculus retroflexus.

brain stimulation or administration of dopamine agonists and that lesions of the lateral habenula markedly attenuate methamphetamine-induced inhibition of substantia nigra cells.

The finding that continuous amphetamine and cocaine have markedly dissimilar effects in caudate but very similar effects in lateral habenula and fasciculus retroflexus suggest that alterations in these pathways may at least partially underlie the very similar effects which develop during and following amphetamine or cocaine binges in humans, i.e., progressive paranoia and a rebound depression.

CONTINUOUS STIMULANTS, NEUROTOXICITY AND PSYCHOSIS

From these observations, we conclude that it is some unique property of several days of continuous stimulants, and not just the damage to dopamine terminals, which eventually leads from the motor stereotypy phase to the distinctive "late stage" behaviors. Continuous cocaine rats dissociate the two phenomena: they are quite spectacular in their "late stage" behaviors, yet they apparently have minimal, if any, neurotoxic effects on dopamine terminals. This necessitates a reevaluation of what these continuous stimulant models of paranoid psychosis have to tell us.

What are the neurochemical underpinnings of this "late-stage"? Clearly there is apparently a highly important, and perhaps decisive aspect in the incessant hyperstimulation of dopamine systems, which eventually leads to a destruction of dopamine circuitry (in the case of AMPH), or to receptor alterations in other cells which are possibly post-synaptic to dopamine (in the case of cocaine). It is also possible that this leads to the degeneration of axons in fasciculus retroflexus with both drugs. During this incessant dopamine hyperstimulation, there is a depletion and down-regulation of dopamine receptors. An animal showing "late-stage" behaviors can always be immediately brought out of these by one of two opposite manipulations: a higher dose of a dopamine agonist (which will immediately induce motor stereotypies and a cessation of all social and hallucinatory behaviors), or discontinuation of the stimulant or administration of a dopamine blocker (which will produce the "crash" and eliminate all behaviors). This leads to the hypothesis that the "paranoid stimulant late-stage model" is a unique reflection of this cumulative stage of neurotransmission in dopaminergic and related systems—when they are becoming depleted and receptor number is falling, but their stimulation continues.

These findings may lead to a new, more complex but much more interesting theory of psychosis involving dopamine dysregulation. If it turns out that the axons from lateral habenula which are degenerating after continuous amphetamine or cocaine binges are the same as those which mediate the negative feedback from forebrain dopamine-rich and limbic structures onto midbrain dopamine-secreting cells, an extraordinarily interesting theory about paranoid and perhaps other psychotic behaviors would follow, involving the eventual failing of the major outputs from a structure evolutionarily quite primitive, yet highly integrative, and one with important inhibitory feedback control over dopamine. This inhibitory control, in the case of habenula, would not be just the simple autoreceptor feedback over the terminal, or the direct inhibition of the input cell by the output cell, but rather one in which other complex brain structures could also regulate the gating of dopamine release. This conception may further enrich previous notions by relating psychotic behavior to the loss of inhibitory control over dopamine by higher brain structures, and this makes for a rich and appealing theory.

Whatever neurochemical alterations ultimately prove to be responsible, it seems clear that the late-stage of continuous stimulants such as AMPH or cocaine represents a highly distinctive state of great relevance to paranoid schizophrenia and a novel model of hallucinatory behaviors. It may also be of theoretical importance that both drugs, when given in a regimen which induces a hallucinatory "late-stage" have profound neurotoxic effects in brain.

REFERENCES

Angrist, M., & Gershon, S. (1970). The phenomenology of experimentally induced amphetamine psychosis—preliminary observations. *Biol. Psychiat., 2*, 95-107.

Angrist, B., Sathananthan, G., Wilk, S., & Gershon, S. (1974). Amphetamine psychosis: Behavioral and biochemical aspects. *J. Psychiat. Res., 11*, 13.

Bell, D.S. (1965). Comparison of amphetamine psychosis and schizophrenia. *Am. J. Psychiat., 111*, 701-707.

Bell, D.S. (1973). The experimental reproduction of amphetamine psychosis. *Arch. Gen. Psychiat., 29*, 35-40.

Bowers, M. (1968). Pathogenesis of acute schizophrenic psychosis. *Arch. Gen. Psychiat., 19*, 348.

Connell, P. (1958). *Amphetamine psychosis.* Maudsley Monographs No. 5. London. Oxford University Press.

Eison, M.S., Eison, A.S., & Ellison, G. (1981a). The regional distribution of amphetamine in rat brain is altered by dosage and prior exposure to the drug. *J. Pharmacol. Exp. Ther., 218*, 237-241.

Eison, M.S., Ellison, G., & Eison, A.S. (1981b). The regional distribution of d-amphetamine and local glucose utilization in rat brain during continuous amphetamine administration. *Exp. Brain Res., 43*.

Ellinwood, E.H. Jr. (1967). Amphetamine psychosis: I. Description of the individuals and the process. *J. Nerv. Ment. Dis., 144*, 273-283.

Ellinwood, E.H., & Kilbey, M. (1977). Chronic stimulant intoxication models of psychosis. In I. Hanin & E. Usdin (Eds.), *Animal models in psychiatry and neurology.* (pp. 61-74).

Ellison, G. (1992). Continuous amphetamine and cocaine have similar neurotoxic effects in lateral habenula nucleus and fasciculus retroflexus. *Brain. Res. 598*, 353–356.

Ellison, G.D., & Eison, M.S. (1983). Continuous amphetamine intoxication: An animal model of the acute psychotic episode. *Psychol. Med., 13*, 751-761.

Ellison, G., & Morris, W. (1981). Opposed stages of continuous amphetamine administration: Parallel alterations in motor stereotypies and in vivo spiroperidol accumulation. *Eur. J. Pharmacol., 74*, 207-214.

Ellison, G., & Ratan, R. (1982). The late stage following continuous amphetamine administration to rats is correlated with altered dopamine but not serotonin metabolism. *Life Sci., 31*, 771-777.

Ellison, G.D., Eison, M.S., & Huberman, H. (1978a). States of constant amphetamine intoxication: Delayed appearance of abnormal social behaviors in rat colonies. *Psychopharmacology, 56*, 293-299.

Ellison, G., Eison, M., Huberman, H., & Daniel, F. (1978b). Structural and biochemical alterations in dopaminergic innervation of the caudate nucleus following continuous amphetamine administration. *Science, 201,* 276-278.

Ellison, G.D., Nielsen, E.B., & Lyon, M. (1981). Animal models of psychosis: Hallucinatory behaviors in monkeys during the late stage of continuous amphetamine intoxication. *J. Psychiat. Res., 16,* 13-22.

Fuller, R., & Hemrick-Luecke, S. (1980). Long-lasting depletion of striatal dopamine by a single injection of amphetamine in iprindole-treated rats. *Science, 209,* 305-306.

Gawin, F.H. (1986). Neuroleptic reduction of cocaine-induced paranoia but not euphoria? *Psychopharmacology, 90,* 142-143.

Gold, M.S., & Bowers, M. Jr. (1978). Neurobiological vulnerability to low-dose amphetamine psychosis. *Am. J. Psychiat., 135,* 1546-1548.

Griffith, J., Cavanaugh, J., Held, N., & Oates, J. (1972). D-amphetamine: Evaluation of psychotomimetic properties in man. *Arch. Gen. Psychiat., 26,* 97-100.

Hanson, G. R., Matsuda, L., & Gibb, J.W. (1987). Effects of cocaine on methamphetamine-induced neurochemical changes: Characterization of cocaine as a monoamine uptake blocker. *J. Pharmacol. Exp. Ther., 242,* 507-513.

Huberman, H., Eison, M., Byran, K., & Ellison, G. (1977). A slow-release silicone pellet for chronic amphetamine administration. *Eur. J. Pharmacol., 45,* 237-242.

Kilbey, M.M., & Ellinwood, E.H. (1977a). Reverse tolerance to stimulant-induced abnormal behavior. *Life Sci., 20,* 1063-1076.

Kilbey, M.M., & Ellinwood, E.H. (1977b). Chronic administration of stimulant drugs: Response modification. In E.H. Ellingwood & M.M. Kilbey (Eds.), *Cocaine and Other Stimulants.* New York: Plenum Press.

Kleven, M.S., Woolverton, W., & Seiden, L. (1988). Lack of long-term monoamine depletions following repeated or continuous exposure to cocaine. *Brain Res. Bull., 21,* 233-237.

Kramer, J.C. (1969). Introduction to amphetamine abuse. *J. Psychedelic Drugs, 2,* 8-13.

Lesko, L.M., Fischman, M., Javaid, J., & Davis, J. (1982). Iatrogenous cocaine psychosis. *N. Engl. J. Med., 307,*1153.

Lipton, J., Zeigler, S., Wilkins, J., & Ellison, G. (1991). Silicone pellet for continuous cocaine administration: Heightened late-stage behaviors compared to continuous amphetamine. *Pharmacol. Biochem. Behav., 38,* 927-930.

Manschreck, T.C., Laughery, J.A., Weisstein, C.C., Allen, D., Humblestone, B., Neville, M., Podlewski, H., & Mitra, N. (1988). Characteristics of freebase cocaine psychosis. *Yale J. Biol. Med., 61,* 115-122.

Nelson, L., & Ellison, G. (1978). Enhanced stereotypies after repeated injections but not continuous amphetamines. *Neuropharmacology, 17,* 1081-1084.

Nielsen, E., & Ellison, G.D. (1980). A silicone pellet for long-term continuous administration of amphetamine. *Comm. Psychopharmacol., 4,* 17-20.

Nielsen, E., Lee, T., & Ellison, G.D. (1980a). Following several days of continuous administration of d-amphetamine acquires hallucination-like properties. *Psychopharmacology, 68,* 197-200.

Nielsen, E.B., Neilsen, M., Ellison, G., & Braestrup, E. (1980b). Decreased spiroperidol and LSD binding in rat brain after continuous amphetamine. *Eur. J. Pharmacol., 66,* 149-154.

Nwanze, E., & Jonsson, G. (1981). Amphetamine neurotoxicity on dopamine nerve terminals in the caudate nucleus of mice. *Neurosci. Lett., 26,* 163-168.

Post, R.M. (1975). Cocaine psychoses: A continuum model. *Am. J. Psychiat., 132,* 225-231.

Post, R.M., & Rose, H. (1976). Increasing effects with repetitive cocaine administration in the rats. *Nature, 260,* 731-732.

Ricaurte, G.A., Schuster, C.R., & Seiden, L.S. (1980). Long-term effects of repeated methylamphetamine administration on dopamine and serotonin neurons in the rat brain: A regional study. *Brain Res., 193,* 153-163.

Robinson, T., & Becker, J. (1986). Enduring changes in brain and behavior produced by chronic amphetamine administration: A review and evaluation of animal models of amphetamine psychosis. *Brain Res. Rev., 11,* 157-198.

Ryan, L. J., Martone, M., Linder, J., & Groves, P.M. (1988). Cocaine, in contrast to d-amphetamine, does not cause axonal terminal degeneration in neostriatum and agranular frontal cortex of long-evans rats. *Life Sci., 43,* 1403-1409.

Scheel-Kruger, J. (1971). Behavioral and biochemical comparison of amphetamine derivatives, cocaine, benzotropine and tricyclic anti-depressant drugs. *Eur. J. Pharmacol., 18,* 63.

Siegel, R. (1978). Cocaine hallucinations. *Am. J. Psychiat., 135,* 309-314.

Slater, E. (1959). Amphetamine psychosis. *Br. Med. J., 1,* 488.

Smith, R.C. (1969). The world of the Haight-Ashbury speed freak. *J. Psychedelic Drugs, 2,* 77-83.

Snyder, S.H., Bannerjee, S., Yamamura, H., & Greenberg, D. (1974). Drugs, neurotransmitters and schizophrenia: Phenothiazines, amphetamine and enzymes synthesizing psychotomimetic drugs and schizophrenia research. *Science, 184,* 1243-1253.

Steranka, L., & Sanders-Bush, E. (1980). Long-term effects of continuous exposure to amphetamine on brain dopamine concentration and synaptosomal uptake in mice. *Eur. J. Pharmacol., 65,* 439-443.

Stripling, J.S., & Ellinwood, E.H. (1976). Cocaine: Physiological and behavioral effects of acute and chronic administration. In S.J. Mule (Ed.), *Cocaine: Chemical, biological, clinical, social and treatment aspects.* Cleveland: CRC Press.

Stripling, J.S., & Ellinwood, E.H. (1977). Sensitization to cocaine following administration in the rat. In E.H. Ellingwood & M.M. Kilbey (Eds.), *Cocaine and other stimulants.* New York: Plenum Press.

Trulson, M.E., Babb, S., Joe, J., & Raese, J. (1986). Chronic cocaine administration depletes tyrosine hydroxylase immunoreactivity in the rat brain nigral striatal system: Quantitative light microscopic studies. *Exp. Neurol., 94,* 744-756.

Waldorf, D., Murphy, S., Reinarman, C., & Joyce, B. (1977). *Doing coke: An ethnography of users and sellers,* Washington, D.C.: Drug Abuse Council.

Wesson, D.R., & Smith, D.E. (1977). Cocaine: Its use for central nervous system stimulation including recreational and medical uses. In R.C. Petersen & R.C. Stillman (Eds.), *Cocaine 1977,* Washington, D.C.: U.S. Government Printing Office.

Zeigler, S., Lipton, J., Toga, A., & Ellison, G. (1991). Continuous cocaine administration produces persisting changes in brain neurochemistry and behavior. *Brain Res., 552,* 27-35.

24

Persistent Sensitizing Effects of Drugs on Brain Dopamine Systems and Behavior: Implications for Addiction and Relapse

TERRY E. ROBINSON

Much of our knowledge about addictive drugs comes from studies in which animals (or biological tissues) are exposed to a drug only once. If people took a drug only once, however, we would not be faced with an enormous drug abuse problem. Unfortunately, given the opportunity, some people, as well as some animals, tend to administer certain drugs repeatedly and compulsively, leading to dependence and addiction. It is this repeated, compulsive use of drugs that creates the abuse problem. Thus, it is important to understand that the actions of most psychoactive drugs *change* when they are administered repeatedly.

Of course, it has been known for a long time that tolerance often develops with repeated drug administration. Tolerance refers to the decreased effect of a drug with continued administration, so that higher and higher doses are required to produce the same effect (Jaffe, 1980). The role of tolerance in the development of physical dependence and the role of physical dependence and withdrawal in sustaining drug use have been central foci of research on addiction for the last 20 to 30 years (Jaffe, 1980; Koob & Bloom, 1988). It is less well appreciated, however, that the action of drugs can also change in a very different manner. This second type of alteration in drug action produced by repeated drug use is known as *sensitization* or *reverse tolerance*. Sensitization refers to the fact that some effects of addictive drugs do not decrease, but rather *increase* with repeated administration of a constant dose. Therefore, lower and lower doses are required to produce the same effect. Sensitization-related changes in behavior can be extremely persistent, in some instances persist indefinitely. Relative to tolerance, the role of sensitization in maintaining compulsive drug use has received very little attention.

This chapter focuses on the persistent, sensitizing effects of addictive drugs. It is argued that the persistent neuroplastic adaptations to repeated drug

This work was supported by a grant from the NIDA (DA 04294).

use, which are responsible for behavioral sensitization, play a major role in the development of addiction and especially in the high rate of relapse seen in drug addicts even after very long periods of abstinence. The phenomenon of sensitization has been studied most thoroughly after the repeated administration of amphetamine (AMPH), and therefore many of the examples presented here come from studies using AMPH (Robinson & Becker, 1986). There is evidence to suggest, however, that studies of AMPH sensitization may be relevant to other drugs—not only closely related psychomotor stimulants, such as cocaine and methylphenidate but also drugs from diverse classes, including opiates, phencyclidine (PCP), nicotine and methylenedioxymethamphetamine (MDMA).

SENSITIZATION TO AMPHETAMINE

The behavioral sensitization produced by repeated AMPH treatment has been well characterized over the last decade, and the most interesting features of the phenomenon are only briefly summarized here (for more comprehensive reviews, Kalivas & Stewart, 1991; Kuczenski & Segal, 1988; Robinson, 1991; Robinson & Becker, 1986). In many studies of AMPH sensitization, a constant dose of the drug is given repeatedly, and the behavioral response to successive injections is quantified. With this type of treatment regimen, there is a *progressive* enhancement in the psychomotor stimulant effects of AMPH. For example, there is a progressive increase in the ability of AMPH to induce locomotor hyperactivity or stereotyped behavior (Segal & Mandell, 1974). To produce a sensitized response to AMPH, however, the drug must be administered *intermittently*. The continuous administration of AMPH for many days via a Silastic pellet or osmotic minipump does not produce sensitization to a subsequent challenge. Furthermore, injections that are widely spaced in time (e.g., 3–7 days) produce more rapid sensitization than a similar number of injections given close together in time, e.g., daily or twice daily. Although repeated AMPH treatment produces a progressive enhancement in many AMPH-induced behaviors, even a *single injection* of a relatively moderate dose (1–3 mg/ kg) is sufficient to sensitize an animal to the psychomotor stimulant effects of a second injection given up to 1 month later (Robinson et al., 1982).

Probably the most striking characteristic of sensitization is how long it persists after the discontinuation of drug treatment. In rats, enhanced behavioral responsiveness to AMPH has been reported as long as 1 year after the discontinuation of AMPH pretreatment (Paulson et al., 1991), and in humans, former AMPH addicts are reported to remain hypersensitive to the psychotogenic effects of AMPH even after years of abstinence (Sato et al., 1983).

Several variables influence the development of sensitization, including the age and sex of the animal. For example, AMPH is capable of producing an acute motor stimulant effect in very young rats (2–6 days postnatal), but repeated treatment with AMPH does not produce behavioral sensitization until after weaning, which occurs about 21 days postnatally in rats (Fujiwara et al.,

1987). Also, there are sex differences in AMPH sensitization. Female rats show more rapid and robust behavioral sensitization to AMPH than do males, even after controlling for sex differences in the metabolism of AMPH (Camp & Robinson, 1988a & b; Robinson, 1984), and a similar sex difference is found with cocaine (Post & Contel, 1983). The sex difference in AMPH sensitization seems to be due to the action of circulating levels of endogenous gonadal hormones, because male rats gonadectomized as adults show a pattern of sensitization identical to females, whereas ovariectomy of females has no effect on AMPH sensitization (Camp & Robinson, 1988a & b; Robinson, 1984). This finding suggests that some endogenous testicular substance or some gonadal steroid-induced substance decreases the susceptibility to sensitization in males, although the nature and mechanism of action of such a substance are unknown.

One last variable that can have a marked influence on the expression of sensitization is the amount of time elapsed since the discontinuation of drug pretreatment. The influence of this variable may be subtle if injections are widely spaced in time (e.g., every 3–7 days), but it becomes increasingly evident if injections are given relatively close together in time. This point is perhaps best illustrated by a study in which an escalating dose pretreatment regimen was used. This dose regimen mimics to some extent the pattern of drug use seen in addicts; that is, runs of escalating AMPH use interspersed with "crashes" (Paulson et al., 1991). During the first week after the discontinuation of escalating dose AMPH pretreatment, Paulson et al. (1991) found no difference between AMPH pretreated and control animals in their locomotor response to an AMPH challenge (Fig. 24-1). That is, despite a full 6 weeks of AMPH pretreatment, animals did not seem to be behaviorally sensitized. By 2 weeks after the discontinuation of AMPH pretreatment, however, animals were markedly hyperresponsive to an AMPH challenge. Furthermore, this sensitized behavioral response to an AMPH challenge persisted undiminished for one year after the last pretreatment injection. This latter observation suggests, of course, that not only did AMPH pretreatment produce behavioral sensitization but also that sensitization may persist indefinitely, perhaps for the life of the animal (Paulson et al., 1991).

Yet, why did the animals not seem to be sensitized when challenged with AMPH during the first week after the discontinuation of AMPH pretreatment (Paulson et al., 1991)? In addressing this question, it is important to note that, during this early withdrawal period, when animals were not hyperresponsive to an AMPH challenge, they showed abnormalities in spontaneous locomotor behavior across the day-night cycle. For the first 3 days after the discontinuation of AMPH treatment, the animals were hypoactive during the day and at night. By 1 week, locomotor activity during the day was not significantly different from control, but AMPH-pretreated animals were still markedly hypoactive at night (see Segal & Mandell, 1974). Interestingly, this nocturnal hypoactivity was not a simple disturbance in motor function, because AMPH-pretreated animals showed a normal large increase in locomotor activity when the lights first went off at night. As the night progressed, however, they did not sustain the high levels of locomotor activity characteristic of controls. This post-

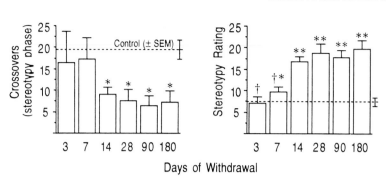

Figure 24-1. Summary of the effect of pretreatment with saline or escalating doses of amphetamine (AMPH) on the behavioral response to a challenge injection of AMPH (2.6 mg/kg, i.p.) given 3, 7, 14, 28, 90, or 180 days after the discontinuation of pretreatment. **Left,** Amount of locomotor activity induced by an AMPH challenge, as indicated by the number of cage crossovers during the stereotypy phase, i.e., between 10 and 60 minutes postinjection. With this measure, a low crossover score indicates high levels of focused stereotyped behavior. Each bar represents the average (+SEM) number of crossovers for independent groups of animals pretreated with AMPH and then challenged 3-180 days later. Dashed horizontal line, average number of crossovers for saline-pretreated control animals; vertical range bar to the right of the dashed line, ±SEM for the controls; asterisks, AMPH-pretreated animals withdrawn for 14-180 (but not 3-7 days) show a significant decrease in stereotypy phase locomotor activity relative to controls. **Right,** Average ratings for stereotyped head and limb movements for each group, accumulated over the entire test session, using the same format as in the left panel. Asterisks, AMPH-pretreated rats withdrawn for 7-180 days (but not 3 days) have significantly higher stereotypy ratings than controls; daggers, animals withdrawn for 3 to 7 days have significantly lower stereotypy ratings than those withdrawn for 14-180 days. In summary, AMPH-pretreated animals are markedly hyperresponsive (sensitized) to a challenge injection of AMPH when tested between 14 and 180 days after the discontinuation of AMPH pretreatment, but not when tested 3-7 days after the discontinuation of pretreatment. (From Paulson et al., 1991, with permission.)

AMPH withdrawal behavioral depression was transient, because by 28 days after the discontinuation of AMPH pretreatment spontaneous locomotor activity was normal across the entire light-dark cycle (Fig. 24-2).

As mentioned above, the behavioral depression seen early after the discontinuation of AMPH pretreatment is not a simple motor deficit, and it is probably related to more complex changes in motivational and affective state. This idea is supported by reports of alterations in reactivity to novelty and in rewarded behavior during withdrawal from AMPH or cocaine (Carroll & Lac, 1987; Schreiber et al., 1976). Changes in intracranial electrical self-stimulation (ICSS) behavior have been particularly well characterized. For at least a few days after withdrawal from chronic treatment with AMPH or cocaine, rats show a depression in the rate of responding and an elevation in the reinforcing threshold for ICSS in a variety of brain structures (Kokkinidis, 1988; Markou & Koob, 1991). It is suggested therefore that the behavioral depression seen initially after the discontinuation of repeated AMPH pretreatment in animals (Kokkinidis, 1988;

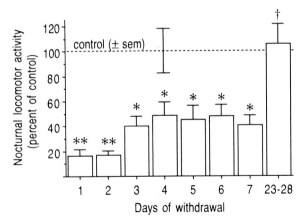

Figure 24-2. Average (+SEM) spontaneous locomotor activity (crossovers) during the last 1.5 hours of the daily lights-off period in AMPH-pretreated animals (*bars*) withdrawn for 1-7 days or 23-28 days. Horizontal dashed line, the average for saline-pretreated control animals; the range line over the dashed line, ±SEM for the controls. The marked depression in nocturnal locomotor activity seen in AMPH-withdrawn animals is most pronounced toward the end of the lights-off period (see Paulson et al., 1991), which is why this period is illustrated here. A one-way ANOVA comparing all groups was significant (F = 7.01, P < 0.001). Subsequent post-hoc tests (Fishers PLSD) showed that animals withdrawn for 1-7 days are significantly less active than controls (P < 0.05) and than animals withdrawn for 23-28 days. Animals withdrawn for 23-28 days are not significantly different from controls. Also, animals withdrawn for 1-2 days are significantly less active than those withdrawn for 3-7 days. These data show therefore that for at least the first week after the discontinuation of repeated AMPH pretreatment rats show decreased levels of spontaneous nocturnal locomotor activity, and this behavioral depression recovers within a month. (Data are replotted from Paulson et al., 1991.)

Paulson et al., 1991) may be related to the withdrawal or abstinence syndrome seen in humans, which is characterized by psychomotor alterations, dysphoria, anxiety, anhedonia, and anergia (Gawin & Ellinwood, 1988). In both rats and humans this withdrawal syndrome is relatively transient, and the symptoms dissipate over a period of a few weeks. The persistent consequences of AMPH pretreatment (sensitization) becomes evident only after transient behavioral depression dissipates.

It is not clear whether the emergence of sensitization after the discontinuation of repeated drug treatment is delayed because time is required for sensitization to develop or because the expression of sensitization is masked by neural alterations underlying transient behavioral depression. As discussed above, if a constant dose of AMPH is given repeatedly and intermittently, there is a *progressive* increase in the motor stimulant effects of AMPH after successive treatments (Robinson & Becker, 1986), supporting the latter interpretation. Perhaps sensitization can only be expressed as the neural adaptations responsible for behavioral depression dissipate. For example, the behavioral depression associated with AMPH withdrawal is accompanied by a transient decrease in the postmortem tissue concentration of hypothalamic norepinephrine (Paulson et al., 1991), and cocaine withdrawal is accompanied by a decrease in basal extracellular dopamine in the ventral striatum (Parsons et al., 1991; Robertson et al., 1991). Whatever the case, the first week or so after the discontinuation of AMPH treatment is clearly a rapidly evolving, dynamic period, which may make it difficult to dissociate neural changes associated with transient post-AMPH withdrawal behavioral depression from those associated with persistent behavioral sensitization at this time.

SENSITIZATION TO OTHER DRUGS OF ABUSE

Although sensitization to AMPH has been studied more thoroughly than sensitization to other addictive drugs, the phenomenon is by no means unique to AMPH. There have been many studies on the sensitization produced by cocaine (Post & Contel, 1983), and several related psychomotor stimulants have been reported to produce sensitization as well, including methylphenidate (Shuster et al., 1982), fencamfamine (Aizenstein et al., 1990) and the endogenous trace amine, phenylethylamine (Borison et al., 1977).

Of even more interest to the present discussion are reports that addictive drugs other than psychomotor stimulants are also capable of producing sensitization. Drugs from other classes obviously have a very different spectrum of action than do psychomotor stimulants, such as AMPH or cocaine, but in addition to their unique effects, many addictive drugs share psychomotor stimulant properties. Evidence that abused drugs from very diverse classes share psychomotor stimulant properties has been reviewed by Wise and Bozarth (1987), who incorporated this evidence into "a psychomotor stimulant theory of addiction." They argue, for example, that even nominal CNS depressants, such as opiates, barbiturates, benzodiazepines, phencyclidine, and alcohol, have psychomotor stimulant properties. The stimulant properties of these latter agents are often masked by their depressant effects, especially at high doses, and presumably the expression of their stimulant versus depressant effects is due to their action on different neural systems. The neural systems involved, however, are not well understood and have only begun to be characterized in a few cases. Nevertheless, brain dopamine (DA) systems have been implicated (Wise & Bozarth, 1987), which is consistent with recent studies showing that a wide variety of addictive drugs share the ability to increase the extracellular concentration of dopamine in both the dorsal and ventral striatum (Di Chiara & Imperato, 1988; Robinson & Camp, 1990).

Of particular interest here is evidence that not only may many addictive drugs share the ability to produce *acute* psychomotor activation and to elevate extracellular DA, but also with repeated administration their ability to produce psychomotor activation progressively increases; i.e., they induce sensitization.

Morphine

The behavioral sensitization produced by repeated treatment with the narcotic analgesic morphine has been well characterized (for reviews, see Kalivas et al.,

1988; Kalivas & Stewart, 1991; Stewart & Vezina, 1988). Although morphine has pronounced CNS depressant effects, it also can produce heightened locomotor activity. After a low dose of morphine, locomotor activity predominates. Only after higher doses is locomotor activity depressed. With high doses of morphine, the locomotor stimulant effects emerge after an initial period of hypoactivity (Babbini & Davis, 1972). When morphine is administered repeatedly and intermittently, its ability to produce locomotor activation is progressively enhanced (Babbini & Davis, 1972; Schnur, 1985; Shuster et al., 1975a & b), and this enhanced responsiveness (sensitization) to the stimulant effects of morphine persists for very long periods of time after the discontinuation of drug treatment (Bartoletti et al., 1983; Shuster et al., 1975a). For example, Babbini et al. (1975) have reported that sensitization to the locomotor activating effects of morphine persists for up to 8 months after ceasing pretreatment. Furthermore, the degree of behavioral sensitization produced by morphine is dependent on the pretreatment dose, with high pretreatment doses producing greater sensitization to a low challenge dose than low pretreatment doses (Bartoletti et al., 1987; Shuster et al., 1975a). However, even doses of morphine below those required to produce overt dependence may produce sensitization (Bartoletti et al., 1987).

Not only do systemic injections of morphine produce sensitization but local injections of morphine (and related compounds) into the ventral tegmental area (VTA) do so as well (Kalivas et al., 1988; Stewart & Vezina, 1988). An acute injection of morphine into the VTA produces marked locomotor hyperactivity, and with repeated intermittent injections there is a progressive enhancement of this effect (Joyce & Iversen, 1979; Vezina & Stewart, 1984). Finally, many examples of cross-sensitization between morphine and other drugs have been reported, including cross-sensitization to fentanyl (Bartoletti et al., 1987), methadone (Bartoletti et al., 1985), and AMPH (Stewart & Vezina, 1988). Cross-sensitization to meperidine or pentazocine has not been found (Bartoletti et al., 1985).

The similarities between the sensitization produced by morphine and AMPH are quite striking. Both agents produce a progressive enhancement of their psychomotor stimulant effects, which persists for long periods of time after the discontinuation of pretreatment. In addition, Shuster and his colleagues (1975a & b) have reported there are other characteristics of morphine sensitization in mice that are very similar to the most salient characteristics of AMPH sensitization:

Repeated injections of morphine produce a progressive increase in its locomotor stimulant effects, and a *single injection* is sufficient to produce persistent sensitization.

The sensitization produced by morphine is greater when injections are spaced in time than when they are given close together in time, and if injections are given too close together in time, tolerance to the locomotor activating effects of morphine occurs.

Sensitization to morphine does not occur in young mice (<15 days old), but does occur if injections are given after mice are 15 days old.

The development of morphine sensitization is prevented by DA antagonism (Vezina & Stewart, 1984, 1989) or by concurrent treatment with a
protein synthesis inhibitor, as is sensitization to AMPH or cocaine (Robinson, 1991; Shuster et al., 1977).

Lastly, Shuster et al. (1975a & b) suggest that sensitization of the locomotor response to morphine does not occur indirectly via tolerance to its depressant effects, a suggestion that is consistent with the results of more recent
studies involving the intracerebral application of morphine (for review, see
Stewart & Vezina, 1988).

Phencyclidine (PCP)

PCP was originally developed as a dissociative anesthetic, and although not
used clinically, it has become a popular drug of abuse known on the streets as
"angel dust." The pharmacology of PCP is very complex, because it shares
properties with many other agents, including barbiturates and psychotomimetic
opioids that bind to the so-called sigma receptor (Balster, 1987). Of most relevance here, however, is that PCP also shares a number of properties with
AMPH. The sympathomimetic effects of PCP were noted very early, and like
AMPH, it is psychotogenic and produces marked locomotor activation (Balster, 1987). The motor stimulant effects of PCP are thought to involve its action
on the mesostriatal DA system (Balster, 1987), which is consistent with reports
that PCP increases the overflow of radiolabeled DA from striatal tissue in vitro
(Vickroy & Johnson, 1982) and increases the extracellular concentration of DA
in vivo (Chapman et al., 1990).

It is now well documented that some of the motor stimulant effects of PCP
are progressively enhanced (sensitized) by repeated intermittent treatment with
PCP (Greenberg & Segal, 1986; Iwamoto, 1986; Nabeshima et al., 1987). For
example, repeated injections of either PCP or the prototypical sigma receptor
agonist, N-allylnormetazocine (SKF-10,047), result in sensitization of locomotor activity, rearing, and nonfocused sniffing (Greenberg & Segal, 1986). In
addition, there is reciprocal cross-sensitization between PCP and SKF-10,047,
so that pretreatment with one agent enhances the behavioral response to a
subsequent challenge injection of the other (Greenberg & Segal 1986; Iwamoto,
1986). On the other hand, Greenberg & Segal (1985) report asymmetric cross-
sensitization between PCP and AMPH. That is, animals pretreated with AMPH
are hyperresponsive to a subsequent challenge with PCP (see Nabeshima et al.,
1989), but animals pretreated with PCP are not sensitized to AMPH. In contrast, Nabeshima et al. (1987) report that animals pretreated with PCP do show
an increased incidence of sniffing, rearing, and licking when subsequently challenged with AMPH. Differences between studies may be due to differences in
the exact nature of the behaviors quantified in different experiments, because
this is clearly a crucial variable (Greenberg & Segal, 1985, 1986). Nevertheless,
there is no doubt that at least some of the motor stimulant effects of PCP are
sensitized by repeated PCP treatment, and as with AMPH, these effects do not
seem to be attributable to either conditioning (Greenberg & Segal, 1986) or
pharmacokinetic factors (Greenberg & Segal, 1986; Nabeshima et al., 1987).

Other Drugs

There are very few studies on sensitization to other addictive drugs, but a few reports suggest that it does occur. For example, Spanos and Yamamoto (1989) reported that repeated intermittent treatment with MDMA (methylenedioxymethamphetamine; "ecstasy") sensitized both its locomotor stimulant effects and the "serotonin behavioral syndrome." There are also a few reports suggesting that the locomotor stimulant effects of caffeine and nicotine may be enhanced with repeated intermittent treatment. For example, Meliska et al. (1990) reported sensitization of wheelrunning in rats given intermittent, but not continuous, treatment with caffeine, although this effect seemed to be context dependent (Meliska et al., 1985). In addition, Clarke (1990, p. 159) has noted that, "although acute administration of nicotine increases locomotor activity in a dose-related manner in rats pre-exposed to the drug on a daily basis . . . , chronic (two week) infusion of nicotine via osmotic minipumps reduced locomotor activity" (also see Ksir et al., 1985). Marked sensitization to nicotine has also been described following its local infusion into the VTA or nucleus accumbens (Kita et al., 1992).

To summarize, it is clear that (1) the motor stimulant effects of a diverse group of addictive drugs are progressively enhanced (sensitized) if these drugs are administered repeatedly and intermittently and (2) this enhanced sensitivity to their motor stimulant properties persists for very long periods of time after the discontinuation of drug treatment. The remainder of this chapter explores two aspects of this phenomenon: its neurobiological basis (with a focus on AMPH sensitization) and the possible relationship of sensitization to addiction and relapse.

NEUROBIOLOGY OF SENSITIZATION

The neurobiological basis of sensitization to AMPH has probably received the most attention, but even this is not well understood. Nevertheless, significant progress has been made. For example, many recent studies on the neurobiological basis of sensitization have explored the idea that sensitization is due to persistent neuroplastic adaptations in those systems that mediate the psychomotor stimulant effects of addictive drugs, and most of these studies have focused on brain DA systems (for more detailed reviews, see Kalivas et al., 1988; Kalivas & Stewart, 1991; Kuczenski & Segal, 1988; Robinson, 1991; Robinson & Becker, 1986; Stewart & Vezina, 1988). There are a number of reasons why AMPH sensitization in particular may be due to enduring alterations in brain DA systems. First, the behaviors sensitized by AMPH (and by other addictive drugs) are thought to be produced in large part by the activation of DA systems (Wise & Bozarth, 1987). Second, the activation of DA systems is necessary for the induction of sensitization. The co-administration of DA antagonists prevents the development of sensitization to AMPH, cocaine, or morphine (Kuczenski & Leith, 1981; Vezina & Stewart, 1989; Weiss et al., 1989), and a 6-OHDA lesion of the nucleus accumbens prevents sensitization to

AMPH (Segal et al., 1979). Also, the selective blockade of DA D_1 receptors (but not D_2 receptors) is reported to be sufficient to prevent AMPH sensitization (Vezina & Stewart, 1989), although others have found that AMPH sensitization is prevented by blockade of either D_1 or D_2 receptors (Akiyama et al., 1991). Nevertheless, these studies are all consistent with the idea that activation of DA receptors is necessary for the induction of sensitization.

Although the activation of DA receptors seems to be necessary to produce AMPH sensitization, there is no compelling evidence that AMPH sensitization is accompanied by persistent alterations in DA receptor binding in forebrain DA terminal regions or in behavioral responsiveness to the DA receptor agonist, apomorphine (for review, see Robinson & Becker, 1986). This leads to the conclusion that AMPH sensitization is probably not due to postsynaptic DA receptor supersensitivity (Robinson & Becker, 1986). However, most of the studies reviewed earlier by Robinson and Becker (1986) involved binding to DA D_2 receptors, which would not detect sensitization-related changes in DA receptor-coupling to second-messenger systems (Roseboom & Gnegy, 1989). A recent report that cocaine pretreatment produces a persistent increase in the sensitivity of nucleus accumbens neurons to iontophoretically applied SKF 38393, a DA D_1 receptor agonist (Henry & White, 1991; White et al., 1992), suggests that the contribution of a postsynaptic change, perhaps specific to DA D_1 receptors, warrants further consideration. Nevertheless, several reports have found that neither DA-stimulated adenylate cyclase activity nor [^{3}H] cis-flupenthixol binding to DA D_1 receptors is changed in AMPH-sensitized animals, at least in the absence of an AMPH challenge (Barnett et al., 1987; Roberts-Lewis et al., 1986; Roseboom & Gnegy, 1989; see Robinson & Becker, 1986 for additional references). The ability of an AMPH challenge to *desensitize* DA-stimulated adenylate cyclase activity is enhanced in AMPH-sensitized animals (Barnett et al., 1987; Roberts-Lewis et al., 1986; Roseboom & Gnegy, 1989). On the other hand, it is possible that not all DA D_1 receptors are coupled to adenylate cyclase (Mahan et al., 1990), and therefore, the effects reported by White et al. (1991) could be due to effects on non-adenylate-cyclase-linked DA D_1 receptors. In addition, AMPH pretreatment has been shown to alter the "interaction among calmodulin, stimulatory guanyl nucleotide-regulatory protein, dopamine receptors and adenylate cyclase as well as calmodulin content" (Roseboom & Gnegy, 1989, p. 197; see also Gnegy et al., 1991), although it is not known whether these effects are presynaptic or postsynaptic. It is concluded that, at this time, the relationship between postsynaptic changes in AMPH-sensitized animals and behavioral sensitization remains unclear.

On the presynaptic side, however, evidence is accumulating for a persistent increase in the releasibility of DA in sensitized animals. Robinson & Becker (1982) first reported that AMPH pretreatment produces a long-lasting enhancement in AMPH-stimulated DA release from striatal tissue in vitro, and there have now been a number of such reports (see Robinson, 1991 for references). Furthermore, Castañeda et al. (1988) found that striatal DA release stimulated by AMPH, potassium, and electrical field stimulation was enhanced in AMPH-sensitized animals, and Kolta et al. (1989) reported a sensitization-related enhancement of AMPH-stimulated DA release from nucleus accumbens tissue in vitro. More recently, sensitization-related changes in DA release have been assessed in vivo using the technique of intracerebral microdialysis (Fig. 24-3). AMPH sensitization is accompanied by an increase in the ability of AMPH to elevate the extracellular concentration of DA in both the caudate nucleus (Ichikawa, 1988; Kazahaya et al., 1989; Patrick et al., 1991; Robinson,

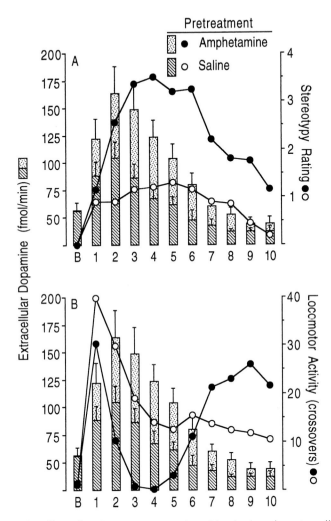

Figure 24-3. The effect of AMPH pretreatment (sensitization) on the extracellular concentration of dopamine (DA) in the nucleus accumbens and on behavior (stereotypy, locomotion) before (B-Baseline) and after (intervals 1-10) a challenge injection of 2.0 mg/kg of AMPH given 15-21 days after the discontinuation of AMPH pretreatment. The bars represent the average (+SEM) extracellular concentration of DA over 20-minute intervals in AMPH (*stippled*) and saline (*stripes*) pretreated animals, and the same data are plotted in both the upper and lower panels. **Top,** Average stereotypy ratings in AMPH (*solid circles*) and saline (*open circle*) pretreated animals, during each 20-minute interval, are overlaid on the neurochemical data. **Bottom,** Symbols representing the average amount of locomotor activity (crossovers) during each 20-minute interval in AMPH- and saline-pretreated animals are overlaid on the neurochemical data. (Data are redrawn from Figures 2 and 3 in Robinson et al., 1988.)

1991) and the nucleus accumbens (Robinson, 1991; Robinson et al., 1988; cf., Segal & Kuczenski, 1992a). It is interesting to note that the *basal* extracellular concentration of DA is not altered in AMPH-sensitized animals, nor is basal DA efflux in vitro. Rather, it is the response to a challenge that is enhanced.

The increased releasibility of DA seen in AMPH-sensitized animals parallels the most salient characteristics of the behavioral phenomenon, some of which were mentioned above (Robinson, 1991). For example, a single injection of AMPH not only produces behavioral sensitization but also enhances AMPH-stimulated DA release in vitro for at least 1 month (Robinson & Becker, 1982). As with behavioral sensitization, the increase in AMPH-stimulated DA release is very persistent, being evident for months after the discontinuation of pretreatment (Robinson, 1991). The enhancement in DA release is influenced by the passage of time since the discontinuation of drug treatment in a manner similar to behavioral sensitization. Kolta et al. (1985) found that AMPH pretreatment increased AMPH-stimulated DA release from striatal tissue in vitro when testing took place long after the discontinuation of pretreatment (15–30 days), but not when testing took place only 3 days after the discontinuation of pretreatment. Parallel time-dependent changes in behavioral sensitization were reported by Kolta et al. (1985). The influence of sex and gonadal hormones on sensitization-related changes in DA release has not been studied, but sensitization-related changes in DA metabolism are influenced by sex and circulating gonadal hormones in a manner similar to behavioral sensitization (Camp & Robinson, 1988a).

It is not at all clear at this time whether the sensitization produced by different agents is due to common neurobiological adaptations. Nevertheless, an increase in stimulated DA release in DA terminal regions (or more accurately, in the ability to enhance the extracellular concentration of DA) has also been reported after pretreatment with cocaine (Akimoto et al., 1989; Kalivas & Duffy, 1990; Keller et al., 1992; Peris & Zahniser, 1987; cf., Segal & Kuczenski, 1992b) or the endogenous trace amine, phenylethylamine (Kuroki et al., 1990). Reciprocal cross-sensitization of DA release between AMPH and cocaine has been reported as well (Akimoto et al., 1990; Kazahaya et al., 1989).

In contrast to the increase in stimulated DA release seen in DA terminal regions of cocaine-sensitized animals, Kalivas and Duffy (1988) report that somatodendritic DA release is decreased. They suggest that this decrease in somatodendritic DA release may be responsible for sensitization-related increases in extracellular DA in DA terminal fields in the forebrain because of decreased negative feedback inhibition.

The role of the DA cell body region in the midbrain and DA terminals in the forebrain in the induction versus expression of sensitization is particularly interesting. It seems that, with AMPH and morphine, drug action at the level of the DA cell bodies is necessary to *induce* behavioral sensitization (Kalivas et al., 1988; Robinson, 1991; Vezina et al., 1987; see Vezina & Stewart 1990 for references). For example, the local infusion of either AMPH or morphine into the VTA is sufficient to sensitize the behavioral response to a subsequent challenge injection given systemically. This occurs despite the fact that an acute intra-VTA infusion of AMPH does not elicit behavioral hyperactivity. In contrast, a local infusion of AMPH or morphine into the nucleus accumbens does not induce sensitization to a subsequent systemic challenge, even though such treatments do elicit acute locomotor hyperactivity. Furthermore, a local microinjection of a DA D_1 receptor antagonist into the VTA is sufficient to prevent the sensitization to systemic AMPH treatment (Stewart & Vezina, 1989).

Although an action of AMPH at DA cell bodies may be required to induce sensitization, this may not be required for the *expression* of AMPH sensitization. This idea is supported by reports that animals pretreated with systemic injections of AMPH are behaviorally hyperresponsive to a local challenge injection of AMPH into the nucleus accumbens (Kolta et al., 1989; Paulson & Robinson, 1991). Furthermore, a sensitization-related enhancement of DA release is seen in striatal and nucleus accumbens tissue slices, a preparation in which DA cell bodies are not present (Kolta et al., 1985, 1989; Robinson & Becker, 1982; Robinson et al., 1982). It is suggested, therefore, that an action of AMPH on DA cell bodies may be required to induce long-term changes in DA neurons, perhaps because changes in protein synthesis are required, but that these changes are later expressed "upstream" in the DA terminal fields. Consistent with this interpretation are reports that AMPH, cocaine, and morphine sensitization are all prevented by co-administration of a protein synthesis inhibitor (Robinson, 1991; Shuster et al., 1975a, 1977).

In summary, there is now considerable evidence showing that experience with a variety of addictive drugs can produce very long-lasting enhancement of the responsiveness of mesostriatal DA neurons to stimuli that increase DA neurotransmission. Although such changes in brain DA systems may be responsible, at least in part, for behavioral sensitization, much more research will be required to establish a definite causal relationship. Nevertheless, much of the available evidence is consistent with such a hypothesis. The exact nature of the change in DA neurons that results in enhanced releasibility of DA in sensitized animals has been the topic of much speculation, and several hypotheses have been formulated (Kalivas & Stewart, 1991; Robinson, 1991; Robinson & Becker, 1986, for reviews). There is, however, very little solid evidence for or against any particular hypothesis at this time.

It also needs to be emphasized that none of the studies on sensitization-related changes in DA systems discussed here rules out contributions by other neurotransmitter systems (Robinson & Becker, 1986). Indeed, there is accumulating evidence implicating noncatecholamine systems in the development of sensitization. For example, behavioral sensitization to AMPH and cocaine is attenuated not only by the co-administration of DA antagonists but also by co-administration of NMDA receptor antagonists (Karler et al., 1989, 1990; Wolf & Rhansa, 1991), suggesting that activity at glutamate synapses may be necessary. Also, there is indirect evidence that GABA neurotransmission in the substantia nigra is altered 45 days after the discontinuation of pretreatment with AMPH (Perez-de la Mora et al., 1990).

The role of conditioning factors in sensitization has not been discussed here, but they are very important variables in the development and expression of sensitization-related changes in behavior produced by addictive drugs

(Stewart, 1992). In many studies, especially if a drug is repeatedly administered in a unique test environment, drug-environment conditioning may play a major role in the enhanced responsiveness seen when the drug is given again in that environment (Post et al., 1987; Stewart & Vezina, 1988). That is, if environmental stimuli are consistently associated with drug use, these environmental stimuli can acquire the properties of conditioned stimuli and can exert a great deal of control over the expression of sensitization. However, sensitization and drug-environment conditioning can be dissociated, and therefore, drug-environment conditioning is not necessary for the development of sensitization (Mazurski & Beninger, 1987; Robinson & Becker, 1986; Vezina & Stewart, 1990). The role of conditioning in sensitization has been reviewed recently by Stewart (1992), and therefore is not discussed further here.

Finally, the possible contribution of pharmacokinetic changes to sensitization deserves mention. Although there is considerable evidence to suggest that pharmacokinetic changes do not account for AMPH sensitization (Demellweek & Goudie, 1983; McCown & Barrett, 1980; Robinson & Becker, 1986), it has been reported recently that brain levels of cocaine are enhanced in cocaine-pretreated rats given a challenge injection of cocaine (Pettit et al., 1990). However, this effect may not persist (Reith et al., 1987), as does behavioral sensitization, and therefore, it remains to be determined whether pharmacokinetic factors can account for the behavioral sensitization to cocaine seen many months after the discontinuation of drug pretreatment.

IMPLICATIONS OF SENSITIZATION FOR ADDICTION AND RELAPSE

To summarize thus far, it has been established that the psychomotor stimulant effects of a variety of addictive drugs are progressively enhanced (sensitized) when these drugs are administered repeatedly and intermittently. Sensitization is very persistent. For example, animals remain sensitized to the motor stimulant properties of AMPH and morphine for 8–12 months after the discontinuation of pretreatment. Mesotelencephalic DA systems seem to be hyperresponsive in sensitized animals. A drug challenge induces greater DA release (or greater accumulation of extracellular DA) in sensitized than in drug-naive control animals.

Because mesotelencephalic DA systems are known to be critical in mediating the psychomotor stimulant effects of many addictive drugs, it is reasonable to suggest that the enhancement of DA neurotransmission seen in sensitized animals may contribute to behavioral sensitization. Yet, what does sensitization to the psychomotor stimulant effects of these agents have to do with their abuse liability? The answer, of course, is that DA systems are thought to mediate not only the psychomotor stimulant effects of many addictive drugs but also their rewarding effects (Wise & Bozarth, 1987). Wise and Bozarth (1987, also p. 475) have even argued that "the locomotor effects and the positive reinforcing effects of these drugs are homologous"; that is, "they derive from activation of a common mechanism." The common mechanism to which they refer is activation of mesostriatal DA systems, in particular, the so-called mesolimbic DA projections from the ventral tegmental area to the ventral striatum, e.g., nucleus accumbens. If both the psychomotor stimulant effects and rewarding effects of addictive drugs are mediated by the same or very closely overlapping DA systems and if the psychomotor stimulant effects of these drugs are sensitized by repeated drug treatment, it follows that their rewarding effects must be sensitized as well.

Sensitization of Drug Reward

There has been very little research on the role of sensitization on subsequent drug reward. Nevertheless, there is accumulating evidence to suggest that prior experience with AMPH, cocaine, or morphine sensitizes drug reward. For example, Lett (1989) recently examined the influence of pretreatment with AMPH, cocaine, or morphine on drug reward using the conditioned place preference (CPP) paradigm. Rats were sensitized with five or six injections of either AMPH, cocaine, or morphine given 24–72 hours apart. A few days after the last pretreatment injection, the animals underwent CPP training, consisting of one to three pairings of a drug with a unique test environment. Control animals were pretreated with saline, and then some of these underwent CPP training and others did not. With this paradigm the strength of drug reward is inferred by the strength of the CPP, assessed on a drug-free test day. For all drugs, pretreated (sensitized) animals showed a significantly greater CPP than did saline-pretreated control animals. Furthermore, cross-sensitization occurred. That is, animals sensitized to AMPH showed an enhanced CPP for morphine, animals pretreated with morphine showed an enhanced CPP for AMPH, and animals pretreated with morphine showed an enhanced CPP for cocaine. These latter findings are consistent, of course, with many reports of cross-sensitization to the psychomotor stimulant effects of stimulants and opiates (Kalivas et al., 1988; Stewart & Vezina, 1988).

There is also evidence from self-administration experiments of sensitization of drug reward. For example, Woolverton et al. (1984) found that a low dose of methamphetamine supported self-administration in rhesus monkeys only *after* they received a series of noncontingent injections of methamphetamine. That is, after methamphetamine pretreatment the threshold dose necessary to maintain self-administration behavior was lowered. In a similar vein, Piazza et al. (1989, 1990) recently found that a sensitizing regimen of AMPH injections increases the probability of acquisition of AMPH self-administration in a subgroup of animals that otherwise would not acquire a self-administration habit. Comparable results have been obtained with cocaine. Horger et al. (1990) reported that rats sensitized with noncontingent injections of cocaine show a higher rate of drug-specific lever-pressing for i.v. cocaine than do saline-pretreated control animals when both groups were later tested for the acquisition of drug self-administration behavior using very low doses of cocaine, doses below those normally required to reliably maintain self-administration behavior. It was suggested that prior exposure to cocaine enhanced cocaine self-administration because "the reinforcing effectiveness of the drug had increased." AMPH pretreatment also facilitates the acquisition of cocaine self-administration (Horger et al., 1991). Although I am not aware of a similar study on opiate self-administration, Gaiardi et al. (1986) report that noncontingent treatment with morphine produces a long-lasting (3 months) increase in sensitivity to the discriminative stimulus properties of morphine and facilitates the acquisition of a morphine conditioned place preference (Guiardi et al., 1991). Finally, it is relevant that sensitization to AMPH can facilitate ICSS reward (Kokkinidis, 1988).

In summary, not only are the psychomotor stimulant effects of addictive drugs sensitized by past drug treatment, but recent studies suggest that their rewarding effects are sensitized as well. Animals pretreated with AMPH, cocaine, or morphine later show an enhanced preference for an environment associated with drug administration, and animals sensitized to AMPH or cocaine show enhanced vulnerability to acquire a self-administration habit. Obviously, sensitization of drug reward would be expected to enhance the development of addictive behaviors, because with more and more drug experience the rewarding impact of these drugs would become progressively enhanced. By definition, this would serve to progressively increase the probability of repeating drug-seeking and drug-taking behaviors in the future.

However, the fact that addicts usually take progressively higher doses of drugs may seem to some readers to be inconsistent with the sensitization of drug reward. It might be argued, for example, that sensitization of drug reward should lead to the intake of lower, not higher, doses of a drug. This issue is discussed later in this chapter, after first discussing how sensitization may increase the likelihood of relapse.

Role of Sensitization in Relapse

Even if an addict managed to remain abstinent, the persistence of the neural adaptations underlying sensitization may render him or her highly susceptible to relapse. It is well known that, in animals trained to self-administer a drug but in which the behavior has been extinguished, noncontingent re-exposure to a low dose of the drug will rapidly reinstate responding (Stewart et al., 1984; Stewart & Wise, 1992). This "priming" phenomenon and its role in relapse have been discussed extensively by Stewart et al. (1984), who argued "that compulsive drug use . . . is maintained by appetitive motivational processes, that is, by the generation of positively affective motivational states" (p. 252) and that priming reinstates drug use because "the presence of the drug in the body (not its absence) activates appetitive motivational mechanisms that are involved in the reinitiation of drug-seeking behavior" (p. 253). Not only can an i.v. injection of a drug prime responding but the application of AMPH or morphine locally into the VTA is sufficient to prime responding for i.v. AMPH or morphine, respectively. For this and other reasons (Stewart et al., 1984), the priming effect is thought to be mediated by the action of drugs (and other stimuli) on mesotelencephalic DA systems.

Of course, sensitization of mesotelencephalic DA systems could greatly facilitate this priming process. If past experience with addictive drugs enhances the responsiveness of mesotelencephalic DA systems, this could increase the ability of low priming doses of a drug to enhance dopaminergic activity, which would increase the positive incentive properties of the priming exposure. Thus, in drug-experienced subjects re-exposure to the drug would be more likely to reinstate compulsive drug-seeking behavior (relapse) than in less experienced subjects. Furthermore, because sensitization represents such an enduring change in responsiveness, an enhanced sensitivity to the priming effects of drugs would be expected to persist even after very long periods of abstinence. As pointed out by Stewart et al. (1984, p. 257),

> The idea that ingestion of a formerly abused drug induces a strong motivational state or craving for the drug and that it retains the ability to reinstate this craving over an indefinite period of abstinence from the drug is not new. One of the basic tenets of Alcoholics Anonymous is that people who have at one time shown uncontrolled drinking and physical dependence are permanently unable to drink moderately; one drink is said to elicit an urge to have another.

It is suggested here that this phenomenon may be, at least in part, a consequence of sensitization of mesotelencephalic DA systems or related neural systems that mediate the positive incentive effects of drugs.

In addition, not only may re-exposure to a drug induce relapse but also there is a considerable body of evidence showing that environmental stimuli associated with drug use can become secondary reinforcers and may also prime responding (Stewart et al., 1984). Thus, the ability of drug-associated environmental stimuli to precipitate relapse may also become enhanced because of sensitization-related changes in the nervous system (see Stewart, 1992 for a more complete discussion of this point).

As an aside, it is also interesting to point out that *intermittency* is not only important in producing behavioral sensitization, as discussed above (Post, 1980; Robinson & Becker, 1986) but is also thought to play an important role in the development of persistent and excessive habitual behaviors, including drug-taking behavior (Falk & Feingold, 1987). Falk and Feingold (1987) have argued eloquently that the reinforcing properties of drugs may be greatly enhanced by intermittent schedules and speculate that intermittent schedules may catalyze drug overindulgence in humans. They state, "when life's crucial commodities are in short supply and available only on intermittent, marginal schedules, such as may occur in an impoverished, inner-city environment, drugs can become all-powerful in reinforcing efficacy" (Falk & Feingold, 1987, p. 1506).

Cross-Sensitization

Sensitization is not only seen when the same drug is later readministered but behavioral cross-sensitization and cross-sensitization of drug reward also occur. The implication of cross-sensitization is that exposure to a drug from one class may later enhance the rewarding effects of a drug from another class, potentially facilitating addiction to the second drug. This is consistent with the observation of priming across drug classes. For example, AMPH can prime morphine responding, and morphine can prime cocaine responding. Even a local injection of AMPH into the VTA is sufficient to prime responding for i.v. heroin (Stewart & Vezina, 1988). This action occurs presumably because common neural systems (DA systems?) are involved in mediating the positive incentive properties of many addictive drugs, so that exposure to even a novel drug can prime drug-seeking behavior. Thus, if DA systems are sensitized by use of one drug, it might be expected that a second, novel drug would more readily provoke relapse in subjects who were previously exposed to other. addictive drugs.

However, relapse to compulsive drug use is not always precipitated by reexposure to a drug, but often by ill-defined environmental events. Sensitization may play a role here as well. Although there is not space to review the literature, there is considerable evidence to suggest that sensitization is not unique to the psychopharmacology of addictive drugs. Many studies show that animals previously exposed to such drugs as AMPH, cocaine, or morphine are later hyperresponsive to stress, and animals previously exposed to stress are hyperresponsive to the motor stimulant effects of a subsequent challenge injection of AMPH, cocaine, or morphine (Antelman et al., 1980; Kalivas et al., 1988; Kalivas & Stewart, 1991; Robinson, 1988). That is, repeated intermittent drug treatment can sensitize animals to subsequent stress and vice versa. In fact, it has been suggested that AMPH induces sensitization *because* of its action as a stressor (Antelman & Chiodo, 1983). A relationship between AMPH and stress is further supported by reports that activation of the hypothalamo-pituitary-adrenal axis is required for the development of AMPH sensitization (Cole et al., 1990). Rivet et al. (1989) suggest that corticosteroids facilitate AMPH sensitization via their action on type II (glucocorticoid) receptors, although there is some disagreement on this latter point (Cools, 1990). Finally, there is also evidence that sensitization to stress involves changes in catecholamine systems, including mesotelencephalic DA systems (Robinson, 1988; Wilcox et al., 1986) and NE projections to the hippocampus (Nisenbaum et al., 1991).

The implication of cross-sensitization between addictive drugs and stress, of course, is that former drug addicts may be hyperresponsive not only to the motor stimulant and incentive properties of drugs themselves but also to the priming effect of subsequent stress. Stress is known to increase DA release in mesotelencephalic DA systems. If the ability of stress to induce DA release were enhanced by past exposure to drugs, it might be expected that environmental or physical stress would be better able to prime drug-seeking behavior in drug-experienced subjects than in drug-naive subjects. The converse may also be true. That is, prior experience with stress could predispose susceptible individuals to drug addiction by sensitizing those neural systems that mediate the positive incentive effects of drugs—presumably mesotelencephalic DA systems. An increase in the positive incentive effects of the initial drug experience would be expected to increase the probability of drug-seeking behavior. There is some experimental evidence in support of this kind of relationship between prior stress and the acquisition of drug self-administration. Piazza et al. (1990) report that in rats, not only does sensitization to AMPH facilitate the acquisition of AMPH self-administration but so does sensitization to stress (repeated tail pinch).

ON THE RELATIONSHIP BETWEEN SENSITIZATION OF
DRUG REWARD AND TOLERANCE TO THE SUBJECTIVE,
EUPHORIC EFFECTS OF ADDICTIVE DRUGS

Evidence that the incentive motivational properties of addictive drugs are sensitized by repeated intermittent drug treatment, as discussed above, seems to be contradictory to the common assumption derived from clinical observations that the euphoric effects of these agents show tolerance (Jaffe, 1980). In fact, it may be that sensitization of drug reward has received relatively little attention because it is generally accepted that addicts progressively increase their dose to overcome tolerance to the euphoric effects of drugs. The apparent contradiction between sensitization of drug reward and tolerance to euphoria requires a reappraisal of widely held assumptions regarding the relationship between the pleasurable sensations produced by addictive drugs and their incentive motivational properties.

The first commonly held assumption is that tolerance develops to the euphoric effects of addictive drugs (Jaffe, 1980). The evidence typically cited in support of this claim is the well-documented observation that addicts usually escalate their dosage with repeated drug use. As stated by Falk et al. (1983, p. 81), "One of the most insidious aspects of drug abuse is the seemingly inexorable tendency for addicts to increase their drug consumption over time." There is, however, very little objective evidence linking this escalation in dose with tolerance to the reinforcing effects of drugs. Falk et al. (1983, p. 81) note, "It is commonly presumed that . . . as tolerance develops, more drug must be ingested to satiate the addict's need for the drug. It is fascinating that there is little experimental data relevant to this assumption and that which does exist does not support." For example, McAuliffe and Gordon (1974) documented that addicts continue to experience euphoria even after years of drug use, and there is even some evidence to suggest an *increase* in the pleasurable effects of morphine in long-term addicts. Lasagna et al. (1955) studied the subjective effects of an acute drug challenge in drug-naive volunteers versus institutionalized "postaddicts." Nearly all of the naive subjects rated the effects of morphine as very unpleasant (cf., McAuliffe & Gordon, 1975). "Postaddicts", on the other hand, overwhelmingly rated the morphine experience as pleasant and scored it high on a dysphoria-euphoria scale. Thus, the ability of morphine to induce euphoria seems to be enhanced in addicts. However, this change in the subjective effects of morphine probably does not reflect sensitization to its positive reinforcing effects, but rather tolerance to its aversive effects, because "postaddicts" also reported a lower incidence of nausea and vomiting than naive subjects.

On the other hand, short-term tolerance may play a role in the escalation of dose seen when drugs are administered in a "run," as is often the case with AMPH or cocaine. If a large supply of AMPH or cocaine is readily available, addicts frequently readminister the drug as soon as the effects of the previous treatment begin to dissipate. However, if successive administrations are given too close together in time, the positive effects of the drug may be masked or suppressed by a transient depression of brain reward systems, as discussed above (Gawin & Ellinwood, 1988; Kokkinidis et al., 1986; Paulson et al., 1991). Therefore, dose may be escalated *within a run* to overcome this apparent short-term tolerance to the rewarding effects of the drug. Yet, this action may not be relevant to the escalation of dose seen over the long-term; that is, *between runs*.

Why then do addicts also typically escalate their dose over the long term? A possible alternative explanation to tolerance of euphoria is that addicts increase their dose to achieve the more intense (and more desirable) "high" associated with large doses and are able to do so because tolerance develops to the *aversive* side effects of drugs. That is, addicts increase their dose because they can do so, without feeling the dire negative effects experienced by naive users. Doses that might be unpleasant or even life-threatening in inexperienced users are tolerated by experienced users, because of tolerance to many of the drug's negative effects, including effects on the autonomic nervous system.

In summary, although there is no strong experimental evidence for tolerance to the euphoric effects of drugs, neither is there any evidence that the euphoric effects of drugs show sensitization. We are still left, therefore, with the paradox that animal studies involving two different paradigms for assessing the incentive rewarding properties of drugs (conditioned place preference and self-administration), and three different drugs (amphetamine, cocaine and morphine), suggest the incentive rewarding effects of drugs are sensitized. How do we resolve the apparent discrepancy between these animal studies and the clinical observations of either tolerance or no change in the euphoric effects of drugs in addicts?

The answer may lie in a second assumption that underlies much of the thinking in this field, which is that the subjective, pleasurable effects of drugs are directly responsible for their incentive motivational effects; i.e., euphoria = reward. This assumption may be invalid. The subjective feelings of pleasure (euphoria) derived from drugs of abuse may be only secondarily or indirectly related to their incentive rewarding properties; i.e., euphoria ≠ reward. Perhaps it is only because these events occur in close association in time that the subjective pleasurable effects of drugs seem to underlie the desire for more drug compulsive and thus compulsive drug-seeking and drug-taking behavior. The idea that the subjective effects of drugs are dissociable from their incentive rewarding properties is not new. For example, Falk et al. (1983) review evidence that "the subjective effects produced by a drug do not necessarily predict whether the drug actually will be self-administered" (p. 58), and note that drug self-administration is often "maintained in the face of various, strong negative consequences" (p. 100). They argue that further research will be required "to determine the conditions under which subjective effects are the basis of the reinforcing effects of the drug" (p. 58). For example, as mentioned above, many people report that morphine initially has very unpleasant, dysphoric effects (Lasagna et al., 1955), although at the same time it clearly has strong positive incentive motivational properties. Similarly, Katz and Goldberg (1988) describe experiments that suggest that "the reinforcing effects and the subjective reports by human volunteers are not functionally equivalent entities" (p. 24).

Lamb et al. (1991) recently reported an especially striking dissociation between the incentive rewarding effects of morphine and its subjective pleasurable effects. These researchers found that in former heroin addicts low doses of morphine maintained responding on a second order schedule of reinforcement (i.e., it acted as a positive reinforcer), despite the fact that 4 of 5 subjects could not distinguish the subjective effects of the lowest dose of morphine from the placebo, which did not maintain responding. Lamb et al. (1991) concluded that, "the reinforcing effects of morphine can occur in the absence of self-reported subjective effects and thus, do not appear to be causally-related to drug-liking or euphoria" (p. 1172). These findings strongly support the hypothesis that euphoria $\neq$ reward.

The hypothesis that euphoria does not equal reward would require, of course, that different neural systems mediate the subjective, pleasurable versus incentive motivational effects of drugs. Yet, Wise and his colleagues have argued that mesotelencephalic DA systems, especially the DA projections to the nucleus accumbens and related output systems from the accumbens, are critical for *both* the incentive rewarding properties and the subjective, pleasurable (hedonic) effects of drugs of abuse and natural reinforcers (Wise, 1982; Wise & Bozarth, 1987). This view is not consistent with the idea that the incentive rewarding effects of drugs are dissociable from their subjective pleasurable (hedonic) effects. However, recent experiments by Kent Berridge at the University of Michigan suggest that the neural systems responsible for the subjective, pleasurable (hedonic) effects of drugs may in fact be dissociable from those responsible for their incentive motivational properties.

Berridge et al. (1989) have found that the mesostriatal DA system, which is so strongly linked with drug reward (Wise & Bozarth, 1987), is not necessary for normal hedonics. They tested the ability of control rats and of rats depleted of mesostriatal DA by an injection of 6-hydroxydopamine (6-OHDA), to make hedonic judgments, using a well-characterized taste reactivity test. With this paradigm it is possible to quantify the ability of animals to assess the positive and aversive qualities of gustatory stimuli, independent of food intake. Interestingly, animals rendered aphagic by a large 6-OHDA lesion of the mesostriatal DA system showed normal taste reactivity. That is, despite a marked feeding deficit, which has been interpreted as a dysfunction in hedonics (Wise, 1982), 6-OHDA—lesioned rats made normal hedonic judgments. However, in this experiment the average DA depletion was only 85%, and the nucleus accumbens was relatively spared. It is possible, therefore, that changes in hedonics would occur with an even larger lesion that did not spare the accumbens. Yet, in subsequent unpublished experiments Berridge and I have found that rats with a >95% depletion of DA in both the caudate nucleus and the nucleus accumbens also had a normal capacity for hedonic judgments, as assessed by taste reactivity. Furthermore, animals in which the affective response to a preferred taste was altered using conditioned taste aversion procedures showed normal hedonics even after a >95% DA depletion. Consistent with these experiments, Berridge & Valenstein (1991) recently reported that feeding evoked by electrical stimulation of the lateral hypothalamus, which has been hypothesized to involve activation of mesostriatal DA systems and to produce a "hedonic sensory experience," does not potentiate the hedonic value of taste stimuli assessed by taste reactivity.

The experiments by Berridge and his colleagues suggest that DA is not necessary for normal hedonics; that is, for experiencing pleasure. On the other hand, there is considerable evidence that DA is involved in mediating drug reward (Wise & Bozarth, 1987). It would seem therefore that the neural systems responsible for the subjective pleasurable effects of drugs are dissociable from those responsible for their incentive motivational properties. Although the mesostriatal DA system may be necessary for the incentive motivational effects of drugs (drug reward), it may not be involved in evaluating the pleasantness of stimuli (hedonics), including drug-related stimuli. Thus, it is possible that with repeated drug use the incentive motivational effects of drugs are progressively sensitized due to enhanced DA neurotransmission, in the absence of changes in the ability of the drug to produce euphoria.

SUMMARY AND CONCLUSIONS

There is now considerable evidence to support the thesis that repeated intermittent exposure to a variety of addictive drugs produces persistent neural adaptations manifested as behavioral sensitization, and that these neural adaptations involve, at least in part, sensitization of mesostriatal DA systems. These persistent sensitization-related changes in mesostriatal DA systems may play a central role in the development of addictive behaviors, and especially in the high rate of relapse that occurs even after long periods of abstinence. The hypothesis that mesostriatal DA may mediate the incentive rewarding properties of drugs, but not their subjective pleasurable effects, also has interesting implications for understanding the role of sensitization in addiction. The implication, of course, is that the incentive rewarding properties of addictive drugs may be progressively increased (sensitized) with repeated drug use, in the absence of persistent changes in their hedonic effects. Sensitization to the incentive motivational effects of drugs, due to adaptations in DA systems, may account for why drug-seeking and drug-taking behaviors become increasingly more compulsive and all important in addicts. The craving for drugs and the lengths to which addicts will go to obtain drugs, even in the face of strong negative consequences, seem out of proportion with the pleasure derived from drugs. It is suggested that this state of affairs may develop with repeated drug use because the neural systems responsible for the incentive motivational effects of drugs are progressively sensitized, even though their ability to engender positive affect (hedonics) may not change.

Despite the efforts to date, relatively little is known about the neurobiology of sensitization, and its role in addiction remains speculative. Nevertheless, there is good reason to believe that further research on this topic will provide valuable new insights into the neurobiology of addiction. Furthermore, attempts to minimize the consequences of sensitization may lead to novel therapeutic strategies in the treatment of addiction.

ACKNOWLEDGMENTS

I thank Kent Berridge, Jill Becker, Dianne Camp, Jane Stewart, and Elliot Valenstein for their helpful comments on an earlier draft of this chapter.

REFERENCES

Aizenstein M.L., Segal, D.S., & Kuczenski, R. (1990). Repeated amphetamine and fencamfamine: Sensitization and reciprocal cross-sensitization. *Neuropsychopharmacology, 3*, 283-290.

Akimoto, K., Hamamura, T., Kazahaya, Y., Akiyama, K., & Otsuki S. (1990). Enhanced extracellular dopamine level may be the fundamental neuropharmacological basis of cross-behavioral sensitization between metamphetamine and cocaine—an in vivo dialysis study in freely moving rats. *Brain Res., 507*, 344-346.

Akimoto, K., Hamamura, T., & Otsuki, S. (1989). Subchronic cocaine treatment enhances cocaine-induced dopamine efflux, studied by in vivo intracerebral dialysis. *Brain Res., 490*, 339-344.

Akiyama, K., Hamamura, T., Ujike, H., Kanzaki, A., & Otsuki, S. (1991). Methamphetamine psychosis as a model of relapse of schizophrenia—a behavioral and biochemical study in the animal model. In T. Nakazawa (Ed.), *Taniguchi Symposia on brain sciences, Vol. 14, Biological basis of schizophrenia* (pp. 169-184). Tokyo: Japan Scientific Societies.

Antelman, S.M., & Chiodo, L.A. (1983). Amphetamine as a stressor. In I. Creese (Ed.), *Stimulants: Neurochemical, behavioral and clinical perspectives* (pp. 269-299). New York: Raven Press.

Antelman, S.M., Eichler, A.J., Black, C.A., & Kocan, D. (1980). Interchangeability of stress and amphetamine in sensitization. *Science, 207*, 329-331.

Babbini, M., & Davis, W.M. (1972). Time-dose relationships for locomotor activity effects of morphine after acute or repeated treatment. *Br. J. Pharmacol., 46*, 213-224.

Babbini, M., Gaiardi, M., & Bartoletti, M. (1975). Persistence of chronic morphine effects upon activity in rats 8 months after ceasing the treatment. *Neuropharmacology, 14*, 611-614.

Balster, R. L. (1987). The behavioral pharmacology of phencyclidine. In H.Y. Meltzer (Ed.), *Psychopharmacology: A third generation of progress* (pp. 1573-1579). New York: Raven Press.

Barnett, I.V., Segal, D.S., & Kuczenski, R. (1987). Repeated amphetamine pretreatment alters the responsiveness of striatal dopamine-stimulated adenylate cyclase to amphetamine-induced desensitization. *J. Pharmacol. Exp. Ther., 242*, 40-47.

Bartoletti, M., Gaiardi, M., Gubellini, G., Bacchi, A., & Babbini, M. (1983). Long-term sensitization to the excitatory effects of morphine. A motility study in post-dependent rats. *Neuropharmacology, 22*, 1193-1196.

Bartoletti, M., Gaiardi, M., Gubellini, C., Bacchi, A., & Babbini, M. (1985). Cross-sensitization to the excitatory effect of morphine in post-dependent rats. *Neuropharmacology, 24*, 889-893.

Bartoletti, M., Gaiardi, M., Gubellini, C., Bacchi, A., & Babbini, M. (1987). Previous treatment with morphine and sensitization to the excitatory actions of opiates: Dose-effect relationship. *Neuropharmacology, 26*, 115-119.

Berridge, K.C., & Valenstein, E.S. (1991). What psychological process mediates feeding evoked by electrical stimulation of the lateral hypothalamus? *Behav. Neurosci. 105*, 3-14.

Berridge, K.C., Venier, I.L., & Robinson, T.E. (1989). Taste reactivity analysis of 6-hydroxydopamine-induced aphagia: Implications for arousal and anhedonia hypotheses of dopamine function. *Behav. Neurosci., 103*, 36-45.

Borison, R.L., Havdala, H.S., & Diamond, B.I., (1977). Chronic phenylethylamine stereotypy in rats: A new animal model for schizophrenia? *Life Sci., 21*, 117-122.

Camp, D.M., & Robinson, T.E. (1988a). Susceptibility to sensitization. I. Sex differences in the enduring effects of chronic d-amphetamine treatment on locomotion, stereotyped behavior and brain monoamines. *Behav. Brain Res., 30*, 55-68.

Camp, D.M., & Robinson, T.E. (1988b). Susceptibility to sensitization. II. The influence of gonadal hormones on enduring changes in brain monoamines and behavior produced by the repeated administration of D-amphetamine or restraint stress. *Behav. Brain. Res., 30*, 69-88.

Carroll, M.E., & Lac, S.T. (1987). Cocaine withdrawal produces behavioral disruptions in rats. *Life Sci., 40*, 2183-2190.

Castañeda, E., Becker, J.B., & Robinson, T.E. (1988). The long-term effects of repeated amphetamine treatment in vivo on amphetamine, KCl and electrical stimulation evoked striatal dopamine release in vitro. *Life Sci., 42*, 2447-2456.

Chapman, C.D., Gazzara, R.A., & Howard, S.G. (1990). Effects of phencyclidine on extracellular levels of dopamine, dihydroxyphenylacetic acid and homovanillic acid in conscious and anesthetized rats. *Neuropharmacology, 29*, 319-325.

Clarke, P.B.S. (1990). Mesolimbic dopamine activation—the key to nicotine reinforcement? In *Ciba Foundation Symposium 152: The biology of nicotine dependence* (pp. 153-168). Chichester: Wiley.

Cole, B.J., Cador, M., Stinus, L., Rivier, C., Rivier, J., Vale, W., Le Moal, M., & Koob, G.F. (1990). Critical role of the hypothalamic pituitary adrenal axis in amphetamine-induced sensitization of behavior. *Life Sci., 47*, 1715-1720.

Cools, A.R. (1990). Amphetamine-induced behavioral sensitization of the mesolimbic noradrenergic system in rats: Role of corticosteroids. *Soc. Neurosci. Abst., 16*, 585.

Demellweek, C., & Goudie, A.J. (1983). Behavioural tolerance to amphetamine and other psychostimulants: The case for considering behavioural mechanisms. *Psychopharmacology* (Berlin), *80*, 287-307.

Di Chiara, G., & Imperato, A. (1988). Drugs abused by humans preferentially increase synaptic dopamine concentrations in the mesolimbic system of freely moving rats. *Proc. Natl. Acad. Sci. USA., 85*, 5274-5278.

Falk, J.L., & Feingold, D.A. (1987). Environmental and cultural factors in the behavioral action of drugs. In H.Y. Meltzer (Ed.), *Psychopharmacology: The third generation of progress* (pp. 1503-1510). New York: Raven Press.

Falk, J. L., Dews, P.B., & Schuster, C.R. (1983). Commonalities in the environmental control of behavior. In P.K. Levison, D.R. Gerstein, & D.R. Maloff (Eds.), *Commonalities in substance abuse and habitual behavior* (pp. 47-110). Lexington, MA: D.C. Heath and Co.

Fujiwara, Y., Kazahaya, Y., Nakashima, M., Sato, M., & Otsuki, S. (1987). Behavioral sensitization to methamphetamine in the rat: An ontogenic study. *Psychopharmacology* (Berlin), *91*, 316-319.

Gaiardi, M., Bartoletti, M., Gubellini, C., Bacchi, A., & Babbini, M. (1986). Sensitivity to the narcotic cue in non-dependent, morphine-dependent and post-dependent rats. *Neuropharmacology, 25*, 119-123.

Gaiardi, M., Bartoletti, M., Bacchi, A., Gubellini, C., Costa, M., & Babbini, M. (1991). Role of repeated exposure to morphine in determining its affective properties: Place and taste conditioning studies in rats. *Psychopharmacology, 103,* 183-186.

Gawin, F.H., & Ellinwood, E.J. (1988). Cocaine and other stimulants. Actions, abuse, and treatment. *N. Engl. J. Med., 318,* 1173-1182.

Gnegy, M.E., Hewlett, G.H.K., Yee, S.L., & Welsh, M.J. (1991). Alterations in calmodulin content and localization in areas of rat brain after repeated intermittent amphetamine. *Brain Res., 562,* 6-12.

Greenberg, B.D., & Segal, D.S. (1985). Acute and chronic behavioral interactions between phencyclidine (PCP) and amphetamine: Evidence for a dopaminergic role in some PCP-induced behaviors. *Pharmacol. Biochem. Behav., 23,* 99-105.

Greenberg, B.D., & Segal, D.S. (1986). Evidence for multiple opiate receptor involvement in different phencyclidine-induced unconditioned behaviors in rats. *Psychopharmacology* (Berlin), *88,* 44-53.

Henry, D.J., & White, F.J. (1991). Repeated cocaine administration causes persistent enhancement of D1 dopamine receptor sensitivity within the rat nucleus accumbens. *J. Pharmacol. Exp. Ther. 258,* 882-890.

Horger, B.A., Giles, M.K., & Schenk, S. (1992). Preexposure to amphetamine and nicotine predisposes rats to self-administer a low dose of cocaine. *Psychopharmacology 107,* 271-276.

Horger, B.A., Shelton, K., & Schenk, S. (1990). Preexposure sensitizes rats to the rewarding effects of cocaine. *Pharmacol. Biochem. Behav., 37,* 707-711.

Ichikawa, J. (1988). Changes in behavior and central monoaminergic systems in the rat after repeated methamphetamine pretreatment: Presynaptic regulatory mechanism. *Yakubutsu Seishin Kodo, 8,* 389-403.

Iwamoto, E.T. (1986). Comparison of the pharmacologic effects of N-allylnormetazocine and phencyclidine: Sensitization, cross-sensitization, and opioid antagonist activity. *Psychopharmacology* (Berlin), *89,* 221-229.

Jaffe, J.H. (1980). Drug addiction and drug abuse. In A.G. Gilman, L.S. Goodman, & A. Gilman (Eds.), *The pharmacological basis of therapeutics,* pp. 535-584. New York: Macmillan.

Joyce, E.M., & Iversen, S.D. (1979). The effect of morphine applied locally to mesencephalic dopamine cell bodies on spontaneous motor activity in the rat. *Neurosci. Lett., 14,* 207-212.

Kalivas, P.W., & Duffy, P. (1988). Effects of daily cocaine and morphine treatment on somatodendritic and terminal field dopamine release. *J. Neurochem., 50,* 1498-1504.

Kalivas, P.W., & Duffy, P. (1990). Effect of acute and daily cocaine treatment on extracellular dopamine in the nucleus accumbens. *Synapse, 5,* 48-58.

Kalivas, P.W., Duffy, P., Abhold, R., & Dilts, R.P. (1988). Sensitization of mesolimbic dopamine neurons by neuropeptides and stress. In P.W. Kalivas & C.D. Barnes (Eds.), *Sensitization in the nervous system* (pp. 119-143). Caldwell, NJ: Telford Press.

Kalivas, P.W., & Stewart, J. (1991). Dopamine transmission in the initiation and expression of drug- and stress-induced sensitization of motor activity. *Brain Res. Rev., 16,* 223-244.

Karler, R., Calder, L.D., Chaudhry, I.A., & Turkanis, S.A. (1989). Blockade of "reverse tolerance" to cocaine and amphetamine by MK-801. *Life Sci., 45,* 599-606.

Karler, R., Chaudhry, I.A., Calder, L.D., & Turkanis, S.A. (1990). Amphetamine behavioral sensitization and the excitatory amino acids. *Brain Res., 537,* 76-82.

Katz, J.L., & Goldberg, S.R. (1988). Preclinical assessment of abuse liability of drugs. *Agents & Actions, 23,* 18-26.

Kazahaya, Y., Akimoto, K., & Otsuki S. (1989). Subchronic methamphetamine treatment enhances methamphetamine- or cocaine-induced dopamine efflux in vivo. *Biol. Psychiatr., 25,* 903-912.

Keller, R.W., Maisonneuve, I.M., Carlson, J.N., & Glick, S.D. (1992). Within-subject sensitization of striatal dopamine release after a single injection of cocaine: An in vivo microdialysis study. *Synapse, 11,* 28-34.

Kita, T., Okamoto, M., & Nakashima, T. (1992). Nicotine-induced sensitization to ambulatory stimulant effect produced by daily administration into the ventral tegmental area and the nucleus accumbens in rats. *Life Sci., 50,* 583-590.

Kokkinidis, L. (1988). Neurochemical correlates of post-amphetamine depression and sensitization in animals. *Anim. Models Psychiat. Disord., 2,* 148-173.

Kokkinidis, L., Zacharko, R.M., & Anisman, H. (1986). Amphetamine withdrawal: A behavioral evaluation. *Life Sci., 38,* 1617-1623.

Kolta, M.G., Shreve, P., De Souza, V., & Uretsky, N.J. (1985). Time course of the development of the enhanced behavioral and biochemical responses to amphetamine after pretreatment with amphetamine. *Neuropharmacology, 24,* 823-829.

Kolta, M.G., Shreve, P., & Uretsky, N.J. (1989). Effect of pretreatment with amphetamine on the interaction between amphetamine and dopamine neurons in the nucleus accumbens. *Neuropharmacology, 28,* 9-14.

Koob, G.F., & Bloom, F.E. (1988). Cellular and molecular mechanisms of drug dependence. *Science, 242,* 715-723.

Ksir, C., Hakan, R., Hall, D.P., & Kellar, K.J. (1985). Exposure to nicotine enhances the behavioral stimulant effect of nicotine and increases binding of [^{3}H]acetylcholine to nicotinic receptors. *Neuropharmacology, 24,* 527-531.

Kuczenski, R., & Leith, N.J. (1981). Chronic amphetamine: Is dopamine a link in or mediator of the development of tolerance or reverse tolerance? *Pharmacol. Biochem. Behav., 15,* 405-413.

Kuczenski, R., & Segal, D.S. (1988). Psychomotor stimulant-induced sensitization: Behavioral and neurochemical correlates. In P.W. Kalivas & C.D. Barnes (Eds.), *Sensitization in the nervous system* (pp. 175-205). Caldwell, NJ: Telford Press.

Kuczenski, R., & Segal, D. (1989). Concomitant characterization of behavioral and striatal neurotransmitter response to amphetamine using in vivo microdialysis. *J. Neurosci., 9,* 2051-2065.

Kuroki, T., Tsutsumi, T., Hirano, M., Matsumoto, T., Tatebayashi, Y., Nishiyama, K., Uchimura, H., Shiraishi, A., Nakahara, T., & Nakamura, K. (1990). Behavioral sensitization to beta-phenylethylamine (PEA): Enduring modifications of specific dopaminergic neuron systems in the rat. *Psychopharmacology* (Berlin), *102,* 5-10.

Lamb, R.J., Preston, K.L., Schindler, C., Meisch, R.A., Davis, F., Katz, J.L., Henningfield, J.E., & Goldberg, S.R. (1991). The reinforcing and subjective effects of morphine in post-addicts: A dose-response study. *J. Pharmacol. Exp. Ther., 259,* 1165-1173.

Lasagna, L., von Felsinger, J.M., & Beecher, H.K. (1955). Drug-induced mood changes in man. 1. Observations on healthy subjects, chronically ill patients, and "postaddicts." *JAMA, 157,* 1006-1020.

Lett, B.T. (1989). Repeated exposures intensify rather than diminish the rewarding effects of amphetamine, morphine, and cocaine. *Psychopharmacology* (Berlin), *98,* 357-362.

Mahan, L.C., Burch, R.M., Monsma, F.J., & Sibley, D.R. (1990). Expression of striatal D1 dopamine receptors coupled to inositol phosphate production and Ca^{2+} mobilization in Xenopus oocytes. *Proc. Natl. Acad. Sci. USA, 87,* 2196-2200.

Markou, A., & Koob, G.F. (1991). Postcocaine anhedonia: An animal model of cocaine withdrawal. *Neuropsychopharmacology, 4,* 17-26.

Mazurski, E.J., & Beninger, R.J. (1987). Environment-specific conditioning and sensitization with (+)-amphetamine. *Pharmacol. Biochem. Behav., 27,* 61-65.

McAuliffe, W.E. (1975). A second look at first effects: The subjective effects of opiates on nonaddicts. *J. Drug Issues, 5,* 369-399.

McAuliffe, W.E., & Gordon, R.A. (1974). A test of Lindesmith's theory of addiction: The frequency of euphoria among long-term addicts. *Am. J. Sociol., 79,* 795-840.

McCown, T.J., & Barrett, R.J. (1980). Development of tolerance to the rewarding effects of self-administered (+)-amphetamine. *Pharmacol. Biochem. Behav., 12,* 137-141.

Meliska, C.J., Landrum, R.E., & Loke, W.H. (1985). Caffeine effects: Interaction of drug and wheelrunning experience. *Pharmacol. Biochem. Behav., 23,* 633-635.

Meliska, C.J., Landrum, R.E., & Landrum, J.T. (1990). Tolerance and sensitization to chronic and subchronic oral caffeine: Effects on wheelrunning in rats. *Pharmacol. Biochem. Behav., 35,* 477-479.

Nabeshima, T., Fukaya, H., Yamaguchi, K., Ishikawa, K., Furukawa, H., & Kameyama, T. (1987). Development of tolerance and supersensitivity to phencyclidine in rats after repeated administration of phencyclidine. *Eur. J. Pharmacol., 135,* 23-33.

Nabeshima, T., Fukaya, H., Kamei, H., Ishikawa, K., Furukawa, H., & Kameyama, T. (1989). Cross-sensitization between phencyclidine and metamphetamine: Repeated administration of methamphetamine at a low dose. *Res. Comm. Sub. Abuse, 10,* 62-76.

Nisenbaum, L.K., Zigmond, M.J., Sved, A.F., & Abercrombie, E.B. (1991). Prior exposure to chronic stress results in enhanced synthesis and release of hippocampal norepinephrine in response to a novel stressor. *J. Neurosci., 11,* 1478-1484.

Parsons, L.H., Smith, A.D., & Justice, J.B., Jr. (1991). Basal extracellular dopamine is decreased in the rat nucleus accumbens during abstinence from chronic cocaine. *Synapse, 9,* 60-65.

Patrick, S.L., Thompson, T.L., Walker, J.M., & Patrick, R.L. (1991). Concomitant sensitization of amphetamine-induced behavioral stimulation and in vivo dopamine release from the rat caudate nucleus. *Brain Res., 538,* 343-346.

Paulson, P.E., & Robinson, T.E. (1991). Sensitization to systemic amphetamine produces an enhanced locomotor response to a subsequent intra-accumbens amphetamine in rats. *Psychopharmacology* (Berlin), *104,* 140-141.

Paulson, P.E., Camp, D.M., & Robinson, T.E. (1991). The time course of transient behavioral depression and persistent behavioral sensitization in relation to regional brain monoamine concentrations during amphetamine withdrawal in rats. *Psychopharmacology* (Berlin), *103,* 480-492.

Perez-de la Mora, M., Lopez-Quiroz, D., Mendez-Franco, J., & Drucker-Colin, R. (1990). Chronic administration of amphetamine increases glutamic acid decarboxylase activity in the rat substantia nigra. *Neurosci. Lett., 109,* 315-320.

Peris, J., & Zahniser, N.R. (1987). One injection of cocaine produces a long-lasting increase in [^{3}H]-dopamine release. *Pharmacol. Biochem. Behav., 27,* 533-535.

Pettit, H.O., Pan, H.T., Parsons, L.H., & Justice, J.B., Jr. (1990). Extracellular concentrations of cocaine and dopamine are enhanced during chronic cocaine administration. *J. Neurochem.*, *55*, 798-804.

Piazza, P.V., Deminiere, J.M., Le Moal, M., & Simon, H. (1989). Factors that predict individual vulnerability to amphetamine self-administration. *Science, 245*, 1511-1513.

Piazza, P.V., Deminiere, J.M., Le Moal, M., & Simon, H. (1990). Stress- and pharmacologically-induced behavioral sensitization increases vulnerability to acquisition of amphetamine self-administration. *Brain Res., 514*, 22-26.

Post, R. (1980). Intermittent versus continuous stimulation: Effect of time interval on the development of sensitization or tolerance. *Life Sci., 26*, 1275-1282.

Post, R.M., & Contel, N.R. (1983). Human and animal studies of cocaine: Implications for development of behavioral pathology. In: I. Creese (Ed.), *Stimulants: Neurochemical, behavioral and clinical perspectives* (pp. 169-203). New York: Raven Press.

Post, R.M., Weiss, S.R., & Pert, A. (1987). The role of context and conditioning in behavioral sensitization to cocaine. *Psychopharmacol. Bull., 23*, 425-429.

Reith, M.E., Benuck, M., & Lajtha, A. (1987). Cocaine disposition in the brain after continuous or intermittent treatment and locomotor stimulation in mice. *J. Pharmacol. Exp. Ther., 243*, 281-287.

Rivet, J.M., Stinus, L., LeMoal, M., & Mormede, P. (1989). Behavioral sensitization to amphetamine is dependent on corticosteroid receptor activation. *Brain Res., 498*, 149-153.

Roberts-Lewis, J.M., Roseboom, P.H., Iwaniec, L.M., & Gnegy, M.E. (1986). Differential down-regulation of D1-stimulated adenylate cyclase activity in rat forebrain after in vivo amphetamine treatments. *J. Neurosci., 6*, 2245-2251.

Robertson, M.W., Leslie, C.A., & Bennett, J.P., Jr. (1991). Apparent synaptic dopamine deficiency induced by withdrawal from chronic cocaine treatment. *Brain Res., 538*, 337-339.

Robinson, T.E. (1984). Behavioral sensitization: Characterization of enduring changes in rotational behavior produced by intermittent injections of amphetamine in male and female rats. *Psychopharmacology* (Berlin), *84*, 466-475.

Robinson, T.E. (1988). Stimulant drugs and stress: Factors influencing individual differences in the susceptibility to sensitization. In P.W. Kalivas & C. Barnes (Eds.), *Sensitization of the nervous system* (pp. 145-173). Caldwell, NJ: Telford Press.

Robinson, T.E. (1991). The neurobiology of amphetamine psychosis: Evidence from studies with an animal model. In T. Nakazawa (Ed.), *Taniguchi Symposia on Brain Sciences, Vol. 14, biological basis of schizophrenia* (pp. 185-201). Tokyo: Japan Scientific Societies Press.

Robinson, T.E., & Becker, J. B. (1982). Behavioral sensitization is accompanied by an enhancement in amphetamine-stimulated dopamine release from striatal tissue in vitro. *Eur. J. Pharmacol., 85*, 253-254.

Robinson, T.E., & Becker, J.B. (1986). Enduring changes in brain and behavior produced by chronic amphetamine administration: A review and evaluation of animal models of amphetamine psychosis. *Brain. Res. Rev., 396*, 157-198.

Robinson, T.E., Becker, J.B., & Presty, S.K. (1982). Long-term facilitation of amphetamine-induced rotational behavior and striatal dopamine release produced by a single exposure to amphetamine: Sex differences. *Brain Res., 253*, 231-41.

Robinson, T.E., & Camp, D.M. (1990). Does amphetamine *preferentially* increase the extracellular concentration of dopamine in the mesolimbic system of freely moving rats? *Neuropsychopharmacology, 3*, 163-173.

Robinson, T.E., Jurson, P.A., Bennett, J.A., & Bentgen, K.M. (1988). Persistent sensitization of dopamine neurotransmission in ventral striatum (nucleus accumbens) produced by past experience with (+)-amphetamine: A microdialysis study in freely moving rats. *Brain Res., 462,* 211-222.

Roseboom, P.H., & Gnegy, M.E. (1989). Acute in vivo amphetamine produces a homologous desensitization of dopamine receptor-coupled adenylate cyclase activities and decreases agonist binding to the D1 site. *Mol. Pharmacol., 34,* 148-156.

Sato, M., Chen, C.C., Akiyama, K., & Otsuki, S. (1983). Acute exacerbation of paranoid psychotic state after long-term abstinence in patients with previous methamphetamine psychosis. *Biol. Psychiat., 18,* 429-440.

Schnur, P. (1985). Morphine tolerance and sensitization in the hamster. *Pharmacol. Biochem. Behav., 22,* 157-158.

Schreiber, H., Bell, R., Conely, L., Kufner, M., Palet, J., & Wright, L. (1976). Diminished reaction to a novel stimulus during amphetamine withdrawal in rats. *Pharmacol. Biochem. Behav., 5,* 687-690.

Segal, D.S., & Kuczenski, R. (1987). Individual differences in responsiveness to single and repeated amphetamine administration: Behavioral characteristics and neurochemical correlates. *J. Pharmacol. Exp. Ther., 242,* 917-926.

Segal, D.S., & Kuczenski, R. (1992a). In vivo microdialysis reveals a diminished amphetamine-induced DA response corresponding to behavioral sensitization produced by repeated amphetamine pretreatment. *Brain Res., 571,* 330-337.

Segal, D.S., & Kuczenski, R. (1992b). Repeated cocaine administration induces behavioral sensitization and corresponding decreased extracellular dopamine responses in caudate and accumbens. *Brain Res., 577,* 351-355.

Segal, D.S., & Mandell, A.J. (1974). Long-term administration of d-amphetamine: Progressive augmentation of motor activity and stereotypy. *Pharmacol. Biochem. Behav., 2,* 249-255.

Segal, D.S., Kelly, P.H., Koob, G., & Roberts, D.C.S. (1979). Nonstriatal dopamine mechanisms in the response to repeated d-amphetamine administration. In E. Usdin, I. Kopin, & J. Barchas (Eds.), *Catecholamines: Basic and clinical frontiers, Vol. 2* (pp. 1672-1674). New York: Pergamon Press.

Shuster, L., Webster, G.W., & Yu, G. (1975a). Increased running response to morphine in morphine-pretreated mice. *J. Pharmacol. Exp. Ther., 192,* 64-67.

Shuster, L., Webster, G.W., & Yu, G. (1975b). Perinatal narcotic addiction in mice: Sensitization to morphine stimulation. *Addict. Dis., 2,* 277-292.

Shuster, L., Yu, G., & Bates, A. (1977). Sensitization to cocaine stimulation in mice. *Psychopharmacology* (Berlin), *52,* 185-190.

Shuster, L., Hudson, J., Anton, M., & Righi, D. (1982). Sensitization of mice to methylphenidate. *Psychopharmacology* (Berlin), *77,* 31-36.

Spanos, L.J., & Yamamoto, B.K. (1989). Acute and subchronic effects of methylenedioxymethamphetamine [(+/−)MDMA] on locomotion and serotonin syndrome behavior in the rat. *Pharmacol. Biochem. Behav., 32,* 835-840.

Stewart, J. (1992). Conditioned stimulus control of the expression of sensitization of the behavioral activating effects of opiate and stimulant drugs. In I. Gormezano & E.A. Wasserman (Eds.), *Learning and memory: The behavioral and biological substrates* (pp. 129-151). Hillsdale, NJ: Erlbaum.

Stewart, J., & Vezina, P. (1988a). A comparison of the effects of intra-accumbens injections of amphetamine and morphine on reinstatement of heroin intravenous self-administration behavior. *Brain Res., 457,* 287-294.

Stewart, J., & Vezina, P. (1988b). Conditioning and behavioral sensitization. In P.W. Kalivas & C.D. Barnes (Eds.), *Sensitization in the nervous system* (pp. 207-224). Caldwell, NJ: Telford Press.

Stewart, J., & Vezina, P. (1989). Microinjections of Sch-23390 into the ventral tegmental area and substantia nigra pars reticulata attenuate the development of sensitization to the locomotor activating effects of systemic amphetamine. *Brain Res., 495*, 401-406.

Stewart, J., & Wise, R.A. (1992). Reinstatement of heroin self-administration habits: morphine prompts and naltrexone discourages renewed responding after extinction. *Psychopharmacology* (Berlin), *108*, 79-84.

Stewart, J., de Wit, H., & Eikelboom, R. (1984). Role of unconditioned and conditioned drug effects in the self-administration of opiates and stimulants. *Psychol. Rev., 91*, 251-268.

Vezina, P., & Stewart, J. (1984). Conditioning and place-specific sensitization of increases in activity induced by morphine in the VTA. *Pharmacol. Biochem. Behav., 20*, 925-934.

Vezina, P., & Stewart, J. (1989). The effect of dopamine receptor blockade on the development of sensitization to the locomotor activating effects of amphetamine and morphine. *Brain Res., 499*, 108-120.

Vezina, P., & Stewart, J. (1990). Amphetamine administered to the ventral tegmental area but not to the nucleus accumbens sensitizes rats to systemic morphine: Lack of conditioned effects. *Brain Res., 516*, 99-106.

Vezina, P., Kalivas, P.W., & Stewart, J. (1987). Sensitization occurs to the locomotor effects of morphine and the specific mu opioid receptor agonist, DAGO, administered repeatedly to the ventral tegmental area but not to the nucleus accumbens. *Brain Res., 417*, 51-58.

Vickroy, T.W., & Johnson, K.M. (1982). Similar dopamine-releasing effects of phencyclidine and nonamphetamine stimulants in striatal slices. *J. Pharmacol. Exp. Ther., 223*, 669-674.

Weiss, S.R., Post, R.M., Pert, A., Woodward, R., & Murman, D. (1989). Context-dependent cocaine sensitization: Differential effect of haloperidol on development versus expression. *Pharmacol. Biochem. Behav., 34*, 655-661.

White, F.J., Henry, D.J., Hu, X.T., Jeziorsky, M., & Ackerman, J.M. (1992). Electrophysiological effect of cocaine within the mesoaccumbens and mesocortical dopamine systems. In J. Lakoski, M.P. Galloway, & F.J. White (Eds.), *Cocaine: Pharmacology, physiology and clinical strategies* (pp. 261-293). Boca Raton, FL: CRC Press.

Wilcox, R.A., Robinson, T.E., & Becker, J.B. (1986). Enduring enhancement in amphetamine-stimulated striatal dopamine release in vitro produced by prior exposure to amphetamine or stress in vivo. *Eur. J. Pharmacol., 124*, 375-376.

Wise, R.A. (1982). Neuroleptics and operant behavior: The anhedonia hypothesis. *Behav. Brain. Sci., 5*, 39-87.

Wise, R.A., & Bozarth, M.A. (1987). A psychomotor stimulant theory of addiction. *Psychol. Rev., 94*, 469-492.

Wolf, M.E., & Khansa, M.R. (1991). Repeated administration of MK-801 produces sensitization to its own locomotor stimulant effects but blocks sensitization to amphetamine. *Brain Res., 562*, 164-168.

Woolverton, W.L., Cervo, L., & Johanson, C.E. (1984). Effects of repeated methamphetamine administration on methamphetamine self-administration in rhesus monkeys. *Pharmacol. Biochem. Behav., 21*, 737-741.

V

HUMAN GENETICS AND PHARMACOLOGICAL TREATMENT

One of the most pressing questions concerning drugs centers on the genetic factors that may be related to drug use. This controversial and important area is reviewed by Cloninger and Dinwiddie. Related to this issue is the study of the brain electrical activity in subjects at risk for alcoholism; evidence that there are changes without exposure to alcohol is discussed by Begleiter and Porjesz.

The book concludes with three chapters suggesting new approaches to the treatment of substance abuse that grow out of contemporary research in neuroscience. Gawin describes cocaine addiction and promising approaches to pharmacotherapy. Post and his colleagues describe the use of carbamazepine in cocaine abuse, while Mello and Mendelson assess the use of buphrenorphine in cocaine and heroin abuse. In the last chapter, O'Brien and his colleagues assess the effectiveness of different forms of treatment for substance abuse. Over the next few decades, entirely new approaches will probably be developed. Biological approaches, appropriately combined with psychosocial interventions, may provide much needed help for addicted individuals and for society as a whole.

25

Genetic Risk Factors in Susceptibility to Substance Abuse

C. ROBERT CLONINGER AND STEPHEN H. DINWIDDIE

Exposure to psychotropic drugs of abuse varies widely according to such nongenetic factors as socioeconomic status, year of birth, and community location (Cloninger et al., 1981). Even the use of common drugs of abuse, such as alcohol and tobacco in the United States, varies widely according to their availability and social acceptability from one generation to the next. Changes in availability and social attitudes to particular drugs can result in changes in patterns of use across generations (Weiss et al., 1988). Consequently, little is known about the inheritance of substance abuse except alcoholism. Studies of the inheritance of substance abuse can be most informative if they are focused on learning about the inheritance of *susceptibility* to substance abuse, which can be assessed regardless of exposure to drugs of abuse.

Putative susceptibility factors for drug abuse are most informative for family studies if they have specific characteristics. First, they should be identifiable and quantifiable regardless of exposure to drugs. Second, they should be stable so that they can be assessed at different ages and in different generations of the same family. Third, they should be predictive of later drug-related variables, such as drug-seeking, persistence in drug use, or complications of drug use. Fourth, they should be at least moderately heritable. The availability of such quantifiable, stable, and heritable factors that are predictive of substance abuse would permit studies of the inheritance of susceptibility to substance abuse regardless of variation in the availability of drugs.

In this chapter, we examine what is known about the clinical psychiatric characteristics of substance abusers that distinguish them from other individuals. In particular, we focus on psychopathology and personality traits that may be susceptibility factors for substance abuse based on the results of prior clinical, longitudinal, and family studies of substance abuse.

This work was supported in part by grants from the U.S. Public Health Service (AA 08028, AAO 07982, AA 003539, AA 007466, MH 31302, and MH 45019).

PSYCHIATRIC CO-MORBIDITY

In studies conducted throughout this century, substance abusers have been found to have increased risk of associated psychiatric disorders compared to others (Cohen, 1982; Dinwiddie et al., unpublished data). Substance abuse is usually associated with personality disorders, mood and anxiety disorders, and somatoform disorders. In the Epidemiologic Catchment Area study in the United States, 53% of drug abusers in the community had at least one other mental disorder; in order of frequency, the disorders included anxiety disorders, mood disorders, antisocial personality, and schizophrenia (Regier et al., 1990).

The strongest and most consistent co-morbid psychiatric disorder observed in substance abusers is antisocial personality disorder. Among 75 studies that reported on the associations of alcoholism, other drug dependence, and antisocial personality, at least 76% found positive associations among each possible pair of these diagnoses (Grande et al., 1984). Teenage onset of antisocial behavior usually leads to abuse of both alcohol and other prescribed or illicit drugs of abuse that are available (Lewis, 1984). In particular, antisocial personality disorder is usually associated with abuse of multiple drugs (including stimulants, solvents, and hallucinogens) and with intravenous administration of multiple types of drugs (Dinwiddie et al., 1990, 1991a & b; Newcomb et al., 1987; Weiss et al., 1986).

Not all studies of substance abusers find positive associations with antisocial personality, however. An alcoholic who does not have antisocial personality disorder is likely to have adult onset of abuse associated with depression (Hesselbrock et al., 1985; Woodruff et al., 1973), phobias, and other anxiety disorders (Mullaney & Trippet, 1979; Smail et al., 1984; Stockwell et al., 1984), or somatization disorder (Lewis et al., 1982; Martin et al., 1985). There are also high rates of depression among opiate abusers (Croughan et al., 1981; Rounsaville et al., 1982) and abusers of sedative-hypnotics (Allgulander et al., 1984), as well as a combination of antisocial personality and depression among stimulant abusers (Mirin & Weiss, 1986; Weiss et al., 1986).

The observation that antisocial personality is associated with early onset of stimulant or polydrug abuse, whereas mood and anxiety disorders are associated with sedative-hypnotic abuse, lends support to a self-medication hypothesis. Antisocial personality leads to early onset of a variety of behaviors that may be characterized as risk taking, danger seeking, or stimulation seeking. Antisocial individuals are easily bored and need stimulation; they seek novelty, thrills, and other means of stimulation, including polydrug abuse with little concern for its illegal or dangerous complications. Such stimulation and thrill seeking are positively reinforcing to antisocial individuals. In contrast, depressed or anxious individuals do not actively seek exposure to illegal drugs, but if exposed to the antianxiety effects of sedatives and hypnotics, these drugs will be positively reinforcing and lead to continued use and possibly abuse.

Family Studies

Substance abuse, like other psychiatric disorders, is often familial (Cloninger et al., 1979; Hill et al., 1977). When alcoholism is co-morbid with other primary psychiatric disorders, the primary diagnosis of the alcoholic case predicts the primary diagnoses of the family members. In other words, the family pattern varies according to the primary diagnosis of the alcoholic case: The antisocial alcoholic has more antisocial relatives and the depressive alcoholic has more depressed relatives compared to other alcoholics (Cloninger et al., 1979). Therefore, the co-morbid psychiatric disorders give important information about what is being inherited—alcoholism itself is not a homogeneous, discrete disease.

However, the primary psychiatric diagnosis is also not sufficient to predict all that is being inherited in a family. Men with antisocial personality have an excess of both antisocial personality and primary alcoholism in their first-degree relatives (Cloninger et al., 1979). Thus, "primary alcoholism" is not a homogeneous, discrete disease, just as alcoholism in general is etiologically heterogeneous.

Studies of the inheritance of alcoholism in Swedish adoptees (Bohman et al., 1981; Cloninger et al., 1981) and in families in the United States (Gilligan et al., 1987, 1988) reveal two types of alcoholics who differ in their pattern of inheritance, age of onset, alcohol-related symptoms, associated personality traits and psychopathology, and outcome in response to treatment (Cloninger, 1987a; Cloninger et al., 1988a & b). Type 1 alcoholics usually have onset of guilt and fear about their loss of control and binges after age 25 years, whereas type 2 alcoholics usually have earlier onset of fighting and arrests when drinking. Type 2 alcoholics have antisocial personality traits; namely, high novelty seeking (i.e., impulsive, quick-tempered), low harm avoidance (i.e., risk taking, socially outgoing), and low reward dependence (i.e., independent, cold-hearted). However, these traits may not be so severe that the individual qualifies as having a primary diagnosis of antisocial personality disorder. In contrast, the type 1 alcoholic is anxiety prone as a consequence of the opposite personality profile, which is particularly characterized by high harm avoidance, i.e., worried, pessimistic, shy, and fatigable.

Given the information summarized in the section on psychiatric co-morbidity, it is not surprising that the type 2 alcoholic, who has early onset of antisocial behavior, is often found to abuse multiple drugs in addition to alcohol (Cloninger, 1988). Type 1 alcoholics are less likely to abuse illicit drugs than are other alcoholics.

HERITABILITY OF CLINICAL RISK FACTORS

The aspects of personality and psychopathology identified in cross-sectional clinical studies and in family studies of substance abuse seem to be related to susceptibility to antisocial behavior or to anxiety and depression. Hence, we can evaluate the genetics of susceptibility to substance abuse by testing the heritability of personality traits that are related to such motivated behaviors as risk taking or anxiety-proneness. Elsewhere, Cloninger (1987b, 1988) has described a unified biosocial theory of personality and its relationship to susceptibility to substance abuse, personality disorders, and anxiety disorders. This theory is based on three heritable dimensions of temperament that are related to three putative neural systems involved in the regulation of behavioral activation (which motivates novelty seeking), behavioral maintenance (which motivates reward dependence), and behavioral inhibition (which motivates harm avoidance). Each system is complex, involving multiple brain structures and neurotransmitters, but each of the three brain monoamines seems to have a major neuromodulatory role in only one system; specifically, dopamine in behavioral activation, norepinephrine in maintenance, and serotonin in inhibition (Cloninger, 1987a). Recently, a study has been carried out with over 2600 twin pairs in Australia using the Tridimensional Personality Questionnaire to measure novelty seeking, harm avoidance, and reward dependence. This study confirms that the heritability of each of these three dimensions is about 60%; the correlations in monozygotic twins are about 0.45, and those in dizygotic twins are about 0.15 (Andrew Heath, Nick Martin, personal communication, 1991).

Predictive Longitudinal Studies

If these heritable personality features are stable indicators of susceptibility to substance abuse, they should be useful in predicting future substance abuse. Since individuals begin using alcohol and other drugs in adolescence, it is particularly helpful to be able to identify individuals at increased risk for susceptibility during childhood before there is exposure to alcohol and other drugs. Several longitudinal studies have found that childhood and adolescent conduct characteristic of antisocial personality, such as being impulsive, aggressive, overactive, distractable, impatient, and excitable, is predictive of alcohol and drug abuse in young adults (Aronson & Gilbert, 1963; Hagnell et al., 1986; Hoffmann et al., 1974; Jones, 1968; Kammeier et al., 1973; Knop et al., 1985; Loper et al., 1973; MacAndrew, 1979, 1981; McCord, 1972; Robins, 1966; Vaillant, 1983). In addition, two prospective longitudinal studies have followed children into adulthood and used comprehensive quantitative personality measurement in childhood to evaluate the possibility that childhood personality predicts adult substance abuse.

In the Berkeley and Oakland longitudinal studies of child development (Block, 1971), both antisocial and anxious personality configurations were found to increase the risk of later alcoholism. Boys with anxious or passive-dependent traits were called "anomic extroverts" because they tended to cry easily and to worry excessively, even though they were usually friendly and warmly sociable. These boys with anxious personalities had a tendency to drink and smoke cigarettes heavily in middle adulthood, but had few or no behavior problems during adolescence. In contrast, boys with antisocial personality traits were called "unsettled undercontrollers" because they had been impulsive, aggressive, and disorganized since childhood. These antisocial boys were found to have a history of risk taking, including substance abuse, since adolescence (Block, 1971).

Recently, in the Stockholm Adoption Study, Cloninger et al. (1988a & b) confirmed the presence of two different pathways to adult substance abuse. In a study of 431 children followed from birth to age 28 years, they found that quantitative ratings of personality at age 10 to 11 years were predictive of adult substance abuse, which was mainly alcoholism in this population. Childhood ratings of high novelty seeking, low harm avoidance, and low reward dependence were each strongly predictive of alcohol abuse in early adulthood. Extreme deviations in the opposite direction also were associated with increased risk of alcohol abuse, but a longer follow-up to later adulthood will be needed to determine whether most late-onset substance abusers are anxious, rather than antisocial. This study confirms that heritable childhood personality variables are important antecedents of adult substance abuse.

Other Predictors of Susceptibility and Treatment Outcome

Several heritable biological variables have been implicated in the susceptibility to substance abuse (Cloninger & Begleiter, 1990). These include low P3 amplitude in the evoked potential responses of children of type 2 alcoholics to infrequent complex stimuli and low platelet monoamine oxidase activity in type 2 alcoholic men. No biological markers have been identified that are characteristic of type 1 alcoholics.

Many candidate gene loci have been proposed as possible contributors to susceptibility or expression of alcoholism and other substance abuse (Devor & Cloninger, 1989). Possible linkages between alcoholism and genes on chromosomes 4 and 13 have been reported, but not yet replicated (Hill et al., 1988; Tanna et al., 1988). The structural locus for the D_2 dopamine receptor on chromosome 11q has been reported to be associated with increased susceptibility to severe medical complications in alcoholics (Blum et al., 1990). This association has been replicated by several, but not all, subsequent investigators (Cloninger, 1991). However, this locus is not tightly linked to alcoholism (Parsian et al., 1991), suggesting that it is not a sufficient cause of substance abuse but rather modifies expression among substance abusers.

In addition to heritable temperament factors, other aspects of character development have been found to be characteristic of drug abusers. Drug abusers tend to have low self-esteem, low goal directedness, and little sense of meaning and purpose in their life, as reviewed by Frankel (1978). Perhaps surprisingly, such feelings of alienation or low self-directiveness are reported to be partly heritable (Tellegen et al., 1988). Such traits are associated with the individual feeling unable to overcome a craving or reactive impulses to use drugs in order to pursue personally valued long-term goals effectively. Longitudinal studies using both measures of temperament and character have yet to be carried out, but should be even more informative than studies of temperament only.

SUMMARY AND CONCLUSIONS

Substance abusers are clinically heterogeneous and have a variety of psychiatric disorders and personality traits. Studies of psychiatric co-morbidity, longitudinal development, and inheritance all suggest that there are two major pathways to substance abuse. One pathway is taken by children with antisocial personality traits who begin a variety of risk-taking behaviors at an early age, including polydrug abuse. These individuals enjoy drug abuse for its euphoriant or stimulant value, which is positively reinforcing for those who are easily bored. Another pathway is taken by children with anxious or passive-dependent traits who avoid early risk-taking behaviors, but may use alcohol and sedatives for their antianxiety effects. Such antianxiety effects are also positively reinforcing and may lead to persistent substance abuse.

The recent development of quantitative measures of personality traits that are stable, heritable, and predictive of later substance abuse should greatly facilitate future studies of susceptibility to substance abuse. Likewise, identification of specific genes that influence susceptibility or expression of substance abuse should be facilitated by being able to characterize individuals who are susceptible to substance abuse regardless of their exposure to drugs.

REFERENCES

Allgulander, C., Borg, S., & Vikander, B. (1984). A 4-6 year follow-up of 50 patients with primary dependence on sedative and hypnotic drugs. *Am. J. Psychiat., 141,* 1580-1582.

Aronson, H., & Gilbert, A. (1963). Preadolescent sons of male alcoholics: An experimental study of personality patterning. *Arch. Gen. Psychiat., 38,* 235-241.

Block, J. (1971). *Lives through time.* Berkeley, CA: Bancroft Books.

Blum, K., Noble, E.P., Sheridan, P.J., Montgomery, A., Ritchie, T., Jagadesswaran, P., Nogami, H., Briggs, A.H., & Cohn, J.B. (1990). Allelic association of human dopamine D2 receptor gene in alcoholism. *JAMA, 263,* 2055-2060.

Bohman, M., Sigvardsson, S., & Cloninger, C.R. (1981). Maternal inheritance of alcohol abuse: Cross-fostering analysis of adopted women. *Arch. Gen. Psychiat., 38,* 965-969.

Cohen, A. (1982). The "urge to classify" the narcotic addict: A review of psychiatric classification. I. *Int. J. Addict., 17,* 213-225.

Cloninger, C.R. (1987a). Neurogenetic adaptive mechanisms in alcoholism. *Science, 236,* 410-416.

Cloninger, C.R. (1987b). A systematic method for clinical description and classification of personality variants: A proposal. *Arch. Gen. Psychiat., 44,* 573-588.

Cloninger, C.R. (1988). Etiologic factors in substance abuse: An adoption study perspective. *NIDA Res. Monogr., 89,* 52-72.

Cloninger, C.R. (1991). D_2 dopamine receptor gene is associated but not linked with alcoholism. *JAMA, 266,* 1833-1834.

Cloninger, C.R., & Begleiter, H. (Eds.). (1990). *Genetics and biology of alcoholism: Banbury Report 33.* Cold Spring Harbor, NY: Laboratory Press.

Cloninger, C.R., Reich, T., & Wetzel, R. (1979). Alcoholism and the affective disorders: Familial association and genetic models. In D. Goodwin & C. Erickson

(Eds.), *Alcoholism and the affective disorders* (pp. 57-82). New York: Spectrum Press.

Cloninger, C.R., Bohman, M., & Sigvardsson, S. (1981). Inheritance of alcohol abuse: Cross-fostering analysis of adopted men. *Arch. Gen. Psychiat., 38*, 861-868.

Cloninger, C.R., Sigvardsson, S., & Bohman, M. (1988a). Childhood personality predicts alcohol abuse in young adults. *Alcohol. Clin. Exp. Res., 12*, 494-505.

Cloninger, C.R., Sigvardsson, S., Gilligan, S.B., von Knorring, A.-L., Reich, T., & Bohman, M. (1988b). Genetic heterogeneity and classification of alcoholism. *Advances Alcohol Substance Abuse, 7*, 3-16.

Croughan, J.L., Miller, J.P., Koepke, J., & Whitman, B.Y. (1981). Depression in narcotic addicts—A prospective study with a five-year follow-up. *Compr. Psychiat., 22*, 428-433.

Devor, E.J., & Cloninger, C.R. (1989). Genetics of alcoholism. *Annu. Rev. Genet., 23*, 19-36.

Dinwiddie, S.H., Reich, T., & Cloninger, C.R. (1990). Solvent use and psychiatric comorbidity. *Br. J. Addict., 85*, 1647-1656.

Dinwiddie, S.H., Reich, T., & Cloninger, C.R. (1991a). The relationship of solvent use to other substance use. *Am. J. Drug Alcohol Abuse, 17*, 173-186.

Dinwiddie, S.H., Reich, T., & Cloninger, C.R. (1991b). Solvent use as a precursor to intravenous drug abuse. *Compr. Psychiat., 32*, 133-140.

Frankel, V.E. (1978). *The unheard cry for meaning.* New York.: Washington Square Press.

Gilligan, S.B., Reich, T., & Cloninger, C.R. (1987). Etiologic heterogeneity in alcoholism. *Genet. Epidemiol., 7*, 395-414.

Gilligan, S.B., Reich, T., & Cloninger, C.R. (1988). Alcohol-related symptoms in heterogeneous families of hospitalized alcoholics. *Alcohol. Clin. Exp. Res., 12*, 671-678.

Grande, T.P., Wolf, A.W., Schubert, D.S.P., Patterson, M.B., & Brocco, K. (1984). Associations among alcoholism, drug abuse, and antisocial personality: A review of literature. *Psychol. Rep., 55*, 455-474.

Hagnell, O., Lanke, J., Rorsman, B., & Ohman, R. (1986). Predictors of alcoholism in the Lundby Study: II. Personality traits as risk factors for alcoholism. *Eur. Arch. Psychiat. Neurol. Sci., 235*, 192-196.

Hesselbrock, M.N., Meyer, R.E., & Keener, J.J. (1985). Psychopathology in hospitalized alcoholics. *Arch. Gen. Psychiat., 42*, 1050-1055.

Hill, S.Y., Cloninger, C.R., & Ayre, F. (1977). Independent familial transmission of alcoholism. *Alcohol. Clin. Exp. Res., 1*, 335-342.

Hill, S.Y., Aston, C., & Rabin, B. (1988). Suggestive evidence of genetic linkage between alcoholism and MNS blood group. *Alcohol. Clin. Exp. Res., 12*, 811-814.

Hoffmann, H., Loper, R.G., & Kammeier, M.L. (1974). Identifying future alcoholics with MMPI alcoholism scales. *Q. J. Stud. Alcohol., 35*, 490-498.

Jones, M.C. (1968). Personality correlates and antecedents of drinking patterns in adult males. *J. Consult. Clin. Psychol., 32*, 2-12.

Kammeier, M.L., Hoffmann, H., & Loper, R.G. (1973). Personality characteristics of alcoholics as college freshmen and at time of treatment. *Q. J. Stud. Alcohol., 34*, 390-399.

Knop, J., Teasdale, T.W., Schulsinger, F., & Goodwin, D.W. (1985). A prospective study of young men at high risk for alcoholism: School behavior and achievement. *J. Stud. Alcohol., 46*, 273-278.

Lewis, C.E. (1984). Alcoholism, antisocial personality, narcotic addiction: An integrative approach. *Psychiat. Dev., 3*, 223-235.

Lewis, C.E., Helzer, J.E., Cloninger, C.R., Croughan, J., & Whitman, B.Y. (1982). Psychiatric diagnostic predispositions to alcoholism. *Compr. Psychiat., 23*, 451-461.

Loper, R.G., Kammeier, M.L., & Hoffman, H. (1973). MMPI characteristics of college freshmen who later became alcoholics. *J. Abnorm. Psychol., 82*, 159-162.

MacAndrew, C. (1979). On the possibility of the psychometric detection of persons who are prone to the abuse of alcohol and other substances. *Addict. Behav., 4*, 11-20.

MacAndrew, C. (1981). What the MAC Scale tells us about men alcoholics: An interpretive review. *J. Stud. Alcohol., 42*, 604-625.

Martin, R.L., Cloninger, C.R., & Guze, S.B. (1985). Alcohol misuse and depression in women criminals. *J. Stud. Alcohol, 46*, 65-71.

McCord, J. (1972). Etiological factors in alcoholism: Family and personal characteristics. *Q. J. Stud. Alcohol., 33*, 1020-1027.

Mirin, S.M., & Weiss, R.D. (1986). Affective illness in substance abusers. *Psychiat. Clin. North Am., 9*, 503-514.

Mullaney, J.A., & Trippet, C.J. (1979). Alcohol dependence and phobias: Clinical description and relevance. *Br. J. Psychiat., 135*, 565-573.

Newcomb, M.D., Bentler, P.M., & Fahy, B. (1987). Cocaine use and psychopathology: Associations among young adults. *Int. J. Addict., 22*,1167-1188.

Parsian, A., Todd, R.D., Devor, E.J., O'Malley, K.L., Suarez, B.K., Reich, T., Cloninger, C.R. (1991). Alcoholism and alleles of the human D_2 dopamine receptor locus: Studies of association and linkage. *Arch. Gen. Psychiat., 48*, 655-663.

Regier, D.A., Farmer, M.E., Rae, D.S., Locke, B.Z., Keith, S.J., Judd, L.L., & Goodwin, F.K. (1990). Comorbidity of mental disorders with alcohol and other drug abuse. *JAMA, 264*, 2511-2518.

Robins, L.N. (1966). *Deviant children grown up: A sociological and psychiatric study of sociopathic personality*. Baltimore: Williams & Wilkins.

Rounsaville, B.A., Weissman, M.M., Crits-Christoph, K., Wilber, C., & Kleber, H. (1982). Diagnosis and symptoms of depression in opiate addicts. *Arch. Gen. Psychiat., 39*, 151-156.

Smail, P., Stockwell, T., Canter, S., & Hodgson, R. (1984). Alcohol dependence and phobic anxiety states. I. A prevalence study. *Br. J. Psychiat., 144*, 53-57.

Stockwell, T., Smail, P., Hodgson, R., & Canter, S. (1984). Alcohol dependence and phobic anxiety states. II. A retrospective study. *Br. J. Psychiat., 144*, 58-63.

Tanna, V.L., Wilson, A.F., Winokur, G., & Elston, R.C. (1988). Possible linkage between alcoholism and esterase-D. *J. Stud. Alcohol., 49*, 472-476.

Tellegen, A., Lykken, D.T., Bouchard, T.J., Jr., Wilcox, K.J., Segal, N.L., & Rich, S. (1988). Personality similarity in twins reared apart and together. *J. Person. Soc. Psychol., 54*, 1031-1039.

Vaillant, G.E. (1983). Natural history of male alcoholism. V: Is alcoholism the cart or the horse to sociopathy? *Br. J. Addict., 78*, 317-326.

Weiss, R.D., Mirin, S.M., Michael, J.L., & Sollogub, A.C. (1986). Psychopathology in chronic cocaine abusers. *Am. J. Drug. Alcohol. Abuse, 12*, 17-29.

Weiss, R.D., Mirin, S.M., Griffin, M.L., & Michael, J.L. (1988). Psychopathology in cocaine abusers: Changing trends. *J. Nerv. Ment. Dis., 176*, 719-725.

Woodruff, R.A., Guze, S.B., Clayton, P.J., & Carr, D. (1973). Alcoholism and depression. *Arch. Gen. Psychiat., 28*, 97-100.

26

Brain Electrophysiology in Subjects at Risk for Alcoholism

HENRI BEGLEITER AND BERNICE PORJESZ

Recent advances in brain imaging have provided unprecedented spatial resolution concerning the neural loci involved in information processing. However, imaging techniques such as computed axial tomography (CAT scan), magnetic resonance imaging (MRI), positron emission tomography (PET), and single photon emission computed tomography (SPECT) cannot provide the temporal resolution necessary to understand the dynamic properties of information processing in the human brain.

At present, scalp-recorded event-related potentials (ERPs) provide the only available window to the neurophysiological transactions of the human brain as it processes information on a millisecond to millisecond basis. These powerful ERP techniques occupy the interface between cellular neurobiology and the behavioral or cognitive sciences.

The quantitative measurement of salient features extracted from the ERP reflect aspects of brain function related to sensory, perceptual, and cognitive processes and the structural and functional integrity of various neural systems. The ERP techniques are unique in assessing level of brain function in ways that permit the simultaneous observation of neural events and behavior. These ERP techniques typically require the subject to be actively engaged in a task. An ERP consists of early components related to sensory aspects of stimulation, and later components sensitive to more subjective aspects of cognition. While the early components are obligatory exogenous responses to the physical characteristics of stimulus, the late components reflect endogenous events, and are responsive to internal processing demands.

For the past two decades we have used encephalographic (EEG) and ERP techniques to assess CNS anomalies in chronic alcoholic patients (for review, see Begleiter & Platz, 1972; Porjesz & Begleiter, 1983, 1985, 1987). CNS anomalies have been observed consistently in abstinent as well as current alcoholics

This work was supported by National Institute on Alcohol Abuse and Alcoholism grants AA 02686 and AA 05524.

and were assumed to reflect the deleterious effects of alcohol abuse. In the last decade a number of compelling studies have indicated that genetics do play a significant role in some forms of alcoholism (Cloninger et al., 1981; Goodwin, 1976; see Chapter 25).

The most impressive studies dealing with the possible role of genetics in alcoholism come from large adoption studies. The adoption method allows the investigator to assess genetic and environmental factors independently. One compares the relationship of nonadopted siblings, adopted siblings, biological parents, and adoptive parents so that genetic and environmental effects may be estimated separately. Indeed, this particular methodological approach yields the most compelling evidence of genetic and environmental effects.

The initial adoption studies were conducted in Denmark by Goodwin and colleagues (1973). They observed that the rate of alcoholism in biological sons of alcoholics reared by adoptive parents was the same as in the probands, supporting a role of genetics in alcoholism. Moreover, they found no identifiable home environmental factors that contributed to the risk for alcoholism.

Another set of adoption studies were conducted in Sweden by Cloninger and his colleagues (Bohman et al., 1981; Cloninger et al., 1981). These investigators collected data on 862 men and 913 women adopted at a very early age. They used a sophisticated cross-fostering analysis with a discriminant function analysis of the background of both the biological and adoptive parents, as correlated with mild, moderate, severe, or no alcohol abuse in the male adoptees. They identified two distinct types of alcoholics labeled Type 1 and Type 2. Type 1 had a mild genetic predisposition that strongly interacted with environmental factors and resulted in either mild or severe alcohol abuse. Type 2 manifested a very high rate of heritability estimated at .90 and was associated with early onset, extensive treatment in the biological fathers, as well as antisocial behavior in the biological fathers. The authors estimated the relative risks to be nine for Type 2 and two for Type 1. A significant interaction between genetics and environment was observed for Type 1 but not for Type 2.

Other adoption studies of alcoholism were carried out by Cadoret and his colleagues at the University of Iowa (Cadoret & Gath, 1978; Cadoret et al., 1980). This group found evidence for a genetic and an environmental factor in alcoholism, but failed to observe gene-environment interactions. This lack of gene-environment interaction may be due to their small sample size.

In sum, sophisticated adoption studies have observed a genetic influence in the development of some forms of alcoholism. This genetic influence does not appear to be direct but is seemingly manifested in the presence of predisposing factors. This predisposition may only be expressed with the presence of precipitating factors in the form of environmental events. To the extent that genetic factors are related to a set of predisposing variables, it should be possible to study these variables in individuals with a family history of alcoholism. The identification of factors predisposing some individuals to develop alcoholism is of paramount importance in gaining a better understanding of the etiology of alcoholism, in development of reliable phenotypic markers for a genetic analysis of large pedigrees, and in formulating rational preventive strategies.

In a typical high-risk study, individuals with a family history of alcoholism who are not alcoholic themselves are matched with individuals without a family history of alcoholism. Both the high-risk group and the low-risk group are assessed on behavioral, physiological, or biochemical variables in the search for potential trait markers. While a number of psychological, behavioral, and biochemical studies have been conducted in subjects at high risk for alcoholism perhaps the electrophysiological findings using spontaneous EEGs and ERPs are the most interesting.

The resting-state EEG recorded from awake abstinent male alcoholics manifests excessive high-frequency activity (beta) and is deficient in the appropriate production of lower EEG frequency activity, such as alpha (for review, see Begleiter & Platz, 1972). It should be noted that some characteristics of the normal EEG are genetically determined (Propping, 1977; Vogel, 1970; Young et al., 1972). These reliable EEG findings in abstinent alcoholics, coupled with the high heritability of normal EEG characteristics and the population genetics data in alcoholism, suggest that individuals at risk for alcoholism should differ from matched controls. Gabrielli et al. (1982) tested this hypothesis in a sample of 265 Danish children. They selected 27 children of alcoholics and compared them with children of parents without alcohol problems. They noted that male children of alcoholics manifested excessive fast EEG activity compared to male controls. This difference in EEG frequency was only specific to males. The investigators readily acknowledge the lack of control regarding the potential psychiatric classification of either or both parents.

In another study by the same group (Pollock et al., 1983), investigators focused specifically on EEG changes subsequent to a challenge dose of alcohol. High-risk subjects were reported to manifest more slow alpha energy, less fast alpha energy, and a lower mean alpha frequency than did the low-risk subjects. However, the prealcohol EEG findings are quite difficult to understand, as the actual statistical findings of the potential difference between high- and low-risk subjects are not given.

In two recent publications, Ehlers and Schuckit (1990, 1991) recorded the EEG in a population of 21- to 25-year-old family history positive (FHP) and family history negative (FHN) males. In one study (Ehlers & Schuckit, 1991), they observed more energy in the fast alpha band (9-12 Hz) in the FHP than in the FHN subjects. In the other study (Ehlers & Schuckit, 1990), they reported no difference between the two groups (FHP-FHN) in the 12-20 Hz EEG band. However, FHN subjects classified as "moderate" drinkers had significantly more power in the 10-20 Hz band than did those classified as "low" drinkers. This finding was not observed in the FHP subjects. The authors conclude that both genetic factors and drinking history may influence electroencephalographic activity in humans.

A study by Kaplan et al. (1988) examined EEG activity between 2 and 20 Hz. No baseline EEG difference was observed between FHP and FHN subjects. A recent study from our laboratory (Cohen et al., 1991) examined EEG activity in the frequency range between 7.5 and 26 Hz in both FHP and matched FHN subjects. Our findings indicated no difference between FHP and FHN subjects in the EEG frequency range examined, replicating the results of Kaplan et al. (1988), Pollock et al. (1983), and Ehlers & Schuckit (1990).

The fact that most of the EEG studies mentioned above indicate that spontaneous EEG activity does not differentiate between FHP and FHN subjects may be due to a number of factors seldom addressed in the literature. It is important to note that the method of subject ascertainment was different in various studies. The selection criteria used to classify subjects as FHP or FHN were substantially different across laboratories. There were also significant mean age differences in subjects recruited. Furthermore, the dependent variables derived from the spontaneous EEG data were not comparable. Finally, none of the aforementioned EEG studies made an effort to control the mental state of the subjects during EEG recording. Failure to control mentation during EEG studies may well increase the variability of the dependent variables, leading to a spurious lack of statistically significant EEG differences. While studies of spontaneous EEG activity in high-risk and low-risk individuals have yielded rather meager findings, studies of event-related brain potentials (ERPs) in these two populations have resulted in many interesting and compelling results.

The ERP is a sensitive index of the functional integrity of various systems in the brain. ERPs not only reflect sensory processes but they are also useful in indexing neurophysiological concomitants of complex cognitive tasks (Donchin et al., 1978; Hillyard et al., 1978). ERPs can easily be recorded in conjunction with behavior or when no behavioral response is required. They can be recorded to attended and unattended stimuli. ERPs reflect the millisecond-to-millisecond transactions that occur in the brain during information processing.

For the past two decades our laboratory has developed and utilized a variety of ERP methods to assess the integrity of various brain systems in abstinent alcoholics. A number of studies have reported prolonged conduction velocities in the brainstem auditory evoked response (BAER, Begleiter et al., 1981; Chu & Squires, 1980; Chu & Yang, 1987; Chu et al., 1982; Rosenhamer & Silfverskiold, 1980). The increases in transmission time were observed in alcoholics abstinent for a relatively short period of time (3-4 weeks). Improvement in conduction velocity has been observed with prolonged abstinence (Nickel & Ludewig, 1981; Porjesz & Begleiter, 1985).

A number of investigations have also utilized ERPs to assess the functional integrity of higher integrative systems. Target-selection paradigms have been used for recording ERPs in alcoholics in the auditory (Pfefferbaum et al., 1980; Salamy et al., 1980) and visual (Begleiter et al., 1980; Porjesz et al., 1980, 1987a) modalities, as well as bimodally (Patterson et al., 1987; Porjesz & Begleiter, 1979). An information-processing ERP paradigm provides an opportunity to compare neuroelectric and behavioral responses to identical relevant and irrelevant stimuli. Control subjects in our study demonstrated an enhanced N1 component to stimuli in the relevant as opposed to irrelevant modality (Porjesz & Begleiter, 1979). In contrast, alcoholics maintained the same N1 voltage regardless of task relevance.

In other studies we investigated the late positive complex (LPC) of the ERP, which typically contains the P3b component (P3). Specifically, we examined the ability of abstinent alcoholics to differentiate between relevant and irrelevant events and their ability to probability match stimuli in accordance with their frequency of occurrence. We repeatedly observed that P3 amplitudes were low or absent in alcoholic patients to rare target stimuli under conditions optimal for eliciting large P3 voltages. This finding typically differentiates alcoholics from control subjects and is most striking over the parietal area where P3 amplitude is found to be maximal in control subjects.

The decreased P3 voltages in the ERP observed in our alcoholic patients were obtained in a variety of studies in our laboratory (Begleiter et al., 1980; Porjesz & Begleiter, 1979, 1982; Porjesz et al., 1980, 1987a & b) and have been replicated by other investigators (Emmerson et al., 1987; Patterson et al., 1987; Pfefferbaum et al., 1987). The consistent reductions in the P3 voltage of the ERP were assumed to reflect the neurotoxic effects of alcohol on the CNS of alcoholic patients.

Recent studies in genetic epidemiology indicate that alcoholism is a highly familial disease. Sons of alcoholic fathers are four times more likely to develop alcoholism than sons of nonalcoholic fathers even when they are separated from their biological parents. Because of these striking findings, we have initiated a series of investigations over the past decade to examine the possible presence of neurophysiological anomalies in subjects known to be at risk for alcoholism.

In the first study, Begleiter et al. (1984) tested the hypothesis that deficits in P3 voltage of the ERP may antecede the onset of chronic alcohol abuse, and may be present in boys at high risk for alcoholism. ERPs were recorded from 25 young, never-exposed sons of alcoholic fathers and 25 control boys matched for age, socioeconomic status, and school grade, who had no family history of alcoholism. The experimental paradigm consisted of a complex visual mental rotation task to identify the orientation of a target stimulus. The high-risk group showed a significantly reduced amplitude of the late positive component (P3) of the ERP, similar to results obtained in abstinent alcoholics (Porjesz & Begleiter, 1985); this reduced amplitude was originally presumed to be solely the consequence of alcoholism. These findings are particularly interesting because they were obtained in young, nondrinking sons of alcoholics without administering alcohol.

Using the same experimental paradigm as Begleiter et al. (1984), O'Connor et al. (1986) recorded ERPs in an older (20-25 years of age) group of sons of alcoholic fathers and matched controls. None of the subjects manifested signs of problem drinking. These investigators also observed a significantly reduced amplitude of the P3 component of the ERP in the high-risk men, replicating the findings of Begleiter et al. (1984).

Begleiter et al. (1987a) then used the brainstem auditory evoked response (BAER) to assess the auditory pathway in young boys at high risk for alcoholism. The investigators examined 23 sons of alcoholics (7-13 years old) and 23 control boys matched for age, socioeconomic status, and school grade. No significant difference in the BAER was found between high-risk and low-risk boys. These results suggest that the BAER abnormalities observed in abstinent alcoholics are likely to be the consequence of alcoholism, whereas the P3 deficits seen in both abstinent alcoholics and individuals at high risk for alcoholism may be antecedents of alcoholism.

In order to determine if the P3 findings in high-risk individuals were modality specific, Begleiter et al. (1987b) studied auditory evoked potentials in another group of high- and low-risk boys. The subjects were 23 young boys (7-16 years old) who were sons of alcoholic fathers and 23 control boys without a family history of alcoholism matched for age, school grade, and socioeconomic status. The subjects in this study were carefully interviewed to ascertain that they had had no exposure to alcohol or other illicit drugs. Clinical examination of the fathers of these young sons of alcoholics indicated that they met the criteria for male-limited (type 2) alcoholism as proposed by Cloninger (1987). They came from families in which familial alcoholism occurred only in males, was highly heritable, gave rise to severe early-onset alcoholism with a high rate of recidivism requiring extensive treatment, and was accompanied by the occurrence of petty criminality.

An auditory oddball paradigm was developed in which subjects pressed a button to discriminable infrequent stimuli. While the auditory pitch discrimination was a relatively easy sensory discrimination, the three interstimulus intervals (0.5, 1.0, and 5.0 seconds) randomized in the study increased the temporal uncertainty and thus the difficulty of the task. The results indicated that boys at high risk for alcoholism manifested significantly reduced amplitudes of the P3 component of the ERP. This auditory study indicates that P3 reductions in high-risk males are present in the visual and auditory modalities and thus are not modality specific.

More recently, we replicated our original findings of reduced P3 voltages without the administration of alcohol in an older sample (18-23) of sons of male alcoholics (Porjesz & Begleiter, 1990). The sample consisted of 25 male offspring of carefully diagnosed (DSM-III/RDC) male alcoholics and was selected from high-density alcoholic families (mean number of alcoholic family members = 4). Thus, sons of alcoholic fathers were excluded in cases where alcoholism may have been sporadic. Furthermore, individuals with mothers who abused alcohol before, during, or after pregnancy were excluded. Controls were matched to the sons of male alcoholics on the basis of age, education, and socioeconomic status. They were selected from families in which there was no history of alcohol abuse or alcoholism in any first- or second-degree relatives. Family history positive and negative subjects were carefully matched on drinking history, including duration and quantity-frequency information.

We used a visual-spatial paradigm with which we had previously demonstrated that abstinent alcoholics manifested reduced P3 amplitudes. The stimuli consisted of a nontarget (vertical line) and two targets: an easily discriminable target that deviated from vertical by 90 degrees (horizontal line) and a difficult-to-discriminate target that deviated from vertical by only 3 degrees. The subject pressed a button as quickly as possible (RT) to all nonvertical stimuli.

The study indicated that, without alcohol ingestion, P3 amplitude is significantly lower in high-risk subjects compared to controls. This replicates our previous findings (Begleiter et al., 1984, 1987b) of lower voltage P3s in an older sample of high-risk males as well as those of O'Connor et al. (1986, 1987) and Whipple et al. (1988). The largest differences in P3 amplitude between groups occurred to the easy target, to which low-risk subjects manifested extremely high voltages. These results are similar to those we obtained in alcoholics with the same paradigm, where the easy target elicited the greatest significant difference in P3 amplitude between groups (Porjesz et al., 1987a). This P3 amplitude difference between groups was most apparent at Pz and Cz electrodes in both studies.

Thus, P3 amplitudes are reduced in voltage in older and younger high-risk nonalcoholic males both to easy and difficult discriminations, in visual and auditory modalities, and without the administration of alcohol. As these results have now been replicated in four different laboratories—O'Connor et al. (1986, 1987, unpublished data), Steinhauer et al. (1987), Whipple et al. (1988), and Amass et al. (personal communication)—under different experimental conditions, these results seem to be generalizable. The neurophysiological deficits observed in young male offspring of male-limited alcoholics are intriguing in light of neurochemical deficits found only in male-limited alcoholics and high-risk individuals (Von Knorring et al., 1985).

Other investigators have reported differences in P3 between high-risk and low-risk individuals only after the administration of either alcohol or placebo. Elmasian et al. (1982) studied the P3 component as well as the slow-wave component of the ERP in three separate groups of subjects, each consisting of five matched pairs (five high risk and five low risk); one group served as the placebo group, the second group received a low dose of alcohol, and the third group was administered a high dose of alcohol. The subjects were male college students between 20 and 25 years of age who were primarily social drinkers. The investigators observed a significant decrease in the amplitude of the P3 component in the high-risk compared to the low-risk subjects. However, this finding was only observed after the administration of either alcohol or placebo. The investigators suggest that all subjects expected to receive alcohol; however, only high-risk subjects manifested a specific expectancy for alcohol characterized by an unusual brain event. It is also suggested by the investigators that higher-than-normal alcohol intake in the mothers of high-risk individuals may result in altered brain physiology.

Another study conducted in the same laboratory (Neville & Schmidt, 1985) examined the late positive component of the ERP in young adults at risk for alcoholism and low-risk individuals. This study did not involve the ingestion of alcohol or placebo and therefore eliminated expectancy for alcohol as a potential confounding factor. Moreover, the mothers of all subjects were interviewed to determine their use of alcohol and other drugs. Group differences in the late component of the ERP were observed.

In a subsequent study, Schmidt & Neville (1985) recorded ERPs in high- and low-risk men while they performed a visual language task. All subjects were social drinkers. They found that the amplitude of the N430 component was significantly smaller in men at high risk compared to men at low risk for alcoholism. Moreover, the latency of the N430 was directly related to the amount of alcohol consumed per occasion in the high-risk group. These results imply that neuronal function associated with language processes are affected by family history of alcoholism, and the interaction between family history and alcohol consumed per occasion.

We examined the effects of alcohol on ERPs in high- and low-risk subjects selected carefully, as noted above. All individuals were tested one week apart, on three separate occasions. The order of the conditions—placebo, low dose of ethanol (0.5 ml/kg), and high dose (0.8 ml/kg)—were randomized across subjects. At this point, we have tested 50 subjects (25 high-risk and 25 low-risk individuals). On each occasion, each subject was tested once before the administration of one of three liquids, and four times subsequent to liquid ingestion: 30, 60, 90, and 120 minutes after ingestion.

In this experiment the subjects were engaged in the visual line paradigm described earlier in this chapter (Porjesz & Begleiter, 1990). It is a P3 paradigm involving easy and difficult line discriminations. We found that, for both the easy and difficult targets, the high-risk subjects produced a P3 voltage that was significantly ($P < 0.01$) lower than that produced by the low-risk subjects both before (Porjesz & Begleiter, 1990) and after ethanol ingestion.

These results of lower P3 voltages obtained in young adult men at high risk for alcoholism replicate our past findings in young boys at high risk for alcoholism (Begleiter et al., 1984, 1987b) as well as the findings by O'Connor et al. (1986, 1987, unpublished data) and Whipple et al. (1988). Taken together, these findings of reduced P3 amplitudes in high-risk males have now been replicated with many different paradigms in different laboratories. This indicates it is not task or modality specific; it can be obtained both under speed and accuracy conditions, with and without alcohol administration, in different age groups.

It is of interest to note that ERPs appear to be quite heritable; they also seem to be rather similar in abstinent alcoholic fathers and their sons (Whipple et al., 1988). The P3 deficits identified in abstinent alcoholics also discriminate between boys at high and low risks for alcoholism. Therefore, we postulate that the ERP deficits identified in high-risk populations may be quite useful as potential phenotypic markers. Such a reliable and sensitive phenotypic marker may be of great utility in conducting a linkage analysis in large family pedigrees.

Taken together, the neurophysiological studies conducted in populations at high risk for alcoholism indicate rather clear differences between high- and low-risk individuals. While many questions remain unanswered, these preliminary findings seem quite intriguing and merit further neurophysiological investigations.

It is becoming critical to understand the significance of the aforementioned neurophysiological findings in populations at high risk for alcoholism. We need to assess the relationship between neuroelectric deficits in sons of alcoholics and subsequent alcohol abuse and alcoholism. The possible predictive value of electrophysiological deficits in young sons of alcoholics can only be assessed by the use of longitudinal studies in which individuals at high and low risk for alcoholism are tested regularly over several years until they pass through the period of maximum risk for alcoholism.

It is well established that alcoholism is not a homogeneous disorder with a unidimensional etiology. A potential biological marker may be present in subjects at high risk for one type of alcoholism but not for other types of alcoholism. In addition, a biological marker for alcoholism is not necessarily specific to this disorder. Indeed, it may be argued that the addictive behaviors represent a set of behaviors optimizing short-term gratification at the expense of long-term deleterious effects. In this context, the addictive behaviors reflect a failure in behavioral regulation. The failure of self-regulatory systems results in the inability to delay gratification as well as to avoid long-term consequences. All addictive behaviors, including alcoholism, might be interpreted as failures in adaptive self-regulatory processes. Indeed, one may argue that all addictive behaviors represent the natural consequence of behavioral dysregulation. This dysregulation is manifested by a significant deficiency in sensitivity to both exteroceptive and interoceptive stimuli that are critical to self-regulation. Moreover, this insensitivity to external and internal stimuli may be partially under genetic control. It has been argued that internal cue insensitivity is a possible diathesis for self-regulatory difficulties (Tarter et al., 1984). These authors assert that alcoholism is a disorder in the cognitive-physiological integration of information caused by a faulty arousal system. Indeed, alcoholics are well known to manifest problems with impulsivity, socialization, and self-control. The main components of self-regulation, including planning, guiding, and monitoring of one's own behavior, are substantially deficient in all disorders of behavior dysregulation.

It may be conjectured that the neurophysiological markers we have summarized in this chapter reflect behavioral dysregulation. To the extent that this dysregulation involves a set of behaviors common to different adverse outcomes, it may be speculated that alcoholism and other disorders of excess have a genetic predisposition, but may require environmental influences to determine the final pathway for expression of the disorder. Alcoholism may not be a unique biologically determined disease, but may be one of a variety of adverse outcomes shaped by genetically determined predisposing factors and precipitated by environmentally determined factors.

REFERENCES

Begleiter, H., & Platz, A. (1972). The effects of alcohol on the central nervous system in humans. In B. Kissin & H. Begleiter (Eds.), *The Biology of alcoholism, Vol. 2* (pp. 293-343). New York: Plenum Press.

Begleiter, H., Porjesz, B., & Tenner, M. (1980). Neuroradiological and neurophysiological evidence of brain deficits in chronic alcoholics. *Acta Psychiat. Scand.* 62(Suppl. 286), 3-13.

Begleiter, H., Porjesz, B., & Chou, C.L. (1981). Auditory brainstem potentials in chronic alcoholics. *Science, 211,* 1064-1066.

Begleiter, H., Porjesz, B., Bihari, B., & Kissin, B. (1984). Event-related potentials in boys at high risk for alcoholism. *Science, 225,* 1493-1496.

Begleiter, H., Porjesz, B., & Bihari, B. (1987a). Auditory brainstem potentials in sons of alcoholic fathers. *Alcohol. Clin. Exp. Res., 11,* 477-483.

Begleiter, H., Porjesz, B., Rawlings, R., & Eckardt, M. (1987b). Auditory recovery function and P3 in boys at high risk for alcoholism. *Alcoholism, 4,* 315-322.

Bohman, M., Sigvardsson, S., & Cloninger, R. (1981). Maternal inheritance of alcohol abuse: Cross-fostering analysis of adopted women. *Arch. Gen. Psychiat., 38,* 965-969.

Cadoret, R.J., & Gath, A. (1978). Inheritance of alcoholism in adoptees. *Br. J. Psychiat., 132,* 252-258.

Cadoret, R.J., Cain, C., & Grove, W.M. (1980). Development of alcoholism in adoptees raised apart from alcoholic biologic relatives. *Arch. Gen. Psychiat.*, *37*, 561-563.

Chu, N.S., & Squires, K.C. (1980). Auditory brainstem response study in alcoholic patients. *Pharmacol. Biochem. Behav.*, *13*, 241-244.

Chu, N.S., & Yang, S. S. (1987). Somatosensory and brainstem auditory evoked potentials in alcoholic liver disease with and without encephalography. *Alcoholism, 4*, 225-230.

Chu, N.S., Squires, K.C., & Starr, A. (1982). Auditory brainstem responses in chronic alcoholic patients. *Electroenceph. Clin. Neurophysiol.*, *54*, 418-425.

Cloninger, C.R. (1987). Neurogenetic adaptive mechanisms in alcoholism. *Science, 236*, 410-416.

Cloninger, C., Bohman, M., & Sigvardisson, S. (1981). Inheritance of alcohol abuse: Cross-fostering analysis of adopted men. *Arch. Gen. Psychiat.*, *38*, 861-867.

Cohen, H.L., Porjesz, B., & Begleiter, H. (1991). EEG Characteristics in males at risk for alcoholism. *Alcohol. Clin. Exp. Res.*, *15*(3),

Donchin, E., Ritter, W., & McCallum, W.C. (1978). Cognitive psychophysiology: The endogenous components of the ERP. In E. Callaway, P. Tueting, & S.H. Koslow (Eds.), *Event-related brain potentials in man* (pp. 349-411). New York: Academic Press.

Ehlers, C.L., & Schuckit, M.A. (1990). EEG fast frequency activity in the sons of alcoholics. *Biol. Psychiat.*, *27*, 631-641.

Ehlers, C.L., & Schuckit, M.A. (1991). Evaluation of EEG alpha activity in sons of alcoholics. *Neuropsychopharmacology 4*, 199-205.

Elmasian, R., Neville, H., Woods, D., Schuckit, M., & Bloom, F. (1982). Event-related potentials are different in individual at high risk for developing alcoholism. *Proc. Natl. Acad. Sci. USA.*, *79*, 7900.

Emmerson, R.Y., Dustman, R.E., Shearer, D.E., & Chamberlin, H.M. (1987). EEG, visually evoked and event related potentials in young abstinent alcoholics. *Alcoholism, 4*, 241-248.

Gabrielli, W.F., Mednick, S.A., Volavka, J., Pollock, V.E., Schulsinger, F., & Itil, T.M. (1982). Electroencephalograms in children of alcoholic fathers. *Psychophysiology, 19*, 404-407.

Goodwin, D.W. (1976). *Is alcohol hereditary?* New York: Oxford University Press.

Goodwin, D.W., Schulsinger, F., Hermansen, L., et al. (1973). Alcohol problems in adoptees raised apart from alcoholic biological parents. *Arch. Gen. Psychiat.*, *28*,238-243.

Hillyard, S.A., Picton, T.W., & Regan, D. (1978). Sensation, perception and attention: Analysis using ERPs. In E. Callaway, P. Tueting, & S.H. Koslow (Eds.), *Event-related brain potentials in man* (pp. 223-321). New York: Academic Press.

Kaplan, R.F., Hesselbrock, V.M., O'Connor, S., & De Palma, N. (1988). Behavioral and EEG responses to alcohol in nonalcoholic men with a family history of alcoholism. *Neuropsychopharmacol. Biol. Psychiat.*, *12*, 873-885.

Neville, H.J., & Schmidt, A.L. (1985). Event-related brain potentials in subjects at risk for alcoholism. *NIAAA Res. Monogr.*, 15/16.

Nickel, B., & Ludewig, L. (1981). Die Bedeutung der fruhen akustisch evozierten Potentiale fur die klinische Diagnose der alkoholischen Wernicke-Enzephalopathie. *Psychiatrie, Neurologie & Medizinische Psychologie, 33*, 193-198.

O'Connor, S., Hesselbrock, V., & Tasman, A. (1986). Correlates of increased risk for alcoholism in young men. *Prog. Neuropsychopharmacol. Biol. Psychiat., 10*, 211-218.

O'Connor, S., Hesselbrock, V., Tasman, A., & DePalma, N.P. (1987). P3 amplitudes in two distinct tasks are decreased in young men with a history of paternal alcoholism. *Alcoholism, 4,* 323-330.

Patterson, B.W., Williams, H.L., McLean, G.A., Smith, L.T., & Schaeffer, K.W. (1987). Alcoholism and family history of alcoholism: Effects on visual and auditory event-related potentials. *Alcoholism, 4,* 265-274.

Pfefferbaum, A., Horvath, T.B., Roth, W.T., et al. (1980). Acute and chronic effects of ethanol on event-related potentials. In H. Begleiter (Ed.), *Biological effects of alcohol* (pp. 625-640). New York: Plenum Press.

Pfefferbaum, A., Rosenbloom, M., & Ford, J.M. (1987). Late event-related potential changes in alcoholics. *Alcoholism, 4,* 275-282.

Pollock, V.E., Volavka, J., Goodwin, D.W., Mednick, S.A., Garbrelli, W.F., Knop, J., & Schulsinger, F. (1983). The EEG after alcohol administration in men at risk for alcoholism. *Arch. Gen. Psychiat., 40,* 857-861.

Porjesz, B., & Begleiter, H. (1979). Visual evoked potentials and brain dysfunction in chronic alcoholics. In H. Begleiter (Ed.), *Evoked brain potentials and behavior* (pp. 277-302). New York: Plenum Press.

Porjesz, B., & Begleiter, H. (1982). Evoked brain potential differentiation between geriatric subjects and chronic alcoholics with brain dysfunction. In J. Courjon, F. Mauguiere, & M. Revol (Eds.), New York: Raven Press. (pp. 117-124).

Porjesz, B., & Begleiter, H. (1983). *The biology of alcoholism: The pathogenesis of alcoholism,* vol. 7. New York: Plenum Press.

Porjesz, B., & Begleiter, H. (1985). Human brain electrophysiology and alcoholism. In R.E. Tarter & D.H. Van Thiel (Eds.), *Alcohol and the brain* (pp. 139-182). New York: Plenum Press.

Porjesz, B., & Begleiter, H. (1987). Evoked brain potentials and alcoholism. In O.A. Parsons, N. Butters, & P.E. Nathan (Eds.), *Neuropsychology of alcoholism* (pp. 45-63). New York: Guilford Publications, Inc.

Porjesz, B., & Begleiter, H. (1990). Event-related potentials in individuals at risk for alcoholism. *Alcoholism, 7*(5), 465-469.

Porjesz, B., Begleiter, H., & Garozzo, R. (1980). Visual evoked potential correlates of information processing deficits in chronic alcoholics. In H. Begleiter (Ed.), *Biological effects of alcohol,* (pp. 603-623). New York: Plenum Press.

Porjesz, B., Begleiter, H., Bihari, B., & Kissin, B. (1987a). The N2 component of the event-related brain potential in abstinent alcoholics. *Electroenceph. Clin. Neurophysiol., 66,* 121-131.

Porjesz, B., Begleiter, H., Bihari, B., & Kissin, B. (1987b). Event-related brain potentials to high incentive stimuli in abstinent alcoholics. *Alcoholism, 4,* 283-288.

Propping, P. (1977). Genetic control of ethanol action in the central nervous system: An EEG study in twins. *Hum. Genet., 35,* 309-334.

Rosenhamer, H.J., & Silfverskiold, B.I. (1980). Slow tremor and delayed brainstem auditory evoked responses in alcoholics. *Arch. Neurol. 37,* 293-296.

Salamy, J.H., Wright, J.R., & Faillace, L.A. (1980). Changes in average evoked responses during abstinence in chronic alcoholics. *J. Nerv. Ment. Dis., 168,* 19-25.

Schmidt, A.L., & Neville, H.J. (1985). Language processing in men at risk for alcoholism: An event-related potential study. *Alcoholism, 2,* 529-534.

Steinhauer, S., Hill, S.Y., & Zubin, J. (1987). Event-related potentials in alcoholics and their first degree relatives. *Alcoholism, 4,* 307-314.

Tarter, R.E., Hegedus, A.M., Goldstein, G., Shelly, C., & Alterman, A.I. (1984). Adolescent sons of alcoholics: Neurophysiological and personality characteristics. *Alcohol. Clin. Exp. Res., 8,* 216-222.

Vogel, F. (1970). The genetic basis of the normal human electroencephalogram (EEG). *Humangenetik, 10,* 91-114.

Von Knorring, A.L., Bohman, M., & Von Knorring, L. (1985). Platelet MSO activity as a biological marker in subgroups of alcoholism. *Acta Psychiat. Scand., 72,* 51-58.

Whipple, S.C., Parker, E.S., & Noble, E.P. (1988). An atypical neurocognitive profile in alcoholic fathers and their sons. *J. Stud. Alcohol., 49,* 240-244.

Young, J.P., Lader, M.H., & Fenton, G.W. (1972). A twin study on the genetic influences on the electroencephalogram. *J. Med. Genet., 9,* 13-16.

27

Cocaine Addiction: Psychology, Neurophysiology, and Treatment

FRANK H. GAWIN

CLINICAL CHARACTERISTICS OF COCAINE ADDICTION

For the past few years we have been experiencing the largest cocaine abuse epidemic in history. In the United States alone, one to three million cocaine abusers are estimated to be in need of treatment (Adams & Kozel, 1985), up to six times the number of heroin addicts. In the 1880s, 1890s, and 1920s, cocaine use surged, was temporarily considered safe, and declined after its dangers became well known (Freud, 1884; Lewin, 1887; Maier, 1926). In the early 1950s and late 1960s, abuse of the similar stimulants, amphetamine and methamphetamine, followed the same pattern (Ellinwood, 1974). In the 1970s, cocaine was considered a relatively safe, nonaddicting euphoriant (Grinspoon & Bakalar, 1980; National Commission on Marijuana and Drug Abuse, 1973). Historical descriptions of cocaine dependence were dismissed as exaggerations similar to marijuana reports from earlier eras. No clinical research on cocaine abuse using systematic and objective techniques had been done, and it was widely assumed that cocaine dependence did not exist. Then in the 1980s cocaine use exploded. Population data show almost a half of Americans now between 30 and 35 years of age have tried cocaine. A powerful route of administration, cocaine smoked as "crack," is now widespread, and it is as addictive as intravenous injection without its stigma or infectious dangers (Gawin & Kleber, 1986a; Grabowski, 1984; Jekel et al., 1986; Siegel, 1982).

Abusers in treatment typically report that two to four years intervene between initial exposure to cocaine and the development of addiction (Gawin & Kleber, 1985a). This interval delays awareness of adverse effects at the beginning of stimulant epidemics and, combined with reports of apparently controlled initial use, promotes an illusion of cocaine's safety. Early on, the public,

Elements of this chapter were derived from a review by the author in *Science* (Gawin, 1991), copyrighted in 1991 by AAAS and reprinted with permission.

scientists, respected publications, and astute clinicians fall victim to this illusion, thus facilitating the repeated emergence of cocaine abuse.

PSYCHOLOGICAL EFFECTS OF COCAINE

Initial Use

Both reports from abusers and human laboratory investigations (in which cocaine is administered to nonaddicted users) demonstrate that cocaine initially induces a sense of profound well-being and alertness (Ellinwood, 1977; Freud, 1884; Johanson & Fischman, 1989; Lewin, 1924; Van Dyke et al., 1982). Cocaine's fundamental effect is to magnify the intensity of almost all normal pleasures. The environment takes on intensified but not distorted qualities. Emotions and sexual feelings are enhanced (Ellinwood, 1977; Freud, 1884; Van Dyke et al., 1982). Self-confidence and self-perceptions of mastery increase, so anxiety is initially decreased. Social inhibitions are reduced, and interpersonal communication is facilitated. Satiation of appetite occurs, so pleasures associated with eating are not enhanced (Gawin & Kleber, 1985b; Johanson & Fischman, 1989).

Human laboratory studies of cocaine's effects are more reliable than retrospective self-reports of cocaine users, but they are seriously limited as aids in understanding cocaine abuse because there are multiple disparities between the methods employed in such experiments and the characteristics of actual "street" cocaine use. Maximum individual laboratory doses are 10% of the maximum doses typically reported by street abusers (Johanson & Fischman, 1989). The usual maximum duration of administration in human experiments is 5 hours (Scherer et al., 1988), compared to street binges lasting as long as 200 hours. In the street use of cocaine, other drugs (alcohol, heroin, and marijuana) are usually taken to decrease unpleasant components of the cocaine experience, such as anxiety. The co-administration of these other drugs, the effects of relative dosages of them, and the effects of varying the time patterns for their administration relative to cocaine administration have not been studied. Further, because administration of cocaine to a cocaine abuser in need of treatment has been considered unethical, the subjects in such studies have less severe histories of cocaine abuse and may instead have substantial histories of abuse of other substances, raising the possibility that any neuroadaptation pertinent to cocaine dependence might be absent and/or that neuroadaptation to other abused substances might be present. Finally, the effects of nonpharmacological factors interacting with cocaine effects have been largely ignored. Variations in the environmental context of cocaine administration, such as familiarity with the administration environment, the spectrum and pleasantness of available activities, the degree of personal isolation, the degree of perceived safety, the presence and difficulty of tasks, and the perceived medical risk, have not been reported. Such studies are fundamental. For example, whether the attention or distraction required to give investigators mental inventories of the subjective effects of cocaine, a procedure used in all the human experiments conducted thus far, might substantially alter the typical experience of cocaine euphoria has not been assessed.

Addiction and Dependence

Based on National Institute of Drug Abuse estimates, only about 10-15% of those who initially try cocaine intranasally go on to abuse the drug (Adams & Kozel, 1984). Some who experiment with cocaine cease use immediately, typically describing overwhelming anxiety rather than euphoria as cocaine's main effect. Some individuals who do experience intensified euphoria sometimes cease use because of cocaine's extreme expense or fluctuations in its availability. Others, before addiction is fully developed, fear the imminent loss of self-control over cocaine use and are able to cease use.

Individual differences in the progression to addiction could provide crucial insights for prevention and treatment. However, in light cocaine users who have not yet developed addiction, reliable predictors of later heavy abuse have not been found, a cocaine "addictive" personality has not been identified, and no objective, systematic assessments of the natural longitudinal course of cocaine use and abuse exist (Gawin & Ellinwood, 1988, 1989).

As cocaine addiction develops, a transition to high-dose, long-duration bingeing occurs, in which the intensely pleasurable effects are experienced alone and increasingly apparent negative contingencies go unrecognized (Ellinwood & Petrie, 1977; Freud, 1884; Gawin & Ellinwood, 1988, 1989; Gawin & Kleber, 1986a; Grabowski, 1984; Jekel et al., 1986; Siegel, 1982). Users readminister cocaine every 10 to 30 minutes. Such compulsive, uncontrolled, binge use begins when availability and dosage escalate (for example, as a result of increased funds or improved supply sources) or when a switch to rapid, higher intensity administration routes occurs (from intranasal use to smoking or intravenous injection) (Connell, 1970; Ellinwood & Petrie, 1977; Gawin & Ellinwood, 1988, 1989; Gawin & Kleber, 1986a). Such binges produce numerous pulses of extreme euphoria, forming vivid memories that are later contrasted with current dysphorias to produce cocaine craving (Gawin & Ellinwood, 1988, 1989; Gawin & Kleber, 1986a). Several days of abstinence often separate binges; users average one to seven binges per week, lasting from 4 to 24 hours. In distinction to the daily alcohol or opiate dependence pattern, the absence of a daily use pattern in a cocaine user does not indicate decreased impairment, but may in fact indicate the opposite (Gawin & Ellinwood, 1988, 1989; Gawin & Kleber, 1986a).

Continuous, rapid, cocaine self-administration also occurs in animal experiments in which unlimited access to intravenous cocaine is provided (Johanson & Fischman, 1989). Death follows within 14 days. If access is limited, an animal will press a lever thousands of times for a single cocaine dose. Human cocaine addicts report that virtually all thoughts are focused on cocaine during binges; nourishment, sleep, money, loved ones, responsibility, and even survival lose all significance (Gawin & Ellinwood, 1988, 1989; Gawin & Kleber, 1986a). Supplies of cocaine are drawn on until they are exhausted. Limitations on drug access, including the high price of cocaine and legal limitations on distribution, regulate human cocaine use and may prevent it from more frequently mimicking animal free access experiments in producing death. A low-intensity parallel to early, controlled use in humans has not been described in animal self-administration studies, probably because most self-administration experiments in animals employ large boluses and intravenous administration, thereby bypassing an initial low-intensity use phase and the binge transition (Gawin & Ellinwood, 1988, 1989).

COCAINE ABSTINENCE SYMPTOMS

A triphasic cocaine abstinence pattern has been described (Gawin & Kleber, 1986a), which dispels the perception that cocaine use produces no withdrawal. This abstinence sequence, initially based on clinical observations in a consecutive series of 30 outpatients, has been verified in one large-scale outpatient study and in some, but not all, assessments of hospitalized cocaine abusers, as well as in animal models and positron emission tomographic studies in humans (Hollander et al., 1990; Martin et al., 1989; Volkow et al., 1988, 1990; Weddington et al., 1990; Wolverton & Kleven, 1988; Kalsa H, Anglin D, Gawin FH, unpublished data). However, the symptoms are more complex and subtle than those previously associated with drug withdrawal, and certainty regarding the characteristics of cocaine abstinence cannot take place until methodological obstacles, delineated below, can be surmounted.

Phase One: Crash

A "crash" of mood and energy immediately follows cessation of a cocaine binge (Gawin & Ellinwood, 1988, 1989; Gawin & Kleber, 1986a; Grabowski, 1984; Jekel et al., 1986; Siegel, 1982). Cocaine craving, depression, agitation, and anxiety then rapidly intensify, and, in over half of abusers seeking treatment, suspiciousness and paranoia are also prominent (Satel & Gawin, 1991; Scherer et al., 1988). Over approximately 1 to 4 hours, cocaine craving decreases and is supplanted by mounting exhaustion and a craving for sleep; further use is then often strongly rejected, unlike the parallel situation after several hours of opiate, sedative, or alcohol withdrawal (Gawin & Ellinwood, 1988, 1989; Gawin & Kleber, 1986a). Abusers administer marijuana, sedatives, opiates, or alcohol to induce sleep. After sleep occurs, hypersomnolence, with electroencephalographic changes characteristic of sleep deprivation (Watson et al., 1972; Watson, personal communication), follows. During brief awakenings, hyperphagia occurs. The hypersomnolence can last several days. Mood normalizes after the hypersomnolence.

Although the crash has been confused with withdrawal (Ellinwood, 1974; Gawin & Kleber, 1986a; Grabowski, 1984; Jekel et al., 1986; Siegel, 1982), it parallels the alcohol hangover and not the withdrawal associated with chronic drug or alcohol administration. Further, although crash symptoms prolong cocaine binges, they do not maintain long-term cocaine abuse.

Phase Two: Withdrawal

In cocaine addiction, continued use is induced by a protracted dysphoric syndrome characterized by decreased activation, anxiety, amotivation, and boredom, with markedly diminished intensity of normal pleasurable experiences (anhedonia). This syndrome emerges shortly (one-half to 4 days) after the crash. This hedonically limited existence, when contrasted to memories of cocaine-induced euphoria, induces severe cocaine cravings, resumption of use, and unceasing cycles of recurrent binges (Gawin & Ellinwood, 1988, 1989; Gawin & Kleber, 1986a). Because it is directly related to craving and resumption of use, this withdrawal phase parallels withdrawal from other abused substances, except for the absence of gross physiological changes (Gawin & Kleber, 1986a). These symptoms are far more subtle than those of the crash and went unrecognized by early observers. They are not constant or severe enough to meet criteria for major psychiatric mood disorders.

The existence of a withdrawal phase is supported by broad clinical and preclinical observation and consensus (Ellinwood & Petrie, 1977; Gawin & Ellinwood, 1988, 1989; Hollander et al., 1990; Martin et al., 1989; Volkow et al., 1988, 1990; Weddington et al., 1990; Wolverton & Kleven, 1988; Kalsa et al., unpublished data). However, precise and objective research quantitation of anhedonia and similar dysphoric symptoms is problematic. Available psychiatric and psychological rating scales are not sensitive to these subtle mood components. For example, no scale or technique assessing anhedonia has been validated in human substance abusers.

In animals, however, elegant tools involving behavioral or electrophysiological responses to electrical, pharmacological, or behavioral stimulation have been developed that model reward functioning (reviewed below), and complementary preclinical data exist to support the hypothesis that reward dysfunction occurs after chronic cocaine abuse.

Anxiety, in distinction to anhedonia, has established and validated measurement techniques, and both experimental cocaine administration in animal models and anxiety inventory ratings in humans have confirmed the delayed emergence of anxiety during cocaine withdrawal (Hollander et al., 1990; Martin et al., 1989; Volkow et al., 1988, 1990; Weddington et al., 1990; Wolverton & Kleven, 1988; Kalsa et al., unpublished data).

Cocaine abusers desiring to cease use are cognizant, when in withdrawal, of the adverse consequences of continuing cocaine use. They are usually able to withstand transiently this anhedonic dysphoria, until they are presented with a conditioned cue. The cue superimposes a second, more transient dimension of craving—*evoked craving*—upon anhedonic craving, and most often, cocaine use then resumes. Conditioned cocaine craving is described as pulsatile, lasting only hours. Cocaine and the amphetamines are the most potent reinforcing agents known, and as such they produce intense classical and operant conditioning (Johanson & Fischman, 1989). Such cravings thus occur after the appearance of varied, idiosyncratic objects or events that were temporally paired with prior cocaine intoxications and that are experienced as partial memories of cocaine euphoria. Cues can include mood states (positive as well as negative), specific persons, locations, events or times of year, mild alcohol intoxication, interpersonal strife previously soothed by cocaine euphoria, or the presence of abuse objects; for example, money, white powder, glass pipes, mirrors, syringes, single-edged razor blades, among others (Gawin & Ellinwood, 1988, 1989; Gawin & Kleber, 1986; Giannini & Sangdahl, 1985; O'Brien et al., 1988).

Initiation of a cocaine binge thus depends on an interaction among drug availability, environmental stimuli (conditioned cues), and the withdrawal status of the dependent abuser. The time course of binge resumption fluctuates within and between cocaine-dependent individuals to an extent much greater than that occurring in opiate or alcohol withdrawal, depending on the valence held by these three factors. Manipulating these factors has thus become the focus of initial medical and societal interventions to control cocaine addiction. Recent treatment advances focus on decreasing withdrawal dysphoria pharmacologically or on extinguishing conditioned craving using graded exposure, in combination with public policies and advances in law enforcement that would decrease the availability of cocaine.

The cocaine disease process could be precisely reconstructed in animals, particularly its administration patterns and aversive experiences, but animal models designed to mimic human cocaine administration characteristics have simply not been employed. This is ironic since the unavailability of precise animal models that impedes rapid advances in other psychiatric and medical disorders is avoidable in studies of cocaine abuse. For example, potential pharmacotherapies targeted at conditioned cocaine craving have not, as yet, appeared in clinical or preclinical research. Such treatments are nonetheless plausible and could be screened by assessing the effect of pharmacological agents on cocaine-seeking behavior that has been linked to conditioned cues in chronically cocaine pretreated-animals given cocaine in a human-like binge pattern. Similarly, the relative importance of conditioned craving versus withdrawal craving at varied stages and degrees of abstinence, which is currently limited to clinical conjecture, could be modeled. Differential and specific treatment effects are also likely to appear according to the stages and degrees of abstinence at the time a treatment technique (isolation from or exposure to cocaine availability; pharmacotherapy at the time of withdrawal anhedonia) is applied. Optimal intervention timing and interactions between treatments could be modeled precisely and rapidly evaluated. Finally, public policy could be based on experimental findings modeled in animals, but it is not. For example, the effect of decreasing availability on increasing the work needed to obtain cocaine (the human equivalent to this work is often criminal activity) might indicate that crime would increase very substantially with increased cocaine prices and that only implausible increases in price would decrease use, or it might indicate the opposite. Vast government expenditures on law enforcement occur, nonetheless, in the absence of guidance from such plausible experiments.

If cocaine abusers remain abstinent, anhedonic symptoms lift within 2 to 12 weeks (Gawin & Kleber, 1986a). Animal studies show that behavioral depression occurs after stimulant withdrawal for a similar time period (Utena, 1962). Based on clinical observations, both symptom severity and duration seem to depend on the intensity of the preceding months of chronic abuse and on the presence of predisposing psychiatric disorders, which amplify withdrawal symptoms (Gawin & Kleber, 1986a). Conversely, in infrequent cocaine users without psychiatric disorders, withdrawal may not occur. High-intensity "binge" cocaine use and coinciding neuroadaptation may be required before withdrawal occurs.

Phase Three: Extinction

After the resolution of withdrawal anhedonia, intermittent, conditioned cocaine craving can still emerge (Gawin & Kleber, 1986a). It can occur months or even years after the last cocaine use. Maintaining cocaine abstinence requires that intermittent, conditioned craving be experienced without relapse. The previous consistent pairing of cues with cocaine euphoria then does not occur, and extinction of craving follows gradually (Gawin & Kleber, 1986a; Giannini & Sangdahl, 1985; O'Brien et al., 1988). Relapse caused by classically conditioned craving and withdrawal has been described in studies of opiate and nicotine withdrawal. In cocaine dependence, however, conditioned craving may be more intense than in other addictive disorders. This is not unexpected, given cocaine's extreme potency as a reinforcer in animal models and the established linkage in animal experiments between strength of reinforcement and magnitude of classical conditioning.

ACUTE NEUROCHEMICAL ACTIONS OF COCAINE

Cocaine and the amphetamines seem to produce pleasure or reward by increasing neurotransmission in mesolimbic and/or mesocortical dopaminergic tracts in the brain (see Chapters 11, 12, and 22). None of these neurotransmitter actions seems to be singly responsible for cocaine euphoria, since each is also produced by other pharmacological agents that do not produce euphoria, are not self-administered by animals, and are not abused by humans (Gawin & Ellinwood, 1988, 1989). Thus, although cocaine reward clearly involves activation of dopaminergic systems, the exact molecular mechanisms involved and whether activation is due to direct cocaine effects on dopaminergic neurons and/or to simultaneous collateral actions on other neurotransmitters are uncertain (Gawin 1986; Gawin & Ellinwood, 1988, 1989; Spyraki et al., 1982). Several lines of evidence support the hypothesis that a simultaneous interaction between catecholamine and serotonergic systems is fundamental to cocaine reward and euphoria. Cocaine and other abused stimulants, such as the amphetamines and methylphenidate, have numerous structural and neuropharmacological dissimilarities, but all have the common properties of producing, via neurotransmitter reuptake inhibition, activation of dopaminergic and noradrenergic pathways associated with mood and activation of serotonergic systems associated with mood and arousal. Manipulations of serotonergic systems modulate the reward potency of both cocaine and amphetamine in animals, and multiple agents that activate dopaminergic and/or noradrenergic systems but are devoid of strong serotonergic activity (benztropine, trihexyphenidyl, nomifensine, L-dopa/carbidopa), are neither intensively abused by humans nor, when administered systemically rather than directly into the CNS, avidly self-administered by animals (Carrol et al., 1990a & b; Modell et al., 1989). Pure serotonin agonists and antagonists lacking acute dopaminergic activity, including those with selective activity at specific serotonin receptor subtypes, also do not produce reward or abuse. Hence, augmentation of the effects of dopamine reuptake blockade must occur via other inputs to dopaminergic reward pathways to produce sufficient dopaminergic activation to produce stimulant euphoria. For example, serotonergic synapses exist with receptors on the cell body of dopaminergic neurons in the midbrain (A10) that may regulate activation thresholds in reward cells. Cocaine-induced serotonin reuptake inhibition could magnify cocaine-induced perturbations in the dopaminergic reward system to induce euphoria. If so, blockade or perturbation of serotonin or other augmenting systems might block cocaine effects while minimally influencing normal reward transmission and, unlike the dopamine receptor-blocking neuroleptics, averting the exacerbation of anhedonia.

NEUROADAPTATION TO CHRONIC COCAINE ABUSE

The response of the nervous system to persistent, drug-induced neurochemical perturbation is a compensatory adaptation in the perturbed systems. Dysregulation follows adaptation when the drug is not present. Yet, it had been assumed until recently that neuroadaptation does not occur in cocaine abuse. In contrast, several investigators have hypothesized that chronic high-dose cocaine use generates sustained neurophysiological changes in brain systems that regulate only psychological processes, particularly hedonic responsivity or pleasure (Gawin & Ellinwood, 1988, 1989; Gawin & Kleber, 1986a). Changes in these neurophysiological systems produce a true physiological addiction and withdrawal, but with a clinical expression that seems to be solely psychological (Gawin & Ellinwood, 1988, 1989).

Intracranial electrical self-stimulation (ICSS) of brain reward sites in animals provides a model for human pleasure. Chronic cocaine and amphetamine administration seems to decrease ICSS reward indices and to increase the threshold voltage required to elicit ICSS in dopaminergic reward areas, such as the nucleus accumbens (Gawin & Ellinwood, 1988). These ICSS decrements imply that brain reward regions affected by cocaine are subsensitive or down-regulated. These findings are consistent with both clinical observations of protracted anhedonia in abstinent cocaine abusers and with postcocaine behavioral depression in animals.

The neurophysiological dysregulations that would be consistent with these ICSS data have not been clearly established, but could take place at several sites. Central dopaminergic, alpha-adrenergic, and beta-adrenergic receptor supersensitivity have been demonstrated after chronic cocaine administration in animals (Gawin & Kleber, 1984). Receptor alterations could produce ICSS decrements in animals and anhedonia in humans. Reliable differentiation of presynaptic and postsynaptic receptor changes, as well as changes in receptor subtypes, such as D_1, D_2, D_3, D_4, and D_5 dopamine receptors, has occurred only recently, and these different receptor subpopulations were not differentiated in most prior studies. A primary effect of decreased dopaminergic reward transmission would be a secondary increase in postsynaptic receptor sensitivity. Disproportionate D_2 autoreceptor supersensitivity—that is, greater functional autoreceptor supersensitivity than postsynaptic D_2 receptor supersensitivity—would decrease dopaminergic neurotransmission. Such changes in dopaminergic autoreceptor subpopulations have been demonstrated in animals with continuous, but not intermittent subchronic administration of cocaine and amphetamine (Dwoskin et al., 1988; Henry et al., 1989; Kokkinidis & McCarter, 1990; Reith et al., 1987; Satel & Gawin, in press). Alternatively, other feedback mechanisms also exist that could influence firing and activation thresholds or other parameters of transmitter release in dopaminergic reward nuclei. These mechanisms include possible neurotoxic degeneration of dopaminergic reward neurons (Gawin & Ellinwood, 1988, 1989; Trulson et al., 1986; Wyatt et al., 1987), D_1 or D_5 receptor-mediated feedback innervation to the cell bodies of reward neurons, and multiple possible feedback loops involving serotonergic, noradrenergic, enkephalinergic, and GABAergic synapses, among others. Pharmacological interventions with actions at each of these sites have been described as influencing cocaine administration in preliminary preclinical or clinical reports. The predominant pharmacological treatment thus far investigated in the treatment of cocaine addiction—the tricyclic antidepressants—has multiple effects that are opposite to those of chronic cocaine; applied chronically, they increase ICSS reward sensitivity, firing rates, and synaptic dopamine concentrations in dopaminergic reward neurons (Gawin & Ellinwood, 1988, 1989; Gawin & Kleber, 1984). They may also induce dopaminergic autoreceptor subsensitivity and possess antianhedonic effects when applied in unipolar depression (Gawin & Ellinwood EH, 1988, 1989; Gawin & Kleber, 1984, 1989).

The appropriateness of generalization from chronic cocaine administration studies in animals to human cocaine withdrawal anhedonia is uncertain. Almost all animal research on the chronic administration of cocaine or other stimulants has employed drug administration paradigms that do not reflect human abuse patterns.

Neurochemical studies in cocaine abusers seeking treatment are limited. Such studies are also potentially confounded by multiple factors: concurrent medical or psychiatric disorders, the intensity and time course of antecedent cocaine use, other drugs abused, questionable reliability of details of self-reports, diet, duration of abstinence, and genetic heterogeneity.

Despite such limitations, it is noteworthy that both neurochemical studies based on peripheral indices of dopaminergic functioning and electroencephalographic studies in street abusers suggest that neuroadaptation occurs in street cocaine abuse (Carroll & Lac, 1987; Gawin & Kleber, 1985b; Hollander et al., 1990; Martin et al., 1989; Volkow et al., 1988, 1990; Watson et al., 1972; Weddington et al., 1990; Wolverton & Kleven, 1988; Woods & Lal, 1987). Several investigations have assessed peripheral neuroendocrine and neurotransmitter metabolite indices of central dopaminergic functioning in treatment-seeking cocaine abusers. Both homovanillic acid (HVA), the principal metabolite of dopamine in humans, and the neurohormone prolactin (inhibited by tuberoinfundibular dopamine release) have been assessed. Basal prolactin and HVA levels in cocaine abusers are either unchanged or reflect decreased dopaminergic functioning (Kleber & Gawin, 1987). However, multiple studies now indicate that transiently increased dopaminergic functioning is associated with resurgence of craving for cocaine (Carroll & Lac, 1987; Gawin & Kleber, 1985b; Hollander et al., 1990; Martin et al., 1989; Volkow et al., 1988; 1990; Weddington et al., 1990; Wolverton & Kleven, 1988; Woods & Lal, 1987).

In vivo imaging of human brain functioning can directly measure metabolism and neurophysiology in the brains of cocaine abusers. The current spatial and temporal resolution of positron emission tomographic scanning, single photon emission computed tomography, magnetic resonance spectroscopy, and multiple methods of assessing regional cerebral blood flow seem to be insufficient to demonstrate alterations precisely in function of brain nuclei in human abusers.

TREATMENT

Stimulant abuse treatment is divided into two phases: abstinence initiation and relapse prevention. Treatment typically occurs in psychiatric settings or in general drug and alcohol treatment facilities. Because stimulant abuse produces problems, such as anhedonia, that are specific to stimulants, referral to specialized stimulant abuse treatment centers, where available, is optimal. Unfortunately, many cocaine abusers receive alcohol or opiate abuse treatment that is applied without adaptations for stimulant abuse (Kleber & Gawin, 1984).

Co-dependence on other substances occurs with stimulant abusers but less often than the use of other substances to self-medicate acute stimulant effects, and it is very important to differentiate these two types of usage. For example, large amounts of alcohol are often used to induce sleep during the crash, but not at other times. Patterns of use provide a clinical guide to the importance of coexisting nonstimulant substance abuse. Only if other intoxicants are repeatedly used outside of stimulant intoxication (e.g., daily opiates with stimulant binges only twice weekly) is the diagnosis indicated of separate substance dependence. However, substitute abuse of another agent, most often alcohol, to ameliorate withdrawal anhedonia can also produce a new dependence during treatment, despite abstinence from cocaine.

Specialized stimulant abuse treatments, including adaptations of most major types of psychotherapy and pharmacotherapy trials, are now being developed and applied (Anker & Crowley, 1982; Ehrlich & McGeehan, 1985; Gawin, 1987; Grabowski & Dworkin, 1985; Maier, 1926; Rounsaville et al., 1985; Siegel, 1985; Wurmser, 1974). Outpatient treatment is regularly successful. From 50 to 90% of abusers who remain in outpatient treatment programs using different psychotherapeutic orientations cease stimulant use (Anker & Crowley, 1982; Kleber & Gawin, 1984; Siegel, 1982). However, because samples are not comparable between these treatment programs, rigorous study design is usually lacking, and no follow-up is provided on dropouts, there are no clear data to suggest that any one treatment approach is superior or that specific patients should be matched to particular psychotherapies.

Abstinence Initiation: Disrupting the Binge Cycles

The first treatment goal in actively dependent patients is to break the cycles of recurrent, protracted stimulant binges or daily binge use. Immediate relapse is a strong possibility as long as anergia, anxiety, and anhedonia are present.

In accordance with each patient's specific needs, outpatient treatment involves multiple weekly contacts, including combinations of peer support groups (Grabowski & Dworkin, 1985), family or couples therapy, treatment contacts with aversive contingencies (Anker & Crowley, 1982), urine monitoring (Gawin, 1987), education sessions, and individual psychotherapy (Khantzian & Khantzian, 1984; Rounsaville et al., 1985; Siegel, 1982). Practical and concrete measures are used to minimize the abuser's exposure to situations and people that can facilitate stimulant use; such measures include restriction of the patient's access to money, changes in his or her location and/or phone number, and curtailment of social activities. Drug-free significant others, who can monitor behavior and provide support and alternative activities to the patient during periods of high craving, are also incorporated into the treatment plan. If abstinence does not closely follow the initiation of treatment, increased interventions, such as hospitalization or increased treatment contacts, becomes necessary.

Because outpatient treatment is regularly successful and stimulants produce no medically dangerous withdrawal symptoms, hospitalization as a first treatment attempt is usually excessive (Ellinwood, 1967; Ellinwood & Petrie, 1977; Gawin & Ellinwood, 1987). The need for hospitalization should be subjected to ongoing assessment, based on the user's therapeutic support network, access to stimulants, route of drug administration, severity of abstinence symptoms, intensity of cravings and conditioned behaviors, ego strength, and prior and current responses to treatment. If hospitalization is necessary, its length should ensure abstinence through the resolution of withdrawal symptoms.

Relapse Prevention

As must the cigarette smoker or alcoholic, the stimulant abuser must make stimulants "psychologically" unavailable since they cannot be made physically unavailable indefinitely (Kleber & Gawin, 1984). The relapse prevention phase of treatment gradually decreases the external controls placed on the abuser during the initiation of abstinence, with the goal of facilitating the abuser's internal controls but without producing insurmountable temptation in the process. Relapse prevention techniques include predicting situations of high relapse risk and rehearsing avoidance strategies, altering lifestyles and developing drug-free socialization networks, merging memories of negative consequences of abuse to counteract memories of drug euphoria, extinguishing conditioned cues, and reducing external stress (Marlatt & Gordon, 1980). Idiosyncratic needs in the addict's life that the stimulant may have met, albeit dysfunctionally, are explored, and constructive alternatives to meeting these needs are pursued (Rounsaville et al., 1985).

Relapse prevention in stimulant abuse is similar to postwithdrawal treatment used for other substance abuse. In stimulant abuse treatment, extinction emerges as a most crucial component of multifocal relapse prevention strategies. All the outpatient treatment studies cited provide prolonged support to help abusers withstand evoked craving. All include, although not by design, four treatment stages for the hierarchical extinction of conditioned craving (Gawin & Ellinwood, 1988). First, during abstinence initiation, enforced isolation from drug use is linked to strict avoidance of conditioned cues. Second, stimuli and cues are reintroduced in imagery, in the context of developing strategies for managing stimulant temptation. Third, the patient gradually re-enters the cue-rich environment under controlled conditions. Fourth, successful abstinence is supplemented with maintenance therapies (continuous self-help and aftercare groups, resumptions of treatment) to counteract the episodic re-emergence of stimulant craving. These steps are most often implemented using long-term group psychotherapy, modeled on self-help support groups, such as Alcoholics Anonymous. The importance of conditioned cues and relapse prevention efforts may be demonstrated by a recent study by Rawson et al. (1986), in which inpatient-alone treatment produced half the success rate of outpatient-alone treatment. Although this study did have self-selection flaws and more conclusive research is needed, these results indicate that extinction cannot occur in an environment devoid of cues.

Experimental Pharmacotherapies

There is mounting evidence that pharmacotherapy may be effective in the treatment of cocaine abuse by influencing the long-term neuroadaptation to the agent. Extended treatment with tricyclic antidepressants produces effects opposite to those of chronic cocaine. They induce receptor subsensitivity, increase ICSS reward sensitivity and dopaminergic transmission, and reversal of anhedonic symptoms in major depression (Gawin & Kleber, 1984). Clinical cases of antidepressant amelioration of stimulant withdrawal were reported by Ellinwood (1977) during the last amphetamine epidemic, but systematic studies were not conducted. In the 1980s, Gawin and Kleber used desipramine hydrochloride, a tricyclic antidepressant, in open clinical trials in severe, psychotherapy-resistant, outpatient cocaine abusers (Gawin, 1986b; Gawin & Kleber, 1984). To minimize the likelihood that desipramine was acting only as appropriate treatment for depression, subjects who met diagnostic criteria for major depression were excluded. Abstinence occurred in 90% of a desipramine group compared to less than 50% in comparison groups given other agents (lithium and methylphenidate) or who continued in psychotherapy without medication (Gawin, 1986b; Gawin & Kleber, 1984). Chronic desipramine seemed to reverse cocaine-induced anhedonia. Tennant & Tarver (1984) demonstrated that short-term desipramine courses, which do not produce the neurophysiological changes of longer courses, do not facilitate abstinence from cocaine. Rosecan (1983) reported that another tricyclic antidepressant, imipramine, produced similar results in an independent, simultaneous, open trial in an unselected cocaine abuse population. Initial data from double-blind, placebo-controlled studies by three groups recently confirmed these findings. Desipramine substantially increases abstinence rates (Gawin et al., 1985; O'Brien, 1987) and decreases cocaine use, craving, and symptom scores (Giannini et al., 1986). These encouraging results are being further evaluated by systematic studies in three additional centers, which should shortly provide a firm basis to evaluate whether a general pharmacotherapy for cocaine abuse now exists.

Pilot attempts to increase dopaminergic neurotransmission in cocaine abusers in other ways have used antiparkinsonian agents, such as benztropine, amantadine, bromocriptine, tyrosine, and the stimulants, methylphenidate and pemoline. All of these agents have been reported to decrease cocaine craving during short-term open administration (Dackis et al., 1987; Gawin, 1986a; Gawin et al., 1985; Gold et al., 1983; Weiss & Mirin, 1986), but systematic assessments of the effects of these treatments on clinical stimulant abuse are lacking. Single-dose bromocriptine reductions of "evoked" cocaine craving have been reported in a placebo-controlled, double-blind laboratory evaluation (Dackis et al., 1987). Giannini et al. (1987) reported that long-term treatments with bromocriptine reduces withdrawal symptoms. However, one double-blind outpatient treatment trial did not substantiate bromocriptine's clinical efficacy (Tennant & Sagherian, 1987), although it did demonstrate the possible short-term effectiveness of amantadine. Similar reductions of stimulant craving by methylphenidate were transient (<14 days) and ineffective when applied clinically (Gawin et al., 1985a).

Other experimental pharmacological research is underway in an attempt to block stimulant effects. Pilot investigations have used lithium, alpha-methylparatyrosine, fenfluramine, trazodone, imipramine, local anesthetics, and neuroleptics (Gawin, 1986a; Gawin & Kleber, 1984, 1986a; Jonsson et al., 1969; Rosecan, 1983; Rowbotham et al., 1984). These substances have either not yet demonstrated clinical effectiveness or have caused untenable side effects. Monamine oxidase inhibitors (MAOIs) may also be useful in preventing relapse (Resnick & Resnick, 1985); however, theoretical dangers exist in the concurrent use of MAOIs and abused stimulants, both of which increase synaptic monoamine concentrations. Therefore, animal studies should precede any clinical MOAI experimentation.

NEUROTOXICITY AND CHRONIC PSYCHIATRIC DISORDERS

Stimulant toxicity could ensue from single acute insults, multiple acute insults, or long-term cumulative effects of cocaine use. Little data exist to distinguish these causes of toxicity. Escalante and Ellinwood (1970) demonstrated that high-dose amphetamine produces neuronal degeneration. Chronic amphetamine also reduces central catecholamine and serotonin concentrations in brain homogenates (Groppetti et al., 1973; Ricuaurte et al., 1980; Taylor & Ho, 1977; Trulson & Jacobs, 1979). Seiden (1984) demonstrated that amphetamine-induced dopamine reductions are permanent, linking them to specific degeneration of dopamine neurons in primate histopathological studies. These studies employed both chronic amphetamine administration (Ricuaurte et al., 1980) and single bolus doses that are within the range found in high-dose street abuse (Seiden, 1984). They showed that a single stimulant bolus produces the selective dopaminergic neurotoxin, 6-hydroxydopamine, in the synaptic cleft, presumably from auto-oxidation of dopamine after stimulant-induced dopaminergic flooding and inadequate enzymatic degradation (Seiden, 1984). Neuronal degeneration follows, thereby producing irreversible reductions in central dopamine concentration. Obvious behavioral changes seldom appear in these animals, even though permanent loss of 50% of dopamine stores occurs. The absence of overt clinical evidence of CNS damage in humans therefore does not preclude possible subtle irreversible changes, such as mood dysfunction. Since neuronal degeneration is irreversible, dopamine neuronal degeneration in animals raises the specter of possibly irreversible defects in the capacity of stimulant abusers to experience positive feelings. Similar findings have been extended to cocaine recently (Trulson et al., 1986; Wyatt et al., 1987), but they are not yet definitive.

There is general agreement that the anhedonic and anergic symptoms of stimulant withdrawal resolve over time. However, animal neurotoxicity reports are complemented by disturbing anecdotal reports from Scandinavia, Japan, and rare cases in the United States (Ellinwood, 1974; Schuster & Fischman, 1985) that describe chronic high-dose stimulant users with persistent anhedonia, anergia, and stimulant craving that do not remit, even after abstinence for as long as 10 years. In light of these reports, it is possible that some chronically relapsing, high-intensity cocaine abusers are self-medicating a stimulant-induced neurotoxic deficit. This hypothesis is probably applicable only to severe abusers. Systematic long-term follow-up studies in abstinent former abusers have not been done and are thus an essential research opportunity for the current epidemic. They are especially important because aging is associated with loss of dopamine neurons, and psychological or motor symptoms may emerge over time.

Chronic stimulant-induced paranoid psychoses and panic anxiety disorders have also been reported (McLellan et al., 1979), but in the context of the widespread use of stimulants over the last two decades, they occur infrequently and could reflect pre-existent psychiatric disorder (Castellani et al., 1985). A neurophysiological model that relates stimulant local anesthetic effects to progressive seizure activity (termed "kindling") and possible psychopathology is the focus of active preclinical research.

Within one decade cocaine addiction has evolved from virtual nonexistence to a complex disorder with interwoven environmental, psychological, and neurophysiological components. Initial clinical investigations of how the "normal euphoria of a healthy person" (Freud, 1884) becomes transformed into the source of "mad craving" (Lewin, 1887) have now resulted in the promise of advances in pharmacological and psychotherapeutic treatment of cocaine addiction. These advances have been founded in basic animal research, which underscores the value of basic research directed at unraveling the neurophysiological mysteries of human experiences of pleasure and pain.

REFERENCES

Adams, E.H., & Kozel, N.J. (Eds.). (1985). Trends in the prevalence and consequences of cocaine abuse. *NIDA Res. Monogr., 61,* 35-49.

Anker, A.L., & Crowley, T.J. (1982). Use of contingency contracts in specialty clinics for cocaine abuse. *NIDA Res. Monogr., 41,* 452-459.

Carroll, M.E., & Lac, S.T. (1987). *Life Sci., 40,* 2183-2190.

Carrol, M.E., Lac, S., Asencio, M., Kragh, R. (1990a). Cocaine withdrawal produces behavioral disruptions in rats. *Psychopharmacology, 100,* 293-300.

Carrol, M.E., Lac, S., Asencio, M., Kragh, R. (1990b). Intravenous cocaine self-administration is reduced by dietary L-tryptophane. *Pharmacol. Biochem. Behav., 35,* 237-244.

Castellani, S., Petrie, W.M., & Ellinwood, E.H. (1985). Drug-induced psychosis: Neurobiology mechanisms. In A.I. Alterman (Ed.), *Substance abuse and psychopathology* (pp. 173-210). New York: Plenum Press.

Charney, D.S., Menkes, D.B., & Heninger, G.R. (1981). Receptor sensitivity and the mechanism of action of antidepressant treatment. *Arch. Gen. Psychiat., 38,* 1160-1180.

Connell, P.H. (1970). Some observations concerning amphetamine misuse: Its diagnosis, management, and treatment with special reference to research needs. In J.R. Wittenborn, H. Brill, J.P. Smith, & S.A. Whittenborn (Eds.), *Drugs and youth.* Springfield, IL: Charles C. Thomas.

Dackis, C.A., Gold, M.S., Sweeney, D.R., et al. (1987). Single dose bromocriptine reverses cocaine craving. *Psychiat. Res., 20,* 261-264.

Dwoskin, L.P., Peris, J., Yasuda, R., et al. (1988). Repeated cocaine administration results in supersensitivity of striatal D-27 auto receptors to pergolide. *Life Sci., 42,* 255-262.

Ehrlich, P., & McGeehan, M. (1985). Cocaine recovery support groups and the language of recovery. *J. Psychoactive Drugs, 17,* 11-17.

Ellinwood, E.H. (1967). Amphetamine psychosis: I. Description of the individuals and process. *J. Nerv. Ment. Dis., 144,* 273-283.

Ellinwood, E.H. (1974). The epidemiology of stimulant abuse. In F. Josephson & E. Carroll (Eds.), *Drug use: Epidemiological and sociological approaches* (pp. 303-329). Washington, DC: Hemisphere.

Ellinwood, E.H. (1977). Amphetamine and cocaine. In M.E. Jarvik (Ed.), *Psychopharmacology in the Practice of Medicine* (pp. 467-479). New York: Appleton-Century-Crofts.

Ellinwood, E.H., & Petrie, W.M. (1977). Dependence on amphetamine, cocaine and other stimulants. In S.N. Pradhan (Ed.), *Drug abuse: Clinical and basic aspects* (pp. 248-262). New York: CV Mosby.

Escalante, O.D., & Ellinwood, E.H. (1970). Central nervous system cytopathological changes and chronic methedrine intoxication. *Brain Res., 21,* 151-155.

Freud, S. (1884). Über Coca. *Centrabl Gesammt Ther., 2*(289), 300-302.

Gawin, F.H. (1986a). Neuroleptic reduction of cocaine-induced paranoia but not euphoria? *Psychopharmacology, 90,* 142-143.

Gawin, F.H. (1986b). New uses of antidepressants in cocaine abuse. *Psychosomatics, 27*(Suppl.), 9.

Gawin, F.H. (1987). Laboratory assessments in treatments of substance abuse: Utilization and effects on treatment design. *Clin. Chem., 11*(Suppl.), 95B-100B.

Gawin, F.H. (1991). Cocaine addiction: Psychology and neurophysiology. *Science, 251,* 1580-1586.

Gawin, F.H., & Ellinwood E.H. (1988). Cocaine and other stimulants. Actions, abuse, and treatment. *N. Engl. J. Med., 318,* 1173-1182.

Gawin, F.H., & Ellinwood, F.H. (1989). In *Treatment of psychiatric disorders: A task force report of the American Psychiatric Association.* Washington, DC: American Psychiatric Association Press, 2, 1218-1241.

Gawin, F.H., & Kleber, H.D. (1984). Cocaine abuse treatment: Open pilot trial with desipramine and lithium carbonate. *Arch. Gen. Psychiat., 42,* 903-910.

Gawin, F.H., & Kleber, H.D. (1985a). Cocaine use in America: Epidemiologic and clinical perspectives. *NIDA Res. Monogr., 61,* 182-192.

Gawin, F.H., & Kleber, H.D. (1985b). Neuroendocrine abnormalities in chronic cocaine abuse. *Br. J. Psychiat., 147,* 569-573.

Gawin, F.H., & Kleber, H.D. (1986a). Abstinence symptomatology and psychiatric diagnosis in chronic cocaine abusers. *Arch. Gen. Psychiat., 43,* 107-113.

Gawin, F.H., & Kleber, H.D. (1986b). Pharmacological treatment of cocaine abuse. *Psychiat. Clin. North Am., 9,* 573-583.

Gawin, F.H., Riordan, C., & Kleber, H.D. (1985a). Methylphenidate use in non-ADD cocaine abusers—a negative study. *Am. J. Drug Alcohol Abuse 11,* 193-197.

Gawin, F.H., Byck, R., & Kleber, H.D. (1985b, December). *Double-blind comparison of desipramine and placebo in chronic cocaine abusers.* Paper presented at the 24th meeting of the American College of Neuropharmacology, Kaanapali, Hawaii.

Giannini, A.J., & Sangdahl, C. (1985). *Int. J. Psychiat. Med., 15,* 415.

Giannini, A.J., Malone, D.A., Giannini, M.C., Price, W.A., & Loiselle, R.H. (1986). Treatment of depression in chronic cocaine and phencyclidine abuse with desipramine. *J. Clin. Pharmacol., 26,* 211-214.

Giannini, A.J., Baumgartel, P., & DiMarzio, L.R. (1987). Bromocryptine therapy in cocaine withdrawal. *J. Clin. Pharmacol., 27,* 267-270.

Gold, M.S., Pottash, A.L.C., Annitto, W.D., et al. (1983, November). *Cocaine withdrawal: Efficacy of tyrosine.* Paper presented at the Society for Neuroscience, Boston.

Grabowski, J., & Dworkin, S.I. (1985). Cocaine: An overview of current issues. *Int. J. Addict., 20,* 1065-1088.

Grabowski, J. (1984). Introduction. *NIDA Res. Monogr., 50,* 8.

Grinspoon, L., & Bakalar, J.B. (1980). Drug dependence: Non-narcotic agents. In H.I. Kaplan, A.M. Freedman, B.J. Sadock (Eds.), Comprehensive textbook of psychiatry. Baltimore: Williams & Wilkins.

Groppetti, A., Zambotti, F., Biazzi, A., & Mantegazza, P. (1973). Amphetamine and cocaine on amine turnover. In E. Usdin & S. Snyder (Eds.), *Frontiers in catecholamine research* (pp. 917-925). New York: Pergamon.

Henry, D.J., Greene, M., & White, F. (1989). Electrophysiological effects of cocaine in the mesoaccumbens dopamine system: Repeated administration. *J. Pharmacol. Exp. Ther., 251,* 901-908.

Hollander, S., Nunes, N., Quitkin, F., & Klein, D.M. (1990). Dopaminergic sensitivity and cocaine abuse: Response to apomorphine. *Psychiat. Res., 33,* 1611.

Jekel, J.F., et al. (1986). Epidemic cocaine abuse in the Bahamas. *Lancet, 1,* 459.

Johanson, C., & Fischman, M. (1989). The pharmacology of cocaine related to its abuse. *Pharmacol. Rev., 41,* 3-52.

Jonsson, L.E., Gunne, L.M., & Anggard, E. (1969). Effects of alpha-methyltyrosine in amphetamine-dependent subjects. *Pharmacol. Clin., 2,* 27-29.

Khantzian, E.J., & Khantzian, N.J. (1984). Cocaine addiction: Is there a psychological predisposition? *Psychiat. Ann., 14,* 753-759.

Kleber, H.D., & Gawin, F.H. (1984). Cocaine abuse: A review of current and experimental treatments. *NIDA res. Monogr., 50,* 111-129.

Kokkinidis, L., & McCarter, B.D. (1990). Post cocaine depression and sensitization of brain stimulation reward. *Pharmacol. Biochem. Behav., 36,* 463.

Lewin, L. (1924). *Phantastica.* Berlin: Verland von Georg Stilke.

Maier, H.W. (1926). *Der Kokainismus.* Leipzig: Georg Thieme Verlag.

Marlatt, G.A., & Gordon, J.R. (1980). Determinants of relapse: Implications for the maintenance of behavior change. In P.O. Davidson, S.M. Davidson (Eds.), *Behavioral medicine: Changing health lifestyles* (pp. 410-452). New York: Brunner/Mazel.

Martin, S., Yeragani, V., Lohdi, R., & Galloway, M.P. (1989). Clinical ratings and plasma HVA during cocaine abstinence. *Biol. Psychiat., 26,* 356-362.

McLellan, A.T., Woody, G.E., & O'Brien, C.P. (1979). Development of psychiatric illness in drug abusers: Possible role of drug preference. *N. Engl. J. Med., 301,* 1310-1314.

Modell, J.G., Tandon, R., & Beresford, T.P. *J. Clin. Psychopharmacol., 9,* 347-351.

National Commission on Marijuana and Drug Abuse. (1973). *Drug Use in America: Problems in perspective.* Washington, DC: Author.

O'Brien, C. (1987, September). *Controlled studies of pharmacological and behavioral treatments of cocaine dependence.* Paper presented at the North American Conference on Cocaine Abuse, Washington, DC.

O'Brien, C.P., Childress, A.R., Arndt, I.O., et al. (1988). Pharmacological and behavioral treatments of cocaine dependence controlled studies. *J. Clin. Psychiat., 49*(Suppl.), 17-22.

Rawson, R.A., Obert, J.L., McCann, M.J., & Mann, A.J. (1986). Cocaine treatment outcome: Cocaine use following inpatient, outpatient, and no treatment. *NIDA Res. Monogr., 67,* 271-277.

Reith, M., Benuck, M., & Lathja, J. (1987). Cocaine disposition in the brain after continuous or intermittent treatment. *J. Pharmacol. Exp. Ther., 243,* 281-287.

Resnick, R., & Resnick, E. (1985, January). *Psychological issues in the treatment of cocaine abusers.* Paper presented at the Columbia University Symposium on Cocaine Abuse: New Treatment Approaches, New York.

Ricuaurte, G.A., Schuster, C.R., & Seiden, L.S. (1980). Long-term effects of repeated methylamphetamine administration on dopamine and serotonin neurons in rat brain: A regional study. *Brain Res., 193,* 153-163.

Rosecan, J. (1983, July). *The treatment of cocaine abuse with imipramine, L-tyrosine and L-tryptophan.* Paper presented at the Seventh World Congress of Psychiatry, Vienna.

Rounsaville, B.J., Gawin, F.H., & Kleber, H.D. (1985). Interpersonal psychotherapy (IPT) adapted for ambulatory cocaine abusers. *Am. J. Drug Alcohol Abuse, 11,* 171-191.

Rowbotham, M., Jones, R.T., Benowitz, N., & Jacob, P. (1984). Trazodone-oral cocaine interactions. *Arch. Gen. Psychiat., 41,* 895-899.

Satel, S.A., & Gawin, F.H. (1991). Characteristics of cocaine-induced paranoia. *Am. J. Psychiat.,*

Scherer, M., Kumor, K., Cone, E., & Jaffe, J. (1988). Suspiciousness induced by 4 hour intravenous injection of cocaine. *Arch. Gen. Psychiat., 45,* 673-677.

Schuster, C.R., & Fischman, M.W. (1985). Characteristics of human volunteering for a cocaine research project. *NIDA Res. Monogr., 61,* 158-170.

Seiden, L. (1984, December). *Neurochemical toxic effects of psychomotor stimulants.*

Paper presented at the 23rd Annual Meeting of the American College of Neuropharmacology.

Siegel, R.K. (1982). Cocaine smoking. *J. Psychoactive Drugs, 14,* 321-337.

Siegel, R.K. (1985). Treatment of cocaine abuse: Historical and contemporary perspectives. *J. Psychoactive Drugs, 17,* 1-9.

Spyraki, C., Fibiger, H.C., & Phillips, A.C. (1982). Cocaine induced place preference conditioning. *Brain Res., 253,* 195-203.

Taylor, D., & Ho, B.T. (1977). Neurochemical effects of cocaine following acute and repeated injection. *J. Neurosci., 3,* 95-101.

Tennant, F.S., Jr., & Sagherian, A.A. (1987). Double-blind comparison of amantadine and bromocriptine for ambulatory withdrawal from cocaine dependence. *Arch. Intern. Med., 147,* 109-112.

Tennant, F.S.J. & Tarver, A.L. (1984). Double-blind comparison of desipramine and placebo in withdrawal from cocaine dependence. *NIDA Res. Monogr., 55,* 159-163.

Trulson, M.E., Babb, S., Joe, J.C., & Raese, J.D. (1986). Chronic cocaine administration depletes tyrosine hydroxylase immunoreactivity in the rat brain nigral striatal system: Quantitative light microscopic studies. *Exp. Neurol., 94,* 744-756.

Trulson, M.E., & Jacobs, B.L. (1979). Chronic amphetamine administration to cats: Behavioral and neurochemical evidence for decreased central serotonergic function. *J. Pharmacol. Exp. Ther., 211,* 375-384.

Utena, H. (1962). Behavioral aberrations in methamphetamine intoxicated animals and chemical correlates in the brain. *Prog. Brain Res., 21,* 1902.

Van Dyke, C., et al. (1982). Intranasal cocaine: Dose relationships of psychological effects and plasma level. *Int. J. Psychiat. Med., 12,* 1-13.

Volkow, N.D., Mullani, N., Gould, K., Adler, S., & Krajewski, K. (1988). Cerebral blood flow in chronic cocaine abusers. *Br. J. Psychiat., 152,* 641-648.

Volkow, N.D., Fowler, J.D., Wolf, A.P., et al. (1990). Effects of chronic cocaine abuse on post-synaptic receptors. *Am. J. Psychiat., 147,* 719-724.

Watson, R., Hartmann, E., & Schildkraut, J.J. (1972). Amphetamine withdrawal: Affective state, sleep patterns, and MHPG excretion. *Am. J. Psychiat., 129,* 263-269.

Weddington, et al. (1990). Changes in mood, craving, and sleep during short-term abstinence from cocaine. *Arch. Gen. Psychiat., 47,* 861.

Weiss, R.D., & Mirin, S.M. (1986). Subtypes of cocaine abusers. *Psychiat. Clin. North Am., 9,* 491-501.

Wolverton, W., & Kleven, M.S. (1988). Evidence for cocaine dependence in monkeys following prolonged exposure. *Psychopharmacology, 94,* 288-291.

Woods, D.M., & Lal, H. (1987). *Life Sci., 41,* 1431-1436.

Wurmser, L. (1974). Psychoanalytic considerations of the etiology of compulsive drug use. *J. Am. Psychoanal. Assoc., 22,* 820-843.

Wyatt, R.J., Fawcett, R., & Karoum, F. (1987). A persistent decrease in frontal cortex dopamine from cocaine. Paper presented at the 26th Annual Meeting of the American College of Neuropsychopharmacology, San Juan, Puerto Rico.

28

Carbamazepine in the Treatment of Cocaine Abuse

ROBERT M. POST, SUSAN R.B. WEISS, AND THOMAS G. AIGNER

Acute and chronic cocaine administration have varied effects on behavior and physiology, depending on dose, intermittency, chronicity, and duration of administration, as well as a host of other factors. Chronic administration of cocaine seems capable of mimicking a variety of psychiatric syndromes, including euphoric and dysphoric mania (Post & Weiss, 1989; Post et al., 1989) and schizophreniform paranoid psychosis (Post, 1975). Most recently, cocaine has been identified as a potential panicogen, capable of inducing cocaine-related panic attacks at first and then spontaneous ones (Post et al., 1987b). These psychiatric syndromes provide useful models for the evolution of psychiatric illness. The preclinical models discussed in this chapter may be pertinent to understanding some of the mechanisms involved in the induction of these types of psychopathology. Drug treatments of the cocaine syndromes may differentially target cocaine-induced physiological side effects, behavioral psychopathology, or euphoria and craving; the latter may be the substrate underlying cocaine's potential for abuse and addiction. A drug interfering with self-administration of cocaine in animals would be a candidate for the treatment of cocaine addiction. If the drug also blocked associated behavioral and physiological effects of cocaine, it might additionally be useful from the perspectives of efficacy, tolerability, and safety.

In this chapter, we review the impact of the anticonvulsant carbamazepine on different preclinical models of cocaine-induced behavioral effects, convulsant effects, and self-administration. Initial data suggest that, although carbamazepine does not block acute cocaine-induced locomotor activity or behavioral sensitization (Post et al., 1984b; Weiss et al., 1990), chronic administration of carbamazepine potently inhibits cocaine- and lidocaine-kindled seizures and their associated lethality (Weiss et al., 1989c, 1990) and also blocks self-admin-

This work was supported by NIMH with supplemental funds from NIDA.

istration of cocaine in rhesus monkeys (Aigner et al., 1990). As such, it would seem to be a promising drug for further clinical testing in humans. Preliminary findings by Halikas and colleagues (Halikas & Kuhn, 1990; Halikas et al., 1989, 1990) suggest that carbamazepine may indeed have a useful clinical effect on cocaine-induced craving, as evidenced from subjective reports and assessment of the number of cocaine-positive urine samples in open and blind studies.

The historical background that led us to explore the use of carbamazepine in cocaine syndromes is perhaps noteworthy as it illustrates how preclinical animal experimentation may result in the testing of a drug with clinical potential.

HISTORICAL BACKGROUND

We began studies of acute intravenous cocaine administration as a potential euphoriant and antidepressant in the early 1970s, based on its potent blockade of reuptake of catecholamines and its euphoriant effects in humans. Our initial studies, however, indicated that it was not a useful antidepressant in moderately to severely depressed patients when given either orally or in repeated intravenous doses (Post et al., 1974). The literature on the chronic effects of cocaine in animals additionally suggested that it may produce paradoxical increases in behavioral responsivity (behavioral sensitization), as well as increasing likelihood of seizures even in response to the same dose over time. Based on the similarity of the time course for the evolution of seizures induced by cocaine and lidocaine, and by amygdala kindling after repeated intermittent electrical stimulation of the brain, we suggested that the local anesthetics might be producing a "pharmacological kindling" process (Post et al., 1975, 1976).

Carbamazepine was identified as a potent anticonvulsant against seizures thought to emanate from the temporal lobe in complex partial seizures and those kindled from the amygdala (Albright & Burnham, 1980; Ballenger & Post, 1978). Given the amygdala's role in emotional regulation, a sensitization and kindling perspective for the course of affective illness, and empirical data on carbamazepine's positive effects on mood in epileptic patients and in some patients with primary mood disorder, we explored carbamazepine as an alternative to lithium in patients with primary manic-depressive illness. Our studies and a large series of international reports now document the acute and prophylactic efficacy of carbamazepine in the treatment of manic-depressive illness (Post, 1990; Post et al., 1986a, 1987a).

We began to explore carbamazepine's effects on a variety of preclinical models to gain a better understanding of its mechanisms of action. We found that carbamazepine did not block the development of amygdala-kindled seizures in the rat, even though it was a potent anticonvulsant on completed kindled seizures (Post et al., 1986b; Weiss et al., 1989c). We had observed that lidocaine-kindled seizures produced marked alterations in aggressive behavior (Post et al., 1975), and wished to assess whether carbamazepine would attenuate this secondary behavioral component that arose during the course of local anesthetic-kindled seizures.

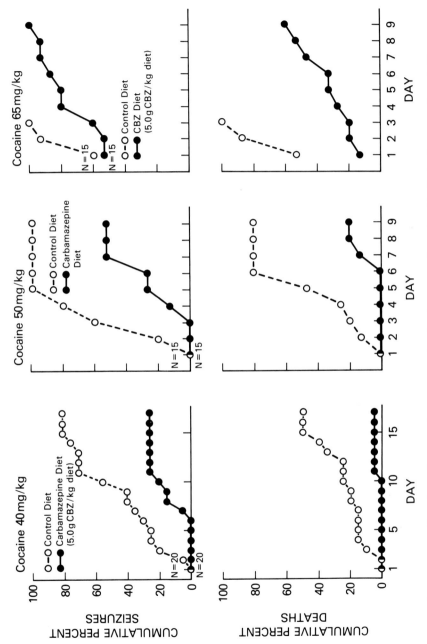

Figure 28-1. Chronic carbamazepine prevents the development of cocaine-kindled seizures and mortality.

In light of carbamazepine's negative effects on the development of amygdala kindling and its potent effects on completed kindled seizures, we were surprised to find that chronic carbamazepine markedly attenuated the development of lidocaine-kindled seizures, but seemed to have no effect on acute high-dose seizures or completed lidocaine-kindled seizures (Post et al., 1986b; Weiss et al., 1989c). Moreover, these data raised the question of whether carbamazepine would also inhibit cocaine-kindled seizures and their associated lethality. As illustrated in Figure 28-1, we found that chronic carbamazepine in the diet did remarkably inhibit the development of cocaine-kindled seizures in the rat (Weiss et al., 1987). However, it had no inhibiting effect on acute high-dose cocaine seizures. Attempts to increase the dose of carbamazepine to achieve a therapeutic effect in this situation were not fruitful and increased seizures and lethality.

The marked inhibition of the development of cocaine-kindled seizures suggested the possible utility of carbamazepine in the treatment of other aspects of the cocaine syndrome, including self-administration and craving. A protocol was submitted to study the effect of carbamazepine on cocaine self-administration in the rhesus primate in November 1987. However, because of a variety of administrative problems, including substantial delays imposed by new animal care regulations, the studies of cocaine self-administration in the primate were not conducted and completed until 1990. Preliminary data do indeed suggest that carbamazepine inhibits cocaine self-administration in the primate (Aigner et al., 1990).

This sequence of preclinical studies was, in part, leap-frogged by Halikas and associates who, on hearing of our data on carbamazepine inhibition of local anesthetic kindling, initiated their clinical studies in the late 1980s.

LACK OF EFFECT OF CARBAMAZEPINE ON COCAINE-INDUCED BEHAVIORAL SENSITIZATION

Initial studies in 1984 and subsequent studies in 1987 indicated that carbamazepine is not able to block the acute psychomotor stimulant effects of cocaine on locomotor activity and cocaine-induced behavioral sensitization (Fig. 28-2) (Post et al., 1984b; Weiss et al., 1989b & c). These data are convergent with the report of Meyendorff et al. (1985) that carbamazepine also does not block methylphenidate-induced euphoria in patients. The acute effects of cocaine on locomotor activity were thought to be mediated by dopaminergic mechanisms, predominantly those in the nucleus accumbens. Thus, this lack of effect on locomotor activity mediated by dopamine in this area of brain is of considerable interest in relationship to carbamazepine's positive effects in inhibiting cocaine self-administration. Self-administration is also thought to be heavily dependent on dopaminergic mechanisms in the nucleus accumbens (Pettit et al., 1984; Roberts et al., 1980), and the dissociation between effects on hyperactivity and self-administration raises a series of issues regarding carbamazepine's mechanisms of action on self-administration.

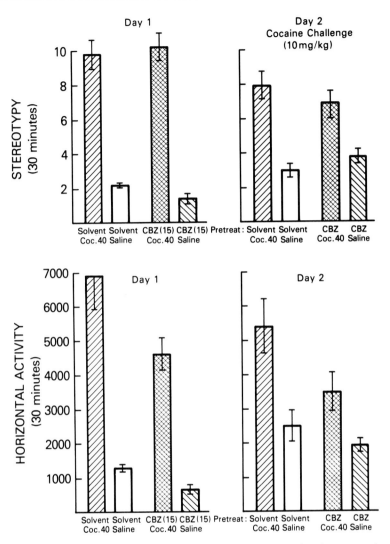

Figure 28-2. Lack of effect of acute carbamazepine on the development of cocaine sensitization.

Cocaine-induced behavioral sensitization presents a model for the progressive induction of behavioral pathology, as well as the role of environmental cues in sensitization and the precipitation of craving. In behavioral sensitization, animals respond with greater increases in locomotor activity after repeated administration of cocaine, in contrast to the traditional view that repeated administration of a drug would most likely be associated with tolerance. An environmental context component or conditioned component of behavioral sensitization seems to be particularly robust. For example, Post et al. (1981) demonstrated that increased response to repeated cocaine administration is only observed when the animals repeatedly demonstrate cocaine-induced hyperactivity in the same test chamber and not when animals are pretreated in a different environment and then tested in the chamber. Number of injections, duration of exposure to the test apparatus, and all other aspects of the research paradigm were controlled, suggesting that it is only the conditioned cues of environmental context that led to behavioral sensitization to cocaine.

This robust effect, achieved with repeated administration of low doses of cocaine (10 mg/kg, i.p.) has now been replicated in a single high-dose cocaine paradigm where, again, behavioral sensitization seems to occur in an entirely context-dependent fashion (Weiss et al., 1989b). Animals injected with a single high dose of cocaine (40 mg/kg) in a Plexiglas test cage show increased locomotor hyperactivity in response to a low-dose challenge (10 mg/kg, i.p.) in that same cage the next day. Remarkably, animals injected with an equal dose of cocaine (40 mg/kg) in a different environmental context on day 1 (e.g., wire home cage) are no more active on day 2 in response to the low-dose challenge than are animals pretreated on day 1 with saline. Weiss and colleagues (1989b) have further demonstrated that the degree of similarity of the testing environment to the environment in which the animals receive cocaine pretreatment determines the degree of cocaine-induced behavioral sensitization. These data are of potential clinical significance, as they reveal an important effect of environmental context and conditioned cues in the locomotor activation and sensitization syndrome. There is increasing recognition of the role of environmental cues in maintaining cocaine-induced behavior and inducing craving and withdrawal reactions (Ellinwood & Kilbey, 1975; O'Brien et al., 1988; Wallace, 1989). As such, the behavioral sensitization paradigm with its important dependence on conditioned effects may be an interesting model of cocaine-induced conditioned phenomena, which may be pertinent to the clinical situation of cocaine-conditioned craving.

As summarized elsewhere (Post & Weiss, 1988; Post et al., 1988, 1991), we have observed that lesions either of the nucleus accumbens or of the amygdala impair cocaine-induced behavioral sensitization. Dopamine depletions in the nucleus accumbens and amygdala or electrolytic lesions of the amygdala, which are insufficient to block cocaine-induced hyperactivity on day 1, are able to inhibit behavioral sensitization. Neuroleptics affect behavioral sensitization in this paradigm in a highly intriguing fashion (Weiss et al., 1989b). Pretreatment with neuroleptics on day 1 blocks the *development* of cocaine-induced behavioral sensitization, but neuroleptics administered before the day 2 challenge are not sufficient to block the *expression* of cocaine-induced behavioral sensitization. These data have been replicated multiple times in our laboratory and in others using a variety of stimulants and neuroleptics. Most recently, Fontana in our laboratory indicated that either a D_1- or a D_2-selective agent was able to produce this same dissociation of effects on sensitization development versus expression.

These data seem to have a dual message of possible clinical importance. To the extent that cocaine-induced behavioral sensitization plays a role in the evolution of behavioral pathology and is a reasonable model for the role of environmental context in acute cocaine reactions, the blockade of dopamine receptors may be an inadequate intervention once the syndrome has already developed. Elsewhere, we have also discussed this phenomenon as an interesting model for neuroleptic-nonresponsiveness in some psychotic states (Post & Weiss, 1989). These data highlight the potential differential impact of pharmacological interventions depending on whether they occur initially early or late in the syndrome (Weiss et al., 1989b). As illustrated in Figure 28-3, carbamazepine is effective early in cocaine kindling development, but is ineffective against acute or fully developed local anesthetic seizures. Conversely, it blocks completed amygdala-kindled seizures, but not their development. To the extent

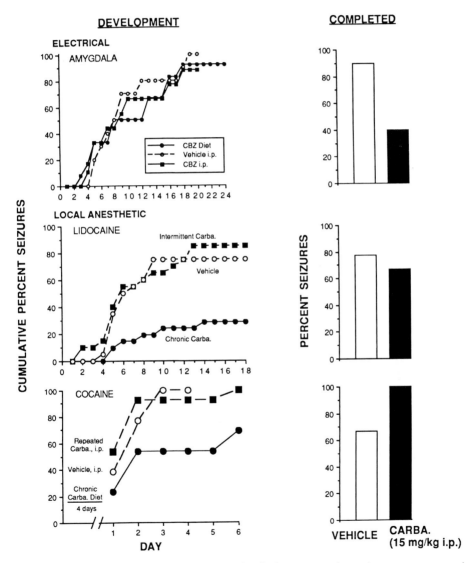

Figure 28-3. Effect of carbamazepine on kindled seizures: dependence on stage and type.

that cocaine abuse syndromes also evolve over time, these data suggest an additional reason for caution in the extrapolation of preclinical data to the clinical situation without taking into account the phase of cocaine syndrome development. Pharmacological approaches that are effective in one phase may not be so in other phases.

As cocaine dose and number of repetitions are increased, behavioral sensitization may demonstrate environmental context-independent components, i.e., pretreatment with cocaine in any environment may become associated with increased motor responses. Repeated high doses of cocaine (40 mg/kg i.p.) also induce increased amounts of stereotypic movements over time. It is of interest that, although carbamazepine does not block the development of sensitization to stereotypy, it does seem to attenuate the peak stereotypy response to cocaine (Weiss et al., 1986, 1990). As such, the biochemical and neural mechanisms seem to shift with the transition from single- to multiple-dose cocaine administrations, and a component of the stereotypic syndrome may become partially responsive to blockade by carbamazepine. These data are of interest since amygdala lesions that inhibited the single-dose cocaine sensitization paradigm no longer seem to be effective in inhibiting sensitization in a multiple-dose paradigm (Weiss et al. and Fontana et al., unpublished observations, 1989-1990). These data provide additional evidence that the biochemical and/or neuroanatomical substrates underlying cocaine-induced behavioral syndromes may shift, in part, after repeated inductions.

CARBAMAZEPINE'S INHIBITION OF COCAINE KINDLING AND ITS ASSOCIATED LETHALITY

Chronic carbamazepine in the diet markedly decreases cocaine-kindled seizures (Fig. 28-1). The kindling effect of cocaine seems to be dependent on its local anesthetic mechanisms since the pure local anesthetic lidocaine, which does not possess psychomotor stimulant properties, also produces pharmacological kindling (Post & Kopanda, 1975; Weiss et al., 1989c). Moreover, the related psychomotor stimulants, such as amphetamine, which are not potent local anesthetics, do not seem to produce the seizure kindling phenomena, even though they produce robust behavioral sensitization. These data suggest that carbamazepine, in its inhibition of cocaine and lidocaine kindling, may be interfering with a local anesthetic-related mechanism, rather than interacting with the dopamine substrate. This interpretation of the data is further supported by the lack of effect of carbamazepine on acute cocaine-induced hyperactivity and behavioral sensitization, in contrast to the potent effects of neuroleptics on at least the acute effects of cocaine and the development of behavioral sensitization (Weiss et al., 1989a).

Data from our laboratory further suggest that chronic oral administration of carbamazepine might be required to block kindling. Not only is acute administration ineffective in blocking acute high-dose cocaine seizures or completed lidocaine-kindled seizures but also repeated intermittent administration of carbamazepine before each cocaine or lidocaine administration is insufficient to block the development of kindling (Weiss et al., 1989c). This ineffectiveness is not caused by an inadequate dose of carbamazepine since increasing the dosage (from 15 mg/kg to 50 mg/kg) potentiates cocaine seizure evolution and lethality (Weiss et al., unpublished observations). We also examined whether pretreatment with repeated i.p. carbamazepine for a period of time before initiation of daily cocaine administration might produce a blockade of cocaine kindling (Weiss et al., 1989a). Administering carbamazepine (15 or 50 mg/kg i.p.) for 22 days before the initiation of cocaine kindling and during kindling was an ineffective treatment. Moreover, even when the dose and timing of i.p. carbamazepine administration were changed to match the blood levels of carbamazepine and its -10,11-epoxide metabolite to those achieved with chronic oral administration, differential efficacy still persisted, suggesting that the absolute blood levels were an unlikely explanation. This supports the view that the chronic administration of drug may have been the important requirement necessary to block the development of cocaine-kindled seizures (Weiss et al., 1989a).

Not only does carbamazepine robustly inhibit cocaine-kindled seizures induced by either 40, 50, or 65 mg/kg (Fig. 28-1), but in instances when animals do show convulsions, carbamazepine also increases the likelihood of survival. Thus, at all doses of cocaine tested in the kindling paradigm, carbamazepine reduces not only the incidence of seizure kindling but also the associated lethality. These data are of considerable interest from several clinical perspectives. Although cocaine may cause death from a variety of mechanisms (including stroke, hyperthermia, cardiac arrhythmia, myocardial infarction, and the like), the mechanism of death after a cocaine-induced seizure is particularly noteworthy. In contrast to animals experiencing a local anesthetic-induced seizure with lidocaine, after which the likelihood of survival is high, animals experiencing seizures with cocaine of a similar time course and severity succumb during or immediately after the seizure. Thus, cocaine-induced seizures may be an important model for sudden death in epileptic patients. Clearly, it is an appropriate model for cocaine-induced lethality in many clinical situations in which cocaine users experience a seizure and then die immediately postictally. The famous sports figures, Len Bias and Don Rogers, and other well-publicized individuals died that way; that mechanism of lethality may be greatly underreported in the general population of cocaine users.

There are also recent data suggesting that cocaine-induced ictal lethality may be relevant to the sudden infant death syndrome (SIDS) (Chasnoff et al., 1989). Children born to cocaine-abusing mothers are eight times more likely to experience respiratory abnormalities and are four times more likely to die of SIDS compared with appropriate controls. Thus, the ability of carbamazepine to block this component of cocaine ictal lethality deserves further study in its own right, independently of whether the drug emerges as a suitable treatment for cocaine addiction.

INHIBITION BY CARBAMAZEPINE OF COCAINE SELF-ADMINISTRATION IN THE RHESUS MONKEY

Aigner and associates (1990) have presented data suggesting that orally administered carbamazepine in the diet produces an attenuation of cocaine self-administration. When the carbamazepine diet is replaced by the conventional diet, self-administration in the rhesus monkey returns to baseline, but again is reduced with the reintroduction of the carbamazepine diet. Such an effect is illustrated in one monkey in Figure 28-4.

For this study, three rhesus monkeys were fitted with chronic indwelling venous catheters and were allowed 2-hour daily access to cocaine. Each animal was placed in a restraint chair in front of a computer monitor that had a touch-sensitive screen so that the animal could obtain a 1-ml infusion of cocaine by touching any location on the screen ten times. As illustrated in Figure 28-4, sequences of alternating 7-day conditions of a control and carbamazepine diet were then evaluated. The carbamazepine diet which contained 5 grams of carbamazepine/kg of food was fed to the animals for 2 hours each day before they were given access to cocaine. Carbamazepine's effect on cocaine self-administration was evaluated at cocaine doses of 100 μg/kg/infusion, 30 μg/kg/infusion, and 10 μg/kg/infusion. Levels of carbamazepine and its -10,11-epoxide (a clinically active anticonvulsant) achieved by the diet in these rhesus monkeys were clinically relevant in the low therapeutic range. The mean levels in the three rhesus monkeys of carbamazepine were 4.41 μg/ml and of epoxide were 0.85 μg/ml, achieving a combined total dose of carbamazepine and epoxide of 5.26 μg/ml.

These doses and blood levels of carbamazepine attenuated cocaine self-administration at the 30 μg/kg/infusion and 10 μg/kg/infusion doses. At these doses (compared with 100 μg/kg/infusion), basal rates of cocaine self-administration were quite high. Under these circumstances, carbamazepine significantly and replicably reduced cocaine intake in all animals tested in the "off-on-off-on" design. In contrast, at the 100 μg/kg/infusion dose (achieving lower rates of cocaine intake), findings were not as reliable in all animals, and the

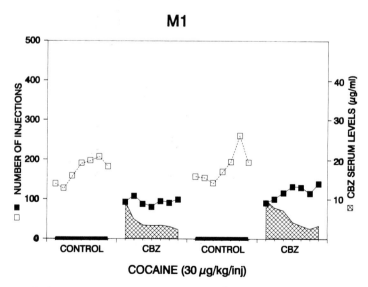

Figure 28-4. Carbamazepine attenuates cocaine self-administration in rhesus monkeys.

overall percentage of reduction achieved by carbamazepine was less than that observed with the lower doses.

MECHANISMS OF ACTION OF CARBAMAZEPINE ON COCAINE KINDLING AND SELF-ADMINISTRATION

To the extent that cocaine self-administration in rhesus monkeys reflects the reinforcing efficacy of cocaine, as others have argued, these findings suggest that carbamazepine may interact with the reinforcing efficacy of cocaine in a manner that leads to reduced intake. It does not seem that carbamazepine is inducing behavioral suppression in these animals, since (similar to the lack of blockade of the stimulant properties of cocaine in the rodent) the rhesus monkeys showing decrements in cocaine self-administration during carbamazepine administration still showed similar degrees of behavioral activation as on the control diet. It also does not seem that carbamazepine is acting like a neuroleptic, since blockade of dopamine receptors should increase rather than decrease cocaine self-administration in these paradigms (Balster et al., 1990). In contrast, dopamine agonists, such as bromocriptine, have been reported to decrease self-administration (Hubner & Koob, 1990), raising the possibility that carbamazepine could have indirect dopamine agonist properties in a similar fashion. Preclinical evidence reviewed elsewhere (Post, 1987, 1988) is consistent with the view that carbamazepine could, by incompletely understood mechanisms, increase the availability of dopamine in extracellular fluid, causing an indirect agonist effect. This, in turn, could downregulate dopamine receptors, potentially resulting in decreased efficacy of cocaine in this system. Arguing against the interpretation is the finding that carbamazepine was equally effective on day 1 of administration as at the end of a week when presumably dopamine receptors would be more robustly downregulated by the putative increases in synaptic dopamine. Although three investigative groups have reported that carbamazepine is able to increase extracellular dopamine in various model systems, the recent data of Pert and Mele in our laboratory (unpublished observations), using in vivo dialysis, indicate that even substantial doses of carbamazepine (up to 50 mg/kg i.p.) are not sufficient to increase extracellular dopamine in the striatum. It is possible, however, that carbamazepine could function as a direct dopamine agonist or as a mixed agonist-antagonist without increasing dopamine release, although dopaminergic-like behavioral effects of carbamazepine have not been reported. Interestingly, we have recently found that chronic carbamazepine, while not affecting dopamine levels on its own, can inhibit cocaine-induced increases in dopamine in the nucleus accumbens (Baptista et al., 1993).

Recent reports suggest that intravenously administered cocaine is capable of increasing serotonin release, as measured by in vivo dialysis (Yan et al., 1990). These data raise the possibility that a serotonergic component of carbamazepine's effect could account for some component of its actions on seizures or self-administration. This view would be bolstered by the suggestion of Yan et al. (1992) that serotonin depletion prevents the anticonvulsant effects of carbamazepine on genetically epilepsy-prone rats subject to audiogenic seizures. However, it is unlikely that a serotonin mechanism is pertinent to carbamazepine's anticonvulsant effects on cocaine-kindled seizures, as preliminary observations by Weiss and associates in our laboratory suggest that depletion of serotonin by the tryptophan hydroxylase inhibitor para-chlorophenylalanine (PCPA) is insufficient to block the inhibition of cocaine-kindled seizure evolution of carbamazepine.

The inhibition by carbamazepine of local anesthetic kindling is also not related to a traditional "tricyclic" effect, as treatment with desmethylimipramine (DMI, 10 mg/kg B.I.D., a regimen that decreases beta receptors in rats) worsens cocaine-kindled seizures and lethality (Fig. 28-5). These data also suggest caution in the clinical use of DMI for cocaine addiction, withdrawal, and craving.

Blockade of α_2-noradrenergic receptors with yohimbine, which is sufficient to block the acute anticonvulsant effects of carbamazepine on amygdala-kindled seizures induced electrically, is not sufficient to block the effects of carbamazepine on cocaine-kindled seizures (Weiss et al., unpublished data). These data suggest that α_2-noradrenergic receptors are not necessary to carbamazepine's effect on cocaine kindling as they are on amygdala kindling.

In contrast to the unsuccessful attempts to manipulate the pharmacological inhibition of cocaine-kindled seizures with PCPA and yohimbine, Weiss et al.

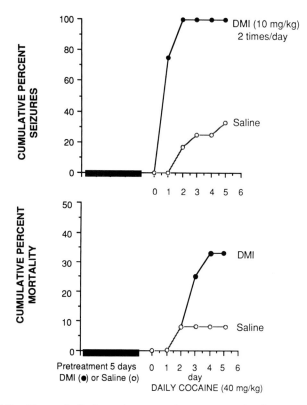

Figure 28-5. Desmethylimipramine potentiates cocaine kindling and lethality.

(unpublished data, 1990) have been able to reverse carbamazepine's inhibition of cocaine-kindled seizures with i.c.v. administration of corticotropin-releasing hormone (CRH). However, the specificity of this effect is in doubt as CRH itself is capable of exacerbating cocaine-kindled seizure evolution in the absence of carbamazepine pretreatment. Nonetheless, these data leave open the possibility that an interaction of carbamazepine with CRH could be related to the ability of carbamazepine to inhibit some components of cocaine syndromes but not others. This possibility was raised by the preclinical data that carbamazepine blocks local anesthetic-induced release of CRH in mouse hypothalamic extract preparation (Calogero et al., 1989). These data are also intriguing from the perspective that blockade of CRH effects using the alpha-helical CRH antagonist attenuated stress-induced cross-sensitization to amphetamine in the studies of Cole and associates (1990). However, in our hands, the alpha-helical CRH antagonist did not inhibit context-dependent cocaine sensitization, and similarly, carbamazepine does not inhibit sensitization. It remains to be seen what part CRH plays in the cocaine kindling phenomenon, but the marked potentiation of cocaine-kindled seizures by CRH suggests a potentially important interaction in this regard.

Although carbamazepine has been postulated to interact with calcium mechanisms at a variety of levels (via adenosine, via $GABA_B$, and via peripheral-type benzodiazepine receptor mechanisms) (Post, 1987, 1988), it is not known whether carbamazepine's effects on calcium could account for its effects on cocaine kindling. Calcium channel blockers do not seem to block cocaine seizures (Derlet & Albertson, 1989), although Trouve et al. (1990) reported that nimodipine does block some of the autonomic effects of cocaine. Although calcium channel blockers are not able to inhibit the acute effects of cocaine, whether they might affect the development of cocaine-kindled seizures remains to be further explored. Recently, carbamazepine has been shown to interact with potassium channels (Zona et al., 1990; Olpe et al., unpublished data) and to alter the dynamics of excitatory amino acids, such as aspartate and glutamate currents (Lampe & Bigalke, 1990; Bernasconi, personal communication, 1987). Whether these effects could be relevant to carbamazepine's profile of effects on kindling and self-administration also remains to be further explored, but is particularly intriguing in light of some suggestions that the glutamate antagonist MK-801 might block not only amygdala-kindled seizure evolution but also cocaine-kindled seizure evolution (Karler et al., 1989). However, preliminary data from Fontana et al. (unpublished observations, 1990) in our laboratory suggest that MK-801 and cocaine may show a cross-sensitization to each other.

Thus, the mechanisms by which carbamazepine exerts its effects on the development of cocaine-kindled seizures and its associated lethality are not adequately delineated. It is possible that the mechanisms involved in this paradigm are also pertinent to those observed in cocaine self-administration, although this remains to be directly explored and established. The inability of carbamazepine to block cocaine-induced acute locomotor hyperactivity or behavioral sensitization suggests that the mechanism underlying these phenomena may not directly extrapolate to the paradigm of self-administration. To the extent that dopaminergic mechanisms have been linked most closely to both stimulant-induced locomotor hyperactivity and self-administration, the dissociation by carbamazepine is particularly intriguing. It clearly indicates that a given drug can affect the self-administration paradigm without affecting activity or sensitization. Whether this dissociative property of carbamazepine will ultimately prove problematic or useful in the clinical realm remains to be further explored. Nevertheless, from a mechanistic perspective, this dissociation may provide important insights into the differential mechanisms underlying these two paradigms.

CLINICAL STUDIES OF CARBAMAZEPINE IN COCAINE ABUSERS

Halikas' initial study of carbamazepine in 35 cocaine abusers, although nonblind and uncontrolled, showed promising results (Halikas et al., 1989; personal communication, 1990). He reported that 13 subjects (37%) achieved a successful treatment response—a decrease from the pretreatment level of cocaine use from 65 days of cocaine use per 100 days to only 3 per 100 days during carbamazepine treatment. Halikas observed a partial response to carbamazepine in another 13 subjects (37%); their use decreased from 78 per 100 days to only 35 per 100 days during carbamazepine treatment. Nine subjects (26%) were unsuccessful. Their pretreatment use of 52 mean days of cocaine use per 100 remained at approximately the same level of 60 per 100 during treatment with carbamazepine. In this study successful outcome was confounded with compliance (possibly reflecting motivation), as the patients in the successful and partially successful groups remained on chronic carbamazepine administration, whereas those in the unsuccessful group did not take the drug in a systematic way. Obviously, further clinical trials are indicated, and these are in progress. Halikas et al. (1990) have completed a blind study, including a 20-day trial with 10 days on carbamazepine and 10 days off, in 32 paid and largely unmotivated subjects. A significant reduction in the number of cocaine-positive urines was observed in those who achieved carbamazepine levels over 4 μg/ml. In addition to this blind trial, D. Gorelick in Baltimore and C. O'Brien in Philadelphia are conducting double-blind clinical trials of carbamazepine in cocaine abusers, and their results are also eagerly awaited. A preliminary study by Hatsukami et al. (1991) in which experience with six patients was reported indicated that carbamazepine (400 mg × 5 days) did not block the subjective effects of inhaled cocaine (40 mg) when compared with placebo. However, promising evidence that carbamazepine might be useful stems from the case report of Sherer et al. (1990) that the drug decreased the cocaine-induced rush.

PROFILE OF EFFECTS OF CARBAMAZEPINE: IMPLICATIONS FOR CLINICAL UTILITY AND ACCEPTANCE

The ultimate utility of carbamazepine must be documented in controlled clinical trials in cocaine abusers, regardless of how promising the preclinical data might be. Nonetheless, the preclinical findings (Weiss et al., 1987, 1989c) were instrumental in the initiation of these clinical studies and the promising neurobiological mechanisms they may help reveal. As we have emphasized throughout this chapter, carbamazepine may play an important role in helping dissect mechanisms of cocaine's psychomotor stimulant properties (where it is ineffective) compared with those involved in kindling, lethality, and intravenous self-administration (where it is effective). Chronic drug administration may be critical to the efficacy of carbamazepine, at least in the cocaine kindling paradigm if not in the self-administration one. This might provide unique leverage for dissecting mechanisms that occur differentially with chronic versus acute intermittent administration. Moreover, in this regard, since chronic administration of carbamazepine seems to be required to produce positive effects on mood and behavior in patients with manic-depressive illness (Post et al., 1986a, 1987a), insights into mechanisms requiring chronic administration may be relevant to the mechanism of action of carbamazepine in affective illness as well.

From the clinical standpoint, there are several other reasons to consider the potential utility of carbamazepine in cocaine abusers. There is an increasing appreciation of the high degree of co-morbidity between affective disorders and cocaine abuse, so that the ability of carbamazepine to potentially target both symptom problems could make it a uniquely useful drug. Although the benzodiazepines seem to decrease cocaine seizures and lethality, even with acute administration, their addiction liability in substance abusers might preclude their clinical utility in chronic administration. Moreover, their use in targeting craving and withdrawal remains to be demonstrated. Carbamazepine has also been reported to be useful in the treatment of benzodiazepine withdrawal itself. These studies have been reported largely using uncontrolled methodologies by Klein and associates (1986), Roy-Byrne (1989), Ries and associates (1989), and Rickels and associates at the University of Pennsylvania (personal communication). These preliminary data suggest that, rather than being a potentially problematic drug of abuse (like the benzodiazepines), carbamazepine in contrast may actually be of use in assisting with other components of drug withdrawal in the poly-substance abuser who is using sedative-hypnotic drugs in addition to cocaine. This problem of co-abuse may not be infrequent, particularly in light of the anxiogenic and stimulant components of cocaine, which often propel the user to co-medicate with other substances to decrease anxiety and assist with sleep.

Elsewhere, we have discussed in detail the potential kindling-like time course of cocaine-induced panic attacks (Post et al., 1987b). To the extent that cocaine-induced panic attacks are related to a local anesthetic mechanism, one could postulate that carbamazepine might also be capable of blocking the development of panic without incurring the liability of the benzodiazepine anticonvulsants. Also consistent with this line of argument is the view that carbamazepine is effective in the treatment of alcohol withdrawal syndromes (Ballenger & Post, 1984, 1990). This effectiveness may be of additional benefit as alcohol tends to be another drug of abuse in a high proportion of cocaine addicts; to the extent that carbamazepine might be effective in the acute and maintenance phases of alcohol withdrawal, this profile could enhance its potential utility as well.

A final rationale for carbamazepine is suggested by its ability to block at least some types of aggression in a variety of preclinical and clinical syndromes (Post et al., 1984a). The potential ability to block local anesthetic-induced aggression was the motivating factor in our initial studies of carbamazepine in cocaine kindling. There is increasing recognition that violence and aggression are secondary effects of cocaine abuse. They might be occurring either on the basis of local anesthetic kindling-like mechanisms in limbic and other structures of the brain or on the basis of cocaine's psychomotor stimulant properties, with its associated induction of paranoia similar to that observed with amphetamine. To the extent that carbamazepine might block some types of aggression and dyscontrol, it might provide an additional rationale for its clinical use in cocaine abusers. One well-controlled study further describes positive effects of carbamazepine on dyscontrol in borderline personality disorder, a syndrome often associated with poly-drug abuse (Cowdry & Gardner, 1988).

These additional clinical rationales are raised with several perspectives in mind. Obviously, if a drug is to be of use in the treatment of cocaine abusers, it must not only be efficacious but also be acceptable, tolerable, and without untoward side effects, including the potential for engendering an additional dependency. As such, carbamazepine may have a useful profile in these secondary areas, and these deserve consideration while its primary efficacy in cocaine abuse and on self-administration and craving in clinical and preclinical studies is being systematically assessed.

In addition, these secondary clinical rationales are also being raised in this context so that appropriate studies can be undertaken to assess whether carbamazepine is having an impact on factors other than cocaine intake. The design of the studies should take into consideration whether patients have co-morbid affective disorder and whether this underlying disorder is being treated successfully. Similarly, in poly-substance abusers, is the drug having an effect on impulsivity, dyscontrol, and on other abused substances, as well as on cocaine itself? In many clinical trials, poly-substance abusers are screened out. Clinical trials with carbamazepine might be designed in such a way that this most problematic subgroup of patients is studied, and the potential differential impact of carbamazepine on the disorder and on different substances of abuse is assessed accurately. Alcohol remains a potent co-morbid condition with many cocaine abusers, and its role in conditioned craving has been highlighted by several investigators, including Childress et al. (1988) and O'Brien et al. (1988). Clearly, an assessment of carbamazepine's impact on co-morbid alcohol abuse remains of considerable interest. Finally, assessment of carbamazepine's impact on the course of cocaine-related symptomatology, such as manic-like behavior and its evolution to dysphoric mania and paranoid psychosis and on aggression and panic attacks, all warrants further study.

Clearly, the utility and clinical impact of carbamazepine in the treatment of cocaine abuse disorders and its associated secondary symptoms and co-morbid conditions are part of a story in process. Although there are promising preliminary preclinical and clinical data, systematic controlled clinical trials remain to be completed in substantial numbers of subjects. Even if the drug proves to be effective, adequate delineation of responsive patient subgroups and symptom target areas will require considerable further investigation. Thus, although the drug holds promise for the treatment of some components of cocaine abuse disorders, much preclinical and clinical research remains to be performed to adequately document its effects and uncover the potential mechanisms of its action.

REFERENCES

Aigner, T., Weiss, S.R.B., & Post, R.M. (1990). Carbamazepine attenuates i.v. cocaine self-administration in rhesus monkeys. *Abst. Am. Coll. Neuropsycopharmacol., 181.*

Albright, P.S., & Burnham, W.M. (1980). Development of a new pharmacological seizure model: Effects of anticonvulsants on cortical- and amygdala-kindled seizures in the rat. *Epilepsia, 21,* 681-689.

Ballenger, J.C., & Post, R.M. (1978). Therapeutic effects of carbamazepine in affective illness: A preliminary report. *Commun. Psychopharmacol., 2,* 159-175.

Ballenger, J.C., & Post, R.M. (1984). Carbamazepine in alcohol withdrawal syndromes and schizophrenic psychoses. *Psychopharmacol. Bull., 20,* 572-584.

Ballenger, J.C., & Post, R.M. (1990). Addictive behavior and kindling: Relationship to alcohol withdrawal and cocaine. In M. Trimble & T.G. Bolwig (Eds.), *The clinical relevance of kindling* (pp. 231-258). West Sussex, England: John Wiley and Sons.

Balster, R.L., Mansbach, R.S., & Gold, L.H. (1990). Pharmacological modification of intravenous cocaine administration. *Abst. Am. Coll. Neuropsychopharmacol. 20.*

Baptista, T., Weiss, S.R.B., & Post, R.M. (1993). Carbamazepine attenuates cocaine-induced increases in the nucleus accumbens: An in vitro dialysis study. *Europ. J. Pharmacol.,* in press.

Calogero, A.E., Gallucci, W.T., Kling, M.A., Chrousos, G.P., & Gold, P.W. (1989). Cocaine stimulates rat hypothalamic corticotropin-releasing hormone secretion *in vitro. Brain Res., 505,* 7-11.

Chasnoff, I.J., Hunt, C.E., Kletter, R., & Kaplan, D. (1989). Prenatal cocaine exposure is associated with respiratory pattern abnormalities. *Am. J. Dis. Child, 143,* 583-587.

Childress, A., Ehrman, R., McLellan, A.T., & O'Brien, C. (1988). Conditioned craving and arousal in cocaine addiction: A preliminary report. *NIDA Res. Monogr., 81,* 74-80.

Cole, B.J., Cador, M., Stinus, L., Rivier, J., Vale, W., Koob, G.F., & Le Moal, M. (1990). Central administration of a CRF antagonist blocks the development of stress-induced behavioral sensitization. *Brain Res., 512,* 343-346.

Cowdry, R.W., & Gardner, D.L. (1988). Pharmacotherapy of borderline personality disorder. *Arch. Gen. Psychiat., 111,* 119.

Derlet, R.W., & Albertson, T.E. (1989). Potentiation of cocaine toxicity with calcium channel blockers. *Am. J. Emerg. Med., 7,* 464-468.

Ellinwood, E.H. Jr., & Kilbey, M.M. (1975). Amphetamine stereotypy: The influence of environmental factors and prepotent behavioral patterns on its topography and development. *Biol. Psychiat., 10,* 2-16.

Halikas, J., Kemp, K., Kuhn, K., Carlson, G., & Creas, F. (1989). Carbamazepine for cocaine addiction? [Letter]. *Lancet, 1,* 623-624.

Halikas, J.A., & Kuhn, K.L. (1990). Reduction of cocaine use among methadone maintenance patients using concurrent carbamazepine maintenance. *Ann. Clin. Psychiat., 2,* 3-6.

Halikas, J.A., Crosby, R.D., Carlson, G.A., Crea, F., Graves, N.M., & Bowers, L.D. (1990). Double-blind cocaine reduction in unmotivated crack users: Carbamazepine versus placebo in a short term crossover design. *Abst., Am. Coll. Neuropsychopharmacol., 217.*

Hatsukami, D., Keenan, R., Halikas, J., Pentel, P.R., & Brauer, L.H. (1991). Effects of carbamazepine on acute responses to smoked cocaine-base in human cocaine users. *Psychopharmacology, 104,* 120-124.

Hubner, C.B., & Koob, G.F. (1990). Bromocriptine produces decreases in cocaine self-administration in the rat. *Neuropsychopharmacology, 3,* 101-108.

Karler, R., Calder, L.D., Chaudhry, I.A., & Turkanis, S.A. (1989). Blockade of "reverse tolerance" to cocaine and amphetamine by MK-801. *Life Sci., 45,* 599-606.

Klein, E., Uhde, T.W., & Post, R.M. (1986). Preliminary evidence for the utility of carbamazepine in alprazolam withdrawal. *Am. J. Psychiat., 143,* 235-236.

Lampe, H., & Bigalke, H. (1990). Carbamazepine blocks NMDA-activated currents in cultured spinal cord neurons. *Neuropharmacol. Neurotoxicol., 1,* 8-10.

Meyendorff, E., Lerer, B., Moore, N.C., Bow, J., & Gershon, S. (1985). Methylphenidate infusion in euthymic bipolars: Effect of carbamazepine pretreatment. *Psychiat. Res., 16,* 303.

O'Brien, C.P., Childress, A.R., Arndt, I.O., McLellan, A.T., Woody, G.E., & Maany, I. (1988). Pharmacological and behavioral treatments of cocaine dependence: Controlled studies. *J. Clin. Psychiat., 49,* 17-22.

Pettit, H.O., Ettenberg, A., Bloom, F.E., & Koob, G.F. (1984). Destruction of dopamine in the nucleus accumbens selectively attenuates cocaine but not heroin self-administration in rats. *Psychopharmacology, 84,* 167-173.

Post, R.M. (1975). Cocaine psychoses: A continuum model. *Am. J. Psychiat., 132,* 225-231.

Post, R.M. (1987). Mechanisms of action of carbamazepine and related anticonvulsants in affective illness. In H. Meltzer & W.E. Bunney, Jr. (Eds.), *Psychopharmacology: A generation of progress* (pp. 567-576). New York: Raven Press.

Post, R.M. (1988). Time course of clinical effects of carbamazepine: Implications for mechanisms of action. *J. Clin. Psychiat., 49,* 35-46.

Post, R.M. (1990). Prophylaxis of bipolar affective disorders. *Int. Rev. Psychiat., 2,* 165-208.

Post, R.M., & Kopanda, R.T. (1975). Cocaine, kindling, and reverse tolerance. *Lancet, 1,* 409-410.

Post, R.M., & Weiss, S.R.B. (1988). Psychomotor stimulant versus local anesthetic effects of cocaine: Role of behavioral sensitization and kindling. *NIDA Res. Monogr., 88,* 217-238.

Post, R.M., & Weiss, S.R.B. (1989). Sensitization, kindling, and anticonvulsants in mania. *J. Clin. Psychiat. 50*(12), 23-30.

Post, R.M., Kotin, J., & Goodwin, F.K. (1974). Effects of cocaine in depressed patients. *Am. J. Psychiat., 131,* 511-517.

Post, R.M., Kopanda, R.T., & Lee, A. (1975). Progressive behavioral changes during chronic lidocaine administration: Relationship to kindling. *Life Sci., 17,* 943-950.

Post, R.M., Kopanda, R.T., & Black, K.E. (1976). Progressive effects of cocaine on behavior and central amine metabolism in rhesus monkeys: Relationship to kindling and psychosis. *Biol. Psychiat., 11,* 403-419.

Post, R.M., Lockfeld, A., Squillace, K.M., & Contel, N.R. (1981). Drug-environment interaction: Context dependency of cocaine-induced behavioral sensitization. *Life Sci., 28,* 755-760.

Post, R.M., Ballenger, J.C., Uhde, T.W., & Bunney, W.E., Jr. (1984a). Efficacy of carbamazepine in manic-depressive illness: Implications for underlying mechanisms. In R.M. Post & J.C. Ballenger (Eds.), *Neurobiology of mood disorders* (pp. 777-816). Baltimore: Williams & Wilkins.

Post, R.M., Weiss, S.R.B., & Pert, A. (1984b). Differential effects of carbamazepine and lithium on sensitization and kindling. *Prog. Neuropsychopharmacol. Biol. Psychiat., 8,* 425-434.

Post, R.M., Uhde, T.W., Roy-Byrne, P.P., & Joffe, R.T. (1986a). Antidepressant effects of carbamazepine. *Am. J. Psychiat., 143,* 29-34.

Post, R.M., Weiss, S.R.B., Szele, F., & Woodward, R. (1986b). Differential anticonvulsant effects of carbamazepine as a function of stage and type of kindling. *Soc. Neurosci. Abst., 374,* 1375.

Post, R.M., Uhde, T.W., Roy-Byrne, P.P., & Joffe, R.T. (1987a). Correlates of antimanic response to carbamazepine. *Psychiat. Res., 21,* 71-83.

Post, R.M., Weiss, S.R.B., Pert, A., & Uhde, T.W. (1987b). Chronic cocaine administration: Sensitization and kindling effects. In A. Raskin & S. Fisher (Eds.), *Cocaine: Clinical and biobehavioral aspects* (pp. 109-173). New York: Oxford University Press.

Post, R.M., Weiss, S.R.B., & Pert, A. (1988). Cocaine-induced behavioral sensitization and kindling: Implications for the emergence of psychopathology and seizures. In P.W. Kalivas & C.B. Nemeroff (Eds.), *Mesocorticolimbic dopamine system* (pp. 292-308). New York: New York Academy of Science.

Post, R.M., Rubinow, D.R., Uhde, T.W., Roy-Byrne, P.P., Linnoila, M., Rosoff, A., & Cowdry, R.W. (1989). Dysphoric mania: Clinical and biological correlates. *Arch. Gen. Psychiat., 46,* 353-358.

Post, R.M., Weiss, S.R.B., & Pert, A. (1991). Animal models of mania. In P. Willner & J. Scheel-Kruger (Eds.), *The mesolimbic dopamine system: From motivation to action* (pp. 443-472). Chichester, England: John Wiley & Sons Ltd.

Ries, R.K., Roy-Byrne, P.P., Ward, N.G., Neppe, V., & Cullison, S. (1989). Carbamazepine treatment for benzodiazepine withdrawal. *Am. J. Psychiat., 146,* 536-537.

Roberts, D.C.S., Koob, G.F., Klanoff, P., & Fibiger, H.C. (1980). Extinction and recovery of cocaine self-administration following 6-hydroxydopamine lesions of the nucleus accumbens. *Pharmacol. Biochem. Behav., 12,* 781-787.

Roy-Byrne, P.P. (1989). Anticonvulsants in anxiety and withdrawal syndromes: Hypotheses for future research. In H.G. Pope & S. McElroy (Eds.), *Use of anticonsulvants in psychiatry: Recent advances* (pp. 155-168). New York: Raven Press.

Sherer, M.A., Kumor, K.M., & Mapou, R.L. (1990). A case in which carbamazepine attenuated cocaine "rush: [Letter]. *Am. J. Psychiat., 147,* 950.

Trouve, R., Nahas, G.G., Manger, W.M., Vinyard, C., & Goldberg, S. (1990). Interactions of nimodipine and cocaine on endogenous catecholamines in the squirrel monkey. *Proc. Soc. Exp. Biol. Med., 193,* 171-175.

Wallace, B.C. (1989). Psychological and environmental determinants of relapse in crack cocaine smokers. *J. Subst. Abuse Treat., 6,* 95-106.

Weiss, S.R.B., Murman, D., Post, R.M., & Pert, A. (1986). Conditioning in cocaine-induced behavioral sensitization. *Soc. Neurosci. Abst., 249.*

Weiss, S.R.B., Costello, M., Woodward, R., Nutt, D.J., & Post, R.M. (1987). Chronic carbamazepine inhibits the development of cocaine-kindled seizures. *Soc. Neurosci. Abst., 262.*

Weiss, S.R.B., Post, R.M., Costello, M., Nutt, D., Tandeciarz, S., Nierenberg, J.,

Lewis, R., & Clark, M. (1989a). Carbamazepine prevents cocaine kindled seizures and lethality but does not interfere with behavioral sensitization. *Abst. Am. Coll. Neuropsychopharmacol., 236.*

Weiss, S.R.B., Post, R.M., Pert, A., Woodward, R., & Murman, D. (1989b). Context-dependent cocaine sensitization: Differential effect of haloperidol on development versus expression. *Pharmacol. Biochem. Behav., 34,* 655-661.

Weiss, S.R.B., Post, R.M., Szele, F., Woodward, R., & Nierenberg, J. (1989c). Chronic carbamazepine inhibits the development of local anesthetic seizures kindled by cocaine and lidocaine. *Brain Res., 497,* 72-79.

Weiss, S.R.B., Post, R.M., Costello, M., Nutt, D.J., & Tandeciarz, S. (1990). Carbamazepine retards the development of cocaine-kindled seizures but not sensitization to cocaine's effects on hyperactivity and stereotypy. *Neuropsychopharmacology, 3,* 273-281.

Yan, O.-S., Jobe, P.C., & Dailey, J.W. (1990). Parenteral carbamazepine: Effect on convulsions and on dialyzable hippocampal serotonin (5-HT) in genetically epilepsy-prone rats. *Soc. Neurosci. Abst., 321.*

Yan, O.-S., Mishra, P.K., Burger, R.L., Bettendorf, A.F., Jobe, P.C., & Dailey, J.W. (1992). Evidence that carbamazepine and antiepilepsirine may produce a component of their anticonvulsant effects by activating serotonergic neurons in genetically epilepsy-prone rats. *J. Pharmacol. Exp. Ther., 261,* 652-659.

Zona, C., Tancredi, V., Palma, E., Pirrone, G.C., & Avoli, M. (1990). Potassium currents in rat cortical neurons in culture are enhanced by the antiepileptic drug carbamazepine. *Can. J. Physiol. Pharmacol., 68,* 545-547.

29

Buprenorphine's Effects on Cocaine and Heroin Abuse

NANCY K. MELLO AND JACK H. MENDELSON

Cocaine abuse has increased among heroin-dependent persons, including those in methadone maintenance treatment programs (Kosten et al., 1986, 1987a & b), and reached epidemic proportions in the general population during the 1980s (Kozel & Adams, 1986). At present, there is no uniformly effective pharmacotherapy for the treatment of cocaine abuse (Gawin & Ellinwood, 1988; Kleber & Gawin, 1984). Although desipramine, a tricyclic antidepressant, reduces cocaine abuse in some patients (Gawin & Ellinwood, 1988; Gawin & Kleber, 1984; Kosten et al., 1987b), it may stimulate relapse in abstinent patients (Weiss, 1988).

Dual dependence on cocaine plus heroin is an even more difficult treatment challenge. Heroin abuse is currently treated with opiate agonists (methadone and l-α-acetylmethadol [LAAM]) and the opiate antagonist naltrexone (Blaine et al., 1981; Dole & Nyswander, 1965; Martin et al., 1973a & b; Mello et al., 1981; Meyer & Mirin, 1979). Yet, opiate agonist pharmacotherapies have not proved useful in treating combined cocaine and heroin abuse (Kosten et al., 1987a). Treatment of cocaine use by heroin abusers with methadone plus desipramine has also yielded inconsistent results (Kosten et al., 1987b; O'Brien et al., 1988). However, naltrexone was more effective than methadone in reducing cocaine abuse by patients who were dually dependent on cocaine and opiates (Kosten et al., 1989a).

Another approach to the pharmacological treatment of opioid abuse is the use of opioid mixed agonist-antagonist drugs, such as buprenorphine. Buprenorphine is a powerful analgesic with minimal capacity to induce physical dependence (Houde, 1979; Jaffe & Martin, 1990; Martin, 1979). Yet, it can antagonize the physiological and subjective effects of high doses of morphine (60 to 120 mg/day) for up to 29.5 hours (Jasinski et al., 1978). Buprenorphine is an oripavine derivative of thebaine and a congener of etorphine, a potent opioid agonist, and diprenorphine, an opioid antagonist (Lewis, 1974). The basic phar-

This work is supported in part by grants from the NIDA (DA 00101, DA 00064, DA 04059, DA 02519, and DA 06116).

macology of buprenorphine has been described elsewhere (Cowan et al., 1977a & b; Lewis et al., 1983). Clinical studies suggest that buprenorphine is potentially useful for the treatment of opioid dependence (Fudala et al., 1990; Mello & Mendelson, 1980, 1985; Mello et al., 1982). Recent studies in the primate model of drug abuse suggest that buprenorphine also may be useful for the treatment of cocaine abuse (Mello et al., 1989, 1990a).

This chapter first reviews studies of the effects of buprenorphine on cocaine self-administration in the primate model. The degree of concordance between findings from these preclinical studies and recent outpatient clinical trials of buprenorphine treatment is discussed. The implications of these data for using primate drug self-administration models to evaluate the effectiveness of new pharmacotherapies are examined. Possible neurobehavioral and pharmacological mechanisms underlying buprenorphine's reduction of cocaine self-administration are described. A more complete discussion of the behavioral pharmacology of buprenorphine appears in Mello and Mendelson (1985, 1992).

PRECLINICAL EVALUATION OF NEW PHARMACOTHERAPIES FOR DRUG ABUSE TREATMENT

Primates will self-administer most drugs that are self-administered by humans; consequently this model has proved valuable for the prediction of drug abuse liability (Brady & Lukas, 1984; Griffiths & Balster, 1979; Thompson & Unna, 1977). Animal models of drug self-administration also can be used to evaluate the potential efficacy of new pharmacotherapies for treatment of drug abuse (Mello, 1991). If medications that significantly reduce drug self-administration in monkeys also prove to be effective in human drug abusers, this could facilitate the rapid identification of promising new pharmacotherapies for the treatment of drug abuse. Concordant findings from preclinical evaluations and clinical studies would significantly reduce the time required to introduce new medications into clinical trials. In the series of studies to be described, the discovery that buprenorphine could reduce cocaine self-administration was based on this primate model (Mello et al., 1989, 1990a). Clinical evaluations of the generality of this observation are now ongoing (Gastfriend et al., 1991; Mendelson et al., 1991) and are described later in this chapter.

BUPRENORPHINE'S EFFECTS ON COCAINE AND FOOD SELF-ADMINISTRATION: PRIMATE STUDIES

In 1989, we examined the effects of daily buprenorphine treatment on cocaine self-administration by five rhesus monkeys (Mello et al., 1989). Two male and three female adult rhesus monkeys with a 262 ± 79 day history of cocaine self-administration were studied. Each monkey was surgically implanted with a double lumen silicon® rubber intravenous catheter under aseptic conditions to permit administration of buprenorphine or saline during cocaine self-administration. The intravenous catheter was protected by a custom-designed tether system that permits monkeys to move freely. Monkeys worked for food (1 g banana pellets) and for intravenous cocaine (0.05 or 0.10 mg/kg/injection) on an FR4 (VR 16:S) operant schedule of reinforcement. An average of 64 responses was required for each food pellet or cocaine injection. Food and cocaine each were available during four 1-hour sessions each day. Food sessions began at 11 A.M., 3 P.M., 7 P.M., and 7 A.M. Cocaine sessions began at 12 noon, 4 P.M., 8 P.M., and 8 A.M. Each food or drug session lasted 1 hour or until 20 drug injections or 65 food pellets were delivered. The total number of cocaine injections was limited to 80 per day to minimize the possibility of adverse drug effects. The nutritionally fortified banana pellet diet was supplemented with fresh fruit, vegetables, biscuits, and multiple vitamins each day.

Daily treatment with buprenorphine (or an equal volume of saline control solution) was administered each day beginning at 9:30 A.M. Buprenorphine and saline were gradually infused at a rate of 1 ml solution every 12 minutes and flushed through the catheter with sterile saline in a volume that exceeded the catheter dead space. Buprenorphine was administered at two doses (0.40 and 0.70 mg/kg/day) that effectively suppressed opiate self-administration in our previous studies in the primate model (Mello et al., 1983). Each dose of buprenorphine and saline was studied for 15 consecutive days (60 sessions). Buprenorphine treatment was abruptly discontinued after 30 days, and daily saline treatment was resumed.

Cocaine Self-Administration During Buprenorphine and Saline Maintenance Treatment

Cocaine and food self-administration during 15 days of baseline saline treatment and six successive 5-day periods of buprenorphine treatment are shown in Figure 29-1. Each of the five monkeys self-administered relatively high doses of cocaine during baseline saline treatment (2.1 to 4 mg/kg/day; group average of 3.07 ± 0.17 mg/kg/day). This dose of cocaine is comparable to that often reported by cocaine abusers; 1 to 2 grams of cocaine per week is equivalent to 2.04 to 4.08 mg/kg/day in a 70-kg man (Mendelson et al., 1988). All monkeys reduced cocaine self-administration during buprenorphine treatment ($P < 0.0001$). During the first 5 days of buprenorphine treatment, average cocaine self-administration decreased by 49% to an average dose of 1.60 ± 0.25 mg/kg/day ($P < 0.01$). Average cocaine self-administration fell to 77% and 83% below baseline during days 6 to 10 and 11 to 15 of buprenorphine treatment, respectively. During 15 days of buprenorphine treatment at 0.40 mg/kg/day, cocaine self-administration averaged 0.98 ± 0.11 mg/kg/day (Mello et al., 1989).

During the second 15 days of buprenorphine treatment at a higher dose (0.70 mg/kg/day), cocaine self-administration decreased to between 91 and 97% below baseline levels (Fig. 29-1). Monkeys self-administered an average of 0.19 ± 0.03 mg/kg/day of cocaine. Analysis of data from individual subjects showed that both the time course and degree of buprenorphine's suppression of cocaine-maintained responding were equivalent in animals that self-administered relatively high (4 mg/kg/day) and low (2.1 mg/kg/day) doses of cocaine during the saline baseline treatment period (Mello et al., 1989).

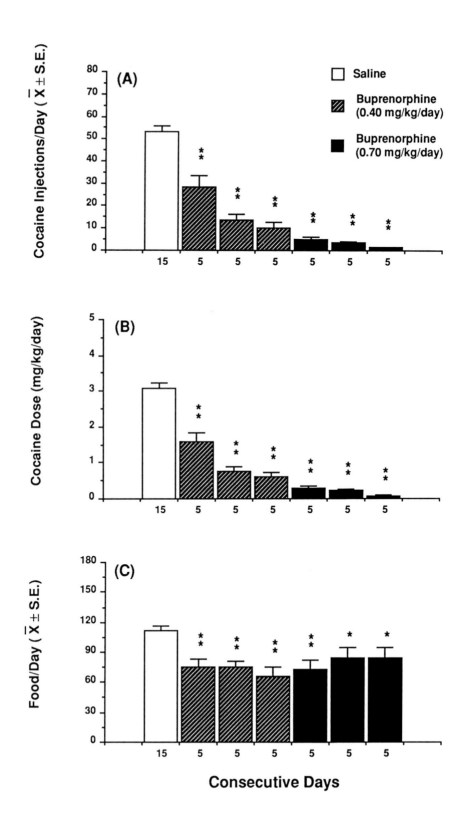

After the abrupt cessation of 30 days of buprenorphine treatment, cocaine-maintained responding remained suppressed for at least 15 days in all animals. Individual monkeys returned to baseline levels of cocaine self-administration at different rates ranging from 15 to 58 days (mean: 30.5 ± 10 days). The prolonged suppression of cocaine self-administration after the termination of buprenorphine treatment in primates is comparable to clinical reports of delayed onset of buprenorphine withdrawal signs and symptoms. For example, peak abstinence signs and symptoms occurred within 15 to 21 days after the abrupt cessation of 54 days of buprenorphine (8 mg/day, s.c.) treatment (Jasinski et al., 1978). After 36 days of sublingual buprenorphine treatment (8 mg/day), mild withdrawal symptoms were reported within 3 to 5 days after the last dose of buprenorphine (Fudala et al., 1989). This sublingual buprenorphine dose is equivalent to 5.3 mg s.c. (R.E. Johnson, personal communication). Differences in the effective dose of buprenorphine and the duration of treatment, as well as the measures of withdrawal, may account for the differences between the two studies (Fudala et al., 1989; Jasinski et al., 1978). The delay (days or weeks) in the appearance of mild buprenorphine withdrawal signs and symptoms probably reflects the slow dissociation of buprenorphine from the opiate receptor (Lewis et al., 1983). Moreover, studies of buprenorphine kinetics in rhesus monkey have shown that multiple doses (1.0 mg/kg every 6 hours) over 4 weeks increase the biological half-life of buprenorphine threefold in comparison to a single 1.0 mg/kg/s.c. injection (Numata et al., 1981).

Food Self-Administration During Buprenorphine and Saline Maintenance Treatment

Food-maintained responding was also suppressed by 31% during the first 15 days of buprenorphine treatment (0.40 mg/kg/day) (Fig. 29-1). During the second 15 days of treatment with a higher dose of buprenorphine (0.70 mg/kg/day), food self-administration gradually recovered to average 20% below baseline. Although these changes in food-maintained responding were statistically significant ($P < 0.05$ to 0.01), it is unlikely that they were biologically significant. There were no correlated changes in body weight, and animals continued to eat daily fruit and vegetable supplements. Four of five animals returned to baseline levels of food-maintained operant responding within 3 to 7 days after cessation of buprenorphine treatment (mean: 8.5 ± 2.9 days).

← ——————————————————————————————

Figure 29-1. Buprenorphine suppresses cocaine self-administration. The effects of single daily infusions of buprenorphine or a saline control solution on cocaine and food self-administration. Saline treatment is shown as an open bar and buprenorphine treatment as a striped bar (0.40 mg/kg/day) and a solid bar (0.70 mg/kg/day). The number of days that each treatment condition was in effect is shown on the abscissa. Each data point is the mean ± SEM of five subjects. **(A)** Average number of cocaine injections self-administered. **(B)** Average dose of cocaine (mg/kg/day) self-administered. **(C)** Average number of food pellets self-administered. The statistical significance of each change from the saline treatment as determined by the analysis of variance for repeated measures, and Dunnett's tests for multiple comparisons are shown by an asterisk (*$P < 0.05$; **$P < 0.01$). (From Mello et al., 1989, with permission.)

Analysis of the pattern of food self-administration by individual monkeys indicated that buprenorphine treatment did not change the overall daily distribution of sessions in comparison to saline treatment. For example, food intake during the first session at 11 A.M. after buprenorphine treatment (9:30 to 10:30 A.M.) was not suppressed in comparison to saline treatment. Moreover, there were no consistent buprenorphine dose effects on patterns of food self-administration. Animals did not appear sedated during buprenorphine treatment, and activity levels were normal. We conclude that buprenorphine treatment suppressed cocaine-maintained responding, but did not produce a generalized suppression of behavior.

Comparison of Buprenorphine's and Naltrexone's Effects on Cocaine and Food Self-Administration

During 1990, we extended our studies of buprenorphine's effects on cocaine- and food-maintained responding to evaluate the effects of a lower buprenorphine dose (0.237 mg/kg/day). We also compared the effects of buprenorphine and the opioid antagonist, naltrexone, on cocaine and food self-administration (Mello et al., 1990a).

This low dose of buprenorphine also significantly suppressed cocaine-maintained responding by 86%, whereas food-maintained responding was suppressed by an average of 34%. Moreover, buprenorphine rapidly reduced cocaine self-administration in all monkeys. Figure 29-2 shows the initial effects of buprenorphine (0.237 and 0.40 mg/kg/day) on daily cocaine self-administration for six individual monkeys. The lower dose of buprenorphine (0.237 mg/kg/day) suppressed cocaine self-administration by 49 to 96% in five monkeys on the first day of treatment. By the second day of treatment, cocaine self-administration fell to 50% or more below baseline in all monkeys. The higher dose of buprenorphine (0.40 mg/kg/day) reduced cocaine self-administration by 50 to 95% in five monkeys on the first day of treatment. The second day of buprenorphine treatment (0.40 mg/kg/day) suppressed cocaine self-administration by 64 to 100% in five monkeys, and one monkey (679C) decreased cocaine self-administration by 50% after 6 days. Cocaine-maintained responding remained 40 to 100% below baseline with three exceptions. On one day, two monkeys (CH-61 and 199C) increased cocaine self-administration to 12 and 22% below baseline, and one monkey (CH-84) exceeded the baseline level by 46% (Fig. 29-2).

Tolerance Does Not Develop to Daily Buprenorphine Treatment

In subsequent studies, we examined whether tolerance develops to the suppressive effects of buprenorphine on cocaine self-administration. Our preliminary findings suggest that tolerance does not develop to the effects of daily treatment with buprenorphine (0.32 mg/kg) on cocaine self-administration over 1 to 4 months. Cocaine self-administration remained suppressed by over 80%. Although food self-administration was suppressed initially, it gradually returned to baseline levels. These data indicate that buprenorphine's effects on cocaine self-administration may not diminish during chronic treatment (Mello et al., 1992).

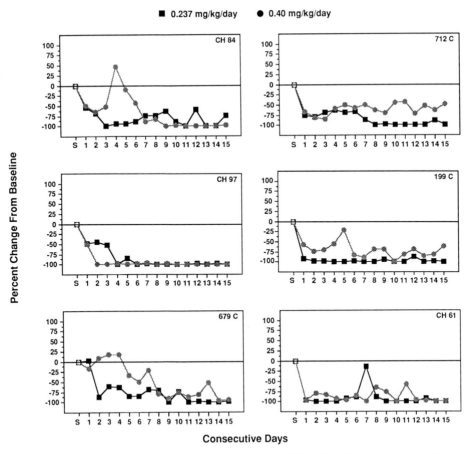

Figure 29-2. Rate of buprenorphine's (0.237 and 0.40 mg/kg/day) suppression of cocaine self-administration by individual monkeys. Data are shown as the percentage of change in cocaine injections from the saline treatment baseline. Saline control treatment (S) and the first 15 days of buprenorphine treatment are shown on the abscissa. Percentage of change from the average number of cocaine injections self-administered during saline treatment (S) is shown on the ordinate. Buprenorphine doses are shown as (*square*) (0.237 mg/kg/day) and (*circle*) (0.40 mg/kg/day). (From Mello et al., 1990a, with permission.)

BUPRENORPHINE'S EFFECTS ON COCAINE AND HEROIN ABUSE: CLINICAL STUDIES

These primate data suggest that buprenorphine may be potentially valuable for the clinical treatment of cocaine abuse and dual addiction to cocaine and heroin because it also suppresses heroin use by heroin abusers (Mello & Mendelson, 1980; Mello et al., 1982). The results of the first open clinical trial of buprenorphine treatment are consistent with the hypothesis that buprenorphine may be efficacious for the reduction of cocaine abuse, as well as heroin abuse (Kosten et al., 1989a). Opioid-dependent patients treated with daily sublingual doses of buprenorphine for 1 month (average: 3.2 mg/day; range: 2 to 8 mg) had significantly fewer cocaine-positive urines than patients treated with methadone (Kosten et al., 1989a & b). In 1990, we began an open trial of the effects of buprenorphine treatment on men with dual cocaine and heroin dependence, and the results thus far are very encouraging (Gastfriend et al., 1991; Mendelson et al., 1991). The trial consisted of a 30-day inpatient phase and a 26-week outpatient phase as described below.

Inpatient Buprenorphine Treatment Program

Men with concurrent opiate and cocaine dependence according to DSM-III-R diagnostic criteria were admitted to the NIDA-supported Treatment Research Unit (TRU) of the Alcohol and Drug Abuse Research Center at McLean Hospital-Harvard Medical School. After methadone detoxification, patients remained on the clinical research ward for 30 days. The first 9 days after detoxification were drug-free. Then patients were given ascending doses of sublingual buprenorphine (1, 2, 4, 6, 8 mg/day) over 5 days. Patients were randomly assigned to a chronic maintenance dose of 4 or 8 mg/day of buprenorphine. The maintenance dose was administered for 16 days until discharge to the outpatient program of the TRU. Patients could elect to remain on their maintenance dose of buprenorphine (4 or 8 mg/day) or transfer to a naltrexone or methadone maintenance clinic or drug-free treatment program.

During the 30-day inpatient phase of this open trial of buprenorphine, studies were undertaken to evaluate the safety and effectiveness of buprenorphine for the treatment of persons with dual intravenous heroin and cocaine dependence (Mendelson et al., 1991). A challenge dose of intravenous morphine (10 mg), cocaine (30 mg), or placebo was administered before and during buprenorphine maintenance. Cardiovascular function, vital signs, and subjective responses were measured.

No significant adverse effects were observed during buprenorphine induction or maintenance. Mild systolic hypotensive episodes were occasionally observed, but no significant systolic or diastolic hypotension occurred. There were occasional reports of nausea or constipation, but no significant changes in dietary or bowel habits were noted. During challenge dose studies, buprenorphine did not significantly accentuate or diminish pulse, blood pressure, or respiration responses after administration of the challenge drug. No adverse effects on cardiovascular function or electrocardiograms (EKGs) were observed when challenge doses were administered during buprenorphine maintenance (Mendelson et al., 1991). These findings confirm and extend our previous observations of buprenorphine's effects in heroin-dependent men (Mello & Mendelson, 1980; Mello et al., 1982).

Outpatient Buprenorphine Treatment Program

The TRU Outpatient Clinic is located at the Massachusetts General Hospital in the center of Boston. The clinic is open 7 days each week. Our outpatient studies of the effects of buprenorphine maintenance treatment on cocaine and heroin abuse are just beginning. Preliminary observations on the first six patients studied over the first 12 weeks of buprenorphine maintenance are summarized here. These men reported a 6.3-year history of *daily* intravenous cocaine use (range: 4 to 15 years) and an 8.7-year history of *daily* intravenous heroin use (range: 1-15 years). Three men also reported current use of benzodiazepines, and two of these men also used marijuana. Drug use history was verified by two or more cocaine- and opiate-positive urines before admission to the treatment unit. All men were tobacco smokers, and four reported the past use of hallucinogens. The mean age of this group was 36 (range: 31 to 42). All were unemployed at the beginning of the study. Five men were skilled laborers (carpenter, roofer), and one was a computer technician. All had failed in previous drug abuse treatment programs.

Four patients were randomly assigned to 4 mg/day of sublingual buprenorphine, but this dose was reduced to 2 mg/day in one man because of hypotensive side effects. When corrected for body weight, the actual dose of 2 mg/day of buprenorphine was 0.027 mg/kg/day. The actual buprenorphine doses of 4 mg/day were 0.044 to 0.060 mg/kg/day. Two patients were randomly assigned to 8 mg/day of buprenorphine, and their actual doses were 0.099 and 0.128 mg/kg/day. These doses were considerably lower than those that effectively reduced cocaine self-administration by monkeys (0.237 to 0.70 mg/kg/day) (Mello et al., 1989, 1990a).

Figure 29-3 summarizes group data from four men maintained on 2-4 mg/day of sublingual buprenorphine for 12 weeks. Data are expressed as the percent of total possible days attended and as the percent of the total number of urines collected that were positive for opiates, cocaine, and other drugs. Urines for drug screens were collected at least once a week and no more than three times a week. Urine collections were scheduled to be unpredictable.

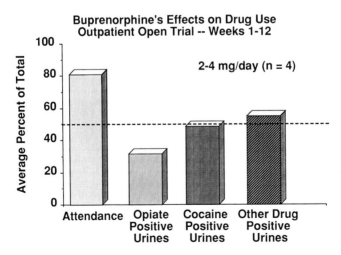

Figure 29-3. Effects of buprenorphine treatment (2-4 mg/day sublingual) on drug abuse. The average of total possible days attended over 12 weeks is shown at the left. The average numbers of the total urine drug screens that were positive for opiates, cocaine, and other drugs are shown in columns 2 through 4. Each point is the average of data from four men who reported daily intravenous use of cocaine and heroin before treatment.

Clinic attendance was high (81%). Only 32% of the urines collected were positive for opiates, and 49% of the urines collected were positive for cocaine. Since these men had a long history of *daily* intravenous use of both drugs, this means that opiate use was reduced by 68% and cocaine use by 51%. Other drug use was primarily accounted for by benzodiazepine abuse and occasional marijuana use. This pattern of polydrug use was consistent with each man's reported history of drug abuse.

The higher dose of buprenorphine (8 mg/day) has been less effective than the 4 mg/day dose in the two subjects studied thus far. Attendance at the clinic was lower (60%), and drug use was higher. Sixty percent of the urines collected were positive for opiates, and 69% were positive for cocaine. Consequently, daily opiate abuse was reduced by 40% and daily cocaine abuse by 31%.

These preliminary data confirm previous findings that buprenorphine reduces opiate self-administration by humans (Mello & Mendelson, 1980; Mello et al., 1982). These data are also concordant with our findings in monkeys that buprenorphine reduces cocaine self-administration (Mello et al., 1989, 1990a). In addition, these findings are consistent with a 30-day outpatient trial of buprenorphine treatment (Kosten et al., 1989a & b). Opiate-dependent patients treated with buprenorphine (average: 3.2 mg/day; range: 2 to 8 mg) had significantly fewer cocaine-positive urines than patients treated with methadone (Kosten et al., 1989a & b).

Pharmacotherapy: What is the Goal?

It is obvious that buprenorphine does not eliminate cocaine and heroin abuse, and it is unlikely that any pharmacotherapy will reduce drug abuse by 100%. Continued use of multiple drugs is common among patients in treatment for drug abuse problems (Kreek, 1987). Yet, during the *relatively* drug-free interval associated with pharmacotherapeutic treatment, the drug abuser is likely to be more receptive to counseling, psychotherapy, job skills training, social service interventions, and the entire armamentarium of the helping professions. In our ongoing outpatient study, cocaine-positive urines were reduced by an average of 31 to 51% compared to the reported pretreatment baseline of *daily* use (100% cocaine-positive urines). Since any reduction in intravenous drug use concomitantly reduces the risk for HIV infection associated with needle sharing, buprenorphine treatment has had a significant positive impact in these patients.

If a medication produced a 30 to 50% reduction in anginal pain or degree of hypertension or in malignant tumor growth, it would be considered highly effective. It is important to maintain this perspective in evaluating the efficacy of pharmacotherapies that reduce drug abuse. In this context, a decrease in daily i.v. cocaine abuse by 31 to 51% is a signifiant change in behavior. If buprenorphine treatment reduces dual cocaine and heroin abuse, the potential benefits to society in terms of reduction of drug abuse problems and the associated risk for HIV infection are incalculable.

Preclinical Evaluation of New Medications for Drug Abuse Treatment

The concordance of data from clinical trials and the primate model of drug self-administration illustrates the potential of this preclinical model for *predicting* the effectiveness of new medications. On the basis of data accumulated thus far on the treatment of opioid and cocaine abuse, there is reason to believe that pharmacotherapies that are maximally effective in suppressing drug self-administration in the primate model are likely to be effective in clinical trials (for review, see Mello, 1991). However, studies of a wider range of new medications with both retrospective and predictive validation with clinical data will be necessary to confirm or refute the hypothesis that the primate drug self-administration model should be as effective for the evaluation of new medications as it has been for the prediction of new drug abuse liability.

MECHANISMS OF BUPRENORPHINE'S SUPPRESSION OF COCAINE SELF-ADMINISTRATION

Since buprenorphine is an opioid mixed agonist-antagonist with affinity for mu receptors and cocaine is a stimulant that acts like a dopamine agonist in most systems, there is no simple explanation for buprenorphine's suppressive effects on cocaine self-administration. The possible contribution of some behavioral and pharmacological factors is described below. Some implications of the apparent interactions between dopaminergic and endogenous opioid peptide systems for drug abuse treatment medication development are also discussed.

Behavioral Interactions Between Cocaine and Buprenorphine

We initially assumed that buprenorphine reduces cocaine self-administration because it attenuates cocaine's reinforcing properties (Mello et al., 1989, 1990a). This assumption was consistent with reports by opioid-dependent men that, during buprenorphine treatment, cocaine use was followed by dysphoria, whereas during methadone treatment, cocaine use was followed by pleasant feelings and somnolence (Kosten et al., 1989b). Kosten and co-workers (1989b) reasoned that since some patients reported that simultaneous heroin + cocaine use (the speedball) decreased any dysphoric effects of cocaine alone, buprenorphine might accentuate cocaine-related dysphoria by antagonizing the effects of heroin. Yet, the pattern of drug use varies, and our patients report sequential use of cocaine first and of heroin first, as well as simultaneous heroin and cocaine use.

However, when we examined the effects of buprenorphine on response to an acute dose of cocaine alone and to an acute dose of morphine alone, both diminished and enhanced drug quality were reported by some subjects (Mendelson et al., 1991; Teoh et al., 1992). Men with a long history of dual dependence on cocaine and opiates were given a challenge dose of cocaine (30 mg i.v.) and morphine (10 mg i.v.) and placebo under double-blind conditions, before and during buprenorphine maintenance. These studies were part of a Phase I inpatient evaluation of buprenorphine safety. Our preliminary findings indicate that buprenorphine (4 and 8 mg/day) completely blocked the effects of morphine, i.e., eight subjects identified morphine as placebo during buprenorphine treatment. The effects of buprenorphine on the perception of cocaine were more complex and appeared to be buprenorphine dose-dependent.

At low doses (4 mg/day), buprenorphine diminished the intensity and quality of the cocaine challenge. But, in some patients, high doses of buprenorphine (8 mg) enhanced the quality and intensity of intravenous cocaine (Mendelson et al., 1991; Teoh et al., 1992). Only eight subjects have been studied so far (Teoh et al., 1992), and these inpatient clinical studies are still in progress.

These emerging clinical findings urge consideration of an alternative hypothesis, i.e., that buprenorphine may reduce cocaine self-administration because it enhances cocaine's reinforcing properties and less cocaine is required to produce positive effects. Some evidence in support of this hypothesis comes from recent studies in squirrel monkeys and in rats. Squirrel monkeys were trained to discriminate cocaine (0.01-1.0 mg/kg) from saline and then were given buprenorphine pretreatment. Lower doses of cocaine were discriminable from saline after buprenorphine treatment (Kamien et al., 1990). Relatively low doses of buprenorphine (0.001-0.01 mg/kg) shifted the cocaine dose-response curve threefold or more to the left. Buprenorphine (0.001-0.01 mg/kg) also potentiated the rate-increasing effects of cumulative doses of cocaine (0.03-0.3 mg/kg) on an FI 3 schedule of shock termination (Kamien et al., 1990). In a conditioned place preference paradigm (CPP), rats were restricted to opposite ends of a shuttle box after administration of saline or a drug. During test conditions, rats had access to the entire shuttle box, and the amount of time spent in the side previously associated with drug or saline administration was measured. Rats spent more time in areas where they received a combination of cocaine (1.5 mg/kg) and buprenorphine (0.01 mg/kg), whereas the same doses of each drug alone failed to elicit CPP (Brown et al., 1991). Higher doses of cocaine (5.0 mg/kg) and buprenorphine (0.075 mg/kg) alone each elicited CPP, but in combination, these drug doses resulted in a longer time spent in the drug compartment of the shuttle box. The possible effects of buprenorphine and cocaine combinations on general activity were not discussed. It was concluded that cocaine and buprenorphine interacted synergistically to elicit CPP, which suggests that buprenorphine may enhance rather than attenuate cocaine's reinforcing properties (Brown et al., 1991). However, it seems unlikely that the reinforcement *enhancement* hypothesis can account for buprenorphine's effects on cocaine self-administration in monkey because monkeys often took no cocaine injections during buprenorphine treatment (see Fig. 29-2; Mello et al., 1990a). A more plausible hypothesis is that buprenorphine may *substitute* for cocaine, perhaps through its dopamine agonist effects. Further clinical and animal studies will be required to clarify buprenorphine's behavioral effects on cocaine self-administration.

Pharmacological Bases of Buprenorphine's Effects on Cocaine Self-Administration

The relative contribution of buprenorphine's opioid agonist and antagonist components to its effects on cocaine's reinforcing properties is unknown. Clinical and primate studies of opioid *agonist* and opioid *antagonist* effects on cocaine self-administration are inconsistent. Neither agonists nor antagonists alone have been as effective as buprenorphine in reducing cocaine self-administration. Consequently, buprenorphine's *combined opioid agonist-antagonist* effects probably are critical for its suppression of cocaine self-administration.

Treatment with the opioid *agonist* methadone did not reduce cocaine-positive urines in heroin-dependent patients (Kosten et al., 1987a, 1989a), but morphine pretreatment suppressed cocaine self-administration in a dose-dependent manner in squirrel monkeys (Stretch, 1977). Clinical and preclinical studies of the effects of opioid *antagonists* on cocaine self-administration have also yielded conflicting results. There is considerable evidence that opioid antagonists, such as naloxone and naltrexone, do not suppress cocaine self-administration in primates or in rodents (Carroll et al., 1986; Ettenberg et al., 1982; Goldberg et al., 1971; Killian et al., 1978; Woods & Schuster, 1972). In rats, naltrexone pretreatment resulted in no change in cocaine self-administration (Ettenberg et al., 1982) or an increase in cocaine self-administration (Carroll et al., 1986). However, in contrast to these studies of opioid antagonist effects on cocaine self-administration in preclinical models, there is one clinical report that naltrexone treatment (100 to 150 mg, three times per week) of opiate-dependent polydrug abusers reduced cocaine-positive urines significantly in comparison to methadone treatment (Kosten et al., 1989a).

We re-examined the effects of *naltrexone* on cocaine- and food-maintained responding in the primate model (Mello et al., 1990a). Naltrexone treatment also reduced cocaine self-administration significantly but to a lesser degree than buprenorphine across the dose range studied. Naltrexone (0.32 mg/kg/day) initially suppressed cocaine self-administration by an average of 28% over 15 days ($P < .0009$). During high-dose naltrexone treatment (3.20 mg/kg/day), cocaine-maintained responding was suppressed by 25% over 15 days ($P < .01$). Cocaine self-administration was not significantly changed by naltrexone in one of the five subjects. Food self-administration decreased by 24% ($P < .05$) after 5 days of 0.32 mg/kg of naltrexone treatment and then exceeded baseline levels during 3.20 mg/kg of naltrexone treatment. These data are shown in Figure 29-4 (Mello et al., 1990a).

Since naltrexone reduced cocaine self-administration by 25 to 28% in monkeys (Mello et al., 1990a) and in opiate- and cocaine-dependent patients (Kosten et al., 1989a), this finding suggests the importance of the antagonist component of buprenorphine in decreasing cocaine use. The long-acting antagonists, naltrexone and diprenorphine (the antagonist constituent of buprenorphine), have a similar duration of action, and both exert antagonist effects at the mu receptor (Jaffe & Martin, 1990). Diprenorphine antagonizes the analgesic actions of buprenorphine (Lewis, 1974).

There is compelling physiological and behavioral evidence that buprenorphine has *kappa antagonist* effects, as well as mu partial agonist and antagonist properties. For example, buprenorphine antagonized the diuretic effects of a kappa agonist bremazocine (Leander, 1987; Richards & Sadee, 1985) and precipitated withdrawal in kappa agonist-dependent monkeys (Gmerek et al., 1987). Buprenorphine also antagonized the effects of a selective kappa agonist (U50, 488) in both a drug discrimination and a shock titration procedure in squirrel monkeys (Negus & Dykstra, 1988; Negus et al., 1991a). However, buprenorphine did not substitute for a selective kappa agonist (U50,

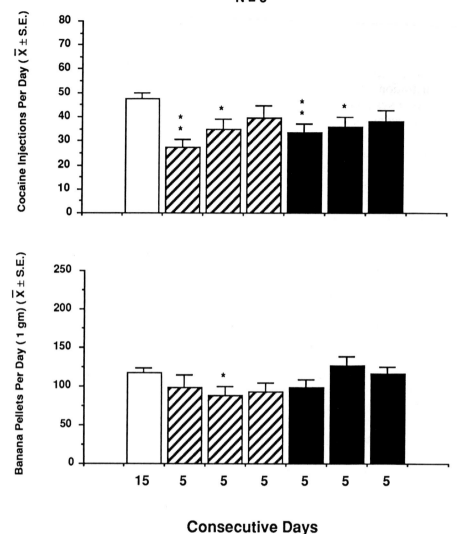

Figure 29-4. Effects of single daily infusions of naltrexone or a saline control solution on cocaine and food self-administration. Saline treatment is shown as an open square and naltrexone treatment as a striped square (0.32 mg/kg/day) and as a closed square (3.20 mg/kg/day). The number of days that each treatment condition was in effect is shown on the abscissa. Each data point is the mean ± SEM of five monkeys. The number of cocaine injections self-administered is shown in the first row. The average number of food pellets self-administered is shown in the second row. The statistical significance of each change from the saline treatment as determined by ANOVA for repeated measures and Dunnett's tests for multiple comparisons is shown by an asterisk (*$P < 0.05$; **$P < 0.01$). □ Saline, ▨ naltrexone (0.32 mg/kg/day), ■ naltrexone (3.20 mg/kg/day). (From Mello et al., 1990a, with permission.)

488) in a drug discrimination procedure, which suggests that it does not have kappa agonist-like properties in that paradigm (Negus et al., 1991a). Similarly, in rats, buprenorphine pretreatment produced dose-dependent antagonism of the discriminative stimulus properties of the kappa agonist U50, 488 (Negus et al., 1991). These data raise the intriguing possibility that buprenorphine's kappa antagonist effects may contribute to its suppressive effects on cocaine self-administration. However, direct evaluation of that hypothesis awaits the availability of a systemically active selective kappa antagonist.

Our recent studies of other opioid mixed agonist-antagonists with a different profile of opiate receptor affinities indicates that these substances affect cocaine self-administration differently than buprenorphine. For example, nalbuphine is an analgesic with kappa agonist and mu antagonist effects. Although nalbuphine also decreases cocaine self-administration, the effect is not selective. Food self-administration was also significantly reduced at nalbuphine doses that decreased cocaine self-administration by rhesus monkeys (Mello et al, 1992).

Dopamine-Endogenous Opioid System Interactions

The mechanisms by which buprenorphine, an opioid mixed agonist-antagonist, and naltrexone, an opioid antagonist, reduce cocaine self-administration are unknown (Figs. 29-1 to 29-4). The reinforcing and discriminative stimulus effects of cocaine are modulated by dopaminergic neural systems (Dackis & Gold, 1985; Fischman, 1987; Kleven et al., 1988; Kuhar et al., 1988; Ritz et al., 1987; Woolverton, 1986; Woolverton & Virus, 1989; Woolverton et al., 1984). Buprenorphine's attenuation of cocaine's reinforcing properties suggests that it may affect dopaminergic neural systems, as well as endogenous opioid systems. This interpretation is consistent with data indicating co-modulatory interactions between endogenous opioid and dopaminergic systems in brain (for review, see Koob & Bloom, 1988; Watson et al., 1988; Yen, 1986).

There is evidence of dopamine and endogenous opioid interactions from neuroendocrine (Kuljis & Advis, 1989; Mello et al., 1990b & c; Mendelson et al., 1986), neuropharmacological (Brown et al., 1991; DiChiara & Imperato, 1988; Hammer, 1989; Ishizuka et al., 1988), and behavioral studies (Blumberg and Ikeda, 1978; Bozarth & Wise, 1981; Kiritsy-Roy et al., 1989; Shippenberg & Herz, 1987). It is intriguing that in rats, chronic cocaine exposure increased opiate receptor density in lateral hypothalamus and other areas thought to be associated with "reward" (Hammer, 1989). Some studies suggest that both cocaine and opioids stimulate increased release of dopamine and activate D_1 receptors in brain (Herz & Shippenberg, 1988). In vivo microdialysis studies in rats (n = 4) showed that both buprenorphine (0.01 mg/kg, i.p.) and cocaine (5.0 mg/kg, i.p.) increased extracellular dopamine in the nucleus accumbens by 100% and 82%, respectively (Brown et al., 1991). Dopamine levels increased rapidly to a peak within 20 minutes after cocaine, then gradually returned to baseline within 120 to 160 minutes. In contrast, buprenorphine administration was followed by a gradual increase in dopamine over 300 minutes. When the same doses of cocaine and buprenorphine were given in combination, dopamine levels increased by 163% within 20 minutes, i.e., a time course similar to that of cocaine alone (Brown et al., 1991).

Neurochemical evidence that buprenorphine can accentuate cocaine-stimulated increases in extracellular dopamine (Brown et al., 1991) is consistent with the hypothesis described earlier that buprenorphine may enhance rather than decrease cocaine's reinforcing properties and therefore decrease cocaine self-administration. Alternatively, stimulation of increased dopamine by buprenorphine alone (Brown et al., 1991) suggests that buprenorphine may *substitute* for cocaine insofar as it also acts like a dopamine agonist. The possible contribution of species differences in the distribution of opioid receptor subtypes to these divergent interpretations of behavioral data in rhesus monkeys (Mello et al., 1989, 1990a) and in rats and squirrel monkeys (Brown et al., 1991; Kamien et al., 1990) remains to be determined. The ways in which endogenous opioid and dopaminergic systems may converge to affect cocaine self-administration are unclear.

We were prompted to study buprenorphine's effects on cocaine self-administration in monkeys in part because our concurrent studies of the effects of cocaine on the neuroendocrine system focused our attention on dopaminergic-endogenous opioid interactions. We examined the effects of an acute dose of cocaine (0.4 and 0.8 mg/kg, i.v.) on basal levels of luteinizing hormone (LH), a gonadotropin that is regulated in part by endogenous opioid inhibitory control of hypothalamic LHRH (luteinizing hormone-releasing hormone) (Mello et al., 1990b). Integrated plasma samples were collected at 10-minute intervals for 40 minutes before and 110 minutes after cocaine administration from follicular phase rhesus females. Cocaine stimulated a significant increase in LH within 20 minutes, and LH remained elevated above baseline levels for 40 to 50 minutes. Group data are shown in Figure 29-5.

Cocaine also significantly decreased prolactin (PRL) below baseline levels (Fig. 29-5). Since cocaine blocks dopamine reuptake, suppression of PRL is consistent with dopaminergic inhibitory control of PRL release from the pituitary (Mello et al., 1990b). We subsequently examined cocaine's effects on anterior pituitary function using synthetic LHRH (100 mcg, i.v.) to mimic the effects of endogenous hypothalamic LHRH, which stimulates the release of pituitary gonadotropins (Mello et al., 1990c). Cocaine (0.4 mg/kg) significantly enhanced LHRH stimulation of LH in comparison to placebo-cocaine or a higher dose of cocaine (0.8 mg/kg). Again, prolactin decreased significantly after cocaine (0.4 and 0.8 mg/kg, i.v.) and LHRH administration, but LHRH alone did not change PRL levels (Mello et al., 1990c).

Cocaine's rapid and significant stimulation of LH release was unanticipated since clinical data suggest that dopamine has an inhibitory effect on LH secretion (Yen, 1986). Insofar as cocaine blocks dopamine reuptake, cocaine should inhibit rather than stimulate LH. Yet, in monkeys dopamine does not suppress basal LH levels or LHRH-stimulated LH at doses that significantly suppress PRL (Pavasuthipaisit et al., 1981; Spies et al., 1980). Our ongoing clinical studies confirm that cocaine (30 mg, i.v.) stimulates a rapid and persistent increase in LH in men with a history of concurrent cocaine and opiate abuse (Mendelson et al., 1991).

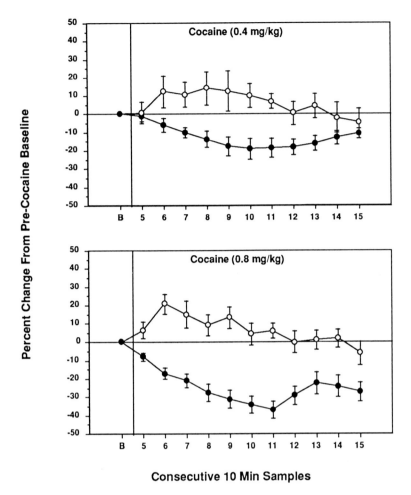

Figure 29-5. Effects of cocaine on basal PRL and LH levels. Integrated plasma samples were collected at 10-minute intervals over 150 minutes. Cocaine (0.4 or 0.8 mg/kg, i.v.) was administered after sample 4 as indicated by the vertical line. Data are expressed as change scores (Δ) from baseline levels. Each PRL data point represents the mean (± SE) of 7 monkeys. Each LH data point represents the mean (± SE) of 9 monkeys. Prolactin ●, luteinizing hormone ○. (Adapted from Mello et al., 1990b.)

Cocaine's stimulation of LH is only one line of evidence supporting the notion that neuroendocrine regulation of LH is co-modulated by both endogenous opioid and dopaminergic systems in brain (Kuljis & Advis, 1989; Yen, 1986). We reasoned that cocaine's reinforcing properties might also involve endogenous opioid peptide as well as dopaminergic regulation. A reduction in cocaine self-administration during daily treatment with the opioid mixed agonist-antagonist buprenorphine and the opioid antagonist naltrexone (Mello et al., 1989; 1990a; Kosten et al., 1989a & b) is consistent with this hypothesis. It is interesting that naltrexone also affects a neuroendocrine system that is co-modulated by dopamine and endogenous opioids. Hypothalamic secretion of endogenous LHRH is controlled by both dopamine and endogenous opioid peptides (Yen, 1986). Naltrexone's stimulation of hypothalamic release of LHRH is inferred from increases in LH (Mendelson et al., 1986; Teoh et al., 1988). Presumably, naltrexone's stimulation of LH reflects its antagonism of endogenous opioid peptide inhibition of the hypothalamic release of LHRH (Mendelson et al., 1986).

One implication of these data is that other treatment agents from the opioid class may also influence cocaine abuse. Evidence of interactions between dopaminergic and endogenous opioid peptide systems in brain may suggest new approaches to the development of pharmacotherapies for the treatment of drug abuse. The convergence of behavioral and clinical data on buprenorphine's effects on cocaine abuse underscores the potential value of the primate drug self-administration model for evaluation of new pharmacotherapies under controlled conditions (Mello, 1991).

ACKNOWLEDGMENTS

We are indebted to our colleagues who made many important contributions to this research program. We especially thank Scott E. Lukas, Ph.D., Jonathan B. Kamien, Ph.D., John Drieze, M.S., and Mark P. Bree from the Behavioral Science Laboratory and David Gastfriend, M.D., Siew Koon Teoh, M.D., Pradit Sintavanarong, M.D., M.P.H., and John Kuehnle, M.D. from the Clinical Research and Treatment Program of the Alcohol and Drug Abuse Research Center, McLean Hospital-Harvard Medical School. We are grateful to Lynne G. Wighton for assistance in data analysis and graphic displays and to Loretta Carvelli for preparation of the manuscript.

REFERENCES

Blaine, J.B., Renault, P., Thomas, D.B., & Whysner, J.A. (1981). Clinical status of methadyl acetate (LAAM). *Ann. N.Y. Acad. Sci., 362,* 101-115.

Blumberg, H., & Ikeda, C. (1978). Naltrexone, morphine and cocaine interactions in mice and rats. *J. Pharmacol. Exp. Ther., 206*(2), 303-310.

Bozarth, M.A., & Wise, R.A. (1981). Heroin reward is dependent on a dopaminergic substrate. *Life Sci., 29,* 1881-1886.

Brady, J.V., & Lukas, S.E. (Eds.). (1984). Testing drugs for physical dependence potential and abuse liability. *NIDA Res. Monogr., 52,* 153.

Brown, E.E., Finlay, J.M., Wong, J.T.F., Damsa, G., & Fibiger, H. (1991). Behavioral and neurochemical interactions between cocaine and buprenorphine: Implications for the pharmacotherapy of cocaine abuse. *J. Pharmacol. Exp. Ther., 256*(1), 119-126.

Carroll, M.E., Lac, S.T., Walker, M.J., Kragh, R., & Newman, T. (1986). Effects of naltrexone on intravenous cocaine self-administration in rats during food satiation and deprivation. *J. Pharmacol. Exp. Ther., 238,* 1-7.

Cowan, A., Doxey, J.C., & Harry, E.J.R. (1977a). The animal pharmacology of buprenorphine, an oripavine analgesic agent. *Br. J. Pharmacol., 60,* 547-554.

Cowan, A., Lewis, J.W., & MacFarlane, I.R. (1977b). Agonist and antagonist properties of buprenorphine, a new antinociceptive agent. *Br. J. Pharmacol., 60,* 537-545.

Dackis, C.A., & Gold, M.S. (1985). Pharmacological approaches to cocaine addiction. *J. Subst. Abuse Treat., 2*, 139-145.

DiChiara, G., & Imperato, A. (1988). Opposite effects of mu and kappa opiate agonists on dopamine release in the nucleus accumbens and in the dorsal caudate of freely moving rats. *J. Pharmacol. Exp. Ther., 244*(3), 1067-1080.

Dole, V.P., & Nyswander, M. (1965). A medical treatment for diacetylmorphine (heroin) addiction: A clinical trial with methadone hydrochloride. *JAMA, 193*, 646-650.

Ettenberg, A., Pettit, H.O., Bloom, F.E., & Koob, G.F. (1982). Heroin and cocaine intravenous self-administration in rats: Mediation by separate neural systems. *Psychopharmacology* (Berlin), *78*, 204-209.

Fischman, M.W. (1987). Cocaine and the amphetamines. In H.Y. Meltzer (Ed.). *Psychopharmacology: The third generation of progress* (pp. 1543-1553). New York: Raven Press.

Fudala, P.J., Johnson, R.E., & Bunker, E. (1989). Abrupt withdrawal of buprenorphine following chronic administration. *Clin. Pharmacol. Ther., 45*(2), 186.

Fudala, P.J., Jaffe, J.H., Dax, E.M., & Johnson, R.E. (1990). The use of buprenorphine in the treatment of opioid addiction. II. Physiologic and behavioral effects of early and alternate-day administration and abrupt withdrawal. *Clin. Pharmacol. Ther., 47*, 525-534.

Gastfriend, D.R., Mendelson, J.H., Mello, N.K., & Teoh, S.K. (1991). Preliminary results of an open trial of buprenorphine in the outpatient treatment of combined heroin and cocaine dependence. *NIDA Res. Monogr., 119*, 461.

Gawin, F.H., & Ellinwood, E.H. (1988). Cocaine and other stimulants, actions, abuse and treatment. *N. Engl. J. Med., 318*, 1173-1182.

Gawin, F.H., & Kleber, H.D. (1984). Cocaine abuse treatment: Open pilot trial with desipramine and lithium carbonate. *Arch. Gen. Psychiat., 41*, 903-909.

Gmerek, D.E., Dykstra, L.A., & Woods, J.H. (1987). Kappa opioids in rhesus monkeys. III. Dependence associated with chronic administration. *J. Pharmacol. Exp. Ther., 242*, 428-436.

Goldberg, S.R., Woods, J.H., & Schuster, C.R. (1971). Nalorphine-induced changes in morphine self-administration in rhesus monkeys. *J. Pharmacol. Exp. Ther., 176*, 464-471.

Griffiths, R.R., & Balster, R.L. (1979). Opioids: Similarity between evaluations of subjective effects and animal self-administration results. *J. Clin. Pharmacol. Ther., 25*, 611-617.

Hammer, R.P. (1989). Cocaine alters opiate receptor binding in critical brain reward regions. *Synapse, 3*, 55-60.

Herz, A., & Shippenberg, T.S. (1988). Neurochemical aspects of addiction. In A. Goldstein (Ed.), *Molecular and cellular aspects of the drug addictions* (pp. 111-140). New York: Springer-Verlag.

Houde, R.W. (1979). Analgesic effectiveness of the narcotic agonist-antagonists. *Br. J. Clin. Pharmacol., 7* (Suppl 3), 297-308.

Ishizuka, Y., Rockhold, R.W., Hoskins, B., & Ho, I.K. (1988). Cocaine-induced changes in 3H-naloxone binding in brain membranes isolated from spontaneously hypertensive and Wistar-Kyoto rats. *Life Sci., 43*, 2275-2282.

Jaffe, J.H., & Martin, W.R. (1990). Opioid analgesics and antagonists. In A.G. Gilman, T.W. Rall, A.S. Nies, & P. Taylor (Eds.), *The pharmacological basis of therapeutics*, 8th ed (pp. 485-521). New York: Pergamon Press.

Jasinski, D.R., Pevnick, J.S., & Griffith, J.D. (1978). Human pharmacology and abuse potential of the analgesic buprenorphine. *Arch. Gen. Psychiat., 35*, 601-616.

Kamien, J., Bergman, J., Madras, B.K., & Spealman, R.D. (1990). Buprenorphine potentiates behavioral effects of cocaine in squirrel monkeys. *FASEB J., 4,* A593.

Killian, A.K., Bonese, K., & Schuster, C.R. (1978). The effects of naloxone on behavior maintained by cocaine and heroin injections in the rhesus monkey. *Drug Alcohol Depend., 3,*243-251.

Kiritsy-Roy, J., Standish, S.M., & Terry, L.C. (1989). Dopamine D-1 and D-2 receptor antagonists potentiate analgesic and motor effects of morphine. *Pharmacol. Biochem. Behav., 32,* 717-721.

Kleber, H.D., & Gawin, F. H. (1984). The spectrum of cocaine abuse and its treatment. *J. Clin. Psychiat., 45*(12), 18-23.

Kleven, M.S., Anthony, E.W., Goldberg, L.I., & Woolverton, W.L. (1988). Blockage of the discriminative stimulus effects of cocaine in rhesus monkeys with the D1 dopamine antagonist Ch 23390. *Psychopharmacology* (Berlin), *95,* 427-429.

Koob, G.F., & Bloom, F.E. (1988). Cellular and molecular mechanisms of drug dependence. *Science, 242,* 715-723.

Kosten, T.R., Rounsaville, B.J., Gawin, F.H., & Kleber, H.D. (1986). Cocaine abuse among opioid addicts: Demographic and diagnostic factors in treatment. *Am. J. Drug Alcohol Abuse, 12,* 1-16.

Kosten, T.R., Rounsaville, B.J., Gawin, F.H., & Kleber, H.D. (1987a). A 2.5 year follow-up of cocaine use among treated opioid addicts. *Arch. Gen. Psychiat., 44,* 281-284.

Kosten, T.R., Schumann, B., Wright, D., Carney, M.K., & Gawin, F.H. (1987b). A preliminary study of desipramine in the treatment of cocaine abuse in methadone maintenance patients. *J. Clin. Psychiat., 48,* 442-444.

Kosten, T.R., Kleber, H.D., & Morgan, C. (1989a). Role of opioid antagonists in treating intravenous cocaine abuse. *Life Sci., 44,* 887-892.

Kosten, T.R., Kleber, H.D., & Morgan, C. (1989b). Treatment of cocaine abuse with buprenorphine. *Biol. Psychiat., 26,* 637-639.

Kozel, N.J., & Adams, E.H. (1986). Epidemiology of drug abuse: An overview. *Science, 234,* 970-974.

Kreek, M.J. (1987). Multiple drug abuse patterns and medical consequences. In H. Meltzer (Ed.), *Psychopharmacology: The third generation of progress.* (pp. 1597-1604). New York: Raven Press.

Kuhar, M.J., Ritz, M.C., & Sharkey, J. (1988). Cocaine receptors on dopamine transporters mediate cocaine-reinforced behavior. *NIDA Res. Monogr., 88,*14-22.

Kuljis, R.O., & Advis, J. P. (1989). Immunocytochemical and physiological evidence of a synapse between dopamine and luteinizing hormone releasing hormone containing neurons in the ewe median eminence. *Endocrinology, 124*(3), 1579-1581.

Leander, J.D. (1987). Buprenorphine has potent kappa opioid receptor antagonist activity. *Neuropharmacology, 26,* 1445-1447.

Lewis, J.W. (1974). Ring C-bridged derivatives of thebaine and oripavine. In M.C. Braude, L.S. Harris, E.L. May, J.P. Smith, & J.E. Villarreal (Eds.), *Narcotic Antagonists. Advances in biochemical psychopharmacology,* Vol. 8 (pp. 123-136). New York: Raven Press.

Lewis, J., Rance, M.J., & Sanger, D.J. (1983). The pharmacology and abuse potential of buprenorphine: A new antagonist analgesic. In N.K. Mello (Ed.), *Advances in substance abuse, behavioral and biological research,* Vol. 3 (pp. 103-154). Greenwich, CT: JAI Press.

Martin, W.R. (1979). History and development of mixed opioid agonists, partial agonists and antagonists. *Br. J. Clin. Pharmacol., 17,* 273S-279S.

Martin, W.R., Jasinski, D.R., & Mansky, P.A. (1973a). Naltrexone, an antagonist for the treatment of heroin dependence effects in man. *Arch. Gen. Psychiat., 28*, 784-791.

Martin, W.R., Jasinski, D.R., Haertzen, C.A., et al. (1973b). Methadone—A re-evaluation. *Arch. Gen. Psychiat., 28*, 286-295.

Mello, N.K. (1991). Pre-clinical evaluation of the effects of buprenorphine, naltrexone and desipramine on cocaine self-administration. *NIDA Res. Monogr., 105*, 189-195.

Mello, N.K., & Mendelson, J.H. (1980). Buprenorphine suppresses heroin use by heroin addicts. *Science, 207*, 657-659.

Mello, N.K., & Mendelson, J.H. (1985). Behavioral pharmacology of buprenorphine. *Drug Alcohol Depend., 14*, 283-303.

Mello, N.K., & Mendelson, J.H. (1992). Primate studies of behavioral pharmacology of buprenorphine. *NIDA Res. Monogr., 121*, 61-100.

Mello, N.K., Mendelson, J.H., Kuehnle, J.C., & Sellers, M.L. (1981). Operant analysis of human heroin self-administration and the effects of naltrexone. *J. Pharmacol. Exp. Ther., 216*(1), 45-54.

Mello, N.K., Mendelson, J.H., & Kuehnle, J.C. (1982). Buprenorphine effects on human heroin self-administration: An operant analysis. *J. Pharmacol. Exp. Ther., 223*(1), 30-39.

Mello, N.K., Bree, M.P., & Mendelson, J.H. (1983). Comparison of buprenorphine and methadone effects on opiate self-administration in primates. *J. Pharmacol. Exp. Ther., 225*(2), 378-386.

Mello, N.K., Mendelson, J.H., Bree, M.P., & Lukas, S.E. (1989). Buprenorphine suppresses cocaine self-administration by rhesus monkeys. *Science, 245*, 859-862.

Mello, N.K., Mendelson, J.H., Bree, M.P., & Lukas, S.E. (1990a). Buprenorphine and naltrexone effects on cocaine self-administration by rhesus monkeys. *J. Pharmacol. Exp. Ther., 254*(3), 926-939.

Mello, N.K., Mendelson, J.H., Drieze, J., & Kelly, M. (1990b). Acute effects of cocaine on prolactin and gonadotropins in female rhesus monkey during the follicular phase of the menstrual cycle. *J. Pharmacol. Exp. Ther., 254*, 815-823.

Mello, N.K., Mendelson, J.H., Drieze, J., & Kelly, M. (1990c). Cocaine effects on luteinizing hormone-releasing hormone-stimulated anterior pituitary hormones in female rhesus monkey. *J. Clin. Endocrinol. Metab., 71*(6), 1434-1441.

Mello, N.K., Kamien, J.B., Lukas, S.E., Drieze J., & Mendelson, J.H. (1993). The effects of nalbuphine and butorphanol treatment on cocaine and food self-administration by rhesus monkeys. *Neuropsychopharmacology, 8*(1), 45-55.

Mendelson, J.H., Mello, N.K., Cristofaro, P., Skupny, A., & Ellingboe, J. (1986). Use of naltrexone as a provocative test for hypothalamic-pituitary hormone function. *Pharmacol. Biochem. Behav., 24*, 309-313.

Mendelson, J.H., Teoh, S.K., Lange, U., et al. (1988). Anterior pituitary adrenal and gonadal hormones during cocaine withdrawal. *Am. J. Psychiat., 145*, 1094-1098.

Mendelson, J.H., Mello, N.K., Teoh, S.K., Kuehnle, J., Sintavanarong, P., & Dooley-Coufos, K., et al. (1991). Buprenorphine treatment for concurrent heroin and cocaine dependence. *NIDA Res. Monogr., 105*, 196-202.

Mendelson, J.H., Mello, N.K., & Teoh, S.K. (1992). Human studies of the biological basis of reinforcement: A neuroendocrine perspective. In C.P. O'Brien & J.H. Jaffe, (Eds.), *Addictive states* (pp. 131-155). New York: Raven Press.

Meyer, R.E., & Mirin, S.M. (1979). *The heroin stimulus*. New York: Plenum Press.

Negus, S.S., & Dykstra, L.A. (1988). Kappa antagonist properties of buprenorphine in the shock titration procedure. *Eur. J. Pharmacol., 56*(1), 77-86.

Negus, S.S., Picker, M.J., & Dykstra, L.A. (1990). Interactions between mu and kappa opioid agonists in the rat drug discrimination procedure. *Psychopharmacology, 102,* 465-473.

Negus, S.S., Picker, M.J., & Dykstra, L.A. (1991). Interactions between the discriminative stimulus effects of mu and kappa opioids in the squirrel monkey. *J. Pharmacol. Exp. Ther., 256*(1), 149-158.

Numata, H., Tsuda, T., Atai, H., Tanaka, M., & Yanagita, T. (1981). Pharmacokinetics of buprenorphine in rats and monkeys. *Jitchuken, Zenrinsho Kenkyu Ho/Central Institute for Experimental Animals Preclinical Report, 3,* 347-357.

O'Brien, C.P., Childress, A.R., Arnt, I.O., McLellan, A.T., Woody, G.E., & Maany, I. (1988). Pharmacological and behavioral treatments of cocaine dependence: Controlled studies. *J. Clin. Psychiat., 49* (Supp.), 17-22.

Pavasuthipaisit, K., Hess, D.L., Norman, R.L., Adams, T.E., Baughman, W.L., & Spies, H.G. (1981). Dopamine: Effects on prolactin and luteinizing hormone secretion in ovariectomized rhesus macaques after transection of the pituitary stalk. *Neuroendocrinology, 32*(1), 42-49.

Richards, M.L., & Sadee, W. (1985). Buprenorphine is an antagonist at the kappa opioid receptor. *Pharmacol. Res., 2,* 178-181.

Ritz, M.C., Lamb, R.J., Goldberg, S.R., & Kuhar, M.J. (1987). Cocaine receptors on dopamine transporters are related to self-administration of cocaine. *Science, 237,* 1219-1223.

Shippenberg, T.S., & Herz, A. (1987). Place preference conditioning reveals the involvement of D-1 dopamine receptors in the motivational properties of μ and k-opioid agonists. *Brain Res., 436,* 169.

Spies, H.G., Quadri, S.K., Chappel, S.C., & Norman, R.L. (1980). Dopaminergic and opioid compounds: Effects on prolactin and LH release after electrical stimulation of the hypothalamus in ovariectomized rhesus monkeys. *Neuroendocrinology, 30,* 249-256.

Stretch, R. (1977). Discrete-trial control of cocaine self-injection behaviour in squirrel monkeys: Effects of morphine, naloxone, and chlorpromazine. *Can. J. Physiol. Pharmacol., 55*(4), 778-790.

Teoh, S.K., Mendelson, J.H., Mello, N.K., & Skupny, A. (1988). Alcohol effects on naltrexone-induced stimulation of pituitary, adrenal and gonadal hormones during the early follicular phase of the menstrual cycle. *J. Clin. Endocrinol. Metab., 66,* 1181-1186.

Teoh, S.K., Sintavanarong, P., Kuehnle, J., et al. (1992). Buprenorphine's effects on morphine and cocaine challenges in heroin and cocaine dependent men. *NIDA Res. Monogr., 119,* 460.

Thompson, T., & Unna, K.R. (Eds.) (1977). *Predicting dependence liability of stimulant and depressant drugs.* Baltimore: University Park Press.

Watson, S.J., Trujillo, K.A., Herman, J.P., & Akil, H. (1988). Neuroanatomical and neurochemical substrates of drug-seeking behavior: Overview and future directions. In A. Goldstein (Ed.), *Molecular and cellular aspects of the drug addictions* (pp. 29-91). New York: Springer-Verlag.

Weiss, R.D. (1988). Relapse to cocaine abuse after initiating desipramine treatment. *JAMA, 260*(17), 2545-2546.

Woods, J.H., & Schuster, C.R. (1972). Opiates as reinforcing stimuli. In T. Thompson & R. Pickens (Eds.), *Stimulus properties of drugs* (pp. 163-173). New York: Appleton-Century-Crofts.

Woolverton, W.L. (1986). Effects of a D1 and a D2 dopamine antagonist on the self-administration of cocaine and piribedil by rhesus monkeys. *Pharmacol. Biochem. Behav., 24*(3), 531-535.

Woolverton, W.L., & Virus, R.M. (1989). The effects of a D1 and D2 dopamine antagonist on behavior maintained by cocaine or food. *Pharmacol. Biochem. Behav., 32,* 691-697.

Woolverton, W.L., Goldberg, L.I., & Ginos, J.Z. (1984). Intravenous self-administration of dopamine receptor agonists by rhesus monkeys. *J. Pharmacol. Exp. Ther., 230*(3), 678-683.

Yen, S.S.C. (1986). Neuroendocrine control of hypophyseal function. In S.S.C. Yen & R.B. Jaffe (Eds.), *Reproductive endocrinology* (pp. 33-74). Philadelphia: WB Saunders Co.

30

Effectiveness of Treatment for Substance Abuse

CHARLES P. O'BRIEN, A. THOMAS McLELLAN,
AND ARTHUR ALTERMAN

A commonly asked question about addiction is whether there is any point in treating it. Almost everyone has personal knowledge of an alcoholic, nicotine addict, or heroin addict who repeatedly returned to his or her drug of choice after periods of abstinence and treatment. There seems to be a general expectation that addiction should be permanently "cured" like pneumonia or a fractured bone. In reality, addictive disorders are more like chronic diseases, such as arthritis or diabetes. By the time patients apply for treatment, many of them have numerous problems in addition to drug taking. These include psychiatric and medical disorders, unemployment, breakdown of social networks, lack of education, and homelessness. Treatment may be considered effective if it only improves the patient's ability to function in society or increases the duration of remission before another relapse to compulsive drug taking. Complete and permanent abstinence from the drug of abuse is, of course, always the desired goal, but much benefit and relief of suffering can be achieved with more modest goals.

There are many different types of substance abuse and many different kinds of treatment available. Therefore to address the question of efficacy, one should ask which type of treatment for which type of patient at which phase of the addiction syndrome. In this chapter we review some of the data on the efficacy of specific treatments used for addictive disorders.

MEASURING SEVERITY

A necessary step in the study of addictive disorders was the development of a measuring instrument that would reliably rate the severity of the disorder.

This work was supported by grants from the U.S. Public Health Service (ROI DA 000586, P50 DA 5186) and the Medical Research Service of the Department of Veterans Affairs.

Table 30-1.
Measurement domains
for alcohol and drug
abuse treatment
evaluations

Alcohol use
Other drug use
Employment, self-support
Crime
Family, social relations
Medical problems
Psychiatric disorders

Simply determining that the condition is present or absent is not helpful in studies of efficacy. Similarly, quantifying the amount of substance used on a daily basis does not adequately describe important psychological and social factors that may determine whether or not a given patient responds to treatment. To characterize the nature and severity of the alcohol, drug, and other problems of patients applying for substance abuse treatment, the Addiction Severity Index (ASI) was developed (McLellan et al., 1980a). The ASI is a structured, 45-minute clinical research interview that is administered by a trained technician. It was designed to assess problem severity in seven areas commonly affected by substance abuse, including alcohol and drug use, medical, legal, employment, family/social, and psychiatric problems (Table 30-1). In each of these areas, verifiable questions are asked, measuring the number, frequency, intensity, and duration of problem symptoms in the patient's lifetime and during the past 30 days. The interview was also designed for repeat administration at points during treatment and after treatment completion. Using data collected on the 30-day periods before admission and the follow-up point, it has been possible to assess the nature and extent of improvements shown by patients in treatment and to compare different types of treatments across all of the seven problem domains. In the remainder of this chapter we review data comparing substance abuse treatment to some of the available alternatives to treatment and comparing different types of treatment. In each case, we do not confine our evaluations simply to the question of substance use after treatment, but attempt to evaluate the efficacy of substance abuse treatment and the available options in terms of the full range of measurement domains available on the ASI. In some cases we review existing reports of evaluation studies that have measured all or most of these domains. In other cases, we report pertinent results from ongoing studies at the Penn-VA Center using comparative data obtained from the ASI on each of these measurement domains.

DEFINING QUANTITY AND TYPE OF TREATMENT

Modern treatment research does not simply compare one treatment with another, but it requires that treatments be defined carefully and administered according to a treatment manual. For example, specific types of psychotherapy have been described and studied in the treatment of heroin addiction using treatment manuals verified by tape recordings of treatment sessions (Woody et al., 1983). Substance abuse treatment is often defined according to programs; thus, we find studies of inpatient versus outpatient, methadone versus drug-free, etc. However, the actual treatment services rendered in these programs have not been defined carefully, and when individual programs have been examined, wide variances in services are found.

Similar types of substance abuse programs often provide significantly different treatments, producing different patient outcomes. In contrast, programs with apparently different intensities and clearly different costs (e.g., inpatient versus outpatient) may provide similar amounts and types of services, resulting in similar patient outcomes. One barrier to research comparing the nature and effects of treatments has been the lack of a valid and reliable instrument to measure treatment services, which is suitable for use across a range of different treatment programs, different treatment settings, and with different patient populations.

The Treatment Services Review (TSR) is a 5-minute, technician-administered interview that provides a quantitative profile of treatment programs in terms of the number and types of services actually provided to the patients (McLellan et al., 1991). The TSR is based on the Addiction Severity Index (ASI), as it also focuses on the same seven treatment problem areas common to substance abusers. However, although the ASI provides a measure of the substance abuser, based on the nature and severity of his or her treatment problems, the TSR measures the treatment *program*, in terms of the nature and number of treatment services provided in those problem areas.

Research measures and instruments have been developed to assess treatment process variables, but these have usually been focused on a single program or modality. The TSR is intended to be a more general measure of treatment and to be suitable for use in alcohol, cocaine, opiate, or "multiple substance" treatment programs and be amenable to inpatient, partial hospital, or outpatient settings. Using this type of measure it may be possible to examine some of the fundamental questions associated with substance abuse treatments as they are presently offered:

- Do patients treated in the same programs receive similar types and amounts of services, and do these services differ for different types of substance abuse problems?
- Do patients who receive more services show more improvement and better posttreatment outcomes?
- Do patients who receive "minimal treatment" as controls in clinical research studies actually get less treatment than the experimental groups?

Test-retest studies indicate satisfactory reliability for the TSR interview when administered either in person or over the phone. Tests of the concurrent validity of the TSR showed the ability to discriminate different levels of treatment services and good correspondence with independent measures of treatment provided. In practice, we have found that the TSR can compare different treatment programs, record changes in the continuity of care provided over time, and examine interpatient differences in treatment effects. Results thus far indicate its promise as a reliable, valid, and useful tool in the evaluation and comparison of substance abuse treatments. Using the TSR, we have been able to quantify the actual services delivered in different treatment settings for each type of problem as measured by the ASI. Contrary to expectations, patients do not necessarily receive more treatment services in an inpatient setting (McLellan et al., 1991).

COMPARISONS WITH UNTREATED SAMPLES

Studies of untreated samples are always difficult for several reasons. First, we are dealing with a potentially fatal disorder, and we cannot ethically deny treatment if it is otherwise available. Second, patients evaluated and then placed on a waiting list when treatment is unavailable may simply find treatment elsewhere. Despite these difficulties, some studies do shed light on what happens to substance abuse and substance abuse-related problems in the absence of treatment. There have been studies of substance abusers out of treatment (Gerstein et al., 1979; Maddux & Desmond, 1986) and substance abusers on waiting lists (Rua, 1989). The issue is reviewed by Sisk and colleagues (1990). Two studies in progress at the Penn-VA Center are presented here.

Treated versus Untreated Heroin Addicts

Metzger et al. (unpublished data) have examined the drug use and needle-sharing practices of two large samples of opiate-addicted patients in the Philadelphia area. One group of subjects was recruited from a methadone maintenance program, and the other sample consisted of opiate-dependent people from the same neighborhood who had been out of all treatments for at least 1 year. Table 30-2 shows drug use and needle sharing data in these two groups

Table 30-2. Opiate-dependent individuals

	Methadone maintenance (n = 152)	Out of treatment (n = 103)
Shared needles	35%	74%[b]
Injected:		
Heroin	29%	64%[b]
Cocaine	21%	58%[b]
"Speedball"	26%	43%[b]
Non-i.v. drug use		
Heroin	5%	4%
Cocaine	9%	23%[a]
Amphetamine	0%	6%[a]
Benzodiazepines	16%	11%
Marijuana	17%	20%

[a] $P < .05$.
[b] $P < .01$.

collected from confidential interviews and questionnaires administered to these subjects by independent research technicians. Some significant levels of opiate and nonopiate drug use and needle sharing remained among treated patients. In this regard, it is important to note that the data for the in-treatment sample contained patients who recently entered treatment. Rates of drug use and needle sharing for those patients who had been in treatment longer than 1 month were significantly lower than for the total group. Regardless, the level of drug use reported by the in-treatment sample was far below that of the out-of-treatment group. For example, although 29% of the methadone maintenance group reported injecting opiates and 21% reported injecting cocaine regularly (defined as more than eight times) during the month before follow-up, corresponding rates among the out-of-treatment sample were 64% and 58%, respectively. Significantly higher rates of use were also noted for injection of heroin and cocaine mixtures (i.e., "speedball"), as well as crack cocaine and amphetamines. Not surprisingly, given these differing rates of use, needle sharing was also reported at a much higher proportion among the out-of-treatment group.

Perhaps the most important findings emerging from this study were on the differential HIV infection rates between the two samples. At the initial assessment point, 10% of the in-treatment sample and 15% of the out-of-treatment sample tested positive for HIV antibodies. Six months later, a follow-up testing showed the positivity rate of the in-treatment sample to be 12%, whereas that of the out-of-treatment sample had increased to 22%. By the 12-month follow-up point, 14% (4% more than at baseline) of in-treatment patients were HIV-positive in comparison to 31% (16% more than at baseline) of the out-of-treatment sample.

The data from this study indicate that i.v. drug users who are not in treatment are at increased risk of continued drug use, needle sharing, and HIV spread relative to a similar cohort of i.v. drug users who are in treatment. At the same time, this study does not prove definitely that treatment is the causal agent responsible for these behavioral differences. For example, it is possible and even likely that the out-of-treatment patients may have lacked the motivation for treatment found among the treated subjects, and this lack, rather than the effects of the treatment itself, may explain the status differences seen. For this reason, it would be important to equate level of motivation, at least at the start of treatment, in order to make any valid judgment regarding the effects of treatment in drug-abusing individuals.

Cocaine-Dependent Patients Assigned to a Waiting List

An ongoing study of male veterans who applied for cocaine abuse treatment at the Philadelphia VA Medical Center compares the relative outcomes of treated versus untreated patients with *approximately* the same level of motivation for treatment. In this 4-week study of waiting list patients, Urschel et al. (unpublished data) are collecting data on three fundamental questions. First, do male veterans seeking treatment at a VA program who have been put on a waiting list get any treatment services outside of the VA setting? Second, do the substance abuse and the related problems of these waiting list patients improve without treatment? Finally, do substance abuse patients on a waiting list actually return to the clinic for treatment once treatment becomes available?

The data for this ongoing study are still preliminary; however, some clear trends have already emerged from the first 26 subjects. First, only 16% of this group of lower socioeconomic, male veterans received any treatment-related services outside of the VA Medical Center. Thus, as expected, these public treatment services may be the only ones available for many uninsured patients. Those patients who did receive some services elsewhere did show at least minor reductions in their alcohol and drug problems and, to a lesser extent, their social problems. The services reported were typically temporary living arrangements in a shelter and temporary medical stabilization within these shelters.

Particularly important was the finding that the majority of these untreated, waiting-list patients showed significant *increases* in the severity of their medical, psychiatric, social, and drug abuse problems over the 4-week waiting period. Specifically, 48% reported increased severity of drug and alcohol problems in contrast to only 18% who reported decreased severity of their substance abuse problems. In addition, 56% of patients reported increased severity of medical problems, 80% reported increased employment and support problems, and 48% had increased problems in psychiatric, family, or social adjustment. Finally, over 40% of patients who were contacted and told that they were eligible for substance abuse treatment at the end of the 4-week waiting period had changed their minds and no longer were willing to accept treatment.

The data from this study still in progress are clear on three points. First, these lower socioeconomic status patients found few treatment options outside the public sector. Second, as has been reported elsewhere, there does seem to be a relatively short "window of opportunity" for substance abuse treatment, and if this opportunity is not taken, there is no guarantee that services will be accepted when they are offered at a later time. Finally, there is no evidence that the drug and alcohol use or other health problems of these patients showed any improvement without treatment. In fact, if the later data continue to show the initial trends, it is likely that there will be significant worsening in the overall drug use and health status of these men who do not receive treatment.

ALTERNATIVES TO SUBSTANCE ABUSE TREATMENT

Less costly alternatives to formal treatment programs have been proposed as treatment for abuse of alcohol and other drugs. There has been substantial work on minimal treatment approaches, such as advice only (Edwards et al., 1977) or "bibliotherapy" (Miller & Taylor, 1980). Bibliotherapy is actually the use of self instruction manuals to provide step-by-step guidelines on how to reduce drinking (Sanchez-Craig, 1984). There is an accumulating body of research in this area, and reviews of the available literature suggest that even these brief interventions can be effective in reducing alcohol use and attendant alcohol-related problems (Heather, 1986). Thus far, these brief interventions have not been studied in patients with high problem severity associated with alcoholism and particularly with other forms of drug dependence, such as heroin and cocaine.

Penal System

Perhaps the most regularly suggested alternatives to substance abuse treatment involve the criminal justice system, with jail, probation, parole, and more recently "boot camp" being the major choices. There are two important points to remember regarding the relative value of addressing substance abuse problems with treatment versus jail. First, jail cells are expensive to build and quite expensive to operate. In 1987 federal, minimum-security prison cells cost approximately $35,000 per cell to build and approximately $27,000 a year to maintain per inmate. Thus, imprisonment alone, even if effective·in reducing alcohol and drug use, is not necessarily a cost-efficient alternative to treatments that may cost as little as nothing for years of care (e.g., Alcoholics Anonymous and similar self-help groups for cocaine and heroin addicts) or as much as $31,000 for 28 days of private inpatient treatment (Saxe et al., 1983). The second point is that correctional interventions through the penal system can be *combined* with treatment interventions delivered on site to improve the effectiveness of imprisonment alone. There are many reports of effective treatments for drug dependence designed for delivery with correctional facilities and still others describing the use of treatments combined with probation and parole. For reviews of legal coercion and treatment, see Inciardi (1988), Wexler et al. (1988), and Anglin and Hser (1990).

An ongoing study at the Penn-VA Center illustrates the combination of medical treatment and the federal probation system in the management of opiate addicts. Metzger, Cornish, and their colleagues (1990) offered treatment with the opiate antagonist naltrexone to federal offenders convicted of opiate-related crimes. Naltrexone is an orally administered, opiate antagonist that has been shown to block the effects of injected opiates for up to 72 hours after ingestion. Although there have been few side effects reported among fully detoxified opiate addicts who have taken the drug, this medication has never been popular with heroin addicts because it provides no chemical reinforcement (pleasure), and it effectively takes away their "freedom to get high." Conversely, naltrexone has been quite useful in the treatment of higher socio-economic strata patients (e.g., addicted physicians, lawyers, etc.) who have been under some externally imposed pressure to take the medication regularly, e.g., loss of license, loss of important job, etc. (O'Brien, 1989). It has been assumed that the external pressure for behavioral change was a major factor in accounting for patient compliance with the naltrexone regimen and thereby in producing and sustaining reductions in opiate abuse and related problems among so-called white collar opiate abusers. There is also substantial external pressure for behavioral change associated with the threat of incarceration or reincarceration among those opiate abusers who have been convicted of opiate-related crimes. Thus, it was reasoned that the threat of incarceration associated with return to opiate use in these subjects might provide the incentive necessary for naltrexone to be an effective adjunct to standard probation/parole. According to figures from the Philadelphia Federal Parole Office, approximately 45% of federal offenders are reincarcerated within 18 months after prison release due to a return to opiate use.

Metzger and colleagues offered probationers and parolees with a history of recent and chronic opiate abuse the opportunity to be assigned randomly to receive either naltrexone administered two times per week (doses of 100 mg and 150 mg) accompanied by standard health care services or to an enhanced probation condition without naltrexone in which they were asked to report to their probation officer twice per week. These two conditions were approximately equal with regard to the total amount of time required for participation and the total amount of contact with a counselor or probation/parole officer. All evaluations were conducted by trained technicians entirely independent of the probation/parole process.

The results from this study indicate that naltrexone is a feasible and effective addition to standard probation/parole. First, although retention rates for naltrexone among many samples of opiate-dependent patients have been poor (averaging less than 20% remaining for 1 month), approximately 45% of the first 50 federal probation/parole subjects who were randomly assigned to receive the medication remained on naltrexone for the entire 6-month study period. Further, while on naltrexone, these subjects provided significantly fewer opiate-positive urines than subjects in the enhanced probation control group (n = 55). Although cocaine use continued to be a problem for both groups, the naltrexone subjects had lower rates of nonopiate drug use than the control subjects, as confirmed by urinalysis.

This study illustrates three important points. First, it is possible to combine a treatment and a correctional approach to the problem of substance abuse; these are not necessarily mutually exclusive interventions. A second and related point is that, as has been shown by most other studies within the criminal justice system, the addition of substance abuse treatment to a correctional intervention can result in better outcomes than those achieved by the criminal justice system intervention alone. In this case not only did the naltrexone treatment seem to enhance the effects of the probation/parole intervention, but also the external pressure applied by the criminal justice system seems to have enhanced the medication compliance and thereby the efficacy of the naltrexone. Third, although this study was focused on a pharmacological intervention used in the treatment of opiate addiction, there is no reason why this paradigm could not be used to evaluate other forms of psychosocial or behavioral treatments (e.g., relapse prevention training for substance abusing parolees) or other pharmacological interventions (e.g., desipramine for cocaine-abusing probationers) for substance abuse combined with criminal justice interventions.

ADDITION OF SERVICES TO METHADONE TREATMENT

A specific question concerning efficacy involves the provision of counseling services along with methadone for opiate addicts. Some have advocated the use of methadone medication alone as a means of saving funds and including more patients in treatment. To address this question, we undertook a prospective, random assignment study of different levels of services within a methadone maintenance treatment program (McLellan et al., 1990). In this study, three groups of voluntary patients were randomly assigned at the beginning of their methadone maintenance treatment to receive different types and amounts of treatment services. All patients received initial physical examinations, laboratory testing, and a short program of AIDS education, the minimum level of services that we felt obliged to provide all patients. Thereafter, Level I patients received methadone maintenance (blocking doses of 60 mg. or more) without additional counseling except in an emergency basis. Level II patients received the same methadone stabilization plus regular counseling by a trained rehabilitation specialist in our program, but no additional services. Level III patients received the same services as Level II patients, but in addition they were also provided family therapy, employment, counseling, and regular medical and psychiatric care as needed.

The TSR was collected weekly to ensure that the designed differences in levels of service actually occurred. The results showed that the protocol was followed and that there were significant differences in the types and amounts of services actually received by patients in these three levels. It is interesting to note that, despite our efforts to provide very few services to the level I patients, they were successful in obtaining some social and counseling services in the methadone program. We next asked whether these differences in the types and amounts of services provided would be associated with differences in the levels of improvement shown by these patients over the course of treatment. To answer this question, ASI interviews were collected by independent technicians at the beginning of the intervention and 6 months later. Improvement scores for each of the seven composite measures were then calculated; t-tests were used to calculate the significance of changes within each of the groups, and analysis of co-variance (ANCOVA) was used to determine whether there were outcome (6-month) differences among the three groups after adjusting for differences at admission.

The analysis showed that there were significant differences in the amounts of improvement shown by patients in these three levels. Those patients in Level I showed some improvement in drug status, as well as modest improvements in employment, but no other changes. In fact, their family and psychiatric problems actually worsened, though not significantly. The simple addition of a counselor to this level of services (i.e., Level II) was associated with significantly enhanced improvement in most areas; the additional services rendered by the family therapists, physicians, employment specialists, and social workers for Level III patients produced still more changes.

These data indicate that the efficacy of methadone treatment can be enhanced by additional services, such as counseling or psychotherapy. Methadone alone has some effects in uncomplicated patients, but it has been shown that substantial numbers of patients with additional disorders will not respond without the addition of other services to methadone. Those patients requiring more than drug counseling can be identified when they apply for treatment by a diagnostic interview (ASI) (McLellan et al., 1980b). For example, patients with coexisting psychiatric disorders respond poorly to drug counseling, but they show significant improvement with the addition of professional psychotherapy (McLellan et al., 1983a & b; Woody et al., 1983).

EVALUATING PATIENTS BEFORE AND AFTER TREATMENT

As discussed above, substance abusers who receive no treatment rarely show improvements and may actually show worsened status. In addition, the available data suggest that substance abuse treatment can be an effective addition to standard criminal justice system interventions, such as jail or probation/parole. There have been many valuable treatment studies comparing the status of a group of patients before and after treatment. Large treatment populations have been examined by Simpson and colleagues (1980), Hubbard and colleagues (1989), DeLeon (1984), Anglin et al. (1989), and Ball et al. (1988). These populations have included therapeutic communities and methadone maintenance samples, and these studies have documented substantial treatment effects.

Similar studies have been conducted at the Penn-VA Research Center using the ASI to measure change across problem areas. Examples of pre to post-treatment comparisons are presented in Table 30-3, which shows the results of studies of male veteran alcohol- and drug-dependent patients evalu-

Table 30-3. Pre- to post-treatment status in alcohol- and drug-dependent patients

	Alcoholics		Drug Dependent	
Variable[a]	Baseline (n = 460)	6 month (n = 460)	Baseline (n = 282)	6 month (n = 282)
Medical factor	.138	.128	.094	.071
Days medical problems	9	8	8	5
Employment factor	.676	.629[c]	.711	.602[c]
Days worked in past 30	8	10[b]	3	11[c]
Employment income	$210.00	$318.00[b]	$80.00	$309.00[c]
Drug factor	.400	.192[b]	.272	.058[c]
Days opiate use	1	<1	12	4[c]
Days stimulant use	<1	0	4	2[b]
Days depressant use	1	1	2	<1
Alcohol factor	.384	.162[c]	.181	.134[b]
Days alcohol use	13	6[c]	8	7
Days drank to intoxication	10	3[c]	5	3[b]
Legal factor	.221	.112	.219	.094[c]
Days illegal activity	1	<1	9	3[b]
Illegal income	$15.00	$11.00	$394.00	$91.00[c]
Family factor	.109	.043[c]	.142	.096[c]
Days family problems	7	3[b]	10	6[b]
Psychiatric factor	.131	.095[b]	.141	.096[b]
Days psychological problems	10	5[b]	11	7[c]

[a] All variables reflect the 30 days before collection. Factor scores vary from 0 to 1 with larger values indicating more serious problems.
[b] $P < .05$ by paired t-test.
[c] $P < .01$ by paired t-test.

ated at the time of treatment admission and again 6 months after treatment discharge (McLellan et al., 1982). The drug abuse treatments studied included methadone maintenance and inpatient therapeutic community programs. Alcohol-dependent patients were treated in inpatient and outpatient 12-step based treatments. The admission and follow-up data were collected by independent technicians who were not part of the treatment process or the clinical staff. Follow-up contact rates averaged 92%, and urine and breathalyzer reports were collected on 20% of patients to verify outcome reports. Comparison data were collected for the 30-day periods preceding admission to treatment and preceding the 6-month follow-up point. Summary measures of overall status in each problem area were calculated by combining unweighted sets of individual items in each problem area. Although these factor or composite scores provide the most statistically reliable measurements possible, they offer little intuitive information. For this reason we have analyzed and presented additional items in Table 30-3 to provide more clinically relevant indications of the changes that occurred.

As can be seen in Table 30-3, there were significant improvements in patient status from admission to 6-month follow-up in both the alcohol- and drug-dependent patient samples. The sample of 460 alcohol-dependent patients showed a 54% reduction in the number of days of drinking and a 67% reduction in the number of days intoxicated from admission to follow-up. Forty-one percent of alcohol-dependent patients were abstinent from all alcohol for the 6-month period. The 282 drug-dependent patients showed a 67% reduction in days of opiate use, a 50% reduction in the days of stimulant use (i.e., amphetamine, cocaine, etc.), and a 42% reduction in depressant use (e.g., barbiturates, sedatives, benzodiazepines) from admission to follow-up. Forty-eight percent of these drug-dependent patients were abstinent from all illicit drugs (except marijuana) during the 6-month period. These improvements were not confined simply to the alcohol and drug use measures, but included significant improvements in psychiatric, employment, family, and criminal status. For example, both patient samples showed increases in days of employment and earned income, as well as reductions in crime, family problems, and psychiatric symptoms.

This pre- to postevaluation of two large samples of male substance abuse patients treated in six VA treatment programs revealed substantial positive changes in their drug and alcohol use patterns at the 6-month follow-up point. Further, the improvements seen in the areas of alcohol and drug abuse were matched by important and pervasive gains in the areas of employment, crime, family/social relationships, and psychiatric status. Additional comparisons of subgroups from these two samples indicated that those patients who had longer periods of treatment showed significantly better outcomes than patients who had received shorter durations of treatment (but favorable treatment discharges) in the same programs. These findings and the substantial body of additional evaluation data available from other treatment outcome studies suggest, but do not prove conclusively, that substance abuse treatments can be quite effective in "producing significant, pervasive and sustained positive change in the lives of these patients" (McLellan et al., 1982, p. 1427).

COMPARISONS BETWEEN TREATMENTS

Another way to approach treatment efficacy is to compare one treatment with another in a defined patient population. The standard design involves a comparison of baseline and follow-up measures using an instrument, such as the ASI (McLellan et al., 1980). It is important to point out that minimal standards for pre- to post-treatment comparisons now include several quality control features. For example, subject interviews and data collection efforts must be completed by independent evaluators who are not associated with the provision of the intervention to reduce the likelihood of "demand effects" commonly seen when patients report their levels of improvement to the clinical staff who helped them. Second, it is now standard in these studies for subjective reports of post-treatment status to be accompanied by breathalyzer and/or urine screening tests and/or collateral reports to validate patient reports. Finally, it has been recognized that a high rate of patient follow-up contact is necessary to ensure that representative information is obtained from the treated sample. In our experience, it is possible to retrieve a minimum of 80-85% of treated patients at a 6-month follow-up point, and studies reporting contact rates lower than this figure should be evaluated critically.

Inpatient versus Outpatient Alcoholism Rehabilitation

Treatments aimed at preventing relapse among recently detoxified alcoholics can be conducted on either an inpatient or an outpatient basis. Since there is a considerable cost discrepancy, it is important to know the relative efficacy of each modality and for each type of patient. Male veterans applying for alcoholism treatment at the Philadelphia Veterans Affairs Medical Center were first detoxified so that they were free of alcohol and other drugs. Those who met study criteria received a full explanation of the study design. If they volunteered, they signed a consent form, and they were assigned randomly either to a day hospital rehabilitation program or an inpatient rehabilitation program. At the time of this interim report, 40 patients were engaged in the study (20 day hospital, 20 inpatient).

This section presents follow-up findings for 32 alcoholic patients who have completed the study so far. Baseline characteristics of the day hospital and inpatient group did not differ from each other. As a group, the subjects were about 41 years of age, had completed almost 12 years of education, and the majority were African-American. They averaged about 16 years of drinking to intoxication, and all met the study criterion of alcohol dependence according to DSM-III. All those with significant cocaine abuse were excluded. There was little evidence of the use of other drugs including marijuana. There were no between-group differences in the degree of substance abuse at baseline.

Treatment Outcome

Although inpatients seemed to be more likely to complete treatment than day hospital patients (87% versus 67%), this difference failed to achieve statistical significance. Patients were re-examined 4 and 7 months after baseline, and a

Table 30-4. Comparison of inpatient and partial hospital treatment of alcohol-dependent patients

| Variables[a] | Day hospital (n = 15) | | Inpatient (n = 17) | | Significant differences | |
	Intake	7 mo.	Intake	7 mo.	Between groups at 7 mo.	Over time
Days alcohol use-past 30	18.6	1.3	19.3	9.2	0.06	<.001
Did not use alcohol (%)	0	73	0	30	NS	0.05
Days intoxicated-past 30	18.4	0.4	18.3	7.3	0.08	<.001
Not intoxicated (%)	0	91	0	40	NS	NS
$ spent on alcohol-past 30	270	4	170	105	NS	0.02
Alcohol factor score	0.733	0.038	0.697	0.287	0.06	<.001

[a] All variables reflect the 30 days before interview. Factor scores vary from 0 to 1 with larger values indicating more serious problems.

portion of the 7-month results are shown in Table 30-4. Seven-month outcomes revealed considerable self-reported reduction of alcohol-related problems for both groups at the post-treatment evaluations and more limited evidence for reductions in drug-related problems. The improvement in alcohol-related problems seems to have been greater for the day hospital than for the inpatients, as can be seen in the significant or near-significant interaction term for the Alcohol Composite score on the ASI at both follow-up evaluations. Thus, 73% of those treated in the day hospital program reported total abstinence in the 30-day period before the 7-month follow-up evaluation as contrasted with 30% for those treated in the inpatient program. With respect to non-substance-related functioning (tables not shown), the ASI data indicate significant improvements for both groups at both follow-up periods in family/social and psychiatric problem levels. Group differences were not generally found in these areas, although there was a trend in favor of the day-hospital-treated patients on two measures of alcohol use.

To examine further the question of differences between day hospital and inpatient treatments, we examined another group of subjects who had agreed to participate in the research only if they were able to choose their own treatment (day hospital, n = 29, and inpatient, n = 13). These patients agreed to undergo all study assessments, but refused to be randomized. The findings on the various ASI measures for the nonrandom patients revealed either no inpatient/day hospital differences or better results for day hospital patients in alcohol-related outcomes, and thus they supported the findings in the randomized group.

Study Conclusions
Alcoholic patients treated either in a 1-month day hospital rehabilitation program or a 1-month inpatient rehabilitation program reported marked improvement in alcohol-related problems and some reduction in drug-related problem levels 4 and 7 months after entry into treatment. The reductions in alcohol-related problems were relatively greater for those treated in the day hospital

setting. Reductions in alcohol-related problems reported at the 4-month evaluation were relatively maintained for both groups at the 7-month evaluation,
although to a greater extent by day hospital patients. Reductions in psychological and family/social problem levels were also reported for both groups at both
follow-up evaluations. Similar findings have been reported by others (Fink et
al., 1985; Miller & Hester, 1986). Since day hospital programs are considerably
less expensive than inpatient programs, this modality should be considered as a
cost-effective alternative to inpatient rehabilitation.

Inpatient versus Day Hospital Treatment of Cocaine Dependence

Cocaine dependence, as it is known in the 1990s, is a new disorder. Until the
mid-1980s, cocaine was not available in quantity so that compulsive use and
other complications that force the user to seek treatment were not commonly
seen. Now, cocaine dependence is the most common presenting problem in our
large city substance abuse treatment programs, and we have had to develop
new treatments, evaluating them as they are being implemented. Early in the
cocaine epidemic we noted that most alcoholics were also using cocaine. Accordingly, we integrated our cocaine-abusing patients into day hospital rehabilitation treatment, a modality that had functioned successfully for many years in
the treatment of alcoholism. Our impression was that the cocaine-dependent
patients generally became engaged in this treatment program and seemed to do
well. To test this impression and determine whether the day hospital modality
was indeed efficacious for cocaine dependence, we decided to conduct a prospective random assignment trial comparing the results of day hospital with
those of standard inpatient treatment for cocaine abuse/dependence.

The research subjects were 94 men seeking treatment for cocaine dependence at the Philadelphia VA Medical Center. Prospective candidates had to be
younger than 50 years of age, willing to accept either inpatient or day hospital
treatment for 1 month, have a relatively stable residence for follow-up contact,
have no present evidence or history of a psychotic disorder, have no indication
of dementia, and have no major medical problems. All met the study criterion
of cocaine dependence by DSM-III criteria. Those with mixed cocaine dependence and alcohol dependence were included in the cocaine category. Forty-
eight subjects were randomized into day hospital treatment, and 46 were randomized into inpatient rehabilitation. The groups did not differ from each other
on sociodemographic and substance abuse history, except that inpatients were
more likely to have had previous drug treatment (54% versus 31%) than subjects assigned to the day hospital group.

As a group, the subjects were men (in keeping with the presenting population at our VA Medical Center), about 33 years of age, had about 12 years of
education, and were almost entirely African-American. They averaged less
than 3 years of cocaine use, although they had been drinking alcohol to intoxication for over 7 years. There was little evidence of use of drugs other than
cocaine, alcohol, or marijuana. On the average, these patients were using cocaine about 13 times a month and were spending about $600 monthly for drugs.
Relatively few of the subjects had not consumed alcohol in the past 30 days.

Both groups had worked about 10 days in the past month and reported having psychological problems 10 days out of the past 30. On substance use characteristics, the day hospital and inpatient groups did not differ significantly at baseline.

Despite the difference in settings, the two programs were quite similar in terms of actual treatments rendered. The day hospital program is in operation for 27 hours during weekdays, while inpatient treatment is obviously residential. Both programs last 28 days. The major therapeutic modality in both programs is group meetings that focus on overcoming denial and helping the patient learn to cope with everyday problems and stresses. Individual counseling and ancillary psychotropic medication are available when needed in both programs. Both programs provide education about the effects of addiction; both provide recreational therapy and encourage participation in a self-help group. The latter is provided on the campus of the inpatient program, whereas attendance in community meetings is required and monitored in outpatient treatment. Both programs offer medical care, although more medical attention is provided, on average, in the inpatient program.

Treatment Outcome

ASI and urine drug screen data comparing baseline and follow-up are presented below. Inpatients (40 of 46, or 87%) were significantly more likely (chi square = 11.81, 1df, $P = .0006$) to complete treatment than day hospital patients (25 of 48, or 52%). Table 30-5 includes data for all patients assigned to a given treatment whether or not they completed the 1 month of rehabilitation treatment. Four-month outcome findings are based on 76 subjects (41 day hospital, 35 inpatient), and 7-month outcomes are based on 56 subjects (28 in each group). The follow-up rates at both time periods are over 90% for each group. The lower numbers available at this time reflect both delays in data entry and data analysis and follow-up time lags. The outcomes reveal considerable self-reported (ASI) improvement in virtually all drug- and alcohol-related behaviors

Table 30-5. Comparison of inpatient and partial hospital treatment of cocaine-dependent patients

| | Day hospital (n = 28) | | Inpatient (n = 28) | | Significant differences | |
| | | | | | Between groups at 7 mo. | Over time |
Variables[a]	Intake	7 mo.	Intake	7 mo.		
Abstinent from alcohol (%)	19	56	7	44	NS	0.05
Days intoxicated-past 30	6.11	2.19	5.67	2.7	NS	0.012
Days cocaine use-past 30	12.8	3.22	11.6	3.27	NS	<.001
Did not use cocaine (%)	0	59	0	46	NS	0.05
Days marijuana use	3.63	2.52	3.89	1.26	NS	NS
$ spent on drugs-past 30	521	79	476	358	NS	0.012
Drug factor score	0.25	0.1	0.24	0.09	NS	<.001

[a] All variables reflect the 30 days before interview. Factor scores vary from 0 to 1 with larger values indicating more serious problems.

both 4 and 7 months after entry into treatment. An example of these improvements is the change in cocaine use. Virtually none of the subjects has been abstinent from cocaine at baseline, but over 60% reported abstinence at the 4-month follow-up and 59% (day hospital) and 46% (inpatient) reported no use at 7 months. The two groups did not differ significantly on any substance abuse variable at either the 4- or the 7-month periods. The reductions reported at 4 months generally seem to have been maintained at 7 months, with one exception. Amount of money spent on drugs seems to have increased at 7 months for the subjects who had received inpatient treatment. It should be noted, however, that this effect did not achieve statistical significance.

Urine drug screen data were available for about two-thirds of the subjects at each of the follow-up periods. Forty-nine (49) urine drug screens (out of 76, or 64.5%) were available at the 4-month follow-up evaluation. Seventeen of 27 (63.0%) of those obtained for day hospital patients were negative for cocaine, as contrasted with 12 of 22 (54.5%) of those obtained from the inpatient subjects. The two groups did not differ significantly in this respect. Thirty-nine urine drug screens (out of 56, or 69.6%) were available at the 7-month follow-up evaluation. Eleven of 19 urine drug screens (57.9%) obtained for the day hospital group were negative for cocaine as contrasted with 13 of 20 (65%) of those for the inpatient group. Again, the groups did not differ significantly. Thus, the ASI (self-report) findings on abstinence from cocaine are generally supported by the urine data. Additionally, the urine data support the ASI finding of little regression in the level of improvement from the 4- to 7-month follow-up evaluation.

The ASI data indicate significant improvements for both groups at both follow-up periods in family/social, psychological, and employment problem levels. The two treatment groups did not differ in degree of improvement. There was little indication of improvement in medical problems at either time period. There was some indication at the 7-month follow-up period of superior employment functioning for the inpatient subjects, as shown in the significant interaction effects for employment income and for the employment composite score.

Study Conclusions

In this study of day hospital versus inpatient rehabilitation for cocaine dependence, our interim findings are that those randomized to inpatient status were more likely to complete the initial 1-month of rehabilitation treatment (87% versus 52%). However, when all patients entering treatment were re-examined 4 and 7 months after beginning treatment, significant reductions in substance-related problem levels were found for both groups at both follow-up evaluations. Over 60% reported no cocaine use during the 30 days before follow-up. There were no significant differences between treatment groups. Improvements shown at 4 months were generally maintained at 7 months. These conclusions were supported by urine drug screen data. Further, significant reductions in legal, family/social, and psychological problem levels were found for both groups at both follow-up periods. There was no reported improvement in medical problems. At the 7-month evaluation, there was some indication of a superior level of employment-related functioning in those subjects who had received inpatient treatment.

This study shows that the majority of the cocaine-dependent patients did well in both treatment programs as measured by ASI improvement at 4- and 7-month follow-up points. There were no significant differences in efficacy between day hospital and inpatient rehabilitation programs. As was stated above in the discussion of alcoholism treatment, the day hospital approach seems to be a cost-effective alternative to inpatient rehabilitation programs. Further research is needed to determine whether a subpopulation of patients can be identified who require an inpatient rehabilitation program.

DEVELOPING NOVEL TREATMENTS FOR ADDICTION

Treatment researchers are constantly striving to develop new ways to prevent relapse to drug use in former addicts. This is a particularly serious problem with cocaine dependence where return to compulsive cocaine use may occur shortly after leaving a treatment program. Both psychosocial and biological factors contribute to the phenomenon of relapse (O'Brien et al., 1986). A critical part of treatment therefore is analyzing those factors that increase the likelihood of relapse after a period of abstinence.

Conditioning as a Possible Mechanism Involved in Relapse

One of these relapse factors may be the presence of Pavlovian conditioned responses produced by repeated drug administration in the presence of specific stimuli. Conditioned responses produced by morphine administration were first reported from Pavlov's laboratory (Pavlov, 1927). Subsequently, numerous drugs have been found to produce conditioned responses in animals and in humans (Grabowski & O'Brien, 1981). These conditioned responses can be classified as drug-like or drug-opposite. The drug-opposite responses in former opiate users can mimic the opiate withdrawal syndrome (O'Brien et al., 1977). If these responses occur just before a dose of the drug is received, they produce attenuation of drug effects. This attenuation of drug effects produced by conditioned responses can be called "tolerance," and it may form a partial explanation for the diminished drug effects commonly seen with repeated administration of the same dose of a drug (Siegel, 1976). Conditioned drug-like responses can also be produced by pairing distinct stimuli with drug administration. After repeated pairing, the stimuli by themselves can produce drug-like effects in the absence of the drug (Lynch et al., 1976). Drug-like responses have been produced in both animal experiments and in human studies (O'Brien, 1975), and they may form a partial explanation for what are known as the "placebo effects" of drugs.

Cocaine Craving in Former Users

The recent upsurge of cocaine use among our patients has given us the opportunity to study and document the kinds of conditioned responses that may occur in chronic cocaine abusers (Childress et al., 1988). Former cocaine users report craving when they are in situations in which cocaine has been used or when they encounter stimuli (sights, sounds, odors, etc.) previously associated with the use of cocaine. It is true that the concept of craving is difficult to define and that it refers to a subjective phenomenon, but the concept has operational value when talking to patients, and studies utilizing craving as a measure have produced consistent results. This craving or strong desire to use cocaine is puzzling to former users because it conflicts with their previous decision to avoid cocaine. Despite their expressed and apparently genuine intention to refrain from returning to cocaine use, these patients find themselves craving the very substance that had recently gotten them into so much trouble. Some report intense craving, arousal, and palpitations when they encounter a white powder, such as talcum or sugar; see a friend with whom they had used cocaine; encounter drug-buying locations; or experience a pharmaceutical odor—almost anything that has been repeatedly associated with getting and using cocaine. These stimuli may precipitate arousal and craving. Thus, a patient leaving a treatment program is likely to encounter numerous stimuli that may provoke craving and increase the risk of relapse. Although many different factors may contribute to the high rate of relapse among users of cocaine, the responses provoked by drug-related stimuli, presumably by way of a conditioning mechanism, are thought to play a role. The learned aspects of drug dependence have recently been reviewed (O'Brien et al., 1991b).

Prevention of Relapse in Former Cocaine Addicts

Our research group has conducted a series of studies on the causes of relapse after treatment for cocaine dependence. Several of these studies investigate the possibility that reducing or eliminating conditioned responses—by a process of systematic exposure to cocaine-related cues with no drug reinforcement (extinction)—may reduce the rate of relapse in abstinent patients who formerly were cocaine dependent. This procedure may be useful when integrated with traditional abstinence-oriented treatment programs. Traditional treatment approaches have intuitively recognized the power of cocaine-related cues. Thus, abstinent patients are warned to avoid "people, places, and things" associated with prior cocaine use. In reality, even when well-motivated patients try to avoid stimuli connected with cocaine use, such avoidance is almost impossible. Patients need additional tools for coping with or reducing drug craving.

Our treatment approach complements attempts at avoidance of cocaine reminders in the natural environment. We give patients repeated exposure to cocaine cues while they are in a safe environment, in an attempt to reduce the craving and arousal often triggered by these stimuli. This treatment approach is based on the view that cocaine cues essentially are classically conditioned stimuli that become associated, by repeated pairings, with cocaine's pharmacological effects over the natural course of a patient's drug use. By repeatedly exposing the patient to cocaine cues without cocaine being available, the power of these cues to produce conditioned responses (arousal, craving, etc.) that could lead to drug use and relapse should be gradually diminished.

A comprehensive treatment program should address all categories of relapse-producing factors, including pharmacological, social, occupational, medical, legal, family, and additional psychiatric disorders, when they are present. Conditioning factors may play an important role in the tendency for some patients to relapse, but it is unlikely that conditioning factors would override all others. The influence of conditioning probably varies with the individual patient, depending on the relative importance of other relapse-producing factors in his or her life. Thus, we have integrated the extinction procedure within the context of a treatment program that addresses a wide range of issues thought to be important to the recovering addict.

Test of the Effect of Adding Extinction to Treatment for Cocaine Dependence

In our pilot studies of techniques to extinguish conditioned responses in patients formerly dependent on cocaine, we developed symptom lists, laboratory measurements, and procedures for systematically presenting drug-related stimuli to patients. During this pilot phase, we found that the subjective responses, such as craving, would decrease with repeated exposure. Physiological responses, such as tachycardia and other signs of arousal, were more resistant to extinction. Although individual patients seemed to benefit from systematic cue exposure or extinction, the only way to determine whether any technique adds significantly to the treatment of an illness is to test its effect in a controlled study. This requires a relatively homogeneous sample of patients who must be assigned randomly to the experimental treatment or to a control condition.

We have studied 50 cocaine-dependent patients in a passive cue exposure paradigm. A preliminary report has been published (O'Brien et al., 1990), and a complete report of that study has been presented elsewhere (Childress, unpublished data). All the subjects were male veterans who entered the Substance Abuse Treatment Unit of the Philadelphia VA Medical Center with a primary problem of cocaine dependence. These patients ranged in age from 28 to 53 and averaged less than 2 years of cocaine use. Although several of these patients also had histories of alcohol and marijuana use, those with a significant history of opiate dependence were excluded. In general, these relatively "pure" cocaine abuse patients tended to have significantly shorter addiction histories and fewer previous treatment episodes than recent admissions presenting for treatment of opiate or polydrug dependence.

Treatment assignment. After pretreatment testing, patients were assigned randomly to one of four treatment conditions: (1) supportive-expressive psychotherapy + extinction (SE-X); (2) supportive-expressive psychotherapy + activities to control for the extra attention received by patients assigned to the extinction condition (SE-C); (3) standard drug counseling + extinction (DC-X), and (4) standard drug counseling + control activities (DC-C). "Control activities" consisted of sessions (equal in length and number to extinction sessions) with self-help tapes featuring suggestions for developing a healthy lifestyle, better relationships, etc. Drug counseling was administered by experienced counselors according to a treatment manual and represented good standard treatment for substance abuse. Supportive-expressive psychotherapy was administered by experienced doctoral-level psychologists; it has been found to be significantly more effective than drug counseling for opioid-dependent patients (Woody et al., 1983). The efficacy of psychotherapy for cocaine dependence has not been previously examined in a controlled study.

Treatment sessions. Inpatients assigned to extinction groups received 15 hour-long sessions of repeated, nonreinforced exposure to cocaine "reminders" during the 2-week period of hospitalization after the initial detoxification from cocaine. Therapy or counseling sessions were administered three times per week during this 2-week period according to a manual developed in our treatment program. The 2-week inpatient treatment phase was followed by a 2-month outpatient phase offering eight additional weekly sessions of extinction *or* control activities, as well as weekly therapy or counseling, depending on group assignment. All these treatment sessions were offered in addition to standard treatment for cocaine dependence at our clinic. The data presented here focus primarily on the 15 inpatient extinction sessions. Each hour-long cocaine extinction session contained three 5-minute audiotape segments, three 5-minute exposures to a cocaine-related videotape, and three simulated cocaine administration rituals. These drug-related stimuli are presented in the sequence—(1) audio, (2) video, (3) activity—and repeated three times. This procedure provides nine drug-related stimulus exposures per session, for a total of 135 exposures over the course of 15 sessions.

Though most inpatient extinction sessions are conducted on the treatment ward, sessions number 1, 8, and 15 are conducted in the laboratory chamber to allow for monitoring of physiological responses over the course of extinction. During the extinction sessions, the patient is first asked to rate the overall intensity of high, craving, and "crash" (withdrawal) using a 1-10 scale for each. The type and intensity of symptoms are then probed through an accompanying list of 50 responses associated with early "high" (euphoria), toxic (e.g., paranoia), and "crash" phases of cocaine use. The entire rating scale developed in our program is administered at the beginning and again at the end of each hour-long extinction session.

Effects of the extinction sessions. A one-way ANOVA with repeated measures was performed for each of the subjective variables of craving, high, and withdrawal/"crash," using sessions as the repeated measure. These analyses revealed a significant effect of sessions on all three subjective variables: craving ($P < .0000$), high ($P < .0001$), and withdrawal "crash" ($P < .0000$). Of these responses, craving was the most prevalent and persistent, reducing gradually over the course of 15 extinction sessions. Reports of high and withdrawal/"crash" were less common and were largely extinguished by the sixth hour of extinction.

As in the laboratory setting, cocaine craving was the most intense and most frequently reported subjective response in the extinction setting. Extinction sessions were effective in significantly reducing conditioned cocaine craving, "high," and withdrawal over the course of 15 extinction sessions ($P < .000$ for all three variables, one-way ANOVA with sessions as the repeated measure). Figure 30-1 illustrates the reduction in reports of subjective high, crav-

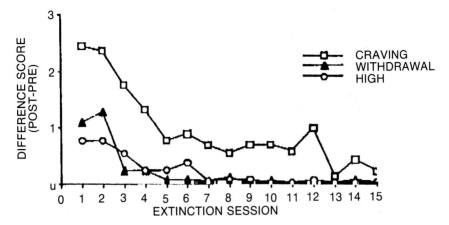

Figure 30-1. Reduction in subjective responding to cocaine-related stimuli as a function of extinction (n = 25). The ordinate shows changes in subjective responses comparing presession to postsession for 15 extinction trials. Means for 25 patients for each of the three subjective responses (craving, withdrawal, high) are plotted.

ing, and withdrawal as a function of extinction sessions in the first 25 patients. The results of the total samples were similar.

Measures of skin temperature and GSR both showed significant reductions as a function of extinction trials. Although these physiological responses were reduced during the extinction trials, their relative persistence is underscored by the fact that arousal was still apparent even after 15 hours of exposure to the same stimuli. Heart rate responses were particularly resistant to extinction. As a whole, there were no significant differences in the heart rate responses to the cocaine-related stimuli from session 1 to session 15.

Treatment outcome. Both extinction groups showed better retention in outpatient treatment and a higher proportion of clean urines than the two control groups. It was noteworthy that the group receiving counseling plus extinction did better than the group receiving SE therapy from a doctoral-level therapist plus the nonextinction control condition. When the two extinction groups were combined, the between-group differences on retention and clean urines were significant at the .05 level. These results were encouraging because the extinction sessions were well accepted by the patients, and the technique can be applied by nonprofessional drug counselors. The effects of this extinction procedure were roughly comparable in magnitude to the effects of available medication in promoting cocaine abstinence (Gawin et al., 1989). Combinations of medication and behavior therapy may produce additive or even synergistic effects, and this approach should be examined in controlled studies.

CONCLUSIONS

Questions about the efficacy of treatment for substance abuse cannot be answered simply. Substance use disorders are a set of chronic disorders comprising biopsychosocial aspects, and all of these aspects influence response to treatment. "Cure" is not a reasonable goal when confronting this type of disorder. When we use reliable instruments to measure the seven problem areas involved in addictive disorders, we can measure treatment effects in comparison to no treatment and we can compare the efficacy of treatments to one another. To advance this field, we must ask precise questions involving a defined patient population and a defined type of treatment.

We can also use these methods to develop novel treatments that may be effective only in a particular situation, such as naltrexone in probationers or extinction in certain cocaine addicts. Because of the many systems involved in substance use disorders, a treatment may not be effective by itself, but incremental efficacy may be demonstrable if the treatment is imbedded in a comprehensive treatment program.

ACKNOWLEDGMENTS

Portions of this chapter were presented at the 1990 meeting of the Association for Research on Nervous and Mental Disease and in O'Brien et al., 1991a.

REFERENCES

Anglin, M.D., Speckart, G.R., & Booth, M.W. (1989). Consequences and costs of shutting off methadone. *Addict. Behav., 14*(3), 307-326.

Anglin, M.D., & Hser, Y. (1990). Legal coercion and drug abuse treatment. In J. Inciardi (Ed.), *Handbook on drug control in the United States*. Westport, CT: Greenwood Press.

Ball, J.C., Meyers, C.P., & Friedman, S.R. (1988). Reducing the risk of AIDS through methadone maintenance treatment. *J. Health Social Behav., 29*(3), 214-226.

Childress, A.R., McLellan, A.T., Ehrman, R., & O'Brien, C.P. (1988). Classically conditioned responses in cocaine on opioid dependence: A role in relapse? *NIDA Res. Monogr., 84*, 25-43.

DeLeon, G. (1984). The therapeutic community: Study of effectiveness. *Treat. Res. Monogr., 84-1286*.

Edwards, G., Orford, J., Egert, S., Guthrie, A., Hawker, C., Hensman, M., Mitcheson, M., Oppenheimer, E., & Taylor, C. (1977). Alcoholism: A controlled trial of treatment and advice. *J. Stud. Alcohol., 38*, 1004-1031.

Fink, E.B., Lonagabaugh, R., McCrady, B.M., Stout, R.L., Beattie, M., Ruggieri-Authelet, A., McNeil, D. (1985): Effectiveness of alcoholism treatment in partial versus inpatient settings: Twenty-four month outcomes. *Addict. Behav., 10*, 235-248.

Gawin, F., Kleber, H., Byck, R., Rounsaville, B.J., Kosten, T.R., Jatlow, P.I., & Morgan, C. (1989). Desipramine facilitation of initial cocaine abstinence. *Arch. Gen. Psychiat., 46*, 117-121.

Gerstein, D., Judd, L.L., & Rovner, S.A. (1979). Career dynamics of female heroin addicts. *Am. J. Drug Alcohol Abuse, 6*(1), 1-23.

Grabowski, J., & O'Brien, C.P. (1981). Conditioning factors in opiate use. In N.K. Mello (Ed.), *Advances in substance abuse*, (pp. 69-121). Greenwich, CT: JAI Press.

Heather, N. (1986). Change without therapists: The use of self-help manuals by problem drinkers. In W.R. Miller & N. Heather (Eds.), *Treating addictive behaviors: Processes of change* (pp. 331-359). New York: Plenum.

Hubbard, R.L., Marsden, M.E., Rachal, J.V., Harwood, H.J., Cavanaugh, E.R., & Ginzburg, H.M. (1989). *Drug abuse treatment: A national study of effectiveness.* Chapel Hill, NC: University of North Carolina Press.

Inciardi, J.A. (1988). Some considerations on the clinical efficacy of compulsory treatment: Reviewing the New York experience. *NIDA Res. Monogr., 86.*

Lynch, J.J., Stein, E.A., & Fertsiger, A.P. (1976). An analysis of 70 years of morphine classical conditioning: Implications for clinical treatment of narcotic addiction. *J. Nerv. Ment. Dis., 163,* 47-58.

Maddux, J.F., & Desmond, D.P. (1986). Relapse and recovery in substance abuse careers. *NIDA Res. 72.*

McLellan, A.T., Luborsky, L., O'Brien, C.P., & Woody, G.E. (1980a). An improved evaluation instrument for substance abuse patients: The Addiction Severity Index. *J. Nerv. Ment. Dis., 168,* 26-33.

McLellan, A.T., Druley, K.A., O'Brien, C.P., & Kron, R. (1980b). Matching substance abuse patients to appropriate treatments. A conceptual and methodological approach. *Drug Alcohol Depend., 5(3),* 189-193.

McLellan, A.T., Luborsky, L., Woody, G.E., & O'Brien, C.P. (1982). Is treatment for substance abuse effective? *JAMA, 247,* 1423-1427.

McLellan, A.T., Luborsky, L., Woody, G.E., Druley, K.A., & O'Brien, C. (1983a). Predicting response to alcohol and drug abuse treatments: Role of psychiatric severity. *Arch. Gen. Psychiat., 40,* 620-625.

McLellan, A.T., Luborsky, L., Woody, G.E., O'Brien, C.P., & Druley, K.A. (1983b). Increased effectiveness of substance abuse treatment: A prospective study of patient-treatment "matching." *J. Nerv. Ment. Dis., 171(10),* 597-605.

McLellan, A.T., Arndt, I.O., Woody, G.E., & O'Brien, C.P. (1990). *Three levels of service provision in methadone maintenance.* Paper presented at the Committee on Problems of Drug Dependence conference, Richmond, VA.

McLellan, A.T., Alterman, A.I., Cacciola, J., Metzger, D., & O'Brien, C. (1992). A new measure of substance abuse treatment: Initial studies of the treatment services review. *Am. J. Psychiat., 180(2),* 101-110.

Metzger, D., Cornish, J., & Woody, G.E. (1990). Naltrexone in federal offenders. *NIDA Res. Monogr., 95.*

Miller, W.R., & Hester, R.K. (1986). Inpatient alcoholism treatment: Who benefits? *Am. Psychol., 41,* 794-805.

Miller, W.R., & Taylor, C.A. (1980). Relative effectiveness of bibliotherapy, individual and group self-control training in the treatment of problem drinkers. *Addict. Behav., 5,* 13-24.

O'Brien, C.P. (1975). Experimental analysis of conditioning factors in human narcotic addiction. *Pharmacol. Rev., 27,* 535-543.

O'Brien, C.P. (1989). The use of antagonists in the treatment of opioid dependence. In T.B. Karasu (Ed.), *Treatments of psychiatric disorders* (pp. 1332-1341). Washington, DC: American Psychiatric Association Press.

O'Brien, C.P., Testa, T., O'Brien, T.J., Brady, J.P., & Wells, B. (1977). Conditioned narcotic withdrawal in humans. *Science 195,* 1000-1002.

O'Brien, C.P., Ehrman, R., & Ternes, J. (1986). Classical conditioning in human opioid dependence. In S. Goldberg & I. Stolerman (Eds.), *Behavioral analysis of drug dependence* (pp. 329-356). San Diego: Academic Press.

O'Brien, C.P., Childress, A.R., McLellan, T., & Ehrman, R. (1990). Integrating systematic cue exposure with standard treatment in recovering drug dependent patients. *Addict. Behav., 15,* 355-365.

O'Brien, C.P., Alterman, A., & McLellan, A.T. (1991a). Developing and evaluating new treatments for alcoholism and cocaine dependence. In M. Galanter (Ed.), *Recent developments in alcoholism.* New York: Plenum.

O'Brien, C.P., Childress, A.R., & Ehrman, R. (1991b). Conditioning models of drug dependence. In C.P. O'Brien & J. Jaffe (Eds.), *Advances in understanding the addictive states.* Association for Research in Nervous and Mental Disease. New York, N.Y.

Pavlov, I.P. (1927). *Conditioned reflexes.* London: Oxford University Press.

Sanchez-Craig, M. (1984). *Therapist's manual for secondary prevention of alcohol problems: Procedures for teaching moderate drinking and abstinence.* Toronto: Addiction Research Foundation.

Saxe, L., Dougherty, D., Esty, K., & Fine, M. (1983). *The effectiveness and costs of alcoholism treatment.* Health Technology Case Study 22. Washington, DC: Office of Technology Assessment.

Siegel, S. (1976). Morphine analgesic tolerance: Its situation specificity supports a Pavlovian conditioning model. *Science, 193,* 323-325.

Simpson, D., & Savage, L. (1980). Drug abuse treatment readmissions and outcomes. *Arch. Gen. Psychiat., 37,* 896-901.

Sisk, J.E., Hatziandreu, E.J., & Hughes, R. (1990). *The effectiveness of drug abuse treatment: Implications for controlling AIDS/HIV infection.* Background Paper No. 6, USGPO No. 052-003-01210-3. Washington, D. C.: Office of Technology Assessment.

Wexler, M.K., Falkin, G.P., & Lipton, D.S. (1988). *A model prison rehabilitation program: An evaluation of the Stay'n Out Therapeutic Community.* New York: NDRI Press.

Woody, G.E., Luborsky, L., McLellan, A.T., O'Brien, C.P., Beck, A.T., Hole, A., & Herman, I. (1983). Psychotherapy for opiate addiction: Does it help? *Arch. Gen. Psychiat., 40,* 639-645.

Index